YALE-G FIRST AID: CRUSH USMLE STEP 2CK AND Step 3

(Fifth Edition)

YALE GONG, MD, MS

Senior Clinical Investigator

Perelman School of Medicine

University of Pennsylvania

Philadelphia, Pennsylvania

Magdalini Tsintou, MD, MS

Neuroscientist

Massachusetts General Hospital

Harvard University

School of Medicine

Boston, Massachusetts

i

Library of Congress Cataloging-in-Publication Data, USA

Gong, Yale

YALE-G FIRST AID: CRUSH USMLE STEP 2CK AND STEP 3 (5th Edition)/ By Yale Gong.

   p. ; cm.

ISBN13: 978-1642552027

The Fifth Edition, August 1, 2018.

Publisher:
www.usmle-yaleg.com and www.amazon.com

Contact: yaleg.usmle@gmail.com

Cover design: www.fiverr.com

Reviewers

Matthew A. Warner, MD
Anesthesiologist
Mayo Medical School & Mayo Clinic
Rochester, Minnesota

Acknowledgments

Genuine thanks to Dr. Ramon Diaz-Arrastia (Presidential Professor of Neurology at the University of Pennsylvania), Dr. Adeleke Adesina, Dr. Mary T. S. Bah, Dr. Angela Pronger, www.smashusmle.com, and other professional friends for their important support of this highly challenging book! Same thanks to www.uptodate.com and www.google.com for all their helpful information!

Preface

This fifth edition of the "Yale-G First Aid: Crush USMLE Step 2CK And Step 3" has been significantly updated from Yale-G's previous versions with the author's persistent efforts for the past eight years, based on **www.usmle.org*, www.uptodate.com, www.uworld.com,** "Current Medical Diagnosis and Treatment", Kaplan medical books, and a large volume of kind, supportive feedbacks from medical students and doctors in the US and around the world. According to those frank feedbacks, this book has indeed collected the most comprehensive clinical knowledge particularly needed for the USMLE Step 2 CK and Step 3 and thus been accepted as the best single resource compared to all similar books in the USMLE market. If you have been looking for the equivalent of "First Aid for the USMLE Step 1" for USMLE Step 2 CK without success, this can be it! This one can be your "bible" for USMLE Step 2 CK and Step 3! All the comprehensive and high-yield materials are in here and presented in an easy-to-digest format. This book is also helpful with Step 2 CS (for differential diagnosis) and your clinical rotations. **Important features of this book include:**

1. **Systematic and refined summaries of all common and uncommon diseases and disorders that are frequently tested in the USMLE Step 2 CK and Step 3.** They are composed mainly of important concepts, etiologies, essentials of diagnoses, differential diagnoses, treatments, and preventive measures.

2. Well-organized contents in easy-to-remember formats and abbreviations; more than **100 tables** for summaries and differential diagnoses, and necessary details of high-yield "orderly steps" in the diagnosis and management of major diseases. **Most important clinical points are in "PEARLS", underlined, and bolded as priorities and with great potential to be seen in the USMLE.**

3. **600 refined, fundamental, and high-yield questions (HYQs) in real-examination format** ("Single best answer" and "Matching") chapter by chapter for application of the key clinical knowledge. All explanations and related topics should be read carefully.

4. **155 selected high-yield clinical images with brief diagnostic features** side by side for deeper digestion and memory of the associated fundamental clinical knowledge.

After a thorough digestion of this book followed by practicing with the best Q-bank at "www.uworld.com" with note-taking, you are ready to crush the USMLE Step 2 CK and Step 3 with high scores! I'm so confident of this that I keep the promise of "money back guarantee" for the book for any rare failure of the Step 2 CK and Step 3.

This book is your ticket to the USMLE and ECFMG certification! It can also be a special aid in medical school education in the US and around the world. I take all feedbacks and contributions constructively with rewarding promises, and will keep monthly updating in the new Kindle version at Amazon to make it better and better!

Yale Gong, MD, MS

*www.usmle.org: "USMLE Step 3: Examinees are seeing increased numbers of items that assess an expanded range of competency-based content, including foundational science essential for effective healthcare; biostatistics, epidemiology, and population health; literature interpretation; medical ethics; and patient safety."

Table of Contents

InfXs

Cardiovascular

Respiratory

GI & Nutrition

Endocrine & Metabolic

Heme One, Dindrene

MSK & connective Tissue

Neurology

Neurology

Dermatology

Gynecology

Obstetrics

Pebs

Surg +trauma

Surg + trauma

Psychiatry

Psychiatry

Biostats n shit

Chapter 1

INFECTIOUS DISEASES

Infectious diseases are among the most common disorders that we encounter in our daily lives. They can affect any organ or system in the body and cause us tremendous losses. However, most of them are preventable and curable. While the major pathogens causing particular diseases have not changed much over time, the sensitivity pattern of these microorganisms to antibiotics has changed significantly in recent years. Thus pathologic culture and drug sensitivity testing (C/S) is still the best clinical guide to treatment of infectious diseases.

PEARLS—HIGH-YIELD CLINICAL POINTS OF ANTIBIOTICS

I. Antibiotics for Gram$^+$ Cocci

—**Staphylococcus (Staph) and Streptococcus (Strep) are the most common organisms.**

1. Drugs of choice

(1) Strep-pneumoniae; Strep-hemolytic group A, B, C, G; Strep-viridans: penicillin (PCN) G, V/K.

(2) Staph, non-penicillinase-producing: PCN; penicillinase-producing Staph: semisynthetic PCN.

(3) Enterococcus faecalis: Ampicillin +/- gentamicin.

(4) Enterococcus faecium: Vancomycin +/- gentamicin.

2. Semisynthetic or penicillinase-resistant penicillins (PRPs):

Mechanisms: Blocking peptidoglycan cross-linking and inhibiting transpeptidases.

IV: Oxacillin, nafcillin, or methicillin (rare); oral (PO): cloxacillin, dicloxacillin, etc. They are highly effective against Staph and Strep, and thus usually used in bacterial skin infections (cellulitis, impetigo), meningitis, endocarditis, osteomyelitis, and septic arthritis. **Main adverse effects:** anaphylaxis (rare), interstitial nephritis (methicillin #1).

Methicillin is rarely used now due to its renal toxicity. Thus, **"Methicillin-resistant Staph-aureus" (MRSA)** actually refers to **"oxacillin- or nafcillin-resistant Staph-aureus", and the drug of choice is vancomycin.** However, for sensitive organisms, oxacillin/nafcillin is preferred to vancomycin.

Beta-lactamase inhibitors — "CAST": Clavulanic acid, Avibactam, Sulbactam, Tazobactam.

3. PCN-G, PCN-V/K, ampicillin, and amoxicillin: Effective against Strep (S. pyogenes, S. viridans, and S. pneumonia) and **Gram$^-$** bacteria, but not against S. aureus. **Ampicillin and amoxicillin are penicillinase sensitive** and only effective against S. aureus when combined with sulbactam or clavulanate; both are effective against Enterococci and Listeria.

4. Replacement for penicillin (PCN) allergy:

(1) Replacement for mild PCN allergy:

Cephalosporins (Cepha-): See below.

(2) Replacement for severe PCN allergy (hypersensitivity):

Fluoroquinolones, clindamycin, and macrolides.

<u>**Fluoroquinolones**</u> (ciprofloxacin, levofloxacin, gatifloxacin, moxifloxacin, ofloxacin):

Mechanisms: Inhibit DNA topoisomerase II and IV → **bactericidal.**

The **new fluoroquinolones** (moxifloxacin, levofloxacin, and gatifloxacin) are strongly effective **against Pneumococcus, Mycoplasma, Chlamydia, and Legionella. They are thus the first-line empiric antibiotics for pneumonia.** Most quinolones are active against the **Enterobacteriaceae. Only ciprofloxacin covers Pseudomonas.**

Adverse effects: Abnormal bone growth and cartilage in children and pregnant women (contraindicated); tendonitis, Achilles tendon rupture, and prolonged QT on ECG. Gatifloxacin is rarely used now due to potentially abnormal glucose metabolism.

<u>**Macrolides**</u> (erythromycin, clarithromycin, azithromycin): Inhibit translocation during protein synthesis → **bacteriostatic.** Mainly used for atypical pneumonia (Mycoplasma, Chlamydia, Legionella), STDs (Chlamydia), B. pertussis, and some patients infected with **Gram$^+$** cocci but severely allergic to PCNs).

<u>**PEARLS:**</u> **For life-threatening Staph-aureus (MRSA) and Strep-B infection with severe PCN allergy, strongest antibiotics are vancomycin, synercid, and linezolid. Macrolides are never used for severe S. aureus infections.**

II. Antibiotics for Gram$^-$ Bacteria

1. Drugs of first choice for Gram$^-$ Cocci

Moraxella catarrhalis: Cefuroxime;

Gonococcus: Cefixime, ceftriaxone;

Meningococcus: PCN or cefotaxime.

2. Drugs of first choice for Gram$^-$ Rods

Pseudomonas-A: It's an opportunistic pathogen that mostly affects immunosuppressed patients. **Drugs of choice: piperacillin-tazobactam (with beta-lactamase inhibition), ceftazidime, or cefepime, or a carbapenem +/- gentamicin.**

Acinetobacter: imipenem, meropenem;

Bacteroids (GI strains): Metronidazole;

Campylobacter jejuni: Erythromycin or azithromycin;

Enterobacter: Ertapenem, imipenem, cefepime;

E. coli: Uncomplicated—fluoroquinolones, nitrofurantoin; sepsis—cefotaxime, ceftriaxone;

Haemophilus: General infection—**TMP-SMX (co-trimoxazole, bactrim)**; central nervous system (CNS) or serious infection—cefotaxime, ceftriaxone;

Helicobacter pylori: Amoxicillin + clarithromycin + proton pump inhibitors (PPI);

Klebsiella: A 3rd-generation cephalosporin;

Legionella species (pneumonia): Azithromycin or fluoroquinolones +/- rifampin;

Proteus mirabilis: Ampicillin.

For most multidrug resistant infections (including P. aeruginosa), colistin (polymyxcin E) is the only option despite its nephrotoxicity and ototoxicity. Cefepime plus amikacin can be the second.

3. PCNs (piperacillin, ticarcillin, azlocillin, mezlocillin):

They are strong against the large Enterobacteriaceae group (E. coli, Proteus, Enterobacter, Citrobacter, Morganella, Serratia, and Klebsiella) and Pseudomonas; usually applied for hospital-acquired pneumonia, intra-abdominal infections (cholecystitis, cholangitis, pyelonephritis), bacteremia, neutropenia with fever, etc.

4. Cephalosporins: See below.

5. Fluoroquinolones: See above.

6. Aminoglycosides (gentamycin, tobramycin, amikacin) and **monobactams** (aztreonam):

Mechanisms: Block transpeptidation at 30S → **bactericidal.** (1) Effective against the same Gram⁻ bacilli as listed above. (2) Synergistic with beta-lactam antibiotics for enterococci and staphylococci. (3) Ineffective against anaerobes. (4) **Kidney and ear toxicity.**

7. Carbapenems (imipenem, meropenem):

These are **broad-spectrum antibiotics on gram⁺ cocci, gram⁻ rods, and anaerobes, strongly active against Enterobacteriaceae and Pseudomonas (EXCEPT ertapenem), plus Staph. Main adverse effects** (S/E) include GI distress, CNS toxicity, and nephrotoxicity, which is mostly prevented by using with cilastatin. Significant adverse effects limit use to life-threatening infections or as a last resort.

III. Cephalosporins

Mechanisms of actions: Block peptidoglycan cross-linking and inhibit transpeptidases.

1ˢᵗ-generation cephalosporins (Cepha-): Cefazolin, cefadroxil, and cephalexin. They have good activity against most **Gram⁺** bacteria (including S. aureus) plus Proteus, E. coli, and Klebsiella.

2ⁿᵈ-generation cephalosporins: Cefuroxime, cefprozil, and cephamycins (cefoxitin, cefotetan).

They are less effective against S. aureus but more against **Gram⁻ bacilli** (H. influenza, Bacteroides, E. coli, P. mirabilis, and Klebsiella) and **beta-lactamase producing** M. catarrhalis and Enterobacteriaceae. **Cefotetan** is the drug of choice for infection with **diabetic ulcerations**, but not Pseudomonas.

3ʳᵈ-generation cephalosporins: Ceftazidime, cefotaxime, and ceftriaxone. They are strong against most **Gram⁻** bacteria including **beta-lactamase producing organisms**. They are the drugs of choice for pneumonia or meningitis caused by PCN-insensitive **Pneumococci** or **Enterobacteriaceae because they can cross the blood-brain barrier. Ceftazidime also covers Pseudomonas.**

4th**-generation cephalosporins: Cefepime**, cefozopran, and cefclidine. They are **stronger** than the 2nd- and 3rd-generation cephalosporins against most **Gram**[-] and some **Gram**[+] bacteria. **Cefepime also covers S. aureus, Strep, and Pseudomonas.**

5th**-generation cephalosporins: Ceftaroline is similar to ceftriaxone but with unique coverage of penicillin-resistant Gram**[+] bacteria **(Strep and MRSA),** not active for Pseudomonas and Enterobacteriaceae. **Ceftobiprole** is active for **penicillin-resistant bacteria** and **Enterobacteriaceae.**

Adverse effects (S/E) of cephalosporins: few, much less hypersensitivity than with PCN; 5-10% cross allergy with PCN; occasional GI symptoms, autoimmune hemolytic anemia, Vit K deficiency, and disulfiram-like reactions.

IV. Antibiotics for Anaerobes

1. **Metronidazole** (Flagyl) is best **for abdominal and genital anaerobes.**

2. **Clindamycin:** Blocks transpeptidation at 50S subunit; **bacteriostatic. It's best for chest anaerobes and invasive Strep-A. S/E:** C. difficile (pseudomembranous) colitis, fever, diarrhea, etc.

3. Other choices: Carbapenems, piperacillin + tazobactam, ticarcillin + clavulanate, ampicillin + sulbactam, and amoxicillin + clavulanate are strong medicines for anaerobes. The 2nd-generation cephalosporins (cefoxitin and cefotetan) are also effective.

V. Antibiotics for Encapsulated Bacteria

These bacteria are **more aggressive, including Pneumococcus (Pneumococ), H. Influenza (Hib), Meningococcus (Meningococ), and Klebsiella. Choices of antibiotics:**

1. **New quinolones (Levo-, Moxi-, and Gati-) or the 3**[rd]**-generation cephalosporins are the best for Pneumococcus, Meningococcus, and Klebsiella.**

2. **Ampicillin is the best choice for H. Influenza (and Listeria).** Other bacteria that ampicillin covers include E coli, Proteus, and Salmonella. Ampicillin is usually a good initial choice for otitis media, preventive use for dental infection or endocarditis, UTI with pregnancy, and limited Lyme disease.

VI. Special Antibiotics

1. **Beta-lactam antibiotics—Penicillins, cephalosporins, carbapenems and aztreonam:** More effective than most others in the same class.

2. **Anti-pseudomonas plus anti-beta-lactamase penicillins: Piperacillin-tazobactam; ticarcillin-clavulanate).**

3. **Vancomycin (a glycopeptide):** Strongly bactericidal against most **Gram positives** (including Staphylococci, MRSA), **anaerobes**, diphtheroids, and clostridium species. It's usually saved for patients

allergic to beta-lactam antibiotics, with MRSA or persistent anaerobic infection. Vancomycin is combined with an aminoglycoside for a complex infection with both Gram$^+$ and Gram$^-$ bacteria.

4. **Doxycycline:** Effective against Chlamydia, limited Lyme disease, Rickettsia, primary and secondary syphilis patients allergic to penicillins, Mycoplasma, Borrelia, and Ehrlichia. **Adverse effects:** tooth discoloration (before age 8), Fanconi syndrome (Type II RTA), photosensitivity, and esophagitis/ulcer.

EYE, EAR, NOSE AND THROAT INFECTIONS

INFECTIONS OF THE EYES

Common eye infections are summarized in Table 1-1.

Table 1-1: Summary of Eye Infections

Disease / Clinical features, diagnosis (Dx), and treatment (Tx)
Infectious conjunctivitis: See Table 1-2.   **Bacterial keratitis**   **Features:** Corneal infection caused by foreign body, contact lens and trauma, etc; **hazy cornea** with central **ulcerations** and adjacent stromal **abscesses**. **Tx:** Refer to an ophthalmologist immediately.
Fungal keratitis   **Features:** Usually seen in **farmers and immunodeficient** patient, with vegetable growth on the cornea with multiple **stromal abscesses**. **Tx:** Refer to an ophthalmologist immediately.
CMV retinitis   **Features: #1 common** viral infection of the eyes with **AIDS or immunodeficiency; painless retinitis** without conjunctivitis or keratitis. **Fundoscopy:** Fluffy/granular retinal lesion with opacity or hemorrhage. Corneal scraping staining (Tzanck test) usually shows multinuclear giant cells. **Tx:** Refer to an ophthalmologist immediately.
HSV retinitis   **Features: Painful, with conjunctivitis or keratitis. Fundoscopy:** Retinal pallor, ulcerations or necrosis. Corneal scraping staining usually shows multinuclear giant cells. **Tx:** Refer to an ophthalmologist immediately.
Orbital cellulitis (Image 18)   **Features:** Peri- or post orbital septum infection; more common in children. Sudden fever, proptosis, painful eyes, decreased eye movement, and red swollen eyelids. **Tx:** Systemic antibiotics.
Dacryocystitis

Features: Infection of the dacryocyst mostly by **Staph-aureus and Strep-B** in > 40 y/o patients; abrupt fever, pain, and redness in the medial canthus, often with purulent discharge and increased WBC. **Tx:** Systemic antibiotics against Staph-aureus and Strep-B.

Chalazion (Image 19)

Features: Also known as **meibomian gland lipogranuloma**, a granulomatous inflammation of the meibomian gland due to obstruction, changing from painless or painful swelling to a firm nodule on the lid. It often co-exists with rosasea or blepharitis. **Dx** is clinical. **Tx:** 1. Cleaning and compression initially; incision and drainage if necessary. 2. If persistent or recurrent, biopsy is required for suspected squamous cell carcinoma (SCC).

Hordeolum (Stye, Image 20)

Features: Mnemonic: **"Horrible Staph"**; mostly an abscess caused by **Staph-aureus** infection. Painful, **tender swelling** localized to the **eyelid**. Risk factors: smoking and unsanitary behavior. **Dx** is clinical. **Tx:** Warm compression and antibiotics against Staph-aureus. If ineffective: incision and drainage.

Infectious Conjunctivitis

It's an inflammation of the conjunctiva mostly caused by bacteria or viruses. Conjunctivitis can also be caused by chemicals, allergy, fungi, or parasites. Thus the etiologic differentiation is crucial for correct diagnosis (**Dx**) and treatment (**Tx**) to avoid possible loss of vision.

Common infectious conjunctivitis by etiology is summarized in Table 1-2.

Table 1-2: Summary of Infectious Conjunctivitis

Cause / Clinical features, diagnosis, and treatment

Viral (Image 21)

Adenovirus is the #1 common virus and occurs in epidemics, with severe ocular irritation, **copious watery discharge** from the pink/red eye, and pre-auricular lymph mode (LN) swelling; highly contagious. **Tx:** Usually self-limited but contagious. A topical corticosteroid is used if it's severe.

Bacterial (Highly contagious)

Staph, Strep, Hib, Pseudomonas: Foreign body sensation and **purulent discharge** from the eye. **Dx:** Gram stain + culture (if severe). **Tx:** Empiric antibiotic drops and ointment.

N. gonococcus: Copious purulent discharge. It may lead to corneal perforation and blindness. **Dx:** Gram stain shows Gram⁻ intracellular diplococci. **Tx:** Emergent IM **ceftriaxone**; oral ciprofloxacin or ofloxacin. Hospitalization if it's severe.

Chlamydial

C. trachomatis A-C is the **#1 cause of chronic** conjunctivitis and preventable **blindness** worldwide. Patient presents with recurrent epithelial keratitis in childhood, with trichiasis, corneal scarring, and entropion. **Dx:** Giemsa stain and culture for Chlamydia. **Tx: Azithromycin**, tetracycline, or erythromycin for 3-4 weeks.

Otitis Media

It's an infection of the middle ear between the eustachian tube and the tympanic membrane. The most common microorganisms are **Pneumococcus**, followed by Hib and Moraxella catarrhalis. This organism type is the same as in bronchitis and sinusitis. Viruses cause most other cases of otitis media.

Essentials of diagnosis

1. History of ear pain, fever, and decreased hearing.

2. **Physical examination (P/E)** reveals a red, bulging tympanic membrane with **immobility (No.1 sign)** and loss of the light reflex, with air insufflations. P/E results determine the diagnosis in most cases. Membrane perforation is a rare complication.

Treatment

1. Oral **amoxicillin** is still the best initial therapy.

2. High-dose amoxicillin-clavulanate is used if there has been recent amoxicillin use or resistance. Other alternatives are 2nd or third-generation cephalosporins.

3. Patient with severe penicillin allergies should avoid cephalosporins and take macrolides instead (azithromycin or clarithromycin).

4. If there are multiple recurrences or if there is no response to multiple antibiotics, **tympanocentesis** should be performed.

Complications and differentiations

1. Membrane perforation or/and hearing loss: It's the most common complication.

2. Recurrent otitis media: Treatment is antibiotics plus myringotomy and ventilating tubes.

3. Otitis media with effusion: With persistent fluid but few symptoms; usually resolves within 3 months. Treatment is antibiotics along with myringotomy and ventilating tubes.

4. Mastoiditis: Redness and tenderness over the mastoid bone, with an outward and forward displacement of the outer ear. Choose the same antibiotics.

5. Cholesteatoma: A pocket of squamous epithelium in the tympanic membrane. It can spread and destroy other temporal bone structures. Treatment is surgical removal.

6. Meningitis or brain abscess: Common intracranial complications, with fever and neurologic deficits.

7. Labyrinthitis: Vertigo, nystagmus, tinnitus, hearing loss, and vomiting.

Otitis Externa

It's also known as "**Swimmer's ear**", inflammation of the skin lining the ear canal and surrounding soft tissue. Continuous wetting of the ear canal and local trauma increase the risk. **Pseudomonas-A** and **S. aureus** are the most common pathogens.

[handwritten: Otitis externa]

Essentials of diagnosis

1. Ear pruritus and pain exacerbated by moving the ear canal, which is inflamed, swollen, and macerated with purulent discharge.

2. Systemic symptoms may or may not be present.

Treatment *[handwritten: - usually self-limiting]*

1. Topical antibiotics: Eardrops with polymyxin B, neomycin, and hydrocortisone are very effective. Dicloxacillin is good for acute infection.

2. Patient with diabetes is at increased risk for malignant otitis externa and skull osteomyelitis, requiring IV antibiotics in hospital.

3. Prevention: For frequent swimming activities, use ear spray with dilute alcohol immediately after swimming.

[handwritten left margin: prev. page | Mastoiditis. URI bugs, ear tubes. - Inflam of mastoid bone, mastoid swelling - anteriorly rotated ear Dx clx TX surg decompression]

[handwritten right margin: viral & bacterial = purulent. bilateral, yellow green discharge, facial tal - pain]

Rhinosinusitis

Rhinitis is a common inflammation of the mucous membrane inside the nose. Non-allergic type can be caused by <u>viruses</u> (Rhinoviruses, Coronaviruses) and <u>bacteria</u> (Pneumococcus, Hib); allergic rhinitis is caused by irritants or allergens.

[handwritten: fever, cough, headache, ear pain, loss of smell.]
[handwritten right margin: - severe ons. if fever ≥3d ᵖ persistan (sx ≥10 days) biphasic (recurrent fev]

Most patients with rhinitis present with <u>stuffy nose, runny nose, and post-nasal drip</u>. Bacterial rhinitis typically shows <u>mucopurulent nasal discharge</u>. Allergic rhinitis is the most common type, typically showing <u>sneezing, nasal itching and watery discharge</u>, and red itchy eyes (See Chapter 3 for details).

Sinusitis is the inflammation of the paranasal sinuses usually due to infection, which is mostly caused by similar organisms as for otitis media such as **Pneumococcus** (No.1), Hib, or Moraxella. Mucosal edema obstructs the sinus openings (ostia), causing sinus secretions being trapped. Most cases of acute sinusitis are rare complications of the common cold or other upper respiratory infections (URIs). Some cases are caused by nasal obstruction due to foreign body, polyps, or deviated septum. **Sinusitis and rhinitis often coexist as rhinosinusitis.**

Essentials of diagnosis

1. **Acute rhinosinusitis**: Based on clinical symptoms and signs—recent history of an URI followed by nasal stuffiness, purulent nasal discharge, and focal teeth pain; sinus pressure or pain that worsens with percussion or bending head down. Cough and fever may be present in 50% of cases. P/E finds specific sinus tenderness. *[handwritten: Dx: XR ~~stain~~ culture]*

2. **Chronic rhinosinusitis**: It may include three subtypes—chronic rhinosinusitis without nasal polyps, with nasal polyps, and allergic fungal rhinosinusitis. Patient usually has a history of recurrent URIs or sinusitis, followed by nasal congestion and postnasal discharge, with mild or absent sinus pain, headache, and fever. Symptoms should be present for > 2-3 months for diagnosis. Patient has increased risk of infection with Staph-aureus and Gram⁻ rods.

Sinus CT scan is the preferred means of diagnosis, showing mucosal thickening with or without nasal polyps. Sinus biopsy or culture is more accurate and necessary if symptoms persist after proper antibiotic treatment.

Treatment *Recurrent bact sinusitis = CT scan foreign bodies*

1. Rhinitis: Treat underlying cause and symptoms. *viral: supportive, NSAIDS, IN saline,*

2. **Acute purulent rhinosinusitis** *NSAIDS*   *Bact: fever/purulent LC,*

(1) Supportive care—smoking avoidance, saline nasal spray (helps drainage), decongestants (pseudoephedrine or oxymetazoline), and nasal steroid or antihistamines (for allergy). *- lot days*
- gets better then worse

(2) Antibiotics—Amoxicillin + clavulanate, TMP-SMX, or levofloxacin is an effective choice. *→ for acute bact. RS.*   *- PCN - Amox-clav*

3. **Chronic rhinosinusitis**

(1) A brief course of oral prednisone (5 days) plus broad-spectrum antibiotics—Amoxicillin + clavulanate; or a penicillinase-resistant penicillin (oxacillin, nafcillin, etc.) for 3-4 weeks.

(2) Long-term macrolide antibiotic treatment.

(3) If symptoms persist, refer to an otolaryngologist for a possible endoscopic drainage or surgery.

Complication

Mucoceles, nasal polyps, orbital cellulitis (from ethmoid sinusitis), cavernous sinus thrombosis, osteomyelitis, etc.

Septic Dural Sinus Thrombosis   *uncontrolled infxn of skin, sinuses, & orbit can spread to the cavernous sinus ↑ICP, HA, fever, peri orbital edema, vomiting, papilledema*

Dural sinus thrombosis encompasses **three subtypes: Cavernous sinus thrombosis (CST), lateral sinus thrombosis, and superior sagittal sinus thrombosis**. The cavernous sinus is the most frequent dural sinus to become infected and thrombosed as septic CST. *CN III, IV, V, & VI frdups.*

Septic CST is a rare, life-threatening suppurative process of the orbit, nasal sinuses, or central face. The cause is usually from a spreading infection in the nose, sinuses, ears, or teeth. **S. aureus and Strep.** are the most commonly associated pathogens, and early antibiotic use is crucial to reduce complications and mortality.

Essentials of diagnosis

1. **Fever and orbital pain** after a recent sinusitis or facial infection.

2. **P/E** usually shows orbital edema, exophthalmos, ophthalmoplegia, slowed pupil reactions, and visual deficits. Changes in mental status (confusion, coma) may indicate complicated CNS infection.

3. **Lab diagnosis:** Elevated WBC; 50% of blood cultures are (+); CSF may be (+) with CNS infection. CT and MRI may support diagnosis. *MRI w MR venography*

Treatment

Take blood for cultures and aggressively treat patient with empiric PCNase-resistant PCN (oxacillin, nafcillin, etc), along with a third or 4th-generation of cephalosporins for 3-4 weeks (broad-spectrum coverage). If severe, surgical drainage may be needed. *prevention/ reversal of cerebral herniation from ↑ICP*

[Handwritten margin notes:]
Cough +1
Exudate +1
Nodes +1
Temp ≥38°C +1
OR ≤14 +1, ≥ -1
Dx: ≤1 = do nothing
2-3, rapid strep - f/u Cx
≥4 Abx

RESPIRATORY TRACT INFECTIONS

Pharyngitis   *odynophagia*

Also known as "Sore throat", it's mostly caused by **viruses** (adenovirus, parainfluenza, rhinovirus, and EBV). However, Group-A **Strep (S. pyogenes)** infections (accounting for up to 15%) are more concerned because of the risk of developing rheumatic fever or glomerulonephritis. Other organisms include Chlamydia, Mycoplasma, Gonococci (from oral sex), Corynebacterium diphtheria, and Candida albicans (immunosuppressed patients).

Essentials of diagnosis

1. Viral pharyngitis mostly shows fever, cough, and rhinorrhea instead of exudates, except EBV.

2. Sore red throat, tonsillar exudates, tender anterior cervical adenopathy, fever and absence of cough are highly suggestive of **Strep pyogenes** (**Image 22**). Mild infections may not show exudates.

3. **Rapid antigen detection test (RADT)** is the best initial testing with high sensitivity and specificity for bacterial pharyngitis. Positive Strep test result means the same as positive throat culture result, whereas a negative Strep test may require a confirmative throat culture if suspicion remains high. A throat culture is the gold-standard (most accurate) test but it takes 24-48 hours to yield results.

Treatment

1. Most cases are viral and treated for symptomatic relief instead of antibiotics. Local therapies such as throat sprays and lozenges (with local anesthetics), a NSAID and a short term of glucocorticoids (if severe) may be helpful.

2. If it's confirmed Strep pharyngitis, oral penicillin V for 10 days is the best treatment. *[handwritten: Amox-Clavulanate]* Macrolides and 2nd-generation cephalosporins are alternatives for penicillin allergy. For the rare case of an erythromycin-resistant strain when patient is unable to tolerate beta-lactam agents, clindamycin is an appropriate choice.

3. If it's mononucleosis, have rest and a NSAID (e.g., ibuprofen).

[handwritten: sore throat ⊕ big spleen = EBV. do monospot]

Laryngitis

It is usually caused by viruses, but maybe also by Moraxella catarrhalis and H. influenza. Patient commonly presents with hoarseness, cough, and other URI symptoms. Laryngitis is mostly self-limited (less than 3 weeks) and only treated for symptomatic relief instead of antibiotics, similar to that for viral pharyngitis. Voice rest is needed.

Important notes: If a patient with voice symptoms has shortness of breath, stridor, persistent cough/hoarseness, hemoptysis, throat pain, difficulty swallowing, unilateral otalgia, or/and weight loss, nasopharyngeal cancer should be suspected.

The Common Cold

The "common cold" is the most common upper respiratory tract infection (URI), mostly by a virus. Susceptibility depends on pre-existing antibody level. Rhinovirus accounts for > 50% of cases and have > 100 antigenic serotypes. Thus, reinfection with another serotype can cause similar symptoms, since there is no cross-immunity among the serotypes.

Clinical features, diagnosis, and treatment

1. Presentations usually include rhinitis (rhinorrhea, nasal congestion), pharyngitis (sore throat), non-productive cough, and malaise. Fever may or may not be present.

2. Most cases resolve in 5-7 days regardless of treatment. Symptomatic and supportive treatment and NSAIDs are adequate therapies in most cases if needed. Avoid abuse of antibiotics.

3. Transmission is mostly by respiratory and hand-to-hand contact. Prolonged infection can lead to secondary bacterial infections such as sinusitis and pneumonia (in immunosuppressed patients). Best prevention is by regular exercise.

Influenza ("Flu")

It's a common systemic viral disease caused by influenza A, B, or C (belonging to the orthomyxovirus family) mainly through respiratory droplet nuclei. It's characterized by strong infectability, rapid transmission, and an epidemic pattern. Influenza can cause damage to the respiratory tract epithelium, leading to complications such as sinusitis, otitis media, bronchitis, and pneumonia. Annual epidemics are due to minor genetic changes in the viral (protein) structure and usually are not life-threatening except in immunocompromised and very young or old patients. Rare large regional or global pandemic outbreaks are due to major genetic reassortment (combination and rearrangement of genetic material causing shifted viruses) and are often fatal.

Essentials of diagnosis

1. Common presentations include systemic symptoms of fever, chills, myalgias, headache, and fatigue, and upper respiratory symptoms of coryza, dry cough, sore throat, and conjunctival injection.

2. **Rapid antigen detection of swabs** or washings is the best initial test for diagnosis. Viral culture is the most accurate test but it takes a few days to show results.

Treatment

1. **Effective specific antiviral drugs for both influenzas A and B are oseltamivir and zanamivir**, and are recommended for all individuals with confirmed or suspected influenza who are severely ill (with dyspnea, tachypnea) or showing signs of rapid deterioration. These antiviral drugs help inhibit the viral replication and spread, and limit the symptomatic duration if **used within 48 hours** after onset. If it's more than 48 hours, only symptomatic treatment is recommended (acetaminophen, antitussives, etc.). Amantadine and rimantadine are no longer recommended due to the high rates of influenza resistance.

2. **All pregnant women** with suspected influenza **should use oseltamivir or zanamivir,** even those who present longer than 48 hours after onset provided that they are not yet improving.

<u>Prevention</u>

1. **Annual influenza vaccination (IIV, inactivated influenza)**: Since 2010, it has been recommended to **everyone from 6 months of age on**. There is also **cross-protection** against some different strains of virus (including novel viruses). It's **contraindicated** in patients with severe allergic reaction (e.g., anaphylaxis) after previous dose or ingestion of egg protein. **Benefits**: Influenza vaccine has been demonstrated to significantly reduce the disease, hospitalization, and death in numerous studies. It's especially beneficial to those with high risk.

2. **Postexposure prophylaxis:** WHO recommends that household contacts of patients with **H_5N_1** avian influenza should receive postexposure prophylaxis with 75-mg **oseltamivir** once daily for 7-10d.

Bronchitis

It is an infection or inflammation of the mucous membranes of the bronchial tree and focal parenchyma. Bronchitis can be classified into acute and chronic forms, each of which has unique etiologies, pathologies, and therapies.

Etiology and classification

1. **Acute bronchitis**: Over 50% of cases are caused by contagious pathogens, mostly by **viruses** (rhinoviruses, adenoviruses, respiratory syncytial virus, and influenza) and bacteria (Pneumococcus, Hib, etc., similar to those for sinusitis). Others include Mycoplasma, Chlamydia, etc.

2. **Chronic bronchitis**: Mostly due to recurrent injury to the airways caused by inhaled irritants. **Cigarette smoking** is the No.1 cause; others include air pollution, occupational exposure to irritants, and cold air. It is a cause of **COPD** (chronic obstructive pulmonary disease) and considered a form of **COPD**.

Essentials of diagnosis

1. **Acute bronchitis**: Usually induced by the common cold or influenza, with cough; sputum may or may not be present. Discolored sputum suggests bacterial infection. Systemic symptoms may occur. P/E may reveal **pulmonary rales while chest X-ray (CXR) is usually normal.** This confirms the diagnosis and also distinguishes it from pneumonia.

2. **Chronic bronchitis ("The blue bloater")**: Patient has hypoxic appearance, hypersecretion of bronchial mucous (sputum), and chronic or recurrent productive cough that last for > 3 months per year for at least 2 years. CXR usually shows thickening of bronchial walls and increased linear markings ("dirty lungs"). The cardiac shadow may be enlarged.

Treatment

1. Most acute infections usually do not require antibiotic but symptomatic treatment (NSAIDs) because of the viral nature.

2. More severe cases with suspected bacterial infections are treated initially with amoxicillin +/- doxycycline or TMP-SMX. If no response, treat with one of amoxicillin-clavulanate, clarithromycin, azithromycin; or with a new fluoroquinolone (gatifloxacin or levofloxacin). Steroids and bronchodilators are usually helpful. For preventive antibiotic use in **chronic bronchitis or COPD, azithromycin** is a good choice.

Pneumonia

if age <5y/o, =>viral

It's a common infection of the pulmonary tissue characterized by inflammation of the lung parenchyma and abnormal filling of alveoli with fluid (consolidation and exudation). **Pneumonia is a leading cause of death from an infectious disease for patients of all ages.**

PEARLS—Important etiologies and drugs of choice

By etiology, pneumonia can be classified as **"Typical"** (lobar or bacterial pneumonia, about 50%) and **"Atypical"** (interstitial pneumonia, caused by Mycoplasma, Chlamydia, Legionella, Rickettsia, viruses, or Pneumocystis, etc). Predisposing factors include smoking, diabetes, alcoholism, malnutrition, lung cancer, and immunosuppression, etc.

1. **S. Pneumococcus:** It's the commonest cause of acute community-acquired pneumonia ("lobar pneumonia"). Choose **Macrolides, new quinolones or 3rd-generation cephalosporins**.

2. **Gram$^-$ bacilli** (E. coli, Pseudomonas or Enterobacter): Mostly hospital-acquired or ventilator-associated pneumonia. Choose **3rd-generation cephalosporins** or/and carbapenems.

3. **Staph-aureus**: Usually following viral infection or bronchitis, especially influenza. Choose **semisynthetic penicillins** (oxacillin, nafcillin, etc.).

4. **Hib** (often in smokers, COPD) and **Klebsiella** (often in alcoholics): Choose a **2nd or 3rd generation of cephalosporins.**

5. **Mycoplasma**: More common in young and healthy patients. Choose **Macrolides**.

6. **Legionella**: A Gram$^-$ bacterium, epidemic infection in older smokers or with special environment such as infected water sources and air-conditioning systems. Choose **Macrolides**.

7. **Pneumocystis carinii (causing PCP):** Often seen in HIV (+) patients with < 200/uL CD4 cells not on antibiotic prophylaxis. Choose **TMP-SMX**.

8. **Coxiella burnetii (Q-fever)**: From exposure to animals, particularly at the time they are giving birth. Treatment of choice is doxycycline; the second option is erythromycin.

9. **Chlamydia psittaci**: From bird's feces and upper respiratory secretions. Choose **Macrolides.**

10. **Viruses**: Influenza A or B, adenovirus, parainfluenza virus, RSV, etc. Amantadine is cost-effective for influenza A, and oseltamivir or zanamivir is effective for both influenzas A and B.

Essentials of diagnosis

consolidation

1. History of **high fever**, cough, chest pain, tachypnea, and dyspnea (if severe). **Typical, bacterial** pneumonia mostly produces **purulent sputum**; **atypical pneumonia** commonly generates a **nonproductive or "dry" cough**. P/E shows respiratory rate increase and pulmonary rales.

2. **Lab diagnosis:**

(1) Leukocytosis with left shift (bandemia); neutrophil dominant for "typical pneumonia" and usually lymphocytosis for "atypical pneumonia".

PNA

(2) **CXR** (**Image 12**) is the most important **initial test** to reveal if it's lobar (bacterial, typically showing lobar consolidation and air bronchograms) or interstitial (other pathogens) pneumonia. The CXR should be considered a sensitive test—if the findings are not suggestive of pneumonia, do not treat patient with antibiotics.

(3) **Sputum Gram stain and culture** is the most specific test to diagnose and distinguish the "typical" and "atypical" pneumonia, and thus should be obtained in all patients.

3. **Special pathogens—Lobar pneumonia**:

Significant purulent sputum indicates **Pneumococcus ("rusty")**, **Klebsiella ("currant jelly")**, or Hemophilus. P/E usually reveals rales, rhonchi, and signs of **lung consolidation**; tachypnea and dyspnea indicate the severity of pneumonia.

4. **Special pathogens— "Atypical pneumonia"**:

(1) **Mycoplasma**: Mild nonproductive dry cough and chest pain. Serologic antibody titer is the specific diagnosis if necessary. Usually it's adequate to make diagnosis on clinical basis and to treat as an outpatient.

(2) **Legionella**: Nonproductive dry cough, CNS symptoms (confusion, headache, and lethargy) plus GI symptoms (diarrhea and abdominal pain). Specific diagnostic test—Urine antigen test is the initial rapid tool; other specific tests (take longer time) include specialized culture with charcoal yeast extract and direct fluorescent antibody (Ab) titers. WBC count can be normal or high with left shift.

(3) **Chlamydia-pneumoniae, Chlamydia-psittaci, Coxiella, and Coccidioidomycoses**: All of these are diagnosed with specific antibody titers.

Treatment

It depends on the pathogen and severity, inpatients or outpatients. Early empiric treatment is crucial since specific pathogens usually cannot be determined at clinical diagnosis.

- MCC = Strep pneumo, HflU an cause CAP

1. **Community-acquired pneumonia**—Empiric treatment against "typical" bacteria and "atypical" pathogens: *Ceftriaxone + azithromycin for CAP*

(1) **Outpatient: First choice--macrolides** (erythromycin) cover pneumococcus, mycoplasma, and chlamydia; azithromycin or clarithromycin also covers Hib. Alternatives—New fluoroquinolones (levofloxacin, moxifloxacin, or gatifloxacin) are also good options.

(2) **Inpatient: New Fluoroquinolones (Levo, Moxi, Gati-)** or 2nd/3rd generation of cephalosporins (cefuroxime or ceftriaxone) combined with doxycycline or a macrolide or beta-lactam/beta-lactamase combination drug (ampicillin + sulbactam; ticarcillin + clavulanate; piperacillin + tazobactam) combined with doxycycline or a macrolide.

- fever Productive cough, pleuritic CP, focal infiltrate on CXR. MCC Pseudomon

2. **Hospital-acquired pneumonia**: Patient has increased risk of **drug-resistant Gram⁻ bacilli** infection if staying > 5 days in the hospital, > age 60, or with COPD, diabetes (DM), cardiovascular diseases (CVD), or renal disease, etc. Give empiric treatment with **3rd-generation cephalosporins** (ceftazidime or cefotaxime), carbapenems (imipenem), or beta-lactam/beta-lactamase inhibitor Combo (e.g., piperacillin + tazobactam).

RNA

3. Supportive therapies: Oxygen (**O₂**) **treatment by degree of severity and hypoxia:** O_2 supply is needed with arterial $PO_2 < 70$, O_2 saturation $< 94\%$ at room air, or RR > 24/min. IV steroids and other medicines in hospital may help patients with serious disease improve further.

Complications

1. Pleural effusion: It can occur in about 50% of patients and usually resolve with antibiotic treatment of the pneumonia. Empyema is rare.

2. Acute respiratory failure: It may occur if the pneumonia is severe.

Preventive pneumococcal vaccination (PCV)

Two types of pneumococcal vaccines are approved for use in the US:

A. **PPSV23**: includes 23 purified polysaccharide antigens, used in adults; B. **PCV13** (pneumococcal protein-conjugate vaccine): used in infants and children.

1. All children should receive four doses of vaccines (**PCV13**)—at 2, 4, 6, and 12-15 months of age.

2. Additional vaccination by **PPSV23** is recommended for people with increased risk of pneumonia: (1) Age 19-64 with intermediate risk (smoking, chronic heart/lung disease, diabetes); (2) Patients with serious underlying disease or immunodeficiency [long steroid use, asplenic state, with cancer, or HIV (+)], PCV13 followed by PPSV23 two months later; (3) All $\geq$ age 65: PPSV23 alone if vaccinated 5 years ago, or PCV13 followed by PPSV23 6-12 months later.

A single dose of PPSV23 is enough to confer life-long immunity for most people > 65 y/a. The efficacy of the vaccine is about 70%. Re-dosing in 5 years is only considered for those with severe immunodeficiency.

Lung Abscess

It's necrosis of the pulmonary parenchyma and formation of suppurative cavities (usually > 2 cm) containing necrotic debris or fluid caused by microbial infection.

Etiology and pathogenesis

90% of the cases have anaerobes (Peptostreptococcus, Prevotella, Bacteroides), and 50% of them also have mixed aerobes (Strep-milleri, Staph-aureus, E. coli, or Klebsiella) involved. 90% of the cases are closely associated with pathological **aspiration** of oropharyngeal contents or foods (with seizures, dysphagia, altered sensorium, etc.). The lower lobes are the commonest sites of aspiration in the upright position, and the posterior segment of the right upper lobe is the most common site in the supine position. Noninfectious causes include pulmonary infarction, vasculitis, and cancer.

Essentials of diagnosis

1. Symptoms of pulmonary infection (fever, cough, sputum, and chest pain), plus typical putrid, **foul-smelling sputum,** and a more chronic course (weeks) with weight loss, anemia, and fatigue.

2. Sputum for Gram stain and culture usually will not show the causative anaerobes. A lung biopsy may be necessary for confirmative diagnosis.

3. CXR mostly shows a thick-walled cavity with air-fluid levels. A chest CT scan helps define the exact extent of the cavitation, and differentiate between abscess and empyema.

Treatment

1. Hospitalize patient and perform postural drainage.

2. Antibiotic treatment:

(1) **Clindamycin** is the best empiric medicine for the "above the diaphragm" anaerobes (without confirmed pathogens).

(2) High-dose amoxicillin +/- clavulanic acid/sulbactam, or vancomycin is effective against most Gram$^+$ cocci (including MRSA).

(3) If Gram$^-$ organisms are suspected, add a fluoroquinolone or ceftazidime.

(4) Antibiotic therapy should be continued for months until CXR shows significant improvement.

Pulmonary Tuberculosis ("TB")

Reds:
- ignore BCG
- <5yo, PPD
- >5yo, IFN-γ assay

TB is an infection with Mycobacterium tuberculosis occurring primarily in the lungs. It's still an important cause of death in many developing countries. About 1/4 of the world's population has PPD (+) if tested. TB is always spread by person-to-person transmission through respiratory droplets. Bacillus Calmette-Guerin (BCG) vaccination is used in many parts of the world except US, with about 50% effect.

New immigrants occupy > 50% TB cases in the US, and the rest predominantly occurs in people with risky behaviors and factors (alcoholism, healthcare professions, homelessness, chronic diseases, etc.). Most of these people have weak T lymphocyte immunity that predisposes them to have TB infection or re-activation.

Essentials of diagnosis

1. History of low fever, night sweats, chronic cough, sputum, weight loss, and an abnormal lung examination. Extrapulmonary TB is < 20% and can affect lymph nodes (LN), GI or GU system.

2. **CXR is the best initial test** for TB, usually showing apical infiltrates, adenopathy, effusion, and chronic cavitations or calcified nodules. **Ghon's complex**—a combination of parenchymal lung calcification and hilar lymphadenopathy—is the pathologic mark of primary TB. It's more common in children with TB. The combination of a primary focus, TB lymphangitis, and hilar TB lymphadenopathy forms a "**dumbbell-shaped**" shadow on a CXR film.

3. **Lab tests**:

(1) Sputum **staining for acid-fast bacilli** supplies **fast and specific diagnosis**. Positive staining is the indication of anti-TB treatment, but the low sensitivity requires three negative smears to rule out.

TB

(2) Sputum **culture is the most specific test**, but is too slow (taking 4-6 weeks to grow) to guide initial treatment; rather, it is necessary for drug sensitivity testing.

(3) Special tests for complicated cases: **Pleural biopsy is the most sensitive** test of pulmonary TB, which will show caseous necrosis. Other tests include examination of thoracic or gastric fluids.

4. **PPD test** (Mantoux test) is used to early screen TB-risky people. The size of the induration (not the erythema) is measured 48-72 hours after the injection; > 15 mm is (+). It is not used to diagnose acute TB because it's neither sensitive nor specific for acute disease.

15: people you shouldn't be testing

10: ① risk pph homeless, prisons healthcare workers.

5: immunosuppr + close contacts

(1) PPD (+) indicates history of TB exposure, and the need of CXR. If CXR is also abnormal, it requires three sputum stains for acid-fast bacilli to see if active TB is present. Acid-fast stain (+) indicates active TB and the need for the treatment of four anti-TB drugs (see Treatment below).

(2) Acid-fast stain (+) with PPD (+) tests but without CXR evidence of active TB indicates the need of 9-month treatment of isoniazid (INH) and Vit-B$_6$ (to prevent peripheral neuritis).

5. **TB in children**: Because the presentations may not be typical, diagnosis is usually based on the presence of the classic triad: (1) recent close contact with an infectious case, (2) a positive TB skin test (TST) or interferon-gamma release assay (IGRA), and (3) suggestive findings on CXR (primary complex) or physical examination.

Differential diagnosis

Pulmonary disease by nontuberculous mycobacteria (NTM, atypical mycobacteria; MAC #1):

(1) Chronic cough, sputum, malaise, and fatigue, usually in an immunodeficient patient; dyspnea, fever, hemoptysis, and weight loss may be present.

(2) CXR shows wide parenchymal infiltrates, often with thin-walled cavities and overlying pleura.

(3) Diagnosis is confirmed by isolation of nontuberculous mycobacteria in a sputum culture.

Treatment *RIPE or INH +B6*
full blown   Latent

1. All TB cases should be **reported to the local health department. All CXR (+) cases** should be **treated with the 4-drugs** (isoniazid, rifampin, pyrazinamide, and ethambutol) for the **first 2 months** (before drug sensitivity results), followed by **INH** (plus Vit-B$_6$) **and rifampin** for **another 4-7 months (totally 6-9 months)**. Ethambutol is added if the sensitivity is not known.

2. The TB conditions that definitely **require over 6-month therapy** are: (1) TB **meningitis** (12 months); (2) TB in **pregnancy** (9 months; avoid pyrazinamide or streptomycin); (3) TB **osteomyelitis**. (4) TB with HIV (+) (6-9 months). Steroids are helpful in TB meningitis or TB pericarditis.

Adverse effects (S/E): All of the TB drugs may have **liver toxicity** except streptomycin (with renal and otic toxicity). INH can also cause peripheral neuritis that can be decreased by Vit-B$_6$ supply. Rifampin can cause benign bodily fluid coloring to orange/red. Ethambutol may cause optic neuritis. Pyrazinamide can cause a benign hyperuricemia (no treatment).

3. <u>**Treatment of latent TB infection on PPD testing**</u> (9-month treatment of INH + Vit-B$_6$, any age):

Peds: only separate mom from baby if you suspect multi-drug resistance in baby + mom follows same tx path

Tuberculosis

(1) **Induration (not erythema) > 5 mm**: Close contacts of active TB patients; abnormal CXR consistent with old, healed TB; steroid use or organ transplantation recipients; HIV (+) persons.

(2) **Induration > 10 mm**: High-risk groups (patients with immunodeficiency, cancer, diabetes, or dialysis; healthcare workers, prisoners, recent immigrants, and homeless people).

(3) **Induration > 15 mm**: Low-risk people and most people.

Prophylaxis

Bacillus Calmette-Guerin (BCG): It's not given routinely because the efficacy is uncertain, and only recommended for disseminated TB (such as TB meningitis).

INFECTIONS OF THE CENTRAL NERVOUS SYSTEM (CNS)

Meningitis

It's an infection and inflammation of the meninges, the connective tissue that covers the brain and spinal cord. Most causes are infectious and non-infectious etiologies (such as medications, SLE, sarcoidosis, and carcinomatosis) are much less. If the course lasts longer than 4 weeks, it's defined as chronic meningitis and is a complex entity with both infectious and noninfectious causes.

<u>**Important etiology**</u>

1. **Pneumococcus**: **#1 common** for all patients **beyond the neonatal period.**

2. **Strep-B or E coli: #1 common in newborns to infants of 6 months in age. Listeria and Klebsiella** are also common for this age group.

3. **Meningococcus: #1 common in adolescents** and spread by respiratory droplets.

4. **Hib**: A very common cause in children in the past but now markedly decreased by the use of the Hib vaccine in children.

5. **Listeria**: More common in **immunodeficient** (particularly T cells or neutrophil deficiency) or **immunocompromised patients**—including with steroid use, alcoholism, chemotherapy, leukemia, lymphoma, HIV (+), **neonates, the elderly** (with lower T-cell function), and pregnancy. However, **pneumococcus** is still the most common pathogen for meningitis with immunodeficiency.

6. **S. aureus**: More common with a history of **neurosurgery**.

7. **Cryptococcus, Toxoplasma, CMV**: More common in patients with markedly low T cells (as in AIDS, **CD4 <100/uL**).

Essentials of diagnosis

1. Patient may have a history of a local infection (otitis media, sinusitis, mastoiditis, and dental infections), or a systemic infection (endocarditis, pneumonia, etc.).

2. Typically presents with high fever, photophobia, headache, nausea, vomiting, confusion, neck stiffness, and positive **Kernig and Brudzinski sign.**

Meningitis

3. **Rash**: Petechial rash suggests Neisseria (may be fulminant); centripetal spreading rash suggests Rocky Mountain spotted fever; "target" erythema migrans and CN7 palsy suggest Lyme disease; vesicular lesions suggest varicella or HSV infection.

4. **Lab tests:** WBC increase with predominant PMNs and bands. A lumbar puncture (**LP**) for cerebrospinal fluid (**CSF**) biochemistry (protein, glucose, etc.), cell count, culture and sensitivity tests is crucial for accurate diagnosis and treatment, but **empiric antibiotics** should be started **while the results are waited for. Special tests include:**

(1) **TB:** Acid fast stain and culture on three high-volume lumbar punctures should be done.

(2) **Cryptococcus:** Cryptococcal antigen is > 95% sensitive and specific.

(3) **Lyme and Rickettsia:** Specific serologic tests, ELISA, etc.

(4) **Virus:** Usually a diagnosis of exclusion.

5. **A head CT is the best initial diagnostic step instead of LP** (which may cause herniation) **if the patient has signs of increased intracranial pressure (ICP)** —vomiting, papilledema, focal motor deficits, or severe confusion. A dose of ceftriaxone prior to the CT scan is recommended (better after a blood sample is taken for culture).

PEARLS—Table 1-3: Differential Points of CSF in Meningitis

Etiology / CSF Biochemistry
1. Bacteria: Pressure > 180 mmH$_2$O, neutrophils increasing, protein > 40 mg/dL, glucose < 40 mg/dL.
2. Virus, syphilis, rickettsia: Pressure normal/increasing, LCs increasing; protein and glucose: mostly normal.
3. TB, fungi (Cryptococcus): Pressure > 180 mmH$_2$O, LCs increasing, protein > 40 mg/dL, glucose < 40 mg/dL.

Treatment (by etiology)

1. **Most cases of bacterial meningitis:** The best empiric treatment is **ceftriaxone or cefotaxime plus vancomycin, which can all pass the blood-brain barrier** against pneumococcus, meningococcus, or Group-B Strep. The antibiotics are usually started while the CT or/and CSF results are waited for.

2. **Resistant cases:** Vancomycin and steroids are added for severe infection with suspected pneumococcal resistance to penicillin, or suspected Staph after neurosurgery.

3. **Immunocompromised patients: Vancomycin plus ampicillin** (against Listeria) **plus cefepime or meropenem**, with very young or old ages, neonates, HIV (+), steroid use, pregnancy, or severe cancer.

4. **Allergy to beta-lactams: Vancomycin plus moxifloxacin** (plus TMP-SMX against Listeria).

5. **Healthcare-associated meningitis: Vancomycin plus ceftazidime or cefepime** to cover both gram-positive and gram-negative rods (Klebsiella P. and P. aeruginosa).

6. **For special pathogens:**

(1) Corticosteroid is added to TB meningitis for possible cerebral edema.

Meningitis

(2) Viral or aseptic meningitis is primarily treated with support.

(3) Lyme disease with CNS infection is best treated with ceftriaxone.

(4) Cryptococcus meningitis is treated initially with amphotericin, followed by lifelong fluconazole in HIV (+) patients.

(5) Aseptic meningitis: It's mostly self-limited and only needs supportive and symptomatic treatment.

Prophylaxis and vaccination

1. Respiratory isolation and rifampin or ceftriaxone for all close contacts of patients with meningococcus. General contacts (such as routine school and work contacts) may not be "close contact".

2. MCV (meningococcal vaccine) is now recommended to all children at 11-12 y/a. Add a booster at 16 y/a or in asplenic or immunocompromised patients.

Encephalitis

It's a diffuse inflammation of the brain parenchyma. Encephalitis is often seen with meningitis and is known as meningoencephalitis. Most of the causes are infectious by viruses. Viral encephalitis can be either primary or postinfectious, which are difficult to differentiate clinically.

Etiology

Viruses are the most common cause, although any bacterial, protozoal, or rickettsial infection can be the etiology. **HSV-1 is the most common one**; other viruses include varicella, CMV, enteroviruses, and arboviruses (Eastern and Western equine, California and St. Louis, etc; see "PEDIATRICS"). Noninfectious causes mostly include metabolic encephalopathies and T-cell lymphoma.

Essentials of diagnosis

1. Obtain a detailed sexual, travel, and exposure history (to both insects and animals). Patient usually has high fever, headache, altered mental status (confusion, lethargy, or coma), and neurologic deficits (focal deficiency, seizure, or neck stiffness).

2. **Lab tests**: (1) **The best diagnostic test is polymerase chain reaction (PCR) for HSV-1 and IgM antibody on CSF and serum for West Nile virus**. CSF-PCR is the new efficient test for etiology with high sensitivity and specificity for HSV, etc. (2) Lymphocytosis (> 5 WBC/uL) with normal glucose is consistent with viral encephalitis or meningitis.

3. A head CT or MRI scan is helpful in differential diagnosis, especially to exclude a focal lesion such as an abscess (usually with confusion and focal neurological deficits), although it may give a non-specific result. **HSV encephalitis usually involves the frontotemporal lobes**, which can be detected by an MRI (increased T2-areas), contrast-CT scan, or EEG (lobal discharges).

Differential diagnosis

Patients with **aseptic meningitis** most commonly present with fever and headache with meningismus on examination; may be lethargic but have a normal sensorium. By contrast, patients with **encephalitis** present with mental status changes. Patients with features of both may be considered to have a **meningoencephalitis**.

Treatment

HSV encephalitis is best **treated with early IV acyclovir** for 2-3 weeks. Famciclovir and valacyclovir are also effective but not available for IV route. **Ganciclovir or foscarnet is effective against CMV. Foscarnet** is also used for **acyclovir-resistant** cases. Other treatment is mainly symptomatic and supportive care (for seizures, cerebral edema, etc.).

Brain Abscess

It's defined as a focal collection of infected and inflammatory materials within the brain parenchyma, mostly after bacterial infections.

Etiology

1. Common pathogens include Strep, Staph, Bacteroides, and Enterobacteria, and are often mixed.

2. Bacteria can spread into the brain from contiguous focal infections such as otitis media, sinusitis, mastoiditis, or dental infections, or cranial trauma/surgery.

3. It may also spread through the bloodstream from endocarditis or pneumonia. Toxoplasmosis can reactivate in patients with severe immunodeficiency or AIDS (when CD_4 counts are < 100/uL).

Essentials of diagnosis

1. Headache and fever are most common symptoms, followed by focal neurologic deficits and seizures. Note that fever and chills may be absent.

2. CT scan with contrast is the initial test (although CNS malignancy also enhances with contrast). MRI is more accurate than is the CT. **A biopsy** of the lesion with **Gram stain and culture** is the definite means of diagnosis and guide for treatment.

3. In HIV (+) patients, about 90% brain lesions will be either toxoplasmosis or lymphoma. Thus, CT or MRI (+) is the strong indication of empiric, diagnostic treatment. If the lesion is smaller after 10-14 days' use of pyrimethamine and sulfadiazine, it is diagnostic and this therapy should be continued.

Treatment

1. Depending on the size of abscess and presence of mass effect, treatment may include IV broad-spectrum antibiotics (4-8 weeks), and /or surgical drainage. Glucocorticoids are used only with evidence of substantial mass effect and significant depression.

2. Because the infection is mostly polymicrobial, it is difficult to have an effective monotherapy. Therapies must be guided by the specific pathogens found. **(1) Empiric antibiotics for hematogenous and post-neurosurgery/trauma brain abscess are vancomycin** (to cover MRSA) **plus nafcillin and cefotaxime or cefepime. (2) For uncertain bacteria or from an oral, otogenic, or sinus source: metronidazole** (for the anaerobes) **plus penicillin G** (for the Strep) or/and **ceftriaxone/cefotaxime** (for Gram⁻ bacilli) are recommended.

3. HIV (+) patient is best treated with pyrimethamine and sulfadiazine as a good application for empiric diagnostic therapy against toxoplasmosis for at least 2 weeks.

GASTROINTESTINAL TRACT INFECTIONS

Infectious Diarrhea and Food Poisoning

Most infectious diarrheas are caused by contaminated foods or water by bacteria or their toxins, often overlapped with food poisoning (with more epidemic cases). The best initial test for diagnosis is to look for blood and/or fecal WBCs—viruses, Giardia, Cryptosporidiosis, Bacillus cereus, Staphylococcus are usually negative for it. Common types of infectious diarrhea by pathogens are summarized below.

PEARLS—Table 1-4: Summary of Infectious Diarrhea and Food Poisoning

Campylobacter jejuni

Sources: Contaminated food, milk, etc; person-to-person. **Features: #1 common bacterial diarrhea/colitis.** Fever, headache, severe RLQ abdominal cramps, and diarrhea with blood/pus (50% cases); occasionally associated with Guillain-Barre syndrome; mostly self-limited. **Tx**: Supportive. If severe, use ciprofloxacin or erythromycin.

Enterotoxigenic E. coli

Sources: From uncooked food and fecal contamination. It is the #1 common **"Traveler's diarrhea"**. **Features**: Abrupt watery diarrhea (rarely bloody); abdominal cramps; rarely vomiting. **Tx**: (1) mostly self-limited, < 3 stools/day: no Tx or use loperamide; (2) If severe, > 3 stools/day: supportive care and ciprofloxacin for 1-3 days.

Enterohemolytic E. coli O157:H7

Sources: From contaminated meat/beef (undercooked) and fruits, etc. **Features**: Abrupt bloody diarrhea, abdominal cramps, looking very sick, possible presentations of hemorrhagic colitis and hemolytic-uremic syndrome **(HUS)**. **Tx**: It's mostly self-limited; supportive care for HUS. Antibiotics are not recommended.

Staph-aureus

Sources: Undercooked **meat, milk,** etc; preformed toxin. **Features:** Abrupt, **intense vomiting** about 2-4 hours after eating; diarrhea is rare. It's mostly self-limited. **Tx:** Mostly support is adequate.

Bacillus cereus

Sources: Reheated rice contaminated with Bacillus spores; preformed toxin. **Features:** Abrupt **vomiting** 2-4 hours after meal followed by **watery diarrhea** later. **Tx:** It's mostly self-limited; supportive care or ciprofloxacin.

Shigella

Sources: Transmitted by **"4Fs"** — "Food, Fingers, Feces, and Flies." **Features**: Hours after eating contaminated food, abrupt lower abdominal cramps followed by inflammatory diarrhea with blood and mucus, tenesmus, nausea, vomiting, fever, and even **HUS** if severe. **Tx: TMP-SMX** or **ciprofloxacin** along with supportive care is usually needed. It usually resolves in a week.

Salmonella

Sources: Poultry—raw/undercooked **chicken or eggs. Features: High fever**, relatively **slow pulses**, nausea, vomiting, and inflammatory diarrhea; usually self-limited and resolves within a week. **Tx:** Mainly supportive. Short-term antibiotics may prolong carrier status and increase relapse rate, and thus prolonged antibiotics (**ciprofloxacin**) should be used if necessary.

Clostridium perfringens and difficile

Sources: C. perfringens—**reheated meat**; contaminated with spores (unrefrigerated); preformed toxin. **C. difficile**—usually due to long-term use of broad-band antibiotics. **Features:** 7-8 hours after eating, abrupt profuse, **watery diarrhea with prominent crampy abdominal pain**. **Dx:** Confirmed by the stool toxin test; WBCs and RBCs in stool. **Tx:** Metronidazole or vancomycin IV.

Clostridium botulinum

Sources: Honey, canned meat; preformed toxin. **Features:** Onset in 1-4 days, flaccid **paralysis**; diarrhea is rare. **Tx: Early specific anti-toxin and penicillin** IV are necessary and effective treatment.

Vibrio cholera

Sources: In **endemic** areas; toxin-induced illness. **Features:** Severe, profuse, **"rice-water diarrhea."**
Tx: Antibiotics and vigorous fluid and electrolyte replacement.

Vibrio parahaemolyticus

Sources: Contaminated **seafood. Features:** Self-limited abdominal cramp and diarrhea. **Tx:** Support. If it's severe with high fever, quinolones should be used.

Yersinia enterocolitica

Sources: Pets; raw/undercooked meat. **Features:** Often causes sporadic ileitis or ileocolitis—fever and RLQ abdominal pain—similar to appendicitis except for inflammatory diarrhea (+/- blood). It may also mimic ulceric colitis or **Crohn** disease; associated with high affinity for iron, hemochromatosis, and blood transfusion. **Dx:** Confirmed by serology and stool culture. **Tx:** Ciprofloxacin is chosen if severe.

Giardia lamblia

Sources: Endemic area, food, contaminated mountain water, and immunodeficiency. **Features:** Watery, foul-smelling diarrhea; abdominal bloating. **Dx:** Stool exam for the parasites or eggs, or by bowel biopsy.
Tx: Oral metronidazole.

Entamoeba histolytica

Sources: Traveling, homosexual behavior, etc. **Features:** RLQ abdominal cramp and diarrhea with blood or pus, accompanied with mass or obstruction. **Dx:** (1) #1 test is stool culture and oval examination. (2) Serology testing for specific antibodies if necessary. **Tx:** Oral metronidazole.

VIRAL HEPATITIS

Definition and pathogenesis

It's a group of acute and chronic infections and inflammation of the liver caused by various hepatitis viruses. They are **all RNA viruses except HBV, which is a DNA virus**. The prevalence is higher in Asian countries. The major **pathogenesis is virus-induced immunologic inflammation and necrosis** of hepatocytes, causing similar manifestations of fever, fatigue, decreased appetite, jaundice (in some), and elevated liver function tests (**LFTs**). **ALT:AST ratio** is mostly >2, opposite to that in alcoholic hepatitis.

Viral hepatitis is divided into five types: Hepatitis A, B, C, D, and E. **Most clinical cases are hepatitis A and B. Hepatitis A and E are mainly spread by digestive tract (restaurants and foods) and tend to be self-limited. Hepatitis B and C are mainly spread by blood (transfusion and IV drug abuse) and body fluids and tend to be chronic.** A minority of them develop cirrhosis or cancer, particularly hepatitis C with chronic progression. Fulminant hepatic necrosis and failure is rare but can occur with any viral hepatitis and acetaminophen sensitivity. Breast-feeding is not contraindicated for infected mothers because the risk of infant infection is very low.

In serology, **IgM** antibody to hepatitis virus A, C, D, or E **indicates acute infection**, whereas **IgG antibody indicates chronic or resolved status**. There is no effective treatment for any acute hepatitis. However, effective treatments of chronic hepatitis B and C in recent years have significantly decreased the morbidities of cirrhosis, liver cancer, etc. Liver transplantation is the last resort of treatment for the late-stage hepatic disease or failure.

Hepatitis A (HA)

HAV is a SS-RNA picornavirus virus, transmitted by **fecal-oral** route and causes predominantly acute hepatitis. It may also be spread sexually. Poor hygiene or contaminated foods are common risk factors. Incubation period is 15-50 days. After infection, it induces life-long immunity. There is **no "chronic hepatitis A."** Risk of fulminant hepatitis is about 1%.

Essentials of diagnosis

1. General symptoms of fever, fatigue, nausea, jaundice, and elevated LFTs. Anti-HAV IgM (+) indicates a recent or acute exposure.

2. Anti-HAV IgG (+) indicates previous exposure or infection, and life-long immunity. Thus anti-HAV IgG (+) does not distinguish between active disease and immunity. IgM (+) specifies acute infection.

Treatment: Most HA resolve spontaneously over a few weeks and only supportive care is needed.

Prophylaxis

(1) Inactivated HAV (vaccine) is recommended for infants at 12-15 months by 2-dose series, patients with a chronic liver disease, and for travellers to endemic areas (e.g., a month before going to Asia or Africa), with 95% effectiveness (active immunization). (2) If one will be travelling to endemic areas within 4 weeks, one needs an HAV-IG vaccination (human gamma (γ)-globulin, passive immunization, protective for 2-3 months).

Hepatitis B (HB)

Mainly a blood-borne infection caused by HBV—a **DNA virus**, identified in all body fluids: blood, saliva, synovial fluid, breast milk, ascites, cerebral spinal fluid, etc. Incubation is 1-6 months. About 50% of fulminant hepatitis is caused by HBV. **For acute hepatitis B, 90% of neonate cases will develop chronic** hepatitis, whereas for **adults, only 10%** will become chronic and 90% will recover. HB is a **major cause of liver carcinoma**. HB is also associated with membrane- and membranoproliferative glomerulonephritis, aplastic anemia, and polyarteritis nodosa.

Essentials of diagnosis

1. General symptoms of fever, fatigue, nausea, jaundice, and elevated LFTs.

2. HBsAg is present in both acute and chronic infection. It is **detectable as early as 1-2 weeks** after infection. It usually persists in **chronic hepatitis (> 6 months)** until the virus is cleared, regardless of symptoms. HBsAg in the acute phase is positive and soon turns negative ("**Window period**"), followed by anti-HBc IgM positive.

3. Anti-HBs IgG is present after vaccination or after clearance of HBsAg—usually detectable 1-3 months after infection. Anti-HBs IgG (+) alone indicates prior immunity via vaccination; anti-HBs IgG (+) plus anti-HBc IgG (+) denotes a previous infection and immunity.

4. HBeAg (+) is an indicator of active HBV replication and infectivity, following HBsAg shortly.

5. Viral load: HBV DNA is measured by PCR. If it persists for > 6 weeks, chronic HB is likely.

PEARLS—**Table 1-5: Important Serological Markers in HBV Infection**

Hbs Ag	Anti-HBs	Anti-HBc	Hbe Ag	Anti-HBe	ALT	Interpretation
+	-	IgM +	+	-	Elevated	Acute HB (Anti-HBc is not protective)
-	-	IgM +	-	-	Elevated	Acute HB, window period
+	-	IgG +	+	-	Persistently Elevated	Chronic HB, with active viral replication
+	-	IgG +	-	IgG +	Normal or mildly elevated	Inactive chronic HB, with low viral replication
+	IgG +	IgG +	+	IgG +	Elevated	Chronic HB, with heterotypic Anti-HBs (10%)
-	IgG +	IgG +	-	IgG +/-	Normal	Recovery from HB, with immunity
-	IgG +	-	-	-	Normal	Vaccination, with immunity

Figure 1-1: Clinical Course and Serology of Hepatitis B Infection (Courtesy of www.gribbles.com)

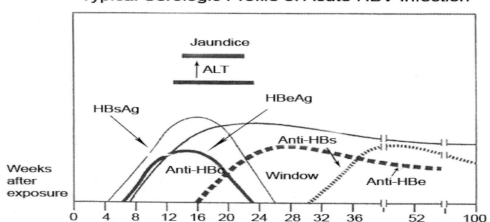

Typical Serologic Profile of Acute HBV Infection

Treatment

1. Acute phase: Supportive therapy is the mainstream of treatment. There is no specific therapy.

2. **Chronic HB:** The new effective antiviral treatment is **6-12 months of entecavir (initially) or tenofovir DF (less risk of resistance). Lamivudine, adefovir, or telbivudine may have more risk of resistance and** alpha-**interferon (PegIFN) has more E/S.** The goal is to reduce the viral load and convert HBeAg (+) state into anti-HBe (+) state. Adverse effects of alpha-interferon include depression, flu-like symptoms, arthralgia, myalgia, leukopenia, and thrombocytopenia.

3. Fulminant HB or liver failure: Liver transplantation is the last resort of treatment.

Important prophylaxis

HBV vaccine (recombinant HBsAg) is the only vaccination that prevents HBV infection and liver carcinoma effectively. Anti-HBc is never seen after the vaccination. It requires a series of three vaccinations for the patient to develop immunity. However, not all patients will have the immunity, and thus testing the titers is necessary.

PEARLS—Recommended vaccination for HBV

1. For all children by 3 doses—at birth, 1-2 months, and 6-18 months and adults who miss it.

2. Indicated for people with high risk—healthcare workers and those with chronic liver disease; repeat every 10 years if still with risk. The efficiency of protection is about 95% for 10 years.

3. If patient was exposed to HBV (by needle puncture, etc.) and received no vaccination before, the patient needs HBIG plus an HBV vaccine within 24 hours, followed by another two vaccines in a few months.

4. If patient has a history of exposure to HBV or previous response—with HbsAb (+) in 9 years [even with HbsAg (+)], then the patient only needs reassurance.

5. If patient was exposed to HBV and no response to previous vaccinations, then the patient needs HBIG in 24 hours.

6. If a pregnant patient has HbsAg (+) and HbeAg (+), the infection risk is 95%. The newborn needs HBIG within 12 hours and the vaccination shortly after delivery, and the patient needs the first HBV vaccination within 24 hours, followed by another two vaccinations later. Combined immunization not only blocks mother-infant spreading, but also enables the mother's breast-feeding with HbsAg (+).

Hepatitis C (HC)

HCV is spread predominantly by blood products, is the **#1 cause of hepatitis among patients with IV drug abuse and blood transfusion**, and accounts for **60% of all hepatitis**. Sexual transmission is much lower than with HB (less than 5%). Perinatal transmission is 5%. Needle-stick transmission is 5-10%. Incubation is 2 weeks to 6 mo and **mostly "silent", asymptomatic, or with mild symptoms**. HCV is rarely acute and it alone rarely leads to severe hepatitis or hepatic failure, which is mostly caused by combined HBV infection. Anti-HCV IgM is diagnostic but not protective in the acute phase. Over **80% of acute HC progresses into chronic hepatitis and is a major cause of cirrhosis (20%) and partial cause of liver cancer. Mnemonic: HC = "4C features"**: "Chronic, Cirrhosis, Carcinoma, and Cryoglobulinemia".

Hepatitis C-associated extra-hepatic diseases   ⇒ OME p. 82

cryoglobulinemic vasculitis, mthgs . FA 547, Path 136

Mixed cryoglobulinemia, ITP, polyarteritis nodosa, leukocytoclastic vasculitis, Sjogren syndrome, Hashimoto thyroiditis and hypothyroidism, membranous and membranoproliferative glomerulonephritis, B-cell lymphoma, plasmacytoma, sporadic porphyria cutanea tarda, lichen planus, and increased risk of diabetes.

Essentials of diagnosis

1. Only 25% of cases have above mild symptoms.

2. **Lab tests**: Elevated LFTs. Anti-HCV is usually (+) and indicative of HCV infection, but not protective. Anti-HCV (-) does not rule out infection because this antibody is sometimes not detectable until months after infection. **HCV RNA load by PCR is the most sensitive and specific diagnostic test**, usually detectable 1-2 weeks after infection. C4 is decreased.

Treatment

1. Most patients are "silent" without symptoms or abnormal LFTs and thus not in need of treatment. Follow-up for LFTs is recommended.

2. Symptomatic chronic HC: Long-term direct acting antagonists (DAAs) have been replacing interferon and ribavirin (due to adverse effects) as the new effective treatment of six genotypes of HC. There are four classes of DAAs.

(1) Nonstructural proteins 3/4A (NS3/4A) protease inhibitors (PIs): Telaprevir and boceprevir, alone or in conjunction with peginterferon and ribavirin for genotype 1 HC. Grazoprevir is newer and more potent, usually in combination with the NS5A inhibitor elbasvir.

(2) NS5B nucleoside polymerase inhibitors (NPIs): Sofosbuvir—high potency across all six genotypes, a very high barrier to resistance.

(3) NS5B non-nucleoside polymerase inhibitors (NNPIs): Dasabuvir—less potent and has a lower threshold for resistance.

(4) NS5A inhibitors: Ledipasvir, ombitasvir, and elbasvir.

If not effective, recommended combinations include elbasvir-grazoprevir, ledipasvir-sofosbuvir, or ombitasvir-paritaprevir-ritonavir. Treatment can decrease the risk of developing chronic infection and cirrhosis. An HCV vaccine is still under development. Preventive principles are similar to HB.

Hepatitis D (HD)

HDV infects either simultaneously **with HBV** or as a superinfection with chronic hepatitis B (more severe). HDV is a defective virus, which requires HBV to supply HbsAg for replication. Thus, HDV cannot infect without HBV and the infection carries the highest risk for fulminant hepatitis. HD with HB is predominantly seen in patients exposed to blood products (transfusion, IVDA, etc). Anti-HBs Ab (+) is protective for both hepatitis B and D. **Mnemonic: "DDV" feature** — "**D**efective & **D**ependent Virus".

Essentials of diagnosis

1. An asymptomatic **HBV carrier suddenly presents with severe symptoms of acute hepatitis**; or chronic HB worsens abruptly to hepatic failure. Then HBV combined with HDV infection should be suspected.

2. **Lab tests**: Elevated LFTs; positive serum or liver HDAg or HDV-RNA (indicating superinfection), or positive serum anti-HDV IgM or IgG (high titers) confirm the diagnosis. Anti-HDV may not be present in acute phase, and thus negative result does not rule out infection (repeating is needed). Liver biopsy showing advanced fibrosis supports chronic HD.

Treatment and prophylaxis

There is no specific therapy for acute HD. Same treatment and prophylaxis as for HB may be tried. Foscarnet as an inhibitor of viral DNA polymerases is under encouraging clinical trial for fulminant HD.

Hepatitis E (HE)

HE is caused by HEV, which has four genotypes and one serum type. It can be a co-infected disease among humans and animals. It's similar to **HA**, with fecal or oral transmission, no chronic form, and usually self-limited, but it can cause **fulminant hepatitis in pregnant patients (20%)** with a high mortality. **Mnemonic**: "Enteric-Fulminant-Maternal" — "**EF-Mom**".

Essentials of diagnosis

1. Most patients have similar symptoms as with HA. It's more severe with pregnant patients.

2. **Lab tests**: Elevated LFTs; serum anti-HEV IgM or/and IgG (+), or/and HEV-RNA (+).

Treatment

Same as for HA—most cases resolve over a few weeks and only need supportive care. Prevention with sanitary procedures is recommended

UROGENITAL INFECTIONS AND SEXUALLY TRANSMITTED DISEASES (STD)

UROGENITAL INFECTIONS

Lower Urinary Tract Infections (Lower UTI)

It's an infection and inflammation of the **urethra (urethritis) or urinary bladder (cystitis, more common). It can be gonococcal and non-gonococcal.**

E. coli is still the most common pathogen, usually associated with sexual activities in female (more common) and prostate hyperplasia in male. Among patients with **multiple sexual partners, Chlamydia or/and Gonococcus** is most common. Other pathogens include Staph-spp., Klebsiella, Proteus, Enterococcus, Mycoplasma, Trichomonas, and HSV. Other risk factors include pregnancy, indwelling urinary catheters, history of UTI, diabetes, and immunocompromised state.

Essentials of diagnosis

1. Irritative voiding symptoms—dysuria, urgency, and frequency in urination. Purulent urethral discharge is usually seen with Gonococcus and mucus discharge with Chlamydia. **Fever is typically absent.** P/E may show suprapubic tenderness. Diagnosis of E. coli UTI is by clinical impression.

2. Urine dipstick: Nitride (+) indicates Enterobacter (+). Esterase (+) indicates polyleukocytes. RBC may be seen in cystitis.

3. Urine Gram stain showing > 10^5 organisms/mL indicates significant bacteriuria, with 90% sensitivity. With **gonorrhea, secretion smear** can show the **Gram⁻, bean-shaped diplococci** inside cells. Culture is the most specific test for gonorrhea.

4. **For Chlamydia** (by C. trachomatis D-K), the new specific testing is polymerase chain reaction **(PCR)** or ligase chain reaction **(LCR)** on either a genital swab or a urine specimen. Other tests include fluorescent antibody **(FA)** examination of a direct smear and Chlamydia culture. However, **pathologic culture sensitivity is low and thus negative result does not exclude Chlamydia.**

Differential diagnosis

<u>Urethritis and cystitis:</u> Both have dysuria and urinary frequency and burning, but cystitis does not give urethral discharge. *Chronic urethritis: due to insuff tx of G&C.*

<u>Interstitial cystitis:</u> (1) Pain with a full bladder or urinary urgency. (2) Submucosal petechiae or ulcers on cystoscopic examination. (3) Diagnosis of exclusion.

Treatment

1. For most complicated urethritis and cystitis (by E. coli, etc): Oral fluoroquinolone such as ciprofloxacin or levofloxacin for 5 to 10 days is the best therapy. Levofloxacin, ceftriaxone, or ertapenem can be used for resistant organisms.

2. For Gonococcal and Chlamydial infections: **A single dose of ceftriaxone and azithromycin, or a single dose of ceftriaxone** IM along with **7-day doxycycline** PO. Gonorrhea can also be treated with a single dose of ciprofloxacin or cefixime PO.

3. The **same** treatment is **for cervicitis and epididymitis**.

Pyelonephritis

It's considered an upper UTI, a diffuse pyogenic infection of the pelvis and parenchyma of the kidney. In adults, it usually ascends from lower UTI and with similar pathogens (**E. coli**, Proteus, Pseudomonas, etc). In children, it is mostly due to bladder-urinary obstruction and recurrence. Recurrent or severe cases may lead to renal scarring, chronic pyelonephritis, emphysematous pyelonephritis, and sepsis (10%).

Essentials of diagnosis

1. **Fever, chill**, nausea, vomiting, **flank pain plus "irritative voiding symptoms."**, malaise
2. P/E demonstrates tenderness on the infected renal site (costovertebral angle).
3. **Lab tests**: Pyuria; urine dipstick—nitride and esterase (+), WBC cast in urine; RBC may be seen with cystitis. CBC: increased WBC with left shift. Urine cultures: obtain in all suspected cases. Blood cultures: obtain in ill-appearing and hospitalized patients.

Treatment

1. Hospitalize patient and take urine or/and blood for bacterial culture and sensitivity (C/S) for suspected cases and potential sepsis.
2. **Empiric therapies:** (1) **Mild to moderate cases**: ceftriaxone, ciprofloxacin or cefepime IV for 7-14 days. (2) **Severe cases with immunosuppression**: ampicillin-sulbactam or ticarcillin-clavulanate or imipenem IV. If no effect in 3 days after changing to proper antibiotics, perform renal ultrasonography or CT/MRI for possible obstruction, abscess, or mass. Treat recurrent cases with antibiotics up to 6 weeks. Repeat urine culture 2-4 days after cessation of antibiotics.

Prostatitis

Bacterial Prostatitis - intraprostatic reflux of pathogens in urine

It is usually caused by the same Gram⁻ organisms found in UTIs (**E. coli**, etc) **in older men**. In young patients with risky sexual behaviour, Gonococcus and/or Chlamydia are more frequent.

Clinical features, diagnosis, and treatment

1. **Acute:** (1) High fever, chill, low back pain, irritative voiding symptoms, and perineal discomfort. *malaise, myalgias   dysuria, urine retention, suprapubic or pelvic pain, frequency, urgency,*
(2) P/E: Digital rectal exam (DRE) reveals prostate swelling, warmth, *anterior* tenderness, and induration; urethral discharge is (-). **Massage is forbidden** for acute infection to avoid spreading to sepsis.
(3) **Lab tests**: Urinalysis shows numerous WBCs; urine culture is mostly (+).   *prostatic abscess?*

Treatment: (1) Hospitalize and monitor patient for sepsis if urinary obstruction exists. *bacteremia/systemic spread.* (2) **TMP-SMX or ciprofloxacin** (4-6 weeks) carries good coverage and prostate penetration. If sepsis is suspected, *levofloxacin* IV ampicillin and gentamycin is indicated.

2. **Chronic:** (1) History of recurrent UTIs with the same organisms; low back pain, testicle pain *– pain w/ ejaculation, bc prostatic fluid is irritative* (epididymitis), irritable voiding symptoms; usually lack of fever or tender /inflamed prostate. (2) **Lab tests**: Three sets of urine culture for chronic disease (may be positive for bacterial prostatitis or negative for nonbacterial prostatitis). Prostate secretion tests give much higher yields of bacteria than the urine.

Treatment: Ciprofloxacin (> 6 weeks) is the drug of choice. Recurrences are common.

PEARLS—Table 1-6: Comparison of Prostatitis by Etiology

Etiology / Clinical features, diagnosis, and treatment
Prostatodynia
Afebrile, irritative voiding symptoms, tender prostate; urinalysis is normal; **secretion smear: WBC < 10/HP, culture (-). Dx:** Ultrasound and urine cytology are done to rule out tumor/mass for elder patient.
Non-bacterial
With similar symptoms but the prostate **secretion WBC is > 10/HP while bacterial culture is (-).** It's the most common type and more common in younger men. **Tx:** Sitz baths, NSAIDs, Anti-cholinergics, azithromycin, etc.
Gonococcal
History of risky sexual behavior, similar symptoms as above, along with purulent secretion, mid-stream **urine WBC > 10/HP, and Gonococcus culture is (+).** Prostate massage is forbidden to avoid bacteremia. **Tx:** Ceftriaxone plus azithromycin (to include Chlamydia).
Chlamydial
Similar to symptoms of Gonococcal prostatitis, with mucous secretion but **bacterial culture is (-).** Positive rate of Chlamydial culture is low, and thus diagnostic treatment is very useful. **Tx: Azithromycin +/- Ceftriaxone** (for possible Gonococcus).

Epididymitis — focal tenderness over the epididymus (posterior testis)

It is the inflammation of the epididymis. Etiology is mostly dependent on age.

Clinical features and diagnosis

1. **Acute epididymitis**: (1) Patient typically has fever, irritative voiding symptoms, unilateral testicular pain and tenderness, hydrocele, and palpable swelling of the epididymis ± testicle; usually < 6 weeks. (2) Among sexually active men < 35 y/a, it is mostly caused by C. trachomatis or N. gonorrhea as an STD. (3) In men aged > 35 years, it is more often associated with bacteriuria secondary to obstructive urinary disease, surgery, systemic disease, or immunosuppression. (4) Potential testicular torsion is a surgical emergency.

— painful ejaculation

2. **Chronic epididymitis**: (1) ≥ 6 week's symptoms of discomfort and/or pain in the scrotum, testicle, or epididymis. (2) It can be subcategorized into inflammatory chronic epididymitis, obstructive chronic epididymitis, and chronic epididymalgia. (3) Chronic infectious epididymitis is most frequently associated with granulomatous reaction (#1 common with TB infection), Assoc w/ gonorrhea & chlamydia, autoimmune ↓2

3. **Lab tests**: (1) It is rapid, sensitive, specific, and preferred to have Gram stain of urethral secretions demonstrating ≥ 5 WBC per oil immersion field. (2) Gonococcal infection is established by the presence of WBC containing intracellular Gram⁻ diplococci on urethral Gram stain. (3) Diagnosis is also confirmed by positive leukocyte esterase test on first-void urine or by microscopic examination of it demonstrating ≥ 10 WBC per high power field. (4) Related tests should be suggested for other possible STDs.

Treatment

Epididymitis

Empiric therapy is indicated before lab results are available. The treatment should target C. trachomatis or N. gonorrhea: (1) **Ceftriaxone plus doxycycline are the best** for the initial therapy of epididymitis. (2) Additional therapy can include a fluoroquinolone if gonorrhoea is basically excluded. (3) Bed rest, scrotal elevation, and analgesics are recommended until fever and local inflammation have subsided.

SEXUALLY TRANSMITTED DISEASES (STD)

Chlamydia

↑WBC, no bacteria bc it is intracellular

It is the **most common STD**. The pathogen is an intracellular organism. The incubation period is 1-3 weeks. Many cases are co-infected with Gonorrhea.

Essentials of diagnosis

1. Approximately 80% in women and 50% in men are asymptomatic.

2. Symptoms in men include dysuria, purulent urethral discharge, scrotal pain & swelling, and fever.

3. Symptoms in women may include dysuria, purulent urethral discharge, and intermenstral or postcoital bleeding.

4. **Lab tests**: Chlamydial culture is low in sensitivity, and has been replaced by PCR as the most sensitive screening test. ELISA is the most specific diagnostic test. Serologic tests are useless.

Treatment

1. Oral **azithromycin one dose or doxycycline for 7 days** is effective.

2. **All sexual partners should be treated**. Asymptomatic, sexually active adolescents should be screened for Chlamydia.

Gonorrhea

It is the **#2 common STD** caused by Neisseria gonorrhea (a **Gram-negative diplococcus**). Gonorrhea is usually symptomatic in men but asymptomatic in women, who carry more complications due to delayed treatment. It is **almost always transmitted sexually**, and **many cases are co-infected with Chlamydia.**

Essentials of diagnosis

1. **Most men have symptoms involving the urethra**—dysuria, frequency of urination, purulent discharge, and erythema and edema of the urethral meatus.

2. **Most women are asymptomatic**. A few cases may show symptoms of cervicitis or urethritis—dysuria, purulent discharge, intermenstral bleeding or dyspareunia.

Neisseria Gonorrhea → purulent monoarthritis or triad of tenosynovitis, dermatitis, migratory polyarthralgia

3. **Disseminated Gonorrhea** is rare (1-2% and more common in women) and may present with fever, skin rash, arthralgia, **migratory/septic arthritis**, or even meningitis. *3rd gen Cephalosporin IV* *wrists*

4. **Lab tests**: (1) **Gram stain of urethral discharge** showing Gram-negative diplococci within WBCs is highly specific for Gonorrhea. (2) Obtain culture in all cases—in men from the urethra and in women from the endocervix. Empiric therapy may be started while culture results are awaited (taking 1-2 days). (3) Consider testing for suspected syphilis and HIV, and blood culture for disseminated Gonorrhea.

Treatment

1. The best therapy is **ceftriaxone** (single dose, IM) to be effectively against Gonococcus and syphilis, **plus azithromycin** (one dose) **or doxycycline** (for 7 days) **to cover frequently coexistent Chlamydia.**

2. Other options for Gonococcus include oral cefixime, ciprofloxacin, or ofloxacin. For disseminated cases, patient is hospitalized and treated with ceftriaxone IV for 7 days. **No vaccination is available due to antigenic variation of pilus proteins.**

Syphilis

It's a systemic contagious disease caused by a spirochete (Treponema pallidum) through sexual contact, characterized by periods of latency and active manifestations. It can be classified as congenital and acquired syphilis.

Essentials of diagnosis

1. **Congenital syphilis**: Infected from the diseased mother at birth. Early disease may be asymptomatic, or with poor feeding and rhinorrhea in infants up to 2 years. Late disease will show Hutchinson teeth, keratitis, scars, and bony abnormity (Saber shins).

2. **Acquired syphilis**:

(1) **Early stage**:

Primary syphilis: Chancre (Image 24) —painless ulcerated papule(s) with clear base and raised borders in genitoanal area (even mouth); **enlarged regional lymph nodes—painless**, rubbery, discrete, and non-tender. It usually appears in 3 weeks and disappears in 3 months,

Secondary syphilis (Images 25-26): Cutaneous rashes (pinkish or pigmented spots) appear in about 2 months, usually symmetric and more marked on the flexor surfaces of the body. Lymph node swellings, papules at mucocutaneous junctions and moist areas (termed **condylomata lata**, extremely contagious), and alopecia are commonly present.

(2) **Latent stage**: Early latent: < 1 year of infection, asymptomatic, serology (+); may persist for life. Late latent: > 1 year, asymptomatic, serology (+/-); 1/3 of cases may develop late syphilis.

(3) **Late or tertiary syphilis** (rare now): mostly known as **neurologic syphilis**. It's rare and characterized by the **Argyll Robertson pupil** (not reacting to light), **Tabes dorsalis** (pain, ataxia, sensory changes, and loss of tendon reflexes), meningovasculitis, and general paresis (memory and personality

changes). **Benign tertiary** with symptoms (non-contagious) may develop 10-20 years after the initial infection. The typical lesion is the **gumma,** which is a chronic granuloma that can occur in any organ and heal spontaneously with a scar.

3. **Screening tests** are **VDRL and RPR**; False (+) VDRL can be with TB, EBV, collagen vascular disease, and subacute bacterial endocarditis. All patients should be tested for HIV infection.

4. **Specific tests** are **FTA-ABS** (fluorescent treponemal antibody-absorption), **MHA-TP** (microhemoagglutination assay for antibodies to Treponema pallidum), and Darkfield exam of the chancre. They are confirmative tests for diagnosis.

Treatment

1. Penicillin (PCN) is the drug of choice for all stages of syphilis. **Primary syphilis** is treated with IM benzathine **PCN 2.4 million IU once**; **secondary syphilis: PCN 2.4 million IU** once a week for **3 weeks**. **Adverse effects: Jarisch-Herxheimer reaction:** Rapid lysis of spirochetes results in endotoxin-like release and reactions 6-12 hours after initial PCN therapy for syphilis. It may occur in > 50% of patients, with fever, headache, sweating, rigors, and temporary exacerbations. It is usually self-limited and treated with NSAIDs.

2. **Tertiary syphilis** is treated with **PCN** 10-20 million IU/d **IV for 10 days**. Patients with severe **PCN allergy** should receive doxycycline (not azithromycin due to resistance) for primary and secondary syphilis, but must be desensitized in tertiary syphilis to use the strong effects of PCN. Pregnant patients must also follow this to be desensitized to use PCN and avoid doxycycline due to its suppression of bone growth and staining of the teeth.

Other Sexually Transmitted Diseases

They are summarized in Table 1-7.

Table 1-7: Other Sexually Transmitted Diseases

Lesion / Clinical features, diagnosis, and treatment
Molluscum Contagiosum (Image 23) 1. In young or immunosuppressed patients, HIV (+), etc; caused by Poxvirus; may or may not be sexually. 2. Single or multiple small, oval, fresh/fleshy, shiny, painless papules on the face, trunk, genital, or extremities. **Dx:** Clinical impression along with KOH smear or Giemsa stain. **Tx: Cryotherapy,** curettage or cantharidin (a topical blistering agent).
Genital Warts (Image 27) 1. Also called **condylomata acuminata,** caused by **HPV** 6 and 11 (16 & 18 are mostly associated with cervical cancer). 2. Soft, tiny, pink papules (1-5mm) on warm, moist genital surfaces; fast growing and pedunculated (**"cauliflower shape"**). **Dx:** Clinical features. **Differential Dx**: "condylomata lata". **Tx: Cryotherapy**, curettage, trichloroacetic acid (TCA), podophyllin, or laser removal.

STDs

Chancroid (Image 28)

1. Acute STD by **H. ducreyi (Gram⁻ bacillus; mnemonic: "Painful cry")**. 2. Irregular, deep, painful genital papules or ulcerations (about 1cm), and inguinal lymph node suppuration, with bad odor. **Dx:** Clinical impression plus smear Gram stain; difficult to culture. **Tx:** Any of **azithromycin** (1 dose), ceftriaxone (1 dose), erythromycin (7 days), or ciprofloxacin (3 days).

Genital Herpes (Image 29)

1. By **HSV-2.** 2. Red, painful, itching vesicles with circular, scarring ulcers on the genital/perineal areas; enlarged inguinal lymph nodes can occur. **Dx: Tzanck test and culture. Tx:** Acyclovir or **valacyclovir** (with enhanced oral absorption). It can relapse with repeated sexual contacts.

Granuloma Inguinale (Donovanosis)

1. **Granulomatis caused by Klebsiella (Calymmatobacterium).** 2. Raised, red, painless papules, with granular ulcerations on the genital or perineum areas; resembles condyloma lata or cancer. **Dx:** Clinical exam with smear/biopsy, or Giemsa/Wright stain (Donovan bodies). **Tx: Doxycycline** for 3 weeks.

Lymphogranuloma Venereum

1. By **Chlamydia** trachomatis (L1-L3). 2. Transient, painless, nonindurated, shallow ulcers. 3. Unilaterally enlarged inguinal lymph nodes with tenderness; development of multiple purulent draining sinuses, buboes, and scars ("Groove sign"). 4. Fever, dysuria, pelvic/joint pains, and headaches may occur. **Dx:** Clinical features and fluorescent Ab stain for Chlamydia. **Tx: Doxycycline**, TMP-SMX, or erythromycin.

Acquired Immunodeficiency Syndrome (AIDS)

AIDS is an acquired immune deficiency syndrome **caused by** the human immunodeficiency virus **(HIV)**. HIV is a retrovirus that particularly **targets and destroys CD4⁺ T-cells, with a subtype HIV-1 (more common globally) and HIV-2 (endemic in West Africa).** HIV can be latent for many years and replicates rapidly, progressively decreases the number of CD4 cells, destroys cell-mediated immunity, and increases the risk of developing dangerous opportunistic infections. HIV does not harm patients directly.

Causes and risk factors

IV drug abuse (IVDA) and unprotected sexual intercourse carry the highest risk of developing AIDS. The risk is 1/100 for each receptive anal intercourse, 1/1000 for vaginal and oral receptive intercourse, and 1/3000-10000 for insertive vaginal intercourse. Other risk factors include blood transfusion, needle sticks (1/300 risk), maternal HIV infection (30% risk without medication), etc.

There is usually a 10-year lag between catching HIV and developing initial symptoms, the time for a normal CD4 level (>700/uL) to the sick level of 200/uL or lower with rapid viral replication.

| PEARLS | Monitoring of the immune system changes |

1. **CD4 T-cell count**: It indicates the degree of immunosuppression, and is the most accurate method of determining what infections or other diseases the patient is risky for, when to start prophylaxis and treatment, and how to adjust them. Without treatment, the CD4 T-cell count drops 50-75 cells per year.

HIV AIDS

CD4 > 700/uL is considered normal. **HIV (+) with CD4 < 200/uL or cervical cancer can be diagnosed as AIDS.**

2. **Viral load testing (RT-PCR RNA level)**: It is used to (1) diagnose HIV in babies; (2) guide antiretroviral therapies, measure response to therapy, and determine the rate of disease progression.

PEARLS—Table 1-8: Important CD4 Counts and Associated Complications

CD4 (count/uL) / Infections and complications
500-700: Lymphadenopathy or recurrent **vaginal candidiasis**; no treatment of AIDS is indicated yet.
200-500: **Oral thrush or vaginal candidiasis**, varicella zoster, herpes simplex, pneumococcal pneumonia, pulmonary TB, Kaposi sarcoma, anemia, lymphoma (non-Hodgkin's), cervical intraepithelial neoplasia (CIN), histoplasmosis, or coccidioidomycosis.
100-200: Pneumocystis carinii pneumonia (**PCP**) or AIDS dementia complex.
<100: **No.1: Toxoplasmosis**; No.2: cryptococcus.
<50: **CMV, Cryptosporidiosis**, Mycobacterium avium complex (**MAC**), progressive multifocal leukoencephalopathy (**PML**), or **CNS lymphoma**.

Essentials of diagnosis

1. **With the above risk factors for months to years**, followed by **recurrent viral or fungal infections**, ill-defined febrile illness, flu-like symptoms (fever, malaise, rash, lymph node swelling), night sweats, weight loss, and cachexia.

2. **Important lab tests**

(1) **HIV screening for risky people—Third generation EIA or ELISA** (enzyme immunoassay) tests detect the presence of HIV-1 or/and HIV-2 antibody as early as three weeks after exposure to the virus. If it's positive, 1-2 times of Western blot (WB) testing is required for confirmation of HIV-1 or/and HIV-2 antibody (IgG antibody to HIV-1 1-2 months after infection). EIA/ELISA has a high sensitivity but moderate specificity for HIV, whereas WB has the highest specificity but moderate sensitivity. A negative EIA/ELISA cannot exclude HIV infection and requires the "fourth generation HIV tests".

(2) **Fourth generation HIV tests—The combination antigen-antibody immunoassay is better able to identify acute or early HIV-1/ HIV-2 infection** (defined as a 6-month period following HIV acquisition), compared with antibody-only (EIA) tests, since they can detect HIV p24 antigen earlier than the antibody. **If it is positive**, an HIV-1/HIV-2 antibody **differentiation immunoassay is performed for confirmation. If the combo-test is negative**, the person is considered HIV-negative and no further testing is needed for most patients in whom acute or early HIV infection is unlikely. However, in patients with a negative combo-test but suspected of having acute or early HIV infection, the viral load testing should be performed.

(3) **Viral load testing**: A recent HIV load test is considered **more sensitive and specificity than EIA/ELISA**. Acute or early HIV infection is diagnosed by a negative immunoassay in the presence of a positive virologic test. However, a viral RNA level < 10,000 copies/mL in a patient with a negative

HIV AIDS

serology may represent a false positive viral test result, as patients with acute or early HIV infection typically have very high levels of viremia. Then the HIV load test should be immediately repeated on a new blood specimen. A second positive viral load test suggests HIV infection, which can be confirmed by a repeat serologic test several weeks later.

If both the immunoassay and virologic test are negative, HIV infection can be mostly excluded.

(4) **Histology**: A type of **giant multinucleate cells called Warthin–Finkeldey cells** are commonly found in hyperplastic **lymph nodes** early in the course of HIV infection and measles.

PEARLS—Important evaluations recommended for HIV (+) persons

1. Detailed history and physical examination!
2. Routine chemistry and hematologic tests.
3. CD4 lymphocyte count and two plasma RNA tests for HIV load.
4. Screen for syphilis (VDRL/RPR) and PPD test. Syphilis (+) patients with AIDS risk factors should take screening HIV-ELISA. If PPD is (+) (induration > 5 mm), it's treated with INH for 9 months.
5. Anti-toxoplasma titer test.
6. Hepatitis tests: HAV and HBV serology tests; if (-), vaccination is given. If HAV or HBV antigen is already (+), vaccination is not needed. If both HBV and HCV tests are (+), only HAV vaccine is given.
7. Pneumococcal vaccine (unless CD4 < 200/uL): Given to all HIV (+) people; boosting per 5 years.
8. Mini mental status exam (MMSE).
9. HIV counselling to possibly infected people.

Differential diagnosis

Mononucleosis (due to EBV or CMV), toxoplasmosis, measles, rubella, syphilis, viral hepatitis, disseminated gonococcal infection, and other viral infections.

Treatment

1. **Drug resistance testing**: For all patients with early HIV infection, drug resistance testing should be performed after the initial diagnosis has been established, regardless of whether treatment is being considered.

2. **Most patients: Start antiviral treatment when CD4 < 500/uL with symptoms; for asymptomatic patient, when CD4 < 350/uL, viral load > 55 x 10^3/uL, or opportunistic infection occurs. Medications**: a combined nucleoside, non-nucleoside, and a protease inhibitor (Inh). The best initial combination is **Atripla** (emtricitabine-tenofovir-efavirenz) or alafenamide-emtricitabine-dolutegravir. **Goal:** Viral load < 400/uL.

New anti-HIV medicines (mostly against HIV-1):

(1) **Nucleoside reverse transcriptase inhibitors (NRTIs):** Tenofovir (TDF), abacavir, lamivudine (3TC), emtricitabine, azidothymidine (AZT)/zidovudine (ZDV), didanosine (DDI), etc. AZT or ZDV can be used for general prophylaxis and during pregnancy to reduce risk of fetal transmission. **Adverse effects** include neuropathy, pancreatitis, anemia, diabetes insipidus, and bone marrow suppression (which can be reversed with G-CSF and erythropoietin).

HIV - AIDS

(2) **Non-nucleoside reverse transcriptase inhibitors (NNRTIs):** Efavirenz (EFV), delavirdine, etc. Adverse effects include CNS toxicity, rash, hyperlipidemia, and elevated hepatic transaminases.

(3) **Protease inhibitors (PIs):** Lopinavir, darunavir, atazanavir, etc., typically administered with an NRTI combination, not alone. Adverse effects include hyperglycemia, GI, liver, and kidney toxicity.

(4) **Fusion inhibitor:** Enfuvirtide (T-20), not effective on HIV-2. **Mnemonic:** EnFUvirtide inhibits Fusion.

(5) **Chemokine coreceptor 5 (CCR5) antagonist:** Maraviroc (MVC).

(6) **Integrase inhibitors:** Raltegravir, elvitegravir and dolutegravir are new drugs with potent anti-HIV-2 activity. Adverse effect: Increasing creatine kinase.

3. **Pregnant patients** *Peds: Vertical transmission, ↓ w AZT @birth.*

- If < 18mos, can't use ELISA bc ELISA uses antibodies & mom gives baby antibodies, no HIV could be there.

All children at birth will carry the maternal HIV antibody and have ELISA (+) testing, but only 25-30% will remain truly infected. Pregnant females with low CD4 or high viral load should be treated fully for their HIV as above. Cesarean delivery for HIV (+) mothers is performed to prevent transmission of the virus if the CD4 is < 350/uL or the viral load is > 1000/uL. Obtain best control of HIV with medications by the time of parturition. *HAART: any HIV⊕ pts*

Baby: Skip ELISA & do DNA-PCR instead.

4. **Post-exposure prophylaxis**

Indications: All persons with direct exposure to the blood or body fluids of HIV (+) patients.

Preventive drugs: zidovudine with and without other three combo-drugs for 4 weeks. Statistic data show that zidovudine alone can decrease the risk by 80%.

Vaccinations: All HIV (+) patients should take vaccines for Pneumococcus, Influenza, and HBV.

*200 PCP
-TMPSMX
-dapsone
-atovaqu
100 TOXO
-TMPSMX
-atovs
80 MAC
-azithro*

OPPORTUNISTIC INFECTIONS (OIs)

OIs are infections that occur more frequently and are more severe in individuals with weakened immune systems (immunodeficiency or immunosuppression), including people with HIV infection.

Clinical features, diagnosis, and treatment of important OIs are summarized below.

Table 1-9: Important Opportunistic Infections with Immunodeficiency or AIDS

Infection / Clinical features, diagnosis, and treatment
Oral and vaginal candidiasis (Image 32)
Also known as **thrush**, it appears as white patches of exudates on the tongue, buccal or vaginal mucosa, causing **burning pain and itching**. It's caused by **Candida albicans** mostly in immunocompromised or HIV (+)/AIDS patients. C. albicans is in most cases a normal oral and vaginal microorganism. **Dx:** Clinical impression. **Tx:** Simple oral/genital candidiasis can be treated with topical –azole (clotrimazole); severe, complicated candidiasis with immunosuppression or HIV is treated with Oral fluconazole +/- topical –azole for 7-14 days. Sexual partners and asymptomatic patients usually do not need treatment.

(Oral) hairy leukoplakia (<u>Image 33</u>)
A whitish, painless patch on the side of the tongue with a corrugated or hairy appearance. It is caused **by E-B virus** and occurs usually in immunocompromised or HIV (+) patients. The white lesion **cannot be scraped off.** The lesion itself is benign and generally needs no treatment but monitoring. **Note: Compare thrush (scrapable) with leukoplakia (precancerous).**

Aspergillosis
1. A **common fungus mostly causing pulmonary diseases by spores** in the air only with immunodeficient status; endemic to Eastern and Central US. Among many species, fumigatus is the No.1, in rotting organic materials. 2. Asthma-like symptoms: Cough, wheezing, fever, etc. 3. Not invasive type: Mycetoma—"**fungal ball**", mainly with hemoptysis. 4. Invasive: More risks with WBC < 500, or cytotoxic drug use. **Dx:** History, abnormal CXR ("**halo sign**"), sputum aspergillus
culture (+), 45^0-**angle branching hyphae**, skin test (+), elevated eosinophil and IgE. **Tx:** 1. Allergic: Steroid dosing and asthma drugs, not antifungals. 2. Mycetoma: surgical removal. 3. Antifungals: **voriconazole** +/- echinocandin first; if intolerant or severe (invasive), amphotericin B or isavuconazole is chosen.

Blastomycosis
1. An **uncommon fungus** in rotting organic material; infected by inhalation. It occurs in both immunodeficient and normal people; may be endemic to Ohio-Mississippi valleys. 2. Starts with respiratory symptoms (fever, cough, chest pain) and spreads mainly to the skin. **Dx:** Isolation of the fungus in sputum, pus, or biopsy. **Tx:** Give prolonged itraconazole or ketoconazole for mild disease (8 months); amphotericin B for severe disease (8 weeks). Most cases of **histoplasmosis** need no treatment.

Coccidioidomycosis
A **pulmonary fungal infection endemic to southwestern US (California, etc.).** It can present as a flu-like disease or as acute pneumonia, and can also involve extrapulmonary organs. **Dx:** Spherules filled with endospores of Coccidioides; confirmed by precipitin antibody increase in IgM (< 2 weeks) or IgG (1-3 months). **Tx:** Only required for disseminated disease or in those with a pulmonary disease or immunodeficiency; moderate cases— fluconazole or itraconazole; life-threatening —amphotericin.

PCP (Pneumocystis Carinii Pneumonia)
1. **A rare yeast-like fungal infection**, found with AIDS when **CD4 < 200**. 2. Mainly as pneumonia: dry cough, marked dyspnea on exertion, fever, and chest pain. **Dx:** Bronchoscopy with bronchoalveolar lavage (**BCL**) for direct visualization of the organism; increased LDH. **Tx:** 1. **TMP-SMX** 14 days for HIV (-) patients; 2. Atovaquone or pentamidine (with S/E of pancreatitis, hyperglycemia, hypoglycemia) 21 days for HIV infected patients. If failed,
clindamycin plus primaquine can be used. Corticosteroids may be added with severe pneumonia. **Prophylaxis (when CD4 < 200):** oral TMP-SMX is most effective. Dapsone or pentamidine also works.

Toxoplasmosis

1. An **intracellular parasite** infection around the world. In the U.S., about 50% of the population is antibody (+) but no symptoms. 2. Usually acquired from cat feces and undercooked meat (pork and lamb most). 3. Most symptoms only show with immunodeficient status or AIDS (when **CD4 <100)**: Headache, fever, nausea, vomiting, and neurol/visual deficiency from a CNS mass. **Dx:** 1. Serology antibody is the #1 method used; direct visualization of the parasite in tissue is the best Dx if available. 2. With AIDS CNS symptoms, contrasted CT or MRI is the best initial test (showing enhanced mass with surrounding edema). **Diagnostic treatment** (10-14 days) with follow-up scan (seeing shrunk lesions) is also good confirmation. **Tx: Pyrimethamine + sulfadiazine** is the best (to avoid single-drug recurrence). **Leucovorin** should be added to prevent pyrimethamine-induced myelosuppression. If sulfadiazine is not tolerated, clindamycin can be used.

Cryptococcosis

A rare **fungal infection when CD4 <100**. Primary infection: meningitis (fever, headache, stiff neck). **Dx:** CSF assay with initial India ink stain and then specific cryptococcal antigen test. A high CSF pressure and antigen titer, and low CSF cell count all imply a worse prognosis. **Tx:** IV Amphotericin B for 10-14 days, followed by life-long oral fluconazole.

CMV

1. Infected with AIDS when **CD4 < 50**. 2. Mainly presenting as retinitis (painful eyes and blurry vision); sometimes with colitis (diarrhea). **Dx:** Fundoscopy for retinitis; colonoscopy with biopsy for colitis. **Tx: Ganciclovir** (S/E: neutropenia); foscarnet or cidofovir (S/E: renal toxicity).

MAC (Mycobaterium avium complex)

1. A rare **non-TB mycobacterium infection with AIDS when CD4 < 50**. 2. Major manifestations: Chronic cough, sputum, fever, bacteremia, wasting, and anemia. **Dx:** Sputum or blood culture for mycobacteria. CXR shows spreading parenchymal infiltrates. **Tx:** Standard regimen—clarithromycin, rifabutin, and ethambutol. **Prophylaxis:** When CD4 < 50, oral clarithromycin, rifabutin, or azithromycin; when CD4 > 100 for a few months, stop.

Cryptosporidiosis

1. A rare **spore-forming protozoa** infection with immunodeficiency when **CD4 < 50**; contracted by fecal-oral route. 2. Typically with severe watery diarrhea. **Dx:** Stool analysis shows oocytes. **Tx:** Supportive care for most cases; **nitazoxanide** for persistent cryptosporidial infection.

HHV8—Kaposi Sarcoma (KS, Image 31): See "Chapter 10: Skin Diseases".

BLOOD INFECTIONS AND RELATED DISEASES

Sepsis

Sepsis is a systemic inflammatory response syndrome (SIRS) caused by overwhelming bacterial infections and their toxins in the blood stream. Septic shock is defined as sepsis-induced hypotension and organ dysfunction due to poor circulatory perfusion.

Etiology

1. Gram⁻ bacterial shock: Usually secondary to vasodilatation caused by endotoxins (lipopolysaccharide) from E. coli, Pseudomonas, Klebsiella, or Proteus, etc. Elderly patients are more often affected.

2. Gram⁺ bacterial shock: Usually secondary to fluid loss caused by exotoxins from Staph, Strep, etc. All adults can be affected.

3. Neonates: Group-B Strep, E. coli, Listeria and Hib are the most common pathogens.

4. Children and asplenic patients: Encapsulated bacteria (Pneumococcus, Klebsiella, Hib, and Meningococcus) are the most common pathogens.

5. IV drug abuse and indwelling lines: S. aureus and S. spp. are the most common organisms.

Essentials of diagnosis

1. Usually with a history of bacterial infection followed by an abrupt onset of fever, chills, tachycardia, tachypnea, and altered mental status.

2. **Septic shock** is defined as sepsis-induced hypotension persisting despite adequate fluid resuscitation, which may be defined as infusion of 30 mL/kg of crystalloids (a portion of this may be albumin equivalent). Early-stage shock is mostly "warm shock" with warm skin and extremities. Late-stage often shows "cold shock" (T <36°C), with hypotension and cool skin and extremities, indicating severe disease. Petechiae or ecchymoses suggest DIC (**Image 34**).

3. **Multiple organ dysfunction syndrome** (**MODS**) refers to progressive organ dysfunction in an acutely ill patient, such that homeostasis cannot be maintained without intervention. It is at the severe end of the severity of illness spectrum of both systemic inflammatory response syndrome (SIRS) and sepsis.

4. **Lab tests**: **Leukocytosis (WBC > 12,000/uL) or leukopenia (WBC < 4,000/uL) with increased bands, decreased platelets (< 100,000/uL in 50% of cases), elevated LFTs and creatinine, and hyperglycemia** (plasma glucose >140 mg/dL or 7.7 mmol/L) in the absence of diabetes. Cultures of the blood, sputum, or urine may be (+). CXR may show lung infiltrates. If DIC is suspected, coagulation tests should be performed, which may show coagulopathy (INR >1.5). Diagnosis is by clinical experience.

Treatment

1. The mainstreams of therapy include securing the airway, correcting hypoxemia, administering aggressive IV fluid, vessel-active agents, empiric antibiotics, surgical drainage of infected fluid collections, removal of infected lines or catheters, and appropriate support for organ dysfunction. The main goal is to maintain BP and perfusion to end organs.

(1) For initial fluid replacement, administer a crystalloid (rather than hyperoncotic) solution by early goal-directed therapy.

(2) For patients who remain hypotensive following intravascular volume repletion, give vasopressors (norepinephrine).

(3) For patients with severe sepsis and septic shock that are refractory to intravenous fluid and vasopressor therapy, additional therapies, such as inotropes, glucocorticoids and blood transfusions (when Hb < 7 g/dL), are administered based on individual assessment.

(4) Antimicrobial regimen: Strong and adequate antibiotics should be administered within the first 6 hours after blood sample is taken for culture and sensitivity testing. Special invasive bacteria such as MRSA and Pseudomonas should be considered.

2. Supportive treatment includes mechanical ventilation in pulmonary dysfunction, hemodialysis in kidney failure, transfusion of blood products, and drug and fluid therapy for circulatory failure. ICU admission may be necessary. Glucocorticoid therapy, nutritional support, and glucose control are beneficial in severe sepsis. Ensuring adequate nutrition is crucial during prolonged illness.

Toxic Shock Syndrome

Staph-aureus strains produce exotoxins that lead to three syndromes: food poisoning (caused by ingestion of S. aureus enterotoxin), scalded skin syndrome (caused by exfoliative toxin), and toxic shock syndrome (TSS) —caused by toxic shock syndrome toxin-1 (**TSST-1**) and other enterotoxins. TSS is characterized by shock and multi-organ dysfunctions mainly due to the TSS toxin rather than the bacteria. It's usually contracted by the use of tampons or sponges during menstruations, or by infected wounds, burns, or insect bites. A minority of cases are caused by Streptococcus.

Essentials of diagnosis

1. Typical **toxic shock manifestations** include fever, headache, tachycardia, hypotension, mucosal changes ("strawberry tongue"), desquamative rash on palms and soles, and GI symptoms (nausea, vomiting, diarrhea). Muscular, renal and hepatic dysfunctions and hypo-Ca can also occur.

2. **Lab tests**: CBC usually reveals leukocytosis with predominant neutrophils. BUN/creatine may be increased. Diagnosis is on clinical basis. Confirmative diagnosis is by isolation of Staph-aureus from vaginal secretion or Strep from oral swab. Blood culture is mostly negative.

Treatment

1. Supportive care: Stabilize patient by correction of hypovolemic shock (with aggressive fluids) and removal of toxin and infected material and tissue.

2. Antibiotics: (1) **For suspected MRSA, clindamycin plus vancomycin** is the best empiric etiologic therapy. (2) If culture shows methicillin-susceptible S. aureus, clindamycin plus oxacillin/nafcillin is the best.

Infectious Mononucleosis

It's a systemic mononucleosis due to **E-B virus (EBV=HHV-4)** infection, mostly transmitted through close contact with body fluid (like saliva). It's also known as the "Kissing disease", more common among young adults. Most adults (90%) have been infected with EBV and are carriers. One infection typically induces lifelong immunity. The incubation period is usually 2-5 weeks.

Essentials of diagnosis

1. Most patients present with high fever (up to 40°C), pharyngitis, enlarged tonsils with exudate, palatal petechiae, cervical lymph node swelling with tenderness; some with bilateral eyelid edema, a generalized maculopapular rash, and hepatosplenomegaly. Up to 30% of cases may be misdiagnosed carriers of Group-A Strep.

2. **Lab tests**: **Lymphocytosis and increased circulating atypical T cells along with a positive Monospot heterophile antibody test support diagnosis** in most cases. Monospot test may be negative in the first few weeks. Measurement of EBV-specific antibodies is usually not necessary since the vast majority of patients are heterophile positive (relatively specific). However, testing for EBV-specific antibodies (IgG and IgM VCA (viral capsid antigen) may be warranted in patients with suspected IM who have a negative heterophile test. Specific IgG and IgM EBV-VCA (-) or IgG EBNA (+) (Epstein-Barr nuclear antigen) excludes acute primary EBV infection. Mild thrombocytopenia and elevation of hepatic enzymes may exist.

3. **Special notes**: (1) Ampicillin use during EBV infection can cause a prolonged, pruritic maculopapular rash, which is not associated with over-sensitivity to beta-lactams and will remit after ampicillin is stopped. (2) CMV may cause an infectious mononucleosis with negative results of Monospot and EBV antibody testing.

Differential diagnosis

Infections by Group-A Strep, CMV, HHV-6, or HIV, etc.

Treatment

1. Most therapies are **supportive and symptomatic**. There is no effective treatment against EBV. Avoid strenuous activities until splenomegaly resolves to prevent splenic rupture.

2. In case of airway obstruction (by swollen tonsils), severe autoimmune hemolytic anemia, or thrombocytopenia, IV steroid is indicated (but not for most cases).

Complications

Group-A Strep pharyngitis (#1, 10%), upper airway obstruction, autoimmune hemolytic anemia, CNS infection (aseptic meningitis, encephalitis, cranial nerve palsies, neuritis), splenic rupture (< 0.5%), and fulminant hepatitis (rare).

Fever of Unknown Origin (FUO)

It refers to a condition in which the patient has an elevated temperature but despite investigations by a physician no explanation has been found. The present criteria are:

(1) Fever higher than 38.3°C (101°F) on several occasions;

(2) Persisting without diagnosis for at least 3 weeks;

(3) At least 1 week's evaluation in hospital (or three outpatient visits and 3-day hospitalization).

Etiology

In adults, **infections and cancer account for > 60% of cases of FUO**, while autoimmune diseases account for about 15%.

1. **Infections**—the most common cause: TB, occult abscesses, UTI, endocarditis, sinusitis, infectious mononucleosis, HIV, malaria, etc.

2. **Occult neoplasms**—#2 common: lymphoma, leukemia, hepatic and renal cell carcinoma, etc.

3. Autoimmune diseases—SLE, Still disease, vasculitis, etc.

4. Others—granulomatous disease, pulmonary embolism, hemolytic anemia, hepatitis, gout, subacute thyroiditis, drug fevers, factitious disorder, etc.

Essentials of diagnosis

1. A detailed history of travel, animal exposure, immunosuppression, drugs and toxins is important.

2. Patient often presents with fever, chills, headache, myalgias, night sweats, and malaise.

3. Confirm the fever and perform the following minimum lab tests:

(1) CBC with differentiation, ESR or C-reactive protein;

(2) Three routine blood cultures drawn from different sites over a period of at least several hours without antibiotic use;

(3) Serum LDH and CPK;

(4) Rheumatoid factor and antinuclear antibodies;

(5) Heterophile antibody test in children and young adults;

(6) Tuberculin skin test (PPD) or interferon-gamma release assay;

(7) HIV antibody assay and HIV viral load for patients at high risk;

(8) Serum protein electrophoresis;

(9) CXR; PET scan; CT scans of chest and abdomen +/- laparoscopy or colonoscopy.

Additional: invasive procedures—biopsy of lymph nodes, bone marrow, or other tissues for suspected tumor or abscess may be necessary to make a diagnosis.

4. Sometimes the cause is determined by observation and excluding all less possible ones. However, undiagnosed cases can be 30-50%. Most adults who remain undiagnosed have a good prognosis. Most children with FUO have treatable or self-limited diseases, with more likelihood of etiologic diagnosis.

Therapeutic guidelines

Try to target the most likely cause. Stop unnecessary medicines. Empirical treatment with anti-inflammatory medications or antibiotics generally should be avoided as diagnostic measures in children with fever of unknown origin (FUO). Exceptions include nonsteroidal agents in children with presumed juvenile idiopathic arthritis (JIA) and anti-tuberculous drugs in critically ill children with possible disseminated TB. Empirical trials of broad-spectrum antibiotics can mask or delay the diagnosis of important infections, such as meningitis, parameningeal infection, infectious endocarditis, or osteomyelitis.

BONE, JOINT AND MUSCLE INFECTIONS

(Pyogenic) Osteomyelitis

It's defined as an **infection and inflammation of any portion of the bone, including marrow, cortex, and periosteum**. It can be acute hematogenous (septic) osteomyelitis, or secondary to chronic infection, decubitus ulcer, trauma, or vascular disease in elder patients.

Etiology—similar to sepsis

1. **Hematogenous osteomyelitis:** Injection drug users, sickle cell disease, children and the elderly, mostly in the long bones of the lower extremities.

2. **Osteomyelitis from a continuous focal infection:** Prosthetic joint replacement, decubitus ulcer, neurosurgery, and trauma.

3. **Osteomyelitis associated with vascular insufficiency:** Patients with diabetes and vascular insufficiency are susceptible to it.

Associated specific microorganisms

1. **Staph-aureus** is still the **#1** common microorganism in most cases. *[handwritten: peds too]*

2. **Salmonella** is more common in osteomyelitis with sickle cell disease (**SCD**). *[handwritten: peds too]*

3. **Pseudomonas** is more common with IV drug abuse, foot puncture, or chronic osteomyelitis.

4. **Staph-epidermidis** is more common with hip replacement.

Essentials of diagnosis

1. Fever, fatigue, localized bone pain, erythema, swelling, and tenderness over the infected bone, usually from hematogenous causes. With a vascular disease, an overlying ulcer or wound/sinus is usually seen. A draining sinus tract through the skin may form in chronic disease.

2. The **earliest sensitive tests are the technetium (T^{99})** bone scan (moderately specific) and **MRI (highly specific, especially for diabetic and vertebral osteomyelitis).** Plain X-ray is usually negative early in the course and later may show periosteal elevation with limited sensitivity. Lab tests usually show leukocytosis, elevated ESR and/or C-reactive protein (CRP). Blood culture and bone biopsy for culture may be needed to guide therapy.

3. **Bone biopsy for culture**: It's **the most accurate test** to guide treatment but is invasive. ESR is increased significantly and non-specifically, and only used for follow-ups after treatment. WBC counts may or may not be elevated and not very helpful in diagnosis.

Treatment

1. **Empiric treatment of S. aureus by Oxacillin or nafcillin plus an aminoglycoside** or a 3rd-generation cephalosporin (for Gram⁻ organisms) for 4-6 weeks for acute osteomyelitis is the best initial therapy until the specific pathogen is isolated. **Vancomycin is best for suspected MRSA and coagulase-negative Staph. Cefepime is best for Pseudomonas. Daptomycin** is an option for the prosthetic origin.

[handwritten notes at bottom: Peds: - If toxic, abx before bx - if not toxic, bx before abx   dx: xray if ⊕ = bx MRI if ⊕ = bx]

Osteomyelitis

2. Chronic osteomyelitis must be treated with specific IV antibiotics for 12 weeks, followed by another 8-12 weeks orally.

3. Surgical debridement of necrotic bone is an important part of treatment.

Infectious Arthritis

blood & synovial cultures

Severe pain, erythema, effusion, ↓, fever

It's also known as **septic arthritis**, a bacterial infection of the joint, and generally divided into **Gonococcal and non-gonococcal arthritis**. Gonococcal arthritis is mostly in young patient and with a history and symptoms of an STD. **Non-gonococcal** arthritis is mostly caused by **S. aureus in elder** patient and with a history of a joint lesion (gout, rheumatoid, or osteoarthritis), artificial joint, previous surgery, IV drug use, or Sickle cell disease (SCD).

Essentials of diagnosis

Tap w arthrocentesis. > 50K WBC = septic Tx Abx

1. <u>Gonococcal arthritis</u>: Prodromal **migratory polyarthralgias and tenosynovitis** are most *sexually active teen* common, along with **characteristic petechiae or purpura** on the skin and purulent monarthritis (in 50% of cases). It is most common in young women during menses or pregnancy. Symptoms of urethritis are frequently absent. **Gonococcus is difficult to culture**, with only 50% (+) from joint aspirates and < 10% (+) from blood cultures; other sites **(cervix, urethra) often have higher positive rate of culture**. Aspirate WBC count is usually > 60-70 x 10^3/uL (mostly PMNs).

2. <u>Non-gonococcal</u>: **Acute** onset of inflammatory **monoarticular arthritis**, mostly in weight- *- Stab wounds* bearing joints and wrists (**knee as #1**), with a swollen, erythematous joint with tenderness and a decreased range of motion. Skin rash is rare. Previous joint damage or drug injection is a risk factor. Infection with causative organisms is commonly found elsewhere in the body. **Joint aspirate assay**: usually yields a large volume of effusions, with **WBC counts mostly > 50 x 10^3/uL** (mostly PMNs) and a low glucose concentration; synovial **bacterial culture has > 90% (+)** rate, and Gram stain is 50% (+).

Treatment   *Arthroscopic lavage with debridement or w/o*

1. If the initial Gram stain of the synovial fluid shows <u>**gram-positive cocci**</u>, **nafcillin/oxacillin plus gentamicin** (to cover most Staph and Strep) or **vancomycin** (to cover possible MRSA and severe infections) should be started.

2. If the initial Gram stain of the synovial fluid shows <u>**gram-negative bacilli**</u>, a 3rd-generation cephalosporin (**ceftriaxone, cefotaxime, or ceftazidime**) is started. If **Pseudomonas is suspected, ceftazidime plus gentamicin** should be given. **If Gonococcus is suspected, ceftriaxone is the best** medication—**patient has dramatic response**.

3. **Dainage:** (1) Daily aspiration of affected joint is necessary until effusion disappears. (2) Surgical drainage may be needed if response to antibiotics is poor, or if the hip or shoulder joint is infected or any joint damage is involved. *debridement & irrigation of the joint space = prevent long-term morbidity*

Gas Gangrene (Clostridial Myonecrosis)

It is the necrotizing destruction of muscle by gas-producing anaerobic organisms (**#1 is Clostridium perfringens**), producing signs of sepsis. It develops either contiguously from an area of deep trauma or

Gas Gangrene

surgical injury (usually due to C. perfringens) or hematogenously from the gastrointestinal tract with muscle seeding (usually due to C. septicum). It's more of a concern during times of war.

Essentials of diagnosis

1. Pain, swelling and edema at the wound site start within 1-4 days of incubation, often followed by fever, hypotension, and tachycardia. Focal crepitation and renal failure are late-stage signs.

2. **Lab tests**: A **Gram stain** of the wound shows **Gram+ rods without WBC**. Culture for C. perfringens may be (+) but not highly sensitive. Gas bubbles on an x-ray are suggestive of this disease, but it may also be caused by Strep. **Direct vision** of pale, dead muscle with a brownish, sweet-smelling discharge is **highly suggestive of the diagnosis**. **Definitive diagnosis** requires demonstration of large, gram-variable rods at the site of injury. Histopathology demonstrates characteristic **absence of acute inflammatory cells**. Gas in the soft tissue may be observed at the bedside and/or radiographically.

Treatment

The main therapy is **high-dose PCN** (24 million IU/day) **plus clindamycin** (especially if allergic to PCN) IV early against **C. perfringens**, followed by surgical **debridement** or amputation. Hyperbaric O_2 therapy may be helpful with the above treatment, but may not always be beneficial.

Tetanus

It's a severe infectious complication of wounds caused by neurotoxins of **Clostridium tetani**, a **Gram+ anaerobic rod with spore**. It usually takes 1-7 days to develop. The neurotoxin is an exotoxin, which can block inhibitory transmitters at the neuromuscular junction and cause extensive muscle spasms.

Essentials of diagnosis

1. History of a deep, dirty wound 1-7 days ago, followed by tonic spasms of voluntary muscles—first by masseter muscles causing **typical "trismus or lockjaw"**, then stiff neck, arm flexion, leg/foot extension, dysphagia, headache, irritability, and eventual respiratory arrest. It carries a high mortality rate.

2. Early diagnosis by clinical experience and immediate treatment are crucial to save life. Wound cultures can be obtained but may not be a reliable means of diagnosis.

Treatment

1. Immediately admit patient to the ICU and provide possible airway and respiratory support. Recommended therapies include IV specific antitoxin IG (to neutralize the unbound tetanus toxin), large doses of PCN (10-14 days) or metronidazole (7-10 days) against C. tetani, control of muscle spasms with neuromuscular blocking agents, and thorough wound debridement to eradicate spores and necrotic tissue.

2. **Prophylaxis**: (1) Tetanus toxoid plus IV IG for patients with any suspected dirty wound beyond 5 years of vaccination. (2) DTaP is recommended at birth, 2, 4, 6, and 15-18 months, and 4-6 years of age. Tetanus toxoid should be boosted every 10 years.

ARTHROPOD-BORNE AND ZOONOTIC INFECTIONS

Lyme Disease

It is an arthropod-borne infection spread **by spirochete Borrelia burgdorferi** from a small (deer) tick bite (Ixodes scapularis, vector for Anaplasma spp. and protozoa Babesia). **Mouse** is the natural reservoir. It's endemic to the **Northeast and Midwest US**, usually in summer. It's **characterized by a fever and a rash**, and can recur as arthritis, cardiac disease, or neurological disease if untreated. "Post-Lyme disease syndrome" refers to the nonspecific symptoms (such as headache, fatigue, and arthralgias) that may persist for months after treatment of Lyme disease.

Essentials of diagnosis

There are three stages—summarized in mnemonic "FACE": Facial palsy, Arthritis, Cardiac block, Erythema migrans.

1. **Early localized infection—erythema chronicum migrans (Image 35)**: Circular and expanding, begining 3-30 days after the tick bite; the rash usually resolves in a few weeks without treatment.

2. Early disseminated infection: 50% of patients have flu-like symptoms, enlarged lymph nodes, migratory joint pain, meningitis, encephalitis, cranial neuritis (often bilateral facial nerve palsy), and cardiac lesion (A-V block, myocarditis, pericarditis).

3. Late persistent infection: Arthritis, chronic polyneuropathy (shooting pains, numbness) or encephalomyelitis (memory, mood changes, psychosis), acrodermatitis chronica atrophicans (rare), etc.

4. **Lab tests**: Typical rash with a fever may not need confirmatory testing. ELISA for IgM (early stage) and IgG followed by a Western Blot (confirmation) are the standard diagnostic methods. A negative result does not necessarily rule out recent infection. Receiving blood transfusion in recent months may cause false positive results.

Treatment

1. Asymptomatic cases may not need treatment, or only need a prophylactic dose of doxycycline with special concerns (e.g. a clear tick bite, endemic area). Limited Lyme disease is treated with oral doxycycline or amoxicillin (with pregnancy).

2. Severe cases and complications (with neurological manifestations, 3rd-grade heart block, arthritis, myocarditis, or encephalitis) are treated with IV ceftriaxone for at least 30 days.

Rocky Mountain Spotted Fever (RMSF)

It's a small-vessel vasculitis caused by R. rickettsii transmitted by the dog/wood tick. It is usually seen in the summer and endemic to the Mideast to Midwest US.

Essentials of diagnosis

1. **Typical triad—abrupt fever, headache, and rash (from palms and soles spreading centripetally)**. Initial diagnosis can be made based on this typical triad in an epidemic area. **Note:** Distinquish palm and sole rashes seen in hand-foot-mouth disease and secondary syphilis.

2. Other symptoms include confusion, lethargy, dizziness, irritability, neck stiffness, and GI upset. Patient may die of a severe complication such as heart failure (from myocarditis), pulmonary edema, or CNS hemorrhage or edema.

3. **Lab tests**: Thrombocytopenia, hypo-Na, and elevated LFTs are common. Direct immuno-fluorescence testing or immunoperoxidase staining for R. rickettsiae in skin biopsy makes a timely diagnosis. Indirect fluorescent antibody (**IFA**) testing makes a retrospective specific diagnosis, usually at the 2nd week.

Treatment

1. Oral **doxycycline** is given for 7 days or more than 3 days after defervescence. Administer by IV route if vomiting is present.

2. **Chloramphenicol** is given for patients with CNS complications or pregnancy.

Malaria

It's a protozoal disease caused by four strains of the genus Plasmodium (P. falciparum, P. vivax, P. ovale, and P. malaria), and transmitted by a female Anopheles mosquito. Among the four strains, **P. falciparum** has the highest morbidity and mortality. Although malaria has been largely eliminated in North America and Europe, it's still endemic in certain areas in Africa and Asia. Thus, chemoprophylaxis and mosquito protection should be used for travellers to the endemic areas.

Essentials of diagnosis

1. History of exposure in an endemic area, with typical periodic attacks of **sequential chills, high fever (> 41ºC), and sweating** over 4-5 hours. Other symptoms include headache, dizziness, malaise, GI upset, myalgias, and arthralgia. Some symptoms may recur every 2-3 days. **P. falciparum** is severe and with parasitized RBCs occlude capillaries in the brain (cerebral malaria), kidneys, and lungs. **P. malaria** has a 72-hour cycle (quartan; fever on 1st and 4th day).

2. **P/E** usually finds **splenomegaly**, rash, and LN swelling 4-5 days after symptoms. If CNS is infected, confusion, neck stiffness, and neurologic signs may be found.

3. **Lab tests**: CBC mostly reveals hemolysis-like anemia with reticulocytosis, and low to normal WBC. **Giemsa/Wright-stained** blood films (thick and thin) are sent for specific diagnosis by experts. Specimens are collected at 8-hour intervals for 3 days, and during and between febrile periods.

Treatment

1. Uncomplicated cases are treated with oral chloroquine or mefloquine. **If chloroquine/mefloquine resistance** is suspected as in many countries, **artemether + lumefantrine/amodiaquine or** quinine plus tetracycline can be used.

2. P. vivax and P. ovale strains are usually resistant to chloroquine, and thus primaquine is added to eradicate the hypnozoites in the liver.

Malaria

3. **Severe**, complicated cases or **P. falciparum** infection are treated by **rectal and IV artesunate** or IV **quinine** (with more adverse effects), followed by doxycycline. Symptomatic and supportive therapies are also important. For a pregnant patient, doxycycline is replaced by clindamycin.

4. Prophylaxis is recommended to travellers to endemic regions. Atovaquone-proguanil or mefloquine is the agent of choice because it also covers chloroquine-resistant cases.

Complications

Cerebral malaria, severe hemolytic anemia (mostly by P. falciparum), acute tubular necrosis and renal failure ("Blackwater fever"), pulmonary edema, bacteremia, and DIC.

Rabies

It is **a rare devastating, deadly viral encephalitis** caused by bites or scratches by infected animals (#1 is **raccoon**, followed by bat or dog). Rabies is only occasionally found in developing countries where rabies vaccination of animals is not widespread. The incubation period ranges from 30-90 days and varies. **Once symptoms appear, it is always fatal!**

Essentials of diagnosis

1. History of a bite by a rabies-suspected animal followed by typical symptoms—sore throat, headache, nausea, vomiting, fever; encephalitis (confusion, combativeness, hyperactivity, seizure); **hydrophobia** (inability to drink, laryngeal spasm with drinking, hypersalivation— **"foaming at mouth"**); almost **always progresses to coma and death**.

2. **Lab diagnosis**: (1) Virus isolated in infected tissue and saliva. (2) 4-fold increase in serum antibody titers. (3) Negri bodies identified in histology. (4) PCR detection of virus RNA.

Treatment and prophylaxis

Rabies is an invariably fatal viral disease that can be prevented with proper wound care and postexposure prophylaxis.

1. Clean the wound thoroughly with soap and prepare for life support care. Ketamine and midazolam may be helpful in symptomatic control. Amantadine may be used for its potential antiviral activity.

2. For a known rabies exposure, both passive and active vaccinations should be given: passive—IV human rabies IG to the patient; active—3 doses of antirabies vaccine IM over a 28-day period.

3. For a wild animal bite (raccoon, bat, or dog), the animal should be captured at best efforts and killed for immunoassay of the brain.

4. For a home dog or cat bite in an endemic area, the animal should be captured and observed for 10 days. The animal most likely does not have rabies if its conditions remain the same.

Other Arthropod-Borne and Zoonotic Diseases

Table 1-10: Summary of Other Arthropod-Borne and Zoonotic Diseases

Disease / Clinical features, diagnosis, and treatment
Cellulitis and Erysipelas (Image 83)
Features: 1. Mostly caused by beta-hemolytic **Streptococcus** (A, B, C, G, and F), **Staph-A (#1) or Pasteurella** multocida through an animal bite (**"Cat-dog-man biting disease"**). 2. Red, hot, swollen and tender skin lesion; with a clear border—erysipelas; without clear border—cellulitis. **Dx**: Clinical manifestations. Cultures are necessary only for extensive or special lesions. **Tx**: Dicloxacillin, augmentin (**amoxicillin + clavulanate**), clindamycin, or cefazolin.
Q-Fever
Features: 1. **Caused by Coxiella burnetii** (Gram⁻) transmitted by inhalation of infected material (aerosol), blood, ingestion of infected milk; found in the placenta of cattle, sheep, and goats. 2. Acute: low fever, headache, myalgias, atypical pneumonia. (3) Chronic (complications): chronic hepatitis or endocarditis. **Dx**: Most cases are self-limited within 2 weeks. Confirmation diagnosis can be made by specific serologic antibody tests if necessary. **Tx**: **Acute, symptomatic cases and prevention—doxycycline.** Chronic/complications: hydroxychloroquine plus doxycycline (> 18 months for endocarditis).
Brucellosis
Features: 1. Also called Undulant Fever, **caused by Brucella Spp**. (a Gram⁻ bacillus) from dairy products or contact with animals. 2. Prolonged fever, sweating, joint pain, enlarged LN, and hepatosplenomegaly. **Dx**: Pathologic culture and serologic tests (+). **Tx**: **Doxycycline plus rifampin.**
Tularemia
Features: 1. Caused **by Francisella tularensis (a Gram- bacillus)** by tick bite, mediated by rabbits, deers, etc. 2. There are different types: ulceration, pneumonia, and typhoid; presenting with fever, painful focal ulceration, papules, or enlarged LN with tenderness. **Dx**: Serologic antibody (+). **Tx**: **Streptomycin/gentamicin/doxycycline.**
"Cat-scratch disease"
Features: 1. Caused by **Bartonella** Hens. (a Gram⁻ bacillus) 2. Fever, painful focal lesion and enlarged cervical LN with or without tenderness. **Dx**: Clinical manifestations. **Tx**: Mostly self-limited. For severe cases, treat with **azithromycin** or **doxycycline.**
Plague
Features: 1. A highly contagious disease caused by **Yersinia pestis** (a Gram⁻ bacillus) through fleabite from rodents (rats, mice, dogs), or respiratory tract. It can be co-infected between humans and animals. 2. Subtypes: (1) By skin wound, it causes bubonic (adenopathic) plague (>80% of cases), with fever, chills, weakness, and headache, followed by intense pain and swelling in a lymph node. (2) By respiratory tract, it causes pneumonic plague. (3) Septicemic plague: may be without a preceding bubo, with high fever, shock, and death if not treated in time. **Dx**: Pathogen isolated or F1 Ab/Ag (+). **Tx**: Immediate supportive care and antibiotics (**streptomycin, gentamicin, or doxycycline**).
Leptospirosis

Features: 1. Caused by Leptospira spp. (spirochetes) through contaminated water by rodents and farm animals. 2. In tropics; flu-like symptoms, myalgias, jaundice, photophobia, etc. 3. **Anicteric**: rash, lymphadenopathy, elevated LFTs; **icteric**: renal or/and hepatic failure, vasculitis. **Dx**: Mainly based on epidemiologic exposure and clinical manifestations; serology or culture may confirm if necessary. **Tx**: Oral **doxycycline, azithromycin**, or amoxicillin. Most cases are mild to moderate.
Ehrlichiosis
Features: 1. Caused by Ehrlichia spp. (Gram⁻) through Amblyomma (lone star tick) bite from deers, etc. 2. Fever, chills, malaise + rash; a few cases may be complicated with GI bleeding, renal injury, or ehrlichial meningitis. **Dx**: Clinical experience. **Tx**: Oral **doxycycline or tetracycline** for a week.

Chapter 1: High-yield Questions (HYQ)

1. A 10 year-old (y/o) girl presents with fever, intermittent abdominal pain, and bloody diarrhea for the past 10 days after a local camping trip. She feels weak and fatigued. Stool analysis reveals some WBCs and RBCs but no bacteria, ova, or parasites. Two stool cultures on enteric pathogens are negative. Physical examination (P/E) finds T = 38.5°C and a soft abdomen with mild RLQ tenderness. CBC results are normal (Nl). What's the most likely diagnosis (Dx)?

A. Traveler's diarrhea   B. Cryptosporidiosis   C. Giardiasis
D. Crohn disease   E. Dysentery

2. A 55 y/o woman presents with malaise, fever, and nausea for the past 2 days. She has been on chemotherapy for breast cancer for the past 3 months. She denies headache, chill, cough, and bone pain. P/E finds T = 38.7°C, HR = 90/min; other results are unremarkable. CBC reveals pancytopenia with WBC = 1,200/uL. Her CXR and urine analysis are normal. Blood and urine samples are taken for pathogen cultures. The best next step of treatment (Tx) is

A. IV ceftazidime and vancomycin   B. IV cefepime and vancomycin
C. IV cefepime   D. IV gentamycin and vancomycin
E. IV piperacillin   F. IV amphotericin B

3. A 65 y/o man presents with an abrupt fever, headache, dry cough, diarrhea, and abdominal pain for the past 10 hours. He lives alone in an old apartment with unsanitary conditions. P/E results are normal except for T = 38.5°C. CXR reveals bilateral infiltrates. WBC = 9,000/uL with left shift (increased ratio of immature neutrophils). There are no other abnormal findings. What's the most likely cause?

A. H. influenzae (Hib)   B. Mycoplasma   C. Legionella
D. Chlamydia   E. TB bacilli

4-5: 4. A 27 y/o woman comes to the clinic one week after a trip to the Northeast (U.S.), and presents with mild fever, headache, and an expanding rash on the right foot. P/E finds T = 38°C, stable vital signs, and a 3-cm circular, erythematous, nontender rash with central clearing on the right foot. ECG reveals I° A-V block. There are no other abnormal findings except for a 3-month pregnancy. What's the most likely diagnosis?

A. Cellulitis

B. Rocky Mountain spotted fever (RMSF)

C. Lyme disease

D. Tularemia

E. "Cat-scratch disease"

5. For the above patient (in Q4) who wishes to stay home after an immediate therapy, the most appropriate antibiotic treatment is

A. oral azithromycin

B. oral doxycycline

C. oral amoxicillin

D. IV PCN

E. IV ceftriaxone

6-8: 6. A 60 y/o woman is brought to the ER with fever, RUQ abdominal pain, and nausea and vomiting for the past 5 hours. P/E results: T = 39.5°C, HR = 90/min, marked RUQ abdominal tenderness on palpation and rebound tenderness. CBC reveals WBC = 18 x 10³/uL with predominant neutrophils and bands. Ultrasonography shows gallstones with dilated bile ducts and fluid. Her vital signs are stable. What's the best initial treatment?

A. Oral quinolones

B. IV quinolones

C. IV ceftazidime

D. IV ampicillin

E. Support and observation in hospital

7. Continued with Q6: The patient still has persistent symptoms after 5 hours of the appropriate antibiotic treatment. What's the best next step now?

A. Fluid and blood cultures

B. IV quinolones

C. IV cefepime

D. IV ampicillin

E. ERCP

8. Continued with Q6-7: For the above patient, the proper tests show mixed Gram⁻ bacteria and anaerobes. At this time, the most appropriate antibiotic to be included is

A. clindamycin

B. quinolones

C. gentamycin

D. ampicillin

E. metronidazole

9-10: 9. A 68 y/o man is brought to the ER for high fever, headache, nausea, vomiting, and confusion. He had a small dental surgery 3 days ago. P/E results: Unclear consciousness, T = 39.5°C, HR = 90/min, RR = 25/min, BP is normal; neck is stiff; Kernig's sign is suspicious. Sensation seems normal. Eye exam shows equal-sized, mildly dilated pupils and papilledema (by fundoscopy). Blood is taken for culture and sensitivity test. What's the most appropriate next step?

A. A head MRI scan

B. Lumbar puncture for CSF assay and culture-sensitivity

C. A head CT scan

D. An empiric antibiotic

E. IV steroid

10. For the above patient, the most appropriate management has been done. Now the best medical treatment is intravenous administration of

A. large-dose PCN

B. ceftazidime + vancomycin

C. ceftriaxone + vancomycin

D. cefotaxime + ampicillin

E. ceftriaxone + ampicillin + vancomycin

11. A 70 y/o man is brought to the ER for fever, headache, and confusion for the past 2 days. He lives alone with poor living conditions. P/E results: Alert, T = 38°C, HR = 88/min, RR and BP are normal; neck is stiff; Kernig's sign is suspicious. Eye exam is normal. CBC: WBC = 15 x 10³/uL, with 50% LC. CSF: Opening pressure = 200 mmH₂O, LC = 60%, neutrophils = 40%, protein = 55 mg/dL, and glucose = 30 mg/dL. This patient most likely has

A. pneumococcal meningitis

B. viral meningitis

C. TB meningitis

D. TB encephalitis

E. viral encephalitis

F. fungal meningitis

12. A 16 y/o girl is brought to the ER for eye pain and blurred vision for the past 12 hours. She uses contact lens daily and follows the sanitary procedures most of the time. Eye exam shows a hazy cornea with central ulceration and adjacent stromal abscesses. Eye movement is normal. What's the most likely diagnosis?

A. Bacterial keratitis   B. Fungal keratitis   C. CMV retinitis
D. HSV retinitis   E. Orbital cellulitis

13. A 40 y/o man complains of (c/o) intermittent abdominal discomfort, decreased appetite, and 5 kg weight loss for the past 3 months. He has a history of smoking and alcohol drinking for 5 years, and two previous blood transfusions. P/E results are mostly normal. Ultrasonography (U/S) shows a normal liver image without any mass. Serology results show that liver function tests (LFTs) are normal; HBsAg, HBeAg, and anti-HBs, anti-HBc, and anti-HBe IgGs are all positive. What's the best explanation?

A. Liver cell carcinoma   B. Chronic Hepatitis B, with low viral replication
C. Chronic Hepatitis B, with active viral replication   D. Recovery from Hepatitis B, with immunity
E. Chronic hepatitis B, with heterotypic Anti-HBs

14. A 25 y/o man suffered from a puncture wound of the right foot 3 days ago and now presents with fever and increased foot pain. P/E shows a swollen wound on the right ankle with tenderness on palpation. T = 39 °C, HR = 90/min, RR = 26/min; BP is normal. CBC shows WBC = 15 x 10^3/uL, with predominant neutrophils and bands. ESR = 120. Tech ^{99} is scheduled and the blood is taken for culture and sensitivity testing. What's the best initial therapy?

A. Oxacillin   B. Vancomycin   C. Ceftriaxone
D. Cefotetan   E. Cefepime

15-16: 15. A 20 y/o sexually active man complains of 2-day's sore throat, fever, swollen neck masses, and abdominal pain. He developed a generalized skin rash after taking ampicillin. He reports having used allopurinol for gout before the onset of these symptoms. P/E shows enlarged tonsils, cervical lymph nodes, and spleen, and a maculopapular rash all over the body. T = 39°C. Vital signs are normal. More tests are scheduled. What's the best explanation for his conditions?

A. Ampicillin allergy   B. Acute upper respiratory infection
C. Allopurinol allergy   D. Infectious mononucleosis
E. AIDS   F. Chlamydia infection

16. CBC for the above patient reports: hematocrits (HCT) = 44%, WBC = 8500/uL with many atypical cells, platelets = 85 x 10^3/uL. Monospot test is (+). Apart from bed rest, what's the most appropriate next treatment?

A. Acyclovir   B. Ganciclovir   C. Steroids
D. PCN-G   E. Early exercise

17. A 20 y/o sexually active female presents with lower abdominal pain, dysuria, and increased, purulent vaginal secretions without odor. She has no fever or other symptoms. Pelvic exam shows a red cervix with mucus, and cervical motion tenderness. Urinalysis (U/A) shows WBC and protein. What's the best next step?

A. Secretion test for chlamydia   B. Thayer-Martin for gonococcus
C. VDRL test for syphilis   D. KOH test for candida
E. Smear for Trichomonas

18. Continued from Q15: Fluorescent antibody test for chlamydia in Q15 has come out with (-), and Thayer-Martin for gonococcus is (+). Given this, the best treatment now is:

A. a single dose of ceftriaxone and azithromycin

B. a single dose of ceftriaxone

C. a single dose of ceftriaxone and doxycycline

D. cefoxitin IV + azithromycin PO

E. Ampicillin + gentamycin + metronidazole + clindamycin for 5 days

19. A 17 y/o girl presents with 3-day's fever, headache, dry cough, and weakness. P/E is normal except for T = 38.5°C. Her urine dipstick testing reveals protein (++) but no bacteria, RBC or WBC. What's the best next step?

A. Serum BUN level testing   B. 24-hour collection of urinary protein

C. Urine culture for pathogens   D. Reassurance: "It's common and benign."

E. Repeating the dipstick test

20. A 60 y/o man presents with increased urinary frequency and urgency, and a sensation of suprapubic fullness but difficulties in voiding for the past 3 days. P/E finds an enlarged urinary bladder and an indurated, enlarged prostate with tenderness. Urinalysis is normal. Analysis for prostatic secretions reveals 18 WBCs/HPF (normal reference is <10), but cultures for bacteria are (-). Other results are unremarkable. A urinary catheter is inserted and 300 mL of urine is removed. What's the most appropriate next step?

A. Repeating the secretion culture   B. Empirical TMP-SMX for E coli

C. Use of an alpha-R blocker   D. Test of prostate specific antigen (PSA)

E. Fine needle aspiration of the prostate

21. A 58 y/o man presents with fever, chills, right flank pain, and dysuria for the past 5 hours. He occasionally smokes and drinks alcohol. P/E finds T = 38.5°C, HR = 110/min, and percussion tenderness over the right renal area. CBC shows WBC = 15 x 10³/uL with left shift. Urinalysis reveals WBC and protein. Urine is sent for culture and sensitivity test. He went home with prescribed oral ciprofloxacin. He comes back 3 days later with T = 38.3°C. What's the most appropriate next step?

A. Increase the dose of oral ciprofloxacin   B. IV ciprofloxacin

C. IV cefepime   D. IV ampicillin + gentamycin

E. Renal CT scan

22. In the same month, a 30 y/o man experiences his second onset of fever, chills, cough with sputum, and chest pain. He has a history of risky sexual behavior with both males and females for "several years." P/E shows T = 39°C, HR = 110/min, and diffuse rales in the lungs. CXR reveals multiple lobar infiltrates. CBC shows WBC = 1200/uL and CD4 = 200/uL. Blood and sputum are taken for examination of pathogens. What's the best initial treatment?

A. Azithromycin or erythromycin   B. Levofloxacin + erythromycin

C. Cefotaxime + imipenem   D. TMP-SMX

E. Ceftazidime + TMP-SMX

23-26: Match the following clinical scenarios with the most likely diagnosis.

A. Bacterial meningitis   B. Subacute sclerosing panencephalitis

C. Viral meningitis   D. AIDS encephalopathy

E. PML   F. Herpes encephalitis

G. CNS abscess   H. Malaria

I. Fulminant viral encephalitis   J. Fulminant hepatitis

23. A 25 y/o man is hospitalized for decreased memory and changes in mood for the past 3 weeks, with occasional right arm clonus. He had a history of fever and headache one month ago, but no trauma. P/E results: T = 39°C, alert. Neurologic exams: decreased recent memory, speech difficulties, and right hemiparesis. Lab tests: increased WBC and LC ratio. CSF: Opening pressure = 220 mmH$_2$O, LC = 60%, neutrophils = 40%; culture is (-). EEG: Spike-and-wave discharges originating from the temporal lobe.

24. A 25 y/o man is hospitalized for a chronic bleeding disease and progressive memory loss. Severely low platelet counts have forced him to receive four times of urgent blood transfusions in a poorly equipped hospital over the past 5 years. Neurologic exams reveal poor recent and remote memory, decreased vision, gait ataxia, limb hyper-reflexia, and changes in mood and personality. T = 38.5°C. Head MRI is unremarkable.

25. A 25 y/o man is hospitalized for a month's history of headache, fever, right arm clonus, memory loss, and changes in mood. He has been HIV (+) for the past 5 months. Neurological exams show decreased recent memory, speech difficulties, and right hemiparesis. T=39°C, CSF-P = 220 mmH2O; culture is (-). CT with contrast reveals a mass in the left temporal lobe.

26. A 45 y/o man is back from a trip to the countryside with malaise, headache, confusion, periodic high fever, chills, and sweating for the past 3 days. P/E reveals T = 41°C, confused status, neck and limb stiffness, generalized rash and lymph node swellings, and hepatosplenomegaly. CBC reveals anemia, leukopenia, and reticulocytosis. Blood samples are taken for special tests.

27. Diagnosis of pathogen for the above patient in Question 23 is confirmed by immunoassay of the CSF. IV acyclovir was administered for the past 3 days and re-examination of the patient shows no changes in his conditions. What's the most appropriate next step now?

A. Increase the dose of acyclovir   B. Change to ceftriaxone

C. Change to foscarnet   D. Change to famciclovir

E. Change to amphotericin B

28. A 65 y/o man has been undergoing 2-week's chemotherapy for lymphoma. P/E finds T = 39°C and other results are (-). CBC shows WBC = 500/uL without bands. The most appropriate next step is to

A. wait for the results of blood culture and sensitivity test to give the correct antibiotics

B. give oral agents to prevent bacterial and fungal infections

C. give IV agents to prevent bacterial and fungal infections

D. give broad-spectrum antibiotics to cover Gram- bacteria, Pseudomonas, and Staph-aureus

E. take blood samples for culture and sensitivity test

29. A 25 y/o female working in a day care center develops a pruritic rash in crops over her whole body except the palms and soles, with fever, headache, cough, and dyspnea for the past 3 days. She claims that she has received all of the appropriate pediatric immunizations. P/E finds T = 39°C, generalized small vesicles on erythematous bases with crusting, and rales heard over the lungs. CBC report is awaited. This patient most likely

A. has about normal CXR result   B. will infect her husband soon

C. has leukocytosis   D. will have life-time immunity after recovery

E. has missed a vaccine in the childhood

30. A 15 y/o girl has just returned from a spring camping trip and presents with irritating red eyes and copious watery discharge from the eyes and nose. P/E reveals a mild fever, tachycardia, and congested conjunctiva and nasal membranes. There are no other abnormal findings. The most likely cause is

A. allergy	B. bacterium	C. chlamydia
D. virus	E. foreign body	

31. A 16 y/o boy has just returned from a spring camping trip and presents with painful red eyes with copious watery discharge. P/E reveals a mild fever, tachycardia, and congested conjunctiva. Fundoscopy shows retinal pallor and ulceration. There are no other abnormal findings. The most likely etiology is

A. CMV	B. HSV	C. chlamydia
D. candida	E. allergy	

32. A 25 y/o man presents with headache and a painful swelling localized to the left eyelid with tenderness, which is not associated with eye movement. There is no conjunctival congestion or discharge, nor other abnormal findings. He claims he has "two girl-friends." The most likely diagnosis is

A. orbital cellulitis	B. post-orbital cellulitis	C. dacryocystitis
D. hordeolum	E. chalazion	

33. A 45 y/o man presents with fever, abdominal pain, nausea, and loose stools of yellowish color for the past 3 days, beginning after he eat a large meal with friends. None of his friends has similar symptoms. He has a 5-year history of smoking, alcohol consumption, and decreased weight. P/E finds a moderate fever and a firm, distended abdomen with decreased bowel sounds, tenderness on deep palpation, and with rebound tenderness. Ascites is (+) and the spleen is enlarged. What's the most important next test to determine the etiology?

A. Abdominal ultrasound	B. CBC	C. Ascites analysis
D. Abdominal CT scan	E. Stool analysis	

34. A 25 y/o female presents with fatigue, decreased appetite, nausea, and yellow urine for the past week. Her last menstrual period (LMP) was 4 weeks ago. P/E finds normal vital signs, jaundice, flat and soft abdomen, and an enlarged liver. Serum ALT and bilirubin are elevated; beta-hCG is (-); anti-HAV IgM and HBsAg are (-); anti-HAV IgG, anti-HBc IgM, and HBeAg are all (+). What's the most likely diagnosis?

A. Acute hepatitis A with HBV carrier	B. Acute hepatitis B with HAV immunity
C. Acute hepatitis A and B	D. Acute hepatitis B with HAV carrier
E. HBV carrier with HAV immunity	

35. A 40 y/o man presents with low-grade fever, sweats, coughs with blood-tinged sputum, right chest pain, and decreased weight for the past month. He has a history of smoking and alcohol use for the past 5 years. P/E finds T = 38°C, normal vital signs, decreased respiratory sounds, and dullness on percussion of the right lower chest. CBC reveals anemia and increased WBC counts and lymphocyte (LC) percentage. CXR shows diffuse infiltrates in the right lower lung. The most appropriate next test for diagnosis is

A. serologic tests	B. chest CT	C. sputum culture
D. PPD test	E. sputum stain for acid fast bacilli	

36-41: Match the following clinical scenarios with the most likely etiology.

A. Klebsiella granulomatis   B. H. ducreyi   C. Chlamydia
D. HSV   E. HPV   F. Poxvirus
G. Candida   H. T. pallidum   I. Gonococcus
J. Allergy

36. A sexually active female presents with multiple soft, fast growing, pedunculated, and pink papules of 3-4 mm in size on the vulva for the past week. There are no other abnormal findings.

37. A sexually active female presents with multiple red, painful, and itchy vesicles with circular, scarring ulcers on the vulva for the past 2 weeks. Tissue is taken for Tzanck test and culture.

38. A sexually active female presents with a week of multiple painless, shallow, circular ulcers on the vulva, with low-grade fever, dysuria, tender swelling of the left inguinal lymph nodes, and a purulent draining sinus. A sample from the ulcer is taken for smear stain and fluorescent tests.

39. A sexually active female presents with a week of multiple painful, irregular, deep papules and ulcers on the vulva with a bad odor, and suppuration of the left inguinal lymph nodes. There are no other abnormal findings. A sample from the ulcer is taken for a Gram stain.

40. A sexually active female presents with a week of multiple raised, red, painless papules (0.5-1cm) with granulomatous ulcers on the vulva. There are no other abnormal findings. A sample from the ulcer is taken for a pathologic stain.

41. A sexually active man presents with low-grade fever, diffuse and symmetric pink papules, and painless lymph node swellings in both inguinal areas. The patient reports finding a small painless smooth ulcer on his penis one month ago, which has now disappeared. Specific serology confirms the diagnosis.

42. A 16 y/o girl is brought to the ER with fever, nausea, vomiting, dizziness, abdominal pain, knee pain, and weakness. She was travelling in another city 5 days ago with her boyfriend and reveals that her LMP occurred during the trip. P/E results: Alert, T = 39°C, HR = 95/min, BP = 90/55 mmHg; soft neck, desquamative rash on hands and feet, and tenderness on the middle abdomen and both knees without swellings. IV fluid is started. Urine sample is taken for analysis and culture. The most appropriate next step is

A. IV nafcillin   B. IV ceftriaxone   C. blood culture and sensitivity test
D. joint fluid aspiration   E. abdominal ultrasound

43. A 30 y/o female with multiple pets presents with fever, dry cough, chest pain, and shortness of breath for the past 3 days. P/E results: Alert, T = 39°C, RR = 28/min, HR = 90/min; BP is normal; rough respiratory sounds. WBC is 12,000/uL. CXR reveals interstitial infiltrates. What's the best initial treatment?

A. Erythromycin   B. Doxycycline   C. Levofloxacin
D. Azithromycin   E. Amoxicillin

44. A 60 y/o female presents with fever, headache, dry cough, and loss of appetite that began after attending a party 3 days ago. Two other friends from the party also have similar symptoms. P/E shows T = 38.5°C and there are no other abnormal findings. What's the most appropriate next step?

A. Amantadine for 4-5 days   B. Oseltamivir for 4-5 days   C. Amoxicillin for 4-5 days
D. Annual flu vaccination   E. Blood culture and sensitivity test

45-50: Match the following clinical scenarios with the most likely cause.

A. Campylobacter jejuni	B. E. coli (O_{157}:H_7)	C. Staph-aureus
D. Shigella	E. Salmonella	F. Enterotoxigenic E. coli
G. Giardia	H. Bacillus cereus	I. Clostridium perfringens
J. Clostridium difficile	K. Clostridium botulinum	L. Vibrio parahaemolyticus
M. Yersinia enterocolitica	N. Proteus	O. Klebsiella

45. A 17 y/o boy has ingested a cup of leftover milk at home. Four hours later, he has severe lower abdominal cramps and loose stools with sparse blood and mucus. There is no vomiting. P/E finds T = 38°C and a soft abdomen with mild RLQ tenderness. Stool analysis reveals WBC and RBC. CBC results are normal.

46. A 10 y/o boy has had a meal of reheated rice in a friend's home. Two hours later, he has severe nausea, vomiting, and upper abdominal cramps. He has one relatively loose stool during the day. P/E finds no fever or other abnormal results. Stool analysis and CBC results are normal.

47. A 16 y/o boy joined a lunch with all kinds of foods (including seafood) in an unsanitary restaurant. In the evening he presents with severe, recurrent lower abdominal cramps and loose stools with blood and mucus for a few hours. He has nausea and sensation of urgently passing stools. There is no vomiting. P/E finds T = 39°C and the lower abdomen is soft with tenderness. Stool analysis shows WBC and RBC. CBC reveals leukocytosis.

48. A 15 y/o boy has had a lunch in an unsanitary restaurant. In the evening, he has abrupt profuse, watery diarrhea. There is no vomiting, abdominal cramp, or fever. He's been using amoxicillin for otitis media for the past 10 days. P/E results are unremarkable. Stool toxin test is (+). CBC is normal.

49. A 17 y/o girl has joined a lunch in a restaurant and had fresh raw fish. In the evening, she has fever, nausea, severe lower abdominal cramps, and diarrhea with blood and mucus. P/E finds T = 38.5°C and a soft abdomen with RLQ tenderness. Stool analysis reveals WBC and RBC. CBC reveals leukocytosis.

50. A 20 y/o newly married female presents with urinary frequency, urgency, and burning sensation for a day. She denies any fever, flank pain, or abnormal vaginal discharge. She also denies any history of UTI or STD. P/E results are about normal. Urine analysis reveals WBC and alkalosis. CBC is normal.

51. A 22 y/o married female comes to the clinic for a general health exam, and found herself about 5-week pregnant confirmed by a positive blood hCG test. She took rubella immunization 6 weeks ago and has been using contraception to her best efforts because the physician has advised her to avoid pregnancy within 3 months. She is generally healthy and concerned about the options of avoiding harm to the fetus. What's your best next step of management?

A. Give advice on abortion	B. Give reassurance	C. Give IV immunoglobulin
D. Perform pelvic ultrasonography	E. Explain the risks and benefits of abortion and let the patient decide	

52. A 30 y/o sexually active man presents with fever, fatigue, and skin rash for the past few days. He was HIV (+) two years ago but has had no obvious symptoms until now. P/E shows T = 38.5°C, normal vital sign, and multiple non-tender, 1-1.5 cm, round, reddish, vascular papules on both arms. What's the most likely diagnosis?

A. Molluscum contagiosum (MC)	B. Common warts	C. Herpes simplex (HS)
D. Kaposi sarcoma (KS)	E. Bacillary angiomatosis	

53. A 25 y/o woman presents with painful, swollen left knee for the past 3 days. She cannot think of any significant events related to it. She denies any abnormal urinary or vaginal discharges, or history of trauma, diseases or drug use. Careful history taking reveals that she has several sexual partners and she uses condoms most of the times. P/E finds low fever, tachycardia, and a swollen left knee with tenderness and limited range of motion. Arthrocentesis: WBC = 85 x 10^3/uL with 88% neutrophils. Gram staining of the joint aspirate is (-). Urinalysis is normal. What's the best next step for diagnosis?

A. Blood culture   B. Urine culture   C. Culture of the joint aspirate
D. Culture of the vaginal discharge   E. Culture of urethral swab

54. A 60 y/o man has been hospitalized for the treatment of diabetes for the past 2 weeks. He has a 10-year history of smoking and alcohol drinking. Symptoms: fever, cough with yellowish sputum, chest pain, tachypnea, and dyspnea. P/E results: T = 38.8°C, RR = 28/min, HR = 90/min; BP is normal; respiratory rales are (+) in both lungs. CBC reveals HCT = 40%, WBC = 12 x 10^3/uL, neutrophils = 88%. CXR shows multiple infiltrates in both lungs. Sputum is taken for Gram stain and culture. Which of the following is **NOT** a common pathogen for this patient?

A. Pneumococcus   B. Staph-aureus   C. E. coli
D. Pseudomonas   E. Hib   F. Klebsiella

55. A 30 y/o man presents with malaise, general muscle pain, and decreased appetite for the past month. He has a 5-year history of smoking, alcohol drinking, and IV drug abuse. P/E results are unremarkable. CBC reveals HCT = 38%, WBC = 6,000/uL, LC = 44%, platelets = 100 x 10^3/uL. Anti-HCV is (+) and LFTs are normal. Test of HCV RNA load by PCR is started. Which of the following is **NOT** commonly associated with the patient's disease?

A. Mixed cryoglobulinemia   B. Polyarteritis nodosa   C. Sjogren syndrome
D. Hashimoto thyroiditis   E. Membrane glomerulonephropathy   F. ITP
G. Plasmacytoma   H. T-cell lymphoma

56. In a pre-term exam, an asymptomatic pregnant patient has been found that the HBsAg, anti-HBe and anti-HBc IgGs are (+), and HBeAg and anti-HBs IgG are (-). There are no other abnormal findings. For this patient's conditions, all the following should be administered immediately after delivery **EXCEPT**

A. IV HBIG to the newborn   B. HBV vaccine to the newborn
C. HBV vaccine to the mother   D. Ribavirin to the mother
E. Alpha-interferon to the mother

57. A 55 y/o man with immunodeficiency presents with malaise, fever, night sweats, and cough with yellow sputum over the past week. He has been on antibiotic prophylaxis for the past 2 months. P/E results: Alert, T = 39°C, RR = 28/min, HR = 90/min; BP is normal; respiratory sounds are rough. CBC reveals HCT = 32%, WBC = 8,000/ul, neutrophils = 85%, LC = 9%. Skin PPD is 9 mm induration. CXR shows left lobe cavitation. Sputum smear reveals weakly acid-fast filamentous branching rods. What's the most likely cause of the disease?

A. Actinomyces   B. Nocardia   C. TB
D. Coccidioides   E. Blastomyces   F. Histoplasma

58. A 10 y/o boy is brought to the clinic an hour after he was bitten by a neighbor's dog due to his provocation. The dog did not get immunization for rabies and is not showing any abnormal symptoms. P/E finds a tender swollen lesion without bleeding on the left forearm of the boy. His wound is cleaned with iodine. The most appropriate next step is

A. observe the dog for 10 days   B. kill the dog and perform the brain biopsy

C. give the boy IV immunoglobulin   D. give the boy active rabies immunization

E. give the boy active and passive immunization   F. give reassurance

59. During a fight at school, a 9 y/o boy received a bite on the right forearm by another boy, and is brought to the clinic an hour later. His records show up-to-date immunizations. P/E finds a swollen tender lesion with tiny bleeding on the right forearm. There are no other abnormal findings. Apart from cleaning the wound, the best next treatment is

A. observation   B. amoxicillin   C. ampicillin and clavulanate

D. amoxicillin and clavulanate   E. clindamycin   F. erythromycin

60. In medical records, human bites have been shown to transmit all the following infections **EXCEPT**

A. hepatitis B   B. hepatitis C   C. herpes simplex

D. syphilis   E. TB   F. actinomycosis

G. tetanus   H. AIDS

Answers and Explanations

1. (D). Regional enteritis (Crohn disease), ulcerative colitis, dysentery and invasive E. coli ($O_{157}:H_7$) may all cause bloody diarrhea and fever. Two negative stool cultures in this case may exclude infections. Traveler's diarrhea, cryptosporidiosis and giardiasis usually cause small bowel infection with watery diarrhea.

2. (C). It's an urgent case of febrile neutropenia induced by chemotherapy that requires immediate antibiotics in hospital. Empiric treatment includes monotherapy of ceftazidime, cefepime, or a carbapenem, or combined therapy of piperacillin plus gentamycin, to cover Gram⁻ bacteria (especially Pseudomonas). Vancomycin is usually added for resistant Staph-aureus or Strep-P or severe skin/mucosa infections. If fever persists despite above treatment, amphotericin B is added to cover suspected systemic fungal infection. Piperacillin alone is inadequate.

3. (C). This is a typical case of legionella pneumonia ("Atypical pneumonia"); WBC count can be normal (Nl) or high with left shift. Mycoplasma pneumonia is similar but more common in young and generally healthy patients, and rarely with diarrhea. Chlamydia psittaci is usually from bird's feces and upper respiratory secretions, and its pneumonia presents with dry cough and chest pain. Choose macrolides for the treatment of "B, C, and D." Hib primarily causes typical-community-lobar pneumonia in elderly and chronically ill patients. TB is rare now and only occurs in patients with poor nutrition or immunosuppression.

4. (C). Lyme disease is caused by B. burgdorferi and transmitted by tick bite. RMSF is caused by R rickettsia, presenting with the triad of fever, headache, and rash (centripetally). Tularemia is caused by Francisella tularensis, with fever, a painful ulcer/papule, or enlarged lymph nodes (LN). "Cat-scratch disease" is caused by Bartonella Hens, with fever, non-tender enlarged lymph nodes, and a painful focal lesion. "B, C, D, and E" can all be treated best with doxycycline. Cellulitis is caused primarily by Staph-aureus (#1) or by Pasteurella via animal bite ("Cat/dog/man biting disease"), presenting with a red, hot, swollen, and tender skin lesion without clear borders. Treatment: Amoxicillin + clavulanate.

5. (E). This is an early disseminated Lyme disease, best treated with IV ceftriaxone (with long effect) or IV PG in hospital (IV/4 hours). For early-localized disease, the #1 choice is usually oral doxycycline without pregnancy or oral amoxicillin with pregnancy. Oral azithromycin is also effective but more expensive.

6. (C). This patient has cholecystitis complicated by biliary duct obstruction and empyema and should be hospitalized and given "C" (3rd-generation cephalosporin) to cover major Gram⁻ bacteria including Pseudomonas; also should be prepared for surgery. Quinolones are the second choice here. Ampicillin is best for Hib and Listeria.

7. (E). "A" should come after "E" because conditions are deteriorating and progressing towards life-threatening sepsis. In this setting even the 4th generation cephalosporins ("C") may not save her life. The patient needs emergent ERCP to remove the stones and drain pus. Combination antibiotics are also required at this point.

8. (E). Metronidazole is best treatment for abdominal and genital anaerobes. Ampicillin is weaker. Clindamycin is best for chest anaerobes (Strep). All these agents are also effective against Gram⁻ bacteria.

9. (D). This is a suspected case of severe meningitis or encephalitis. Usually a lumbar puncture (LP) for CSF analysis and culture and sensitivity test (C/S) followed by "D" (antibiotics) is the best initial step. Because he has signs of increased ICP (nausea, vomiting, and papilledema), lumbar puncture is avoided and an empiric dose of ceftriaxone is given followed by a CT scan of the head. Steroids should be avoided until viral infection has been excluded.

10. (E). For community-acquired adult meningitis, Pneumococcus, Meningococcus and Hib are the commonest pathogens. Pneumococcus is usually resistant to PCN-G. Ceftriaxone plus vancomycin is usually the empiric choice of treatment for a serious bacterial meningitis, but ampicillin should be added to cover the commonly existent Listeria in a patient > 55 y/a or an infant < 3 months.

11. (C). In general, only TB and fungal meningitis have these clinical features and CSF results. Fungal meningitis is rare, typically occurring only in the setting of a chronic or immunodeficient disease. "A" is the #1 common meningitis, usually presenting with more severe manifestations and a predominance of neutrophils in the CSF. Encephalitis is less likely given the symptoms and CSF results.

12. (A). "B" is mostly seen in farmers and immunodeficient patient, with multiple stromal abscesses on the cornea. 'C' is the most common eye infection with immunodeficiency and presents without pain or conjunctivitis. "D" is usually painful with conjunctivitis. "E" is infection of the postorbital septum, with sudden fever, proptosis, painful and decreased eye movements, and red and swollen eyelids.

13. (E). It's important that you fully review and understand Table 1-5. "A" is not very likely given his age and negative ultrasound result.

14. (E). This patient most likely has acute osteomyelitis by Pseudomonas; hence the best treatment choice here is cefepime (a 4th-generation cephalosporin, also covers Staph and Strep). Oxacillin is the initial treatment for Staph-aureus (#1 common for osteomyelitis overall and in IV drug abuse) and Staph-epidermidis (after hip replacement); if resistant or severe, vancomycin +/- gentamycin is the best. Ceftriaxone is a 3rd-generation cephalosporin, good for Gram⁻ bacilli and Pneumococcus but not for Pseudomonas. Cefotetan is a 2nd-generation cephalosporin, good for anaerobes (as in diabetic ulcers) but not for Pseudomonas.

15. (D). This case is more typical of infectious mononucleosis (I-M), which is caused by EBV and best diagnosis by the Monospot test. Ampicillin allergy may have a similar rash but the described rash seen in I-M is a common reaction with ampicillin, allopurinol, and HIV. It is thus not an allergy. "B or E" is less typical.

16. (C). Blood tests confirmed I-M. Splenic rupture is a major complication and patient should be restricted from active exercise or sports until the spleen is no longer palpable. Steroids will be very helpful in reducing tonsil edema and increasing platelet count in this case. Acyclovir is effective against HSV, Ganciclovir against CMV, and PCN against Strep-aureus (sore throat). There is no specific treatment for EBV.

17. (A). Chlamydia is the #1 cause of acute PID in a young female with unsafe sexual behavior, followed by N. Gonococcus. Because it's more difficult to get a (+) test for Chlamydia (than Gonococcus), it should be first checked and treated unless there's strong diagnostic evidence for Gonorrhea (both have similar symptoms). Other choices are less supported.

18. (A). This is a mild case of acute PID. Though Gonococcus has been confirmed, Chlamydia is not yet excluded, and thus "A" is the best choice to cover both. "C" requires doxycycline for 7 days. "D" is the best choice for severe acute PID (high WBC, T > 39°C). "E" works for chronic PID (abscess).

19. (E). It's common to see transient, isolated proteinuria during stress or mild infection, but "E" should be performed to ensure a (-) result before providing reassurance ("D"). If proteinuria is persistent, "A and B" should be performed. "C" may be needed for cases with pyuria.

20. (D). This is nonbacterial prostatitis, also with possible prostate hypertrophy. For his age, prostate cancer needs to be ruled out, initially by "D" then by "E" if still suspected. After cancer is excluded, "C" and NSAIDs can be used. "B" is best for acute bacterial prostatitis and UTI at this age. "A" is unnecessary.

21. (E). This is acute pyelonephritis. As he's been under proper antibiotic treatment for the past 3 days but still has fever, you should suspect UT obstruction (stones, cancer) or abscess. Therefore, he needs immediate renal ultrasound or CT rather than "better antibiotics to cover more Gram⁻ bacteria" ("C and D").

22. (E). This patient most likely has AIDS complicated with lobar pneumonia +/- Pneumocystis (PCP), and thus ceftazidime or cefotaxime plus TMP-SMX is the best choice (for lobar pneumonia and PCP). Anti-HIV drugs should also be started with confirmed HIV and CD4 < 500/uL. "A" is best for outpatient typical and atypical pneumonia (mild). "B" is best for inpatient pneumonia (severe). "C" is best for hospital-acquired pneumonia.

23. (F). Herpes encephalitis—fever, headache, changes in memory, mood and personality, and temporal lesion. Culture (-) is partially supportive.

24. (D). This patient received four times of potentially unsafe blood transfusions in 5 years and thus has a high risk of AIDS encephalitis given this presentation (low fever, progressive dementia and neuropsychological deficits). MS has similar neurologic deficits but MRI usually shows demyelinating plagues scattered in the brain.

25. (G). In HIV (+) patients, 90% of brain lesions will be either toxoplasmosis or lymphoma. In this case, a toxoplasmosis-abscess is the most likely diagnosis. MRI is more accurate. A biopsy of the lesion for Gram stain and culture is essential. Empiric treatment with pyrimethamine and sulfadiazine can be applied.

26. (H). P. falciparum can cause the most severe type of malaria by invading the CNS and mimicking encephalitis or meningitis. History, P/E, CBC, and Giemsa/Wright-stained blood films by experts will confirm the diagnosis. This severe case should be treated with initial IV proguanil + atovaquone, followed by oral mefloquine.

27. (C). Herpes simplex is correctly treated initially with acyclovir. No response to this treatment indicates resistance by HSV. It's rational to change to foscarnet in this case. Increase in acyclovir dose or using a similar

medicine famciclovir will have no better effect here. Ceftriaxone is the choice for pneumococcal meningitis and amphotericin B is for systemic fungal infection.

28. (E). This patient has severe neutropenia and potentially lethal sepsis. Thus, "D" is urgently required after blood is taken for culture and sensitivity test (no waiting). Antifungal treatment is indicated if the antibacterial treatment fails to control the fever, or a fungal infection is suspected or found.

29. (B). This is adult varicella (chickenpox) with pneumonia, which is usually more severe and contagious than the childhood type (infect persons close to her). Vaccination may still leave slight susceptibility to varicella infection. WBC is mostly normal with predominant lymphocytes.

30. (D). This patient most likely has conjunctivitis by adenovirus, which is usually self-limited but contagious. Allergy is more likely if the patient is afebrile, itchy, and with pale membranes. Bacterial conjunctivitis usually causes a foreign body sensation and purulent discharge. C. trachomatis usually cause chronic conjunctivitis with recurrent epithelial keratitis in childhood.

31. (B). This is acute HSV retinitis with conjunctivitis and must be referred to an ophthalmologist ASAP. CMV retinitis is more common with immunodeficiency, usually without pain or conjunctivitis. Fungal keratitis is often seen in farmers and immunodeficient patient; cornea shows multiple stromal abscesses.

32. (D). Mnemonics: "Horrible Staph" abscess, treated with anti-Staph-aureus agents. Chalazion is an obstructive inflammation of the meibomian gland with similar presentation. "C" is mostly caused by Staph-aureus and Strep-B, often with fever, pain, and purulent discharge. "A" usually has sudden fever, proptosis, painful eye movement, and swollen eyelids.

33. (C). This is most likely cirrhosis complicated with ascites and primary peritonitis, and thus "C" is the best method to reveal the potential cause. If the patient is older and the history is longer, hepatocarcinoma needs to be ruled out by "A and D", etc.

34. (B). This is acute HB infection in the "window period". The crucial points are that anti-HBc IgM (+) indicates acute HB infection, and anti-HAV IgG (+) indicates history of HAV infection and long-term immunity. Please grasp the "HBV Serology and Vaccination" well.

35. (E). This is most likely TB pleuritis, and "E" is the fastest test. Though sputum culture for TB bacilli is the most specific test, it has a low sensitivity and is time-consuming. PPD (+) only indicates a history of TB infection or contact, not necessarily present infection. If this patient were older, CT would be indicated to exclude lung cancer.

36. (E). Genital wart is also called condylomata acuminata. It is primarily caused by HPV 6, 11, or 18, and is often shaped as a "cauliflower". Practicing safe sex and cryotherapy are the correct treatment options.

37. (D). Genital herpes is caused primarily by HSV-2. Tzanck test usually confirms the diagnosis. Acyclovir along with safe sex is the treatment of choice.

38. (C). Lymphogranuloma venereum is caused by C. trachomatis, confirmed by (+) fluorescent antibody.

39. (B). Chancroid is an acute sexually transmitted disease (STD) caused by H. ducreyi (Gram⁻ bacillus). The best treatment is 1-dose of azithromycin, along with safe sexual bahavior.

40. (A). Granuloma inguinale (Donovanosis). Giemsa/Wright stain often shows Donovan bodies. Treatment is doxycycline for 3 weeks.

41. (H). Early-stage syphilis—chancre followed by condylomata lata (highly contagious). Specific tests are FTA-ABS and MHA-TP. Treatment is one dose of PCN 2.4 million-IU IM, along with safe sexual behavior.

42. (A). Patient most likely has toxic shock syndrome caused by S. aureus from tampon use. Diagnosis is by clinical impression and treatment is targeted against shock and S. aureus. A sexually active person may have gonococcal arthritis, with a very swollen (knee) joint and marked leukocytosis. It's primarily managed first by "D + C", then "B". "E" is for ectopic pregnancy.

43. (B). This is most likely atypical pneumonia caused by coxiella burnetii (Q-fever), and thus "B" is the #1 choice and "A" is the second. For most atypical pneumonias in outpatients, erythromycin is still the #1 choice, usually with "C or D" added to increase coverage of pathogens.

44. (A). This is most likely a "Flu" case, caused 90% of the time by influenza A. Amantadine is not the most cost-effective medicine. "B" covers both Type A and B but is expensive. "C" is for Gram⁻ bacterial infection. "D" is necessary after recovery. "E" is unnecessary in this case. If the patient has high fever, severe headache, vomiting, and diarrhea that lead you to suspect influenza B or H1N1 infection, oseltamivir ("B") should be used within 48 hrs.

45. (A). This is the most common bacterial diarrhea by Campylobacter jejuni from contaminated food, mostly self-limited. Many other pathogens can also cause bloody diarrhea with mucus. Yersinia enterocolitica usually causes fever, bloody diarrhea with pain and tenderness in the RLQ abdomen. Enterotoxigenic E. coli mostly cause watery diarrhea and is a common pathogen in the "Traveler's disease". E. coli (O157:H7) is usually from contaminated meat or fruits, and it may cause bloody diarrhea and hemolytic-uremic syndrome (HUS).

46. (C). GIT infection of Staph-aureus is usually from undercooked meat, milk. The preformed toxin typically causes abrupt, intense vomiting about 2-4 hours after eating; diarrhea is rare. It's mostly self-limited. If there is typical diarrhea (not "one loose stool") a few hours after vomiting in this case, the pathogen will be most likely Bacillus cereus (from leftover rice)

47. (D). Typical Shigella infection: Fever, lower abdominal cramps and bloody diarrhea a few hours after eating contaminated food. Treatment is ciprofloxacin. Vibrio parahaemolyticus from contaminated seafood can cause self-limited abdominal cramp and (watery) diarrhea.

48. (J). Clostridium difficile toxin often causes profuse watery diarrhea induced by long use of broad-band antibiotics. Treatment is IV metronidazole. C. perfringens can also cause similar watery diarrhea after eating contaminated foods. C. botulinum from contaminated honey, canned meat can produce a very strong bio-toxin and cause flaccid paralysis rather than diarrhea.

49. (M). Yersinia (from pets or raw/undercooked meat) often causes sporadic ileitis or ileocolitis, with fever and RLQ abdominal pain—similar to appendicitis except for inflammatory diarrhea. Treat with ciprofloxacin if severe.

50. (N). Proteus is a common pathogen with UTI when the urine is alkaline. Otherwise most cases of UTIs in the young and old patients are caused by E. coli.

51. (B). It's generally advised that one should avoid pregnancy for 3 months after rubella immunization. However, statistical cases of congenital rubella syndrome in early pregnancy are rare. Thus reassurance is the best answer here rather than any need or advice for a therapeutic abortion. The fetus is in risk when a seronegative female is exposed to a rubella patient. Ultrasound now is too early to show any defects. "C" has not shown to prevent congenital rubella syndrome.

52. (E). It's a complication caused by Bartonella species, a Gram⁻ bacillus. MC is caused by a poxvirus, with non-pruritic, centrally-unbilicated dome-shaped papules. Common warts are caused by HPV, with painless, pruritic, cauliflower-like papules. Herpes simplex typically has painful vesicles. KS typically shows papules that become plaques or nodules later on with color changes from light brown to dark violet, on the face, trunk, and lower limbs.

53. (E). This sexually active young patient is highly suspected of purulent septic arthritis caused by Gonococcus. Systemic symptoms and the listed cultures for Gonococcus are mostly (-), except for culture of the urethral swab, which can give 80% (+) rate.

54. (A). All the listed Gram⁻ bacteria (C, D, E, F) and S. aureus can be common pathogens of pneumonia for patients with chronic disease or prolonged hospitalization, as with this patient's conditions and presentations. They are mainly treated with the 3rd-generation cephalosporins (ceftazidime) and gentamycin. Pneumococcus is the most common pathogen of most community-acquired or lobar pneumonia. It's mostly treated with the new quinolones.

55. (H). It's most likely a hepatitis C. Only 25% of cases have mild symptoms and elevated LFTs. Anti-HCV is usually (+) but not protective. HCV RNA load by PCR is the best diagnostic test. HC is commonly associated with all the listed diseases, membranoproliferative glomerulonephritis, and B-cell lymphoma but not T-cell lymphoma.

56. (D). This patient has chronic active hepatitis B (HB) with low viral replication, and both the risky newborn and mother need immediate vaccinations. 6-12 months of alpha-interferon with lamivudine is effective against chronic HB, whereas ribavirin is the treatment for hepatitis C (HC). The mother also needs another two HBV vaccinations later.

57. (B). All the choices can be opportunistic lung infections induced by immunodeficiency, but only nocardia is a Gram⁺, weakly acid-fast branching rod. Actinomyces is a Gram⁺, branching rod that can be either anaerobic or facultative anaerobic but not acid-fast. Treatment of "B" is TMP-SMX. Other pulmonary fungal infections: Coccidioidomycosis is often endemic to southwestern U.S; blastomycosis and histoplasmosis may be endemic to Ohio-Mississippi valleys.

58. (A). Unimmunized dog bite may transmit the fatal rabies. Postexposure prophylaxis should include passive and active immunizations. Best efforts should be made to catch the dog and kill for brain biopsy. If the dog is caught and does not show any signs of rabies, it is observed for 10 days. If it shows features of rabies at biting or during the observation, it is killed and its brain is taken for biopsy following post-exposure immunizations for the patient.

59. (D). Human bites can be deceptive and are often underestimated and undertreated. Commonly isolated pathogens include Staph, Strep, Corynebacterium, and anaerobes (Bacteroides, Peptostreptococcus). The best prophylactic antibiotics are thus "D" to have the amoxicillin spectrum extended by clavulanic acid.

60. (H). Although evidence suggests that it is biologically possible to transmit AIDS through human bites, there have been no clinical records of the disease transmitted by this way yet. It's also very unlike in reality. All other bite-infections have clinical records.

Chapter 2

DISEASES OF THE CARDIOVASCULAR SYSTEM

Cardiovascular diseases (CVDs) carry a high morbidity and the highest mortality rate among all diseases in most countries. CVDs are closely associated with human life styles and thus can be reduced significantly by regular health examinations, consultations, and life style modifications.

PEARLS—IMPORTANT DIFFERENTIATIONS OF CHEST PAIN

Chest pain is the most common symptom for most CVDs, respiratory diseases, and some upper abdominal disorders. Thus, it's important to grasp the differential points.

Angina and myocardial infarction (MI): See details on the same topics below.

Myocarditis: It is usually **preceded by a viral disease, with a vague chest pain**. Creatine kinase (CK)-MB is often increased. ECG (EKG) will show abnormal conduction or **Q waves**.

Pericarditis: It may be **preceded by a viral illness. Chest pain is sharp, pleuritic, and positional**—worse with lying down and relieved by sitting up. Pericardial rub often exists. ECG usually shows **diffuse ST elevation without Q waves**. CK is mostly normal. It **responds well to anti-inflammatory drugs**.

Pleuritis: Mostly **after lung infection; with sharp chest pain worse on inspiration** and certain position; tenderness, friction rub or dullness may be present. CXR or CT scan is the best diagnostic test.

Pneumonia: Moderate chest pain with **fever, cough, sputum, and hemoptysis. CXR** is the best test.

Pneumothorax: Typically sudden, sharp, pleuritic chest pain and dyspnea; absent breath sounds; mediastinum shifted to the opposite site—suspect of tension pneumothorax—requiring urgent intercostal needle puncture. Non-tension pneumothorax can wait for CXR confirmation and natural relief.

Aortic (aneurysm) dissection: Very severe, sharp, tearing chest pain; typically radiating to the back; loss of pulses, unequal BP between arms, or aortic insufficiency; neurologic signs; mediastinum widened on CXR. MI may occur if dissection extends into coronary artery (Cor-A). Diagnosis is confirmed by transesophageal echocardiography (TEE), CT scan, or aortography.

Pulmonary embolism (PE): Sudden chest pain, dyspnea, tachycardia, cough, and hypoxemia, usually 3-5 days after a surgery or **long immobility**. The chest pain is usually pleuritic but may resemble angina. **CT pulmonary angiography** has supplanted V/Q scanning as **the preferred** means of diagnosis.

Mitral valve prolapse: Transient chest pain with a **typical midsystolic click murmur**.

Pulmonary hypertension (HTN): Dull chest pain with symptoms and signs of right ventricular (RV) failure.

Costochondritis: Chest pain is usually stabbing, localized, and exacerbated with inspiration; reproducible or **worse with chest palpation**. ECG is normal (Nl).

Gastric diseases: **GERD** (burning chest pain, acid reflux, bad taste, relief with antacids); **stomach spasm**; **PUD** (epigastric pain before or after eating).

Pancreatitis: Post-meal persisting sharp epigastric pain radiating to the back, with nausea/vomiting, fever, and increased amylase and lipase levels.

Gallbladder disease: (Mostly post-meal) right upper quadrant (RUQ) abdominal pain with tenderness, nausea/vomiting, jaundice, etc.

Hiatal hernia: Burning chest or epigastric pain; nausea/vomiting; reflux of food; relief with antacids.

ARRHYTHMIAS

Definition: Abnormality (Abnorm) of cardiac rhythm. It can be asymptomatic (Asympt), symptomatic (Sympt), or lethal. Causes of arrhythmia are various and should be treated specifically. Prophylactic antiarrhythmic drugs are generally not recommended because they increase the mortality (especially for ventricular tachycardia, V-Tach). Common cardiac arrhythmias are summarized in Table 2-1 (**Images 1-10**).

Table 2-1, 2-2, 2-3: **Summary of major cardiac arrhythmias.**

Table 2-1: Conduction Block

Type	Etiology	Symptoms/signs	ECG	Treatment (Tx)
1° Atrial-ventricular (A-V) block	Normal status (Nl), aging, digitalis, increased vagal tone	Asymptomatic	PR interval > 0.2s	None
2° A-V block (Mobitz I)	A-V node degeneration, drug effect (β-R blockers, Ca-blockers, digitalis); increased vagal tone	Mostly asymptomatic	**Increased PR interval** until a blocked beat; then PR reset	Cessation of related drug
2° A-V block (Mobitz II)	Abnormal infranodal conduction system by MI, degeneration	Variable symptoms: dyspnea chest pain, or **presyncope;** unstable	**Unexpected blocked** beat w/o PR interval change	1. Ventricular pacemaker; 2. Atropine at hand
3° A-V block (Complete heart block)	Fibrous degeneration (MI, myocarditis, rheumatic fever)	low BP, **CHF, syncope,** Adams-Stokes attack; "A-wave"	No relationship between P and QRS complex	1. Ventricular pacemaker; 2. Atropine at hand
Left bundle branch block	Acute MI, CHF, hypertension (HTN), rheumatic heart disease	Asymptomatic	Wide QRS & invert-T in V5-6 leads	Observation; pacemaker for symptomatic (older) patients

Right bundle branch block	Nl, HTN, CAD, rheumatic heart disease, cardiomyopathy	Asymptomatic	Wide QRS & invert-T in V1-2 leads	Observation; pacemaker for symptomatic cases

Table 2-2: Supraventricular Arrhythmias

Type	Etiology	Symptoms/signs	ECG	Treatment (Tx)
Atrial fibrillation (A-Fib)	CAD, CHF, ethanol, anemia, atrial myxoma, rheumatic fever, COPD, thyrotoxicosis	Asymptomatic; dyspnea, palpitation, chest pain, irregular pulse, system-embolism	Atrial 350-500 bpm, **No discernible P-wave** with baseline; irregular QRS	1. **Warfarin or aspirin** for embolism risk 2. Acute **rate control** (with CHF): amiodarone/sotalo, Ca/β–R blockers, digoxin 3. **Unstable**: Synchronized **e-cardioversion** (50-100j)
Atrial flutter	Similar to A-Fib Rapid fire of an ectopic atrial beat	Asymptomatic; palpitation, lightheaded, syncope	Atrial 250-300bpm, **A-V 2:1**, regular rhythm "Sawtooth" P-wave	1. **Stable**: rate control—**verapamil** is the #1 drug. 2. **Unstable**: Synchronized **cardioversion** (100-369j)
Multifocal Atrial tachycardia (MAT)	Elderly COPD, multiple atrium-pacemaking or re-entry	With or without symptoms	>3 varying P-waves; rate: 100-200bpm	1. Etiologic Tx; 2. Symptomatic: **verapamil**; metoprolol, or adenosine
Paroxysmal Supra-ventricular tachycardia (SVT)	Rapid ectopic arrhythmia from atrium or A-V junction, mostly secondary to re-entry (WPW)	Sudden onset or stop; lightheadedness, palpitation, angina, syncope	Nl QRS, P-wave appeared or hidden in T-wave; rate: 130-230bpm	1. Carotid massage, Valsalva maneuver; 2. **Adenosine** (#1), then verapamil

Table 2-3: Ventricular Arrhythmias

Type	Etiology	Symptoms/signs	ECG	Treatment (Tx)
Premature ventricular contraction (PVC)	Benign ectopic ventricular beats; hypoxia, electrolyte disorders, hyperthyroidism	Mostly asymptomatic; palpitation, syncope	Missing P-waves, early wide QRS, followed by a compensatory pause	Treat symptoms/causes: **β-R blockers** –#1 choice. Flecainide or propafenone is highly effective but contraindicated with CHD.
Nonsustained ventricular tachycardia (NSVT)	#1 CAD or MI; #2 cardiomyopathy, metabolic diseases, drug toxicity (digoxin, etc.)	Skipped beats, hypotension, syncope, CHF, cardiac arrest	>3 consecutive PVCs, ventricular rate >120 bpm, wide & bizarre QRS in regular rapid rhythms, A-V dissociation	1. Most NSVTs: **β- or Ca-blocker** is the initial Tx; 2. For symptomatic, frequent VT: **amiodarone** (drug cardioversion). **Never use lidocaine as prophylaxis!**

Sustained monomorphic ventricular tachycardia (SMVT)	Similar to VT	lightheadedness, palpitation, syncope or hemodynamic collapse within 30″	Regular, wide QRS complex; >100bpm that lasts for >30″ (seconds)	1. **Acute: amiodarone**, procainamide, or lidocaine; 2. **Recurrent**: radiofrequency ablation; 3. **If unstable**: defibrillation.
Ventricular fibrillation (VF)	#1 CAD or MI; PVC, VT	Hypotension, pulselessness, syncope; **electrical storm**: multiple recurrent episodes of VF	Totally erratic tracing or waves	1. **Immediate electrical defibrillation (unsynchronised cardioversion) plus CPR!** 2. **Next: IV amiodarone**, lidocaine, or epinephrine.
Wolff-Parkinson-White syndrome (WPW)	Ebstein anomaly, cardiomyopathy, SVT, AF	Recurrent SVT attacks (>150 bpm), hypotension	Pre-excitation, short PR interval, wide slurred QRS (δ-wave)	1. Initial vagal maneuvers; 2. If it fails, A-V node blocker (**adenosine** or verapamil) IV; 3. Definitive Tx (with AF): radiofrequency ablation (accessory tract)
Torsades de pointes (TdP)	QT syndrome, low K/Mg, overdose of quinidine, procainamide, or disopyramide	Recurrent VT, dizziness, syncope, hearing loss; may cause sudden death	QRS rotations prolonged QT, may lead to VF	1. **First-line: IV MgSO4** (plus KCl, especially with low Mg, K); 2. Isoproterenol followed by transvenous overdrive pacing.

ISCHEMIC HEART DISEASE (IHD)

—CORONARY ARTERY DISEASE (CAD)

Etiology and pathogenesis

The basic mechanisms of CAD are that **coronary O_2 demand surpasses supply due to decreased blood flow secondary to atherosclerotic narrowing of the coronary artery** (Cor-A), leading to cardiac dysfunctioning. It's fatal if there's narrowing of 1-2 major coronary arteries that causes > 75% decrease in cross-sectional area (or 50% decrease in diameter).

Factors that increase O_2 demand: Physical exertion or stress, emotional or mental stress (including anxiety), large meals, etc.

Factors that **lower the O_2-carrying capacity of the blood**: Anemia, carbon monoxide (CO) poisoning, platelet microthrombi at the site of coronary stenosis (local damage).

Major risk factors

CAD

Age (male > 45, female > 55 y/a), **male** gender, **smoking, hypertension, diabetes,** heredity (including race, family history < 55 y/a), **atherosclerosis, hypercholesterolemia** (Hyper-Chol, LDL > 200 mg/dL, HDL < 40 mg/dL), physical inactivity, obesity *abdominal* and overweight, stress, excess alcohol use, and postmenopausal women.

The metabolic syndrome (Insulin resistance syndrome): It refers to any combination of hyperglycemia, hyperlipidemia, hyperuricemia, and hypertension. Genetic predisposition, lack of exercise, and body fat distribution may increase the likelihood of developing diabetes and CVD. *Cardiovascular dz* **(Cardiac) syndrome X:** It refers to angina pectoris (ischemia) occurring in patients with normal coronary arteriogram.

Prognostic indicators

(1) **Left ventricular function—Ejection fraction (EF):** Normal > 50%; if < 50%, associated with increased mortality.

(2) **Severity—Vessels involved:** Left main coronary artery or > 2 arteries indicating worse prognosis.

Angina Pectoris

It mostly refers to "**stable angina**", a paroxysmal chest pain resulting from cardiac ischemia—an imbalance between oxygen supply and demand, and is most commonly caused by the inability of atherosclerotic coronary arteries to perfuse the heart under conditions of increased myocardial oxygen consumption (exercise, stress). **Stable angina** is the type when the chest pain is precipitated by predictable factors (exercise, exertion, etc.). **Unstable angina** is angina that occurs at any time.

Essentials of diagnosis

I. Clinical features –c/i SOB *crushing retrosternal CP, radiates down arm & up jaw*

1. **Nature of the pain**: **Heavy, pressing, or squeezing.**

2. **Location**: Substernal or precordial.

3. **Radiation**: **Commonly to the left jaw or arms.**

4. **Duration**: 15 sec—15 min.

5. **Precipitating factors**: **Exertion, anxiety, meals, and coldness.** Risk factors are the same as above.

   dyspnea, presyncope
6. **Associated symptoms**: Shortness of breath (SOB), anxiety, fatigue, nausea and vomiting (N/V), palpitations, and diaphoresis.

7. **Pain relief**: **Nitroglycerin** (in a few min), resting (standing or sitting).

8. **P/E (Physical examination)**: Tachycardia, diaphoresis, and transient S4 gallop.

9. **ECG: ST-T depression.**

II. Types of angina

Angina Pectoris

1. **Chronic stable angina**: It occurs during exertion, can be relieved by rest or nitrates, and can recur. ECG usually shows evidence of ischemia during pain or stress testing. Angiography mostly demonstrates significant obstruction of major coronary arteries.

2. **Unstable angina: New onset of chest pain that occurs at rest or with less exertion, or requires more medicines to be relieved.** It follows a worsening pattern in frequency, duration, or/and severity of symptoms. It should be considered and managed **as a form of acute coronary syndrome. Diagnosis** is based on presence of severe angina in those patterns **without ST-elevation on ECG.** It often progresses to myocardial infarction, and thus should be stabilized with **aggressive management** (aspirin, beta blockers, LMWH, nitrides, etc.) before stress testing or cardiac catheterization is performed.

3. **Prinzmetal (variant) angina: Chest pain occurs at rest or stress without the usual precipitating factor of exertion, due to coronary artery spasm.** It may result from an altered autonomic neurologic control of the coronary arteries or altered artery contraction. ECG mostly shows **ST-T elevation.** Cardiac catheter will show **no atherosclerosis. Management** is mainly a **diagnostic therapy of a Ca-channel blocker** (the best diagnostic treatment, which usually relieves symptoms immediately), or a nitrate.

III. Lab diagnosis

1. **ECG: It is the best initial test for all forms of chest pain**. It can exclude previous myocardial infarction (MI) or obvious arrhythmia; also to evaluate the use of regular stress test versus thallium testing.

2. **Exercise ECG/echocardiography or treadmill (stress) test: When ECG is normal or inconclusive, stress testing is the best diagnostic test to confirm angina (ischemia), determine the severity of disease, and evaluate post-MI conditions. Echocardiography is more sensitive than ECG.** Stress test is (+) if any of the chest pain, ST-segment depression, hypotension, or significant arrhythmia is induced by exercise.

3. **Thallium (scan)-treadmill test—similar to exercise echocardiography but focusing more on the coronary arteries) —Indications:**

(1) Patients with inconclusive regular treadmill testing.

(2) Patients with mitral valve prolapse.

(3) Patients with **WPW** syndrome.

(4) Patients with left bundle branch block.

(5) Young women with high false positive results on regular stress testing.

(6) Patient with uncertain acute ischemic changes on ECG (nonspecific ST-wave changes, inability to read the ECG, etc.).

(7) Patient requiring quinidine, procainamide, or digitalis.

Ischemia versus infarction: In ischemia, it will show a reversal of the decrease in thallium uptake or wall motion that will return to normal after a period of rest.

Angina Pectoris

4. **For patients unable to exercise**: Perform dipyridamole-thallium, adenosine-thallium, or stress/dobutamine echocardiography (Echo).

5. **Contraindications for stress testing**: Unstable angina, aortic stenosis, idiopathic hypertrophic subaortic stenosis, severe COPD, acute CHF, acute ischemic changes on ECG, aortic dissection, and severe hypertension.

6. **Coronary angiography**: This is the most accurate method of detecting CAD, to detect the presence of narrowing that is best treated with surgery or angioplasty—usually when more than 70% stenosis exists. Coronary angiography is often used when ECG or stress testing results are equivocal.

7. Holter monitoring: It's a continuous ambulatory ECG monitoring that records the rhythm, usually used for arrhythmias and for a 24-hour period (but may extend to 48-72 hours). It does not detect ischemia because it's not accurate for ST segment evaluation.

8. **Cardiac catheterization**: Usually applied in patients poorly controlled with drugs or positive stress test, to help determine the need for angioplasty—triple vessel disease or left main coronary artery disease. Occupational workers for public safety (bus driver, airline pilot) with any CAD symptoms require cardiac catheterization.

Differential diagnosis

See "Important Differentiations of Chest Pain" above.

Treatment

1. **Medical therapies for angina:**

Drugs that can reduce mortality for a patient with chronic angina include aspirin, beta-R blockers, and nitrates (nitrates did not show decreased mortality in acute MI).

(1) **Nitrates**: They are **the first-line therapy for acute angina**. Low doses of nitrates increase vein-dilation and decrease preload; high doses of nitrates increase small-artery and coronary artery dilatation and O_2 supply, and decrease both afterload and preload.

Adverse effects (S/E): Vasodilation can lead to orthostatic hypotension, reflex tachycardia, throbbing headache, and blushing. It's contraindicated if systolic BP < 90 mmHg (to avoid syncope). It's important to have a > 8-hour window-free period to reduce the incidence of tachyphylaxis (usually 12am—6am).

(2) **Beta-R blockers**: They decrease HR, contractility, and blood pressure, and thus decrease myocardial O_2 requirement. They are **contraindicated in severe asthma as well as vasospastic** or variant (Prinzmetal) angina to avoid induction of coronary vasospasm from unopposed alpha-receptor activity. **Long maintenance therapy has been shown to reduce mortality in acute MI and CHF and risk of reinfarction.**

Adverse effects: Fatigue, bronchoconstriction, depression, hallucinations, sexual dysfunction, insomnia, dyslipidemia, Raynaud phenomenon. A nonselective beta-R blocker (propranolol) may mask hypoglycemic symptoms in diabetes (IDDM) and is not routinely used in CAD.

Selective beta1 blockers (with less adverse effects): **Atenolol, metoprolol, or acebutolol is most commonly used in angina pectoris and MI (and CHF).**

Angina Pectoris

New nonselective beta-R blockers: Penbutolol and carteolol are used for hypertension.

(3) **Ca-channel blockers:** They decrease preload and afterload. It may be harmful during the post-infarction period, especially if patient has left ventricular failure. Its efficacy in angina is limited.

Adverse effects: Cardiac—reflex tachycardia, hypotension, and dizziness, CHF; noncardiac—flushing, headache, weakness, nausea, constipation, wheezing, and peripheral edema.

PEARLS—Specific Ca-channel blockers with various selectivity
Strong on heart: Verapamil
Strong on peripheral vessels: Nifedipine
Intermediate: Diltiazem

Verapamil: It causes significant A-V block in ECG; moderate decrease in coronary blood flow and cardiac contractility; hypotension, and ankle edema. It's contraindicated in sick sinus syndrome, A-V node block and ejection fraction (EF) < 35%.

Diltiazem: It causes moderate A-V block and increase in coronary blood flow, mild decrease in contractility, and mild hypotension.

Nifedipine: It has minimal A-V block; mild decrease in cardiac contractility; significant hypotension; increase in coronary blood flow, ankle edema, and headache. It's contraindicated in aortic stenosis and unstable angina.

(4) **Newer therapies: Ranolazine**, a late Na-channel blocker, is used either in combination with a beta blocker or as a substitute in patients who cannot receive one.

2. **Treatment of unstable angina:**

(1) Hospitalize the patient and treat with aggressive medications—aspirin, nitrates, beta-R blockers, heparin, and lipid-lowering agents as described above. Heparin (IV or SC) or low molecular weight heparin (LMWH) is the major therapy because of its high efficacy.

(2) Glycoprotein inhibitors with angioplasty and stent placement are very effective, but thrombolytics are not.

(3) **Revascularization:**

(a) **CBG (Coronary bypass graft)**: Very useful in those with major left coronary disease or 3-vessel disease and left ventricular (LV) dysfunction. It's indicated in cases with symptoms despite medical treatment or with severe adverse effects from therapies. It's more beneficial in those with diabetes or low ejection fraction, although the performance carries more risk.

(b) **PTCA (Percutaneous transluminal coronary angioplasty)**: It is indicated in significant cardiac lesions not eligible for CBG. It's an easier procedure with more risk of re-stenosis. Stent placement is now a standard procedure. Glycoprotein 2b/3a inhibitors (abciximab, tirofiban, or eptifibatide) are usually used with the procedure, followed by aspirin plus ticlopidine or clopidogrel.

3. **Preventive therapies:**

Angina Pectoris

(1) **Lifestyle modification for risk reduction (highly important!)**: Smoking cessation; reduction of stress, weight, and Chol & Trig; regular exercise; treatment of diabetes, hypertension, anemia, COPD, etc.

(2) **Antiplatelet therapy**: **Low-dose aspirin** daily is very effective in prevention of angina. **New antiplatelet drug—ticlopidine or clopidogrel** is an alternative to aspirin in patient who cannot tolerate aspirin. Note that ticlopidine can cause adverse neutropenia.

(3) **Lipid management: See "HYPERLIPIDEMIA"**.

Myocardial Infarction (MI)

MI is ischemic myocardial necrosis as **a result of an abrupt reduction in the coronary blood flow to a segment of myocardium, usually due to a thrombotic occlusion of a coronary artery previously narrowed by atherosclerosis.** MI is associated with a 30% mortality rate and 50% pre-hospital deaths.

Etiology

Atherosclerosis by all causes is the main pathologic basis. Most cases are due to acute coronary thrombosis—atheromatous plaque ruptures into the vessel lumen and thrombosis forms on top of the lesion causing the vascular occlusion.

Risk factors: Same as those for CAD (above).

Non-atherosclerosis causes: Vasculitis, SLE, polyarteritis nodosa, Takayasu arteritis, mucocutaneous lymph node (LN) syndrome (**Kawasaki disease, Image 36**), coronary spasm, variant angina, cocaine abuse, coronary artery embolus, atrial myxoma, atrial or ventricular thrombus, polycythemia vera, thrombocytosis, and anomaly of coronary arteries.

Pathogenesis

Acute MI is mostly "**ST-elevated MI**" and localized to the left ventricle (LV) and in one of the two forms below:

1. **Transmural infarct**: It's more often associated with **Q waves**.

2. **Subendocardial infarct**: It's mostly "**non-Q-wave MI**", confined to the inner 1/2 to 1/3 of the LV wall. The LV subendocardium region is most susceptible to ischemia, because of tenuous oxygen supply. Diltiazem use can reduce the risk of recurrence.

PEARLS—Coronary artery anatomy and MI (**Images 1-10**)

LCA and LAD: They supply most of the **LV and the anterior interventricular septum.** They account for **the most common occlusion in CAD**, causing **LV anterior wall MI.**

CFX: Circumflex artery, supplies the left lateral wall. Its occlusion causes **lateral wall MI.**

RCA: Supplies the SA, AV nodes, and most of the inferior portion of the LV. Its occlusion causes **inferior MI.** St segment elevation II, III, ə, avf.

Essentials of diagnosis

1. **Symptoms:** Characteristic chest pain—**severe, crushing, prolonged (usually > 20min) chest pain, similar in quality to but more severe than angina**; associated with dyspnea, anxiety, diaphoresis, nausea, vomiting, weakness, low fever, sense of **impending doom, and syncope** (in elderly). Painless and atypical MI can be up to 1/3 cases and more likely in postoperative or diabetic patients and the elderly. Sudden cardiac death can occur due to ventricular fibrillation (V-fib).

2. **Signs:** Congestive heart failure (**CHF**) —arrhythmias (mostly tachycardia; inferior MI may have bradycardia), S4 gallop, JVD, and dyskinetic left ventricular (LV) impulse. **Cardiogenic shock signs** are seen with > 40% of myocardial infarction—BP decrease, S3 gallop, and rales. Systolic murmur of papillary muscle or ventricular septal rupture or pericardial friction rub (usually with transmural infarction) on the 3rd-4th day may be heard.

3. **PEARLS**—**ECG (Images 4-10): It's the best diagnostic test within 6 hours of onset** and represented by ventricular wall hypokinesia, **peaked T waves (early), ST-segment elevation (transmural infarct) or depression (subendocardial lesion), new left bundle branch block (LBBB), or Q waves (necrosis, late).**

LV anterior wall MI (#1 common): ST-segment elevation ($\pm$ Q wave) in anterior leads (V$_{1-4}$).

Posterior MI: ST-segment depression (+ large R wave) in inferior leads (V$_{1-2}$).

Inferior MI: ST-segment elevation ($\pm$ Q wave) in inferior leads (II, III, and aVF).

Lateral wall MI: ST-segment elevation ($\pm$ Q wave) in leads I, aVL, and V$_{5-6}$.

4. **Cardiac enzymes (Figure 2-1):**

(1) **CK-MB** is both **highly sensitive and specific** for MI when measured **within 36 hrs** of chest pain. It begins to **elevate at 4-6 hrs after MI**, reaches a **peak at 12-24 hrs** and is back to normal in 72 hrs. CK levels may increase following cardioversion, defibrillation, cardio-pulmonary resuscitation, or muscle trauma, but the MB fraction will only increase with certain extent of **myocardiocyte death**.

(2) **Troponin is most specific** but moderately sensitive; it begins to rise **2-4 hrs after** the start of the chest pain, and **remains high for 7-10 days. It's a more valuable biomarker for MI with the chest pain within 8 hrs and after 36 hrs**.

(3) **Lactate dehydrogenase** (LDH): It's non-specific and not used for diagnosis of acute MI, but **useful for re-infarction**. In acute MI, LDH increases after 12 hrs of chest pain and **peaks in 24-72 hrs and remains high for 10-14 days** after MI. LDH-1/LDH-2 ratio > 1.0 supports of MI.

5. **CBC: Leukocytosis** of 10-20 x 10^3/uL.

6. **Thallium-201 (Tl-201) and Technetium-99m (Tc-99m) scan: Tl-201 scan** is sensitive but not very specific because it cannot distinguish between zones of severe ischemia ("cold spots") and infarction. **Tc-99m scan provides better resolution** for the same function.

7. **Special type of MI:** It may be clinically silent or present as CHF or dysrhythmia in the absence of chest pain, especially in elderly, postoperative, hypertensive, or diabetic patients.

Figure 2-1: Biomarkers of Acute MI (Courtesy of www.circ.ahajournals.org)

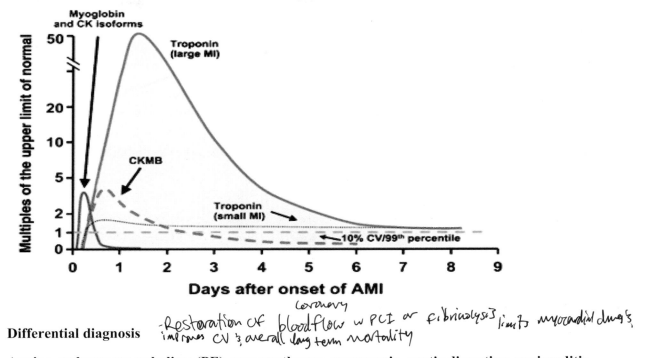

Differential diagnosis

-Restoration of blood flow w PCI or fibrinolysis limits myocardial dmg's, improves CV & overall long term mortality (coronary)

Angina, pulmonary embolism (PE), pneumothorax, pneumonia, aortic dissection, pericarditis, costochondritis, etc.

Treatment

1. **"ABC" first**—airway, breathing, and circulation. Supplemental oxygen has shown a reduction in the risk of death.

2. Treat sustained ventricular arrhythmia or heart failure rapidly.

3. **Beta1-R blockers**: They've clearly shown **reduced post-MI mortality rate** if no contraindications exist (bradycardia, A-V block, hypotension, or COPD). A **beta1 blocker (metoprolol)** is a good **early start** (IV per 5 min) after an acute MI and also good **maintenance therapy**.

4. **Nitrates (PO or IV)**: They can alleviate pain, lung congestion, and left heart failure, but **did not clearly reduce post-MI mortality**.

5. **Antiplatelet therapy: Aspirin (PO)** can reduce coronary reocclusion by inhibiting platelet aggregation on top of the thrombus and **clearly reduce post-MI mortality.** It's used as part of the **maintenance therapy. Clopidogrel, ticlopidine (less S/E), or prasugrel** is indicated in (1) aspirin intolerance (such as allergy); (2) recent angioplasty with stenting. **Prasugrel has more risk of hemorrhagic stroke in elder patients**. Other NSAIDs should be avoided or stopped in MI.

6. **Thrombolytic therapy**: **Best within 6-12 hrs for ST-segment-elevation MI**; the earlier, the better outcome. **Indications** include typical chest pain of acute MI <12 hrs and new LBBB. t-PA (with more tissue selection), streptokinase (with stronger effect), reteplase, or anistreplase is among the good options. **Beyond 24 hrs of symptom onset, it is usually ineffective and contraindicated.**

Complications of thrombolysis:

(1) Overuse: hemorrhage, more common with tissue plasminogen activator.

(2) Re-perfusion arrhythmias.

Contraindications to thrombolytic therapy:

(1) Active bleeding disease;

(2) Dissecting aortic aneurysm (suspect);

(3) Uncontrolled hypertension > 180/110 (First control BP, then give thrombolytics);

(4) Known traumatic CPR;

(5) Recent head trauma or stroke (< 3 months);

(6) History of major trauma or surgery (< 3 years).

7. **Analgesics**: IV opiates (morphine) are important to relieve pain, to supply relaxation and sedation, and to alleviate CVS and respiratory stress effectively.

8. **ACE inhibitors** (Angiotensin-converting enzyme inhibitors, ACE-I): It has shown to **reduce post-MI mortality**. It's best beneficial for post-MI patients **with CHF**, LV dysfunction with an **EF (ejection fraction) < 40%, or regurgitant disease**. It should be started early and in the maintenance therapy. It's also used in any anterior wall MI and should be stopped after 6 weeks. **Dry cough** is the most common S/E. If it's intolerable to the patient, the ACE-Inh should be ceased and another agent be considered.

9. **Hypolipidemic therapy: Atorvastatin** should also be started early and before PCI.

10. **Anticoagulation**: Heparin—IV bolus initially and then continuous infusion to keep the PTT 1.5-2 times the normal value. It's useful for unstable angina and as a follow-up treatment for t-PA use.

11. **Coronary angiography and angioplasty—indications:**

(1) Patients with typical and persistent symptoms with new left bundle branch block; (2) Acute MI when thrombolytics are contraindicated or patient is in a well-equipped hospital; (3) Clinical CHF, post-MI patient with CHF, EF < 40%, recurrent ischemia and ventricular arrhythmias, or failed thrombolytic therapies.

For most patients, clinical trials have demonstrated superiority of primary percutaneous coronary intervention (PCI), irrespective of whether balloon angioplasty or stenting is performed. Bypass surgery —Coronary artery bypass graft surgery (CABG) is infrequently performed in patients with STEMI. The main indications are urgent CABG related to failure of fibrinolysis or PCI, or hemodynamically important mechanical complications.

The benefit of revascularization must be weighed against the increase in mortality associated with CABG in the first three to seven days after STEMI. Thus, if the patient has stabilized, surgery should be delayed to allow myocardial recovery. Patients with the above critical conditions should undergo CABG during the initial hospitalization.

Contraindications to full-dose anticoagulation:

(1) Active bleeding disease;

(2) Recent major surgery;

(3) Severe hypertension (sustained BP > 190/110 mmHg);

(4) Hemorrhagic diathesis (congenital, hepatic, or drug-induced);

(5) Presence of purpura;

(6) Infectious endocarditis;

(7) Anticipated invasive bedside procedures (e.g., thoracentesis, arterial or venous line insertion).

10. **Erythropoietin**: Its non-erythropoietic effects including anti-inflammatory, antiapoptotic, and angiogenic properties may be cardioprotective in patients with acute ST-elevated MI.

11. **Post-MI management:**

(1) Stress testing: All post-MI patients should have a submaximal stress test (70% target load) after 5-7 days or a maximal stress test (85% target load) after 2-3 weeks.

(2) Postinfarction angina or ischemia on stress test: Angiography is recommended to determine the need for angioplasty or bypass surgery.

(3) Medical treatment: A beta-R blocker and aspirin should be given to all post-MI patients without a specific contraindication. ACE-I (inhibitor) should be used in cases with EF < 40%. Lipid lowering drugs should be used to maintain LDL < 100 mg/dL. Smoking and alcohol abstinence is necessary.

Complications of acute MI

1. **Arrhythmias**

(1) Sinus bradycardia: commonly seen in early stages of (inferior) MI due to **sinus or A-V junctional block** and may be protective. Usually no treatment is needed. If it's severe, atropine or temporary pacing can be applied.

(2) Premature atrial or ventricular contractions (PVC): observation.

(3) Tachyarrhythmias: Supraventricular (**SVT**) —**adenosine** is the #1 choice; ventricular tachycardia (**V-tach**)—**lidocaine** is the #1 drug (smaller dose for the elderly, and **never used as prophylaxis** because lidocaine can induce ventricular tachycardia or ventricular fibrillation by itself); ventricular fibrillation (**V-fib**) or asystole—immediate unsynchronized defibrillation and CPR to save life!

(4) **Temporary transvenous pacing**—indications: Complete A-V block; 2nd degree A-V block (type 2); sinus bradycardia despite atropine use; LBBB during MI; new bifascicular block; with hypoperfusion.

2. **Pump dysfunction**: Left or right ventricular or bi-ventricular failure; ventricular aneurysm; infarct expansion. Severe left or bi-ventricular failure is an indication for **intra-aortic balloon counter-pulsation.** This can increase cardiac output and perfusion through the coronary artery.

3. **Mechanical disruption**: Papillary muscle dysfunction or rupture (causing mitral regurgitation, with systolic murmurs at apex radiating to the left axilla), ventricular septal rupture (within 10 days, repairable), free wall rupture (causing cardiac tamponade, with 90% mortality), or pseudoaneurysm (risk of rupture). Treatment requires emergent **surgical repair**.

4. **Acute pericarditis—Dressler syndrome—Post-MI syndrome**: It's immunologically based, with fever, malaise, pericarditis, pleuritis, and leucocytosis; usually late onset, 2-4 weeks post-MI. **Aspirin** is the effective therapy. **Steroids should be avoided** because they may hinder myocardial scar formation.

5. **Thromboembolism**: Mural thrombus with systemic embolism or DVT with prolonged immobilization. Frequent movements are the best prevention and treatment.

6. **Postinfarction angina**: If it's after thrombolytic therapies, it should be treated with angioplasty or bypass surgery.

7. **Recurrent infarction**: It includes extension of existing infarction and re-infarction, with high mortality. Diagnosis is difficult but should be suspected if there is a persistent elevation or re-elevation of ST-segment and high CK-MB after 36 hours. Treatment is repeating thrombolysis or urgent cardiac catheterization and PTCA, along with standard medical therapies for MI.

8. **Sudden cardiac death**: Mostly due to V-fibrillation or/and asystole.

Right Ventricular Myocardial Infarction (RVMI)

No Nitrates!!   *ST↑on II, III, AVF.*

RVMI mainly results from occlusion of the proximal right coronary artery, accompanying about 30% of the inferior LV-MI. The patient usually shows a typical right-sided infarction and heart failure, with the **classic physical triad of hypotension, JVD, and clear lungs** on auscultation. ECG usually reveals ST-segment elevations in an inferior and a posterior distribution (I, III, aVF, and V4R).

Diagnosis: Based on the above "**Triad**", increased cardiac enzymes, and abnormal ECG results (ST-elevation) in right ventricular leads (V4R).

Treatment: The primary treatment is **maintenance of the RV preload—fluids, NOT diuretics;** normal saline but not nitrates or opioids, and augmentation of the cardiac contractility—dopamine. Patients with predominant RVMI usually do not benefit from afterload reducing treatment with either an intraaortic balloon pump or vasodilating agents. It's critical for early effective corrections to restore perfusion.

Acute Coronary Syndrome (ACS)

ACS refers to **any group of symptoms attributed to obstruction of the coronary arteries**. ACS usually occurs as a result of one of three conditions: **ST-elevation myocardial infarction (30%), non-ST-elevation myocardial infarction (25%), or unstable angina (38%)**.

It is difficult to determine the precise etiology from its history and P/E alone. **The risk factors for ACS are the same as for CAD.**

PEARLS—Diagnostic guidelines for ACS

1. The most common symptom prompting diagnosis of ACS is **pressure-like chest pain (> 30 min with infarction)**, often radiating to the left arm, and associated with anxiety, nausea, and diaphoresis.

2. **Lab diagnosis**: (1) **ECG** is abnormal immediately at onset of typical chest pain. **ST-T elevation** progresses to Q-waves or left branch block over up to 7 days. (2) Abnormal myoglobin starts 1-4 hrs after chest pain and lasts 1-2 days; **CK-MB** starts 4-6 hrs and lasts 3 days; troponin starts 2-4 hrs and lasts 7-10 days. **Troponin** cannot distinguish a reinfarction occurring several days after the first onset. Renal inefficiency can result in a false increase in troponin.

3. **Reinfarction**: If a patient presents with a new chest pain within a few days of the first infarction or attack, perform an ECG to detect new ST segment abnormalities. Elevated CK-MB levels after several days indicate new infarction.

PEARLS—Therapeutic guidelines for ACS

1. **ST-elevation MI:** Oxygen, aspirin and beta1 blockers should be started ASAP for best benefits. Primary PCI within 90 min of first medical contact is the goal. Thrombolysis within 30 min in hospital and 6-12 hours of onset of symptoms reduces mortality.

2. **Post-MI take-home medications:** Aspirin (or clopidogrel if aspirin-intolerant), beta1 blockers (metoprolol), ACE-I (or ARB—angiotensin-R blockers if cough-persistent), and statins.

3. **Glycoprotein IIb/IIIa inhibitors (abciximab, tirofiban, eptifibatide):** Useful in ACS with ST depression (non-ST elevation MI) and patients to undergo angioplasty and stenting. tPA is beneficial only with ST elevation MI. Heparin is best for non-ST elevation MI.

4. In **non-ST elevation ACS**, if patient is not better (persistent pain, S3 gallop, worse ECG changes, and rising troponin levels) after using all given medications, urgent angiography and possibly angioplasty (PCI) should be performed.

5. **The No.1 common cause of death is ventricular arrhythmia**—tachycardia and fibrillation. Always get ready to perform immediate electrical cardioversion or defibrillation.

Contraindications: Do not use any "prophylactic antiarrhythmic medications for ventricular tachycardia or fibrillation" because it increases ventricular arrhythmia and mortality.

Do not use nitrates and sildenafil together to avoid severe vascular complications.

Post-MI impotence: Erection problem is mostly due to anxiety. Sexual activity can be recovered when the patient is asymptomatic.

PULMONARY HEART DISEASE (COR PULMONALE)

"Cor pulmonale" is defined as the right ventricular systolic and diastolic failure resulting from pulmonary disease and the attendant hypoxia. It is most commonly cause by COPD or idiopathic pulmonary fibrosis. Less frequent causes include pneumoconiosis, idiopathic pulmonary hypertension, kyphoscoliosis, etc.

Essentials of diagnosis

Cor Pulmonale

1. Common symptoms include dyspnea on exertion, fatigue, lethargy, exertional syncope, and exertional angina. P/E may show signs of pulmonary hypertension (increased S_2 +/- splitting) and right-sided heart failure (hypotension, jugular vein distention, and foot edema).

2. **Lab tests**: (1) CXR typically shows enlarged central pulmonary arteries and right ventricle, and a loss of retrosternal air space. (2) Echocardiography usually demonstrates increased right ventricular pressure with hypertrophy. (3) **Right heart catheterization is the gold standard** for the diagnosis.

Treatment

The three major physiological goals include reduction of right ventricular afterload, decrease of right ventricular pressure, and improvement of right ventricular contractility.

1. Treat underlying cause.

2. Treat "right heart failure" (see the same topic in this chapter)

3. Treat "chronic respiratory failure" (see Chapter 3).

HEART FAILURE (HF)

Heart failure (HF), usually referred to as "Congestive heart failure" (CHF), is a common clinical syndrome resulting from any structural or functional cardiac disorder that impairs the ability of the ventricle to fill with or eject blood and the heart to maintain an adequate output to meet the body's circulatory and metabolic demands under normal conditions. HF due to left ventricular dysfunction is **newly categorized** according to left ventricular ejection fraction (LVEF) into HF with reduced ejection fraction (with LVEF $\leq$ 40 percent, known as HFrEF; also referred to as systolic HF) and HF with preserved ejection fraction (with LVEF > 40 percent; known as HFpEF; also referred to as diastolic HF). CHF is characterized by insufficient oxygen delivery to tissues accompanied by the accumulation of fluid in the lungs and lower body. CHF is mostly from systolic dysfunction, with a low ejection fraction and dilation of the heart.

Etiology

1. The most common cause is primarily abnormal myocardiocytes from MI or ischemia.

2. The second common cause is abnormal myocardiocytes due to prolonged exposure to a hemodynamic burden (primary hypertension, aortic regurgitation, or pulmonary hypertension), myocarditis, cardiomyopathy, alcohol, drug toxicity, or infiltrative disease (sarcoidosis, amyloid, or hemochromatosis).

3. Structural abnormalities: CAD, valvular diseases, congenital heart diseases, pericardial diseases, outflow obstruction, high-output heart failure (hyperthyroidism, pregnancy, Vit-B1 deficiency).

4. Precipitating factors: Increased salt/fluid intake, excess exertion or emotion, arrhythmias, systemic infection, renal failure, cardiac depressants (disopyramide or beta-R blockers), or inappropriate decrease of a drug dose.

Pathogenesis

uF

Heart failure (HF) is pathologically characterized by reduced cardiac output with or without pooling of blood in venous circulation (venous stasis). *can't push blood fwd : leaky, dilated floppy cardiomyopathy, MI, arrhythmias*

1. **Systolic** dysfunction: Impaired myocardial contractility (as from CAD) with decreased EF.

2. **Diastolic dysfunction**: *cant relax to fill* Pressure-volume overload (as from hypertension, valvular dysfunction) with normal or supranormal EF, but decreased total cardiac output. *hypertrophic or restrictive cardiomyopathy infiltrative*

3. Frank-Starling law: (1) In a normal heart, increasing preload results in greater contractility. (2) A failing heart with exertion generates relatively less contractility and significant symptoms.

Essentials of diagnosis

1. **Manifestations of left-sided (LV) heart failure**: Exertional dyspnea, orthopnea, PND (paroxysmal nocturnal dyspnea), cough with frothy or pink sputum, crackles/rales at lung bases, cardiac enlargement and displaced PMI (to the left), S3 (ventricular) gallop, and S4 murmur.

2. **Manifestations of right-sided (RV) heart failure**: Elevated venous pressure, JVD (jugular vein distention), ankle edema, hepatosplenomegaly, and hepato-jugular reflux, ascites, right ventricular heave, and nocturia due to elevated legs and venous return during sleep.

3. Chest X-ray (CXR) reveals fluid retention based on vascular congestion (prominent interstitial markings), cardiac enlargement, Kerley's B lines, and pleural effusion. See **Image 14**.

4. Two-dimensional echocardiography will show the wall motion abnormality and low ejection fraction (EF, usually <40%). Multigated (MUGA) scan or radionuclide ventriculography can also measure EF.

Differential diagnosis

Cardiac dyspnea:

Sudden onset of dyspnea without sputum or history of pulmonary diseases or smoking. Pulmonary function test (PFT) shows restrictive ventilatory defect.

Pulmonary dyspnea:

More gradual onset (except with infections, pneumothorax, or asthma), dyspnea at night, often associated with sputum, history of COPD, smoking, or noxious inhalants. PFT usually shows obstructive or restrictive ventilatory defect.

Treatment

Treatment of HF with reduced EF includes management of contributing conditions such as hypertension, ischemic heart disease, valvular heart disease, diabetes, thyroid dysfunction, and infection, as well as lifestyle modifications including smoking cessation, restriction of alcohol and salt ingestion, and weight control/reduction.

1. **Reduction of cardiac workload:**

(1) Non-medical treatment and correction of reversible causes: Reduce physical and emotional stress and salt/fluid intake; remove exacerbating factors (infection, anemia, heat, obesity, etc); treat vascular lesions, myocardial ischemia, uncontrolled hypertension, etc.

HF   LMWoP

(2) **Medications:** A **diuretic and vasodilator are first-line** therapies (especially with hypertension) **to reduce** preload, afterload, and **mortality. Hydralazine plus spironolactone are recommended for chronic HF. Loop diuretics and nitrides are the best initial medicines for acute left HF with pulmonary edema**, plus O_2-PEEP, morphine, nitroglycerin and dobutamine. **ACE inhibitors (ACE-I)** are more effective in decreasing preload (mainly) and afterload when the **ejection fraction < 40%**, better with spironolactone. Angiotensin II receptor blockers (losartan, valsartan, irbesartan, or candesartan) can be chosen if ACE-I is intolerable. Beta1-blockers are helpful in HF with systolic dysfunction but not with diastolic dysfunction or acute HF; be cautious when the EF is very low.

2. **Improvement of cardiac performance:**

(1) **Positive inotropic agents**: They are indicated with reduced EF or if the above treatment fails. **These can improve symptoms but have not shown to reduce mortality**.

Cardiac glycosides—digitalis: Best for severe CHF with atrial fibrillation or EF < 40% despite treatment with ACE-I and beta-blockers, etc. Mechanisms are inhibition of Na-K-ATPase, resulting in intracellular Na and Ca increase, and thus inotropic effect. Potassium competes with digitalis' binding sites and so hyper-K will decrease its activity, whereas Hypo-K results in higher activity or toxicity (same as by quinidine, Ca-blockers, thiazides, furosemide & bumetanide). Spironolactone can decrease renal clearance of digitalis. Cholestyramine and colestipol can interfere with its GI absorption.

Digitalis intoxication:

Nausea, vomiting, blurred vision with yellow halo, and arrhythmias (#1 is paroxysmal atrial tachycardia with A-V block). **Treatment**: (a) Mild—stop the medication and correct hypo-K. (b) Severe A-V block—choose atropine. (c) If digitalis level is > 10 mg/L, use anti-digitalis fragment. (d) Anti-arrhythmia: use lidocaine or phenytoin.

Other positive inotropic medicines: Intermittent use of **dobutamine** or phosphodiesterase inhibitor (**amrinone, milrinone**).

(2) Correction of underlying arrhythmias and deficiencies.

3. **Surgical correction**: It may be considered for heart failure (HF) due to valve lesions or diastolic dysfunction. Heart transplantation can be the last option for an appropriate patient with end-stage HF.

HYPERLIPIDEMIA

It's defined as total cholesterol **(Chol) level > 200** mg/dL, including increased LDL-C and triglyceride (TG). It's a major **risk factor for CAD** as with age (male > 45, female > 55), smoking, diabetes, hypertension, low HDL (< 40), and history of CAD, etc. **Common causes** include obesity, diabetes, alcoholism, OCP use, familial hypercholesterol, hypothyroidism, hepatic disease, nephritic syndrome, Cushing syndrome, and high-dose diuretic use.

Essentials of diagnosis

1. Most patients have no specific symptoms and are found out by lipid screening testing: total serum **cholesterol levels > 200 mg/dL on two different occasions** is diagnostic.

HLD

2. **LDL-C > 130 or HDL-C < 40 (mg/dL) is diagnostic of dyslipidemia**, regardless of the total cholesterol levels.

3. **TG >100 mg/dL (in children <10 years) and >130 mg/dL (>10 years).**

4. **Hypercholesterolemia appearance: xanthelasmas**—yellowish adipose deposit around the eyelids, etc.

Screening, prevention and treatment

Cholesterol (Chol) monitoring is highly important—it's the best screening test and preventive measure for coronary artery disease (CAD). It should be **started at age 35 in males and 45 in females for most people** (5-10 years earlier if with risk factors for CAD), then every 5 years if results are normal, or evaluation for 10-year risks for CAD. **Treatment is based on risk factors and LDL-C levels mainly,** not on a low HDL or high triglyceride (TG) itself.

1. **The best initial screening test is total fasting cholesterol levels.** If fasting is not practical, non-fasting total cholesterol and HDL can be the screening.

2. If total fasting cholesterol is < 200 and no risk factors, retest in 5 years. If the fasting cholesterol is > 200, patient is treated based on LDL-C levels and risk factors.

3. Patients with LDL of **130-159** mg/dL or triglyceride > 250 mg/mL with 0-1 risk factor: borderline risk, treat with an initial 3-month plan of diet modification and **exercise**.

4. **Indications for starting lipid-lowering medications**:

(1) **Any CAD history (or an equivalent) and LDL > 130** mg/dL (some suggest > 100 mg/dL); **CAD equivalents**: peripheral artery disease, diabetes mellitus, carotid or the aortic artery disease;

(2) **No CAD but LDL > 160 mg/dL with two risk factors**;

(3) **LDL > 190 mg/dL alone. The goal is to keep LDL lower than 100** mg/dL (or < 70 with CAD plus a CAD equivalent). HMG CoA reductase inhibitor (**statins**) is the **first choice** of drugs. Add niacin if the statin alone is ineffective. Use the fibrates if both are intolerable.

(4) For future treatment with **LDL > 100 mg/dL and a history of CAD or CAD equivalent (diabetes, disease of the aota, carotid or peripheral artery), lipid-lowering drugs are started** to lower LDL to less than 100 mg/dL.

(5) If HDL is low (and TG is high): Treat with niacin or gemfibrozil.

PEARLS—Table 2-4: Summary of Lipid-lowering Medications

Drug	Mechanism and Effect	Adverse Effect (S/E)
1. HMG-CoA reductase inhibitors: -statin, lovastatin	**Inh Chol synthesis key enzyme: Decr LDL and TG; effectively lowering mortality! Test liver enzymes before use.**	**Reversible liver enzymes Incr, myositis**; warfarin potentiation
2. Niacin: Niaspan	**Decr fatty acid release and LDL synthesis; Decr LDL, Incr HDL**	Skin flushing (alleviated by aspirin or long-term use; avoid use with

		statins due to increased S/E
3. Lipoprotein lipase stimulators: **Fibrates (gemfibrozil, clofibrate)**	**Incr VLDL and Trig catabolism;** **Decr TG and Incr HDL**	**Myositis, liver enzymes Incr,** GI symptoms, cholelithiasis
4. Bile acid resins: **Cholestyramine/colestipol**	Bind gut bile acids, Decr bile acid stores & LDL; Incr LDL catabolism.	GI symptoms, constipation, Decr other drugs' absorption
5. Chol-absorption inhilevelsbitors: Ezetimibe	**Decr Chol absorption in the** **intestines; Decr LDL.**	Abdominal pain, diarrhea, angioedema
6. PCSK9-Inh/Abs: Evolocumab	Antibodies to proprotein convertase subtilisin kexin 9, **reduce LDL and** **risk of CVD.**	Allergy.

Note: Inh = inhibit or inhibitor; Decr = decrease; Incr = increase; Chol = cholesterol; TG = triglycerides

SYSTEMIC HYPERTENSION

Hypertension (HTN) is defined as a state of repeatedly elevated blood pressure (BP) ⩾ **140/90 mmHg on three occasions**. Both systolic and diastolic pressures are important in determination of the circulation and functions of organs. However, systolic hypertension is a more powerful predictor of cardiovascular conditions and clinical prognosis, especially after 50 y/a when diastolic pressure tends to decrease. By etiology it is generally classified into primary and secondary hypertension.

Conceptions:

Hypertension by office-based blood pressure:
Normal blood pressure: systolic <120 mmHg and diastolic <80 mmHg;
Prehypertension: systolic 120 to 139 mmHg or diastolic 80 to 89 mmHg;
Stage 1 hypertension: systolic 140 to 159 mmHg or diastolic 90 to 99 mmHg;
Stage 2 hypertension: systolic ⩾160 mmHg or diastolic ⩾100 mmHg;
Isolated systolic hypertension: BP ⩾140/<90 mmHg;
Isolated diastolic hypertension: BP <140/⩾90 mmHg.

I. Primary (Essential) Hypertension

It's the hypertension without a definable cause and it accounts for > 95% of all hypertensive cases. It's mostly resulted from either high peripheral resistance or elevated cardiac output. Hypertension is a multi-factorial disease; more factors imply more risk. Screening for hypertension may be started at age 18 or in the middle age. The interval depends on individual's conditions.

Etiology

1. **Sympathetic nervous system hyperactivity**: Mostly in young patients.

2. **Renin-angiotensin system hyperactivity**: Causing increased intracellular Na-Ca-water retention; mostly in young White and Asian populations.

1° essential HTN

3. **Abnormal cardiovascular or renal development**: Abnormal aortic elasticity or reduced micro-vascular network and nephrons numbers (associated with low birth weight).

4. **Defect in natriuresis**: Causing insensitive natriuresis and thus salt-sensitive hypertension.

5. **Risk factors**: About 50% of risk is due to lifestyle factors -- high-Na diet, smoking, obesity, hyperlipidemia, limited exercise, and sleep apnea; and the other half is due to genetics (family history of hypertension or heart disease), advanced age, male gender, the Black population, etc.

Essentials of diagnosis

1. Common symptoms include headaches (typically back of the head and in the morning), lightheadedness, vertigo, tinnitus, altered vision, and fainting episodes. Other possible findings include systolic click, S4 and/or loud S2, increased cardiac size, and retinopathies (copper wires, artery-vein nicking, papilledema, cotton wool spots, hard exudates, and flame hemorrhage; **Image 112**).

2. **Diagnosis**: **Mainly based on physical examination (P/E) results:** BP $\geq$ 140/90 mmHg (either one) on > 3 tests separated by > 30 min.

Classification and management are summarized in Table 2-5.

Treatment

Antihypertensive therapy (BP control) has shown to produce a nearly 50% relative risk (RR) reduction in the incidence of heart failure, a 30-40% RR reduction in stroke, and a 20-25% RR reduction in myocardial infarction. Major mechanisms include decreases in blood volume, cardiac output, and arterial tension. Goals of treatment are BP < 140/90 mmHg for most patients and < 130/80 mmHg for patients with chronic diseases (diabetes, kidney disease, etc.).

1. Nonpharmacologic therapy (lifestyle modification):

This includes exercise, weight reduction, alcohol restriction, and Dietary Approaches to Stop Hypertension (DASH) diet—low in salt, fat, sugar, and red meats, and high in vegetables, fruits, whole grains, poultry, fish, and nuts.

2. Pharmacologic therapy:

Initial monotherapy in uncomplicated hypertension—One of the following four main classes:

(1) Thiazide diuretics (chlorthalidone or indapamide); (2) Long-acting calcium channel blockers (such as amlodipine); (3) ACE inhibitors; (4) Angiotensin II receptor blockers (ARBs).

The main exceptions to modest and gradual BP lowering over the first 24 hours are:

(1) **The acute phase of an ischemic stroke**—The blood pressure is usually not lowered unless it is $\geq$ 185/110 mmHg (candidates for reperfusion therapy) or $\geq$ 220/120 mmHg (non-candidates for reperfusion therapy.

(2) **Acute aortic dissection**—The systolic BP should be rapidly lowered to a target of 100-120 mmHg (to be attained in 20 min).

The best selection of antihypertensive is based on specific conditions of the patient, as summarized in Table 2-6.

Table 2-5: Blood Pressure Classification and Management

Category	Systolic BP (mmHg)	Diastolic BP (mmHg)	Management
Normal levels	<120	<80	Recheck in 2 years
Pre-hypertension (Pre-HTN)	120-139	80-89	lifestyle modification + recheck in 1 year
Stage 1 HTN (mild)	140-159	90-99	Confirmation within 2 months; diuretics
Stage 2 HTN (moderate)	160-179	100-109	Evaluation within 1 month; diuretics + ACE-I mostly
Stage 3 HTN (severe, HTN crisis)	180-209	110-119	Evaluation or referral within 1 week; ≥2 drugs
Stage 4 HTN (urgency)	>210	>120	ACE-I + hydralazine, or immediate referral
Hypertensive emergency or malignant HTN	>220	>120 with end-organ damage (confusion, papilledema, oliguria, renal failure).	Tx: IV nitroprusside plus nitroglycerol/labetalol/nicardipine to reduce BP by 25% in 1-2 hours.

PEARLS—Table 2-6: Selection of Anti-hypertensive Medications

Co-conditions	Drug of Choice	Contraindicated
Angina	1. Metoprolol (β1 blocker); 2. Nicardipine (Ca blocker)	Vessel dilator without a β-R blocker
MI history	Metoprolol (if EF>50%); ACE-I (if EF<40%)	Ca-blocker (if EF<40%)
Heart failure (HF)	Diuretic; ACE-I (if EF<40%)	Ca-blocker or β-R blocker (relatively)
Diabetes, nephropathy	ACE-I (protect renal function); if intolerant: valsartan (Ang-II-R blocker)	β-R blocker (if hypoglycemic); diuretic (if hyperglycemic)
Peripheral vessel disease, coronary artery spasm	Diltiazem	β-R blocker (claudication, COPD)
Asthma	1. Ca-blocker; 2. β2-R agonist	β-R blocker
Migraine	β-R blocker, Ca-blocker	
BPH	Doxazosin (α-R blocker)	
Osteoporosis, elder	Thiazide diuretic	

Pregnancy	1. labetalol; 2. methyldopa; 3. hydralazine	ACE-I; diuretic
Young Whites	**β-R blocker;** ACE-I	
Blacks	**Diuretic;** Ca-blocker	β-R blocker or ACE-I (relatively)

II. Secondary Hypertension

It's defined as hypertension due to an identifiable organic cause; some can be surgically correctable.

Etiology, diagnosis, and treatment

1. **Substance effects**: **Alcohol** is the #1 cause in young male patients; **long OCP (estrogen)** use is the #1 cause in > 35 year-old, obese females. Other substances include cocaine, NSAIDs, cyclosporine, tacrolimus, decongestants, etc. Correction of the original cause is the effective therapy.

2. **Renal disease**: Any primary renal disease can cause hypertension and is generally **the most common cause** of secondary hypertension. ACE-I can alleviate the hypertension and slow the progression of renal diseases.

3. **Renal artery stenosis (RAS)**: (1) More than 90% of cases are caused by artherosclerotic renal ischemia in patients > age 45. (2) Fibromuscular dysplasia (FMD) is a rare cause of RAS and mostly in women < age 50.

Diagnosis: (1) **Clues:** 1) Resistant hypertension with onset < 30 or > 50 y/a without obesity, family history, and other risk factors; 2) Refractory hypertension or newly onset hypertension that is resistant to ≥ 3 medications; 3) There are abdominal/renal artery bruits; 4) There is a history of atherosclerosis; 5) There is abrupt deterioration of the renal function (elevation in the serum creatinine) after the use of ACE Inh; 6) Malignant or accelerated hypertension with signs of end-organ damage.

(2) **The best screening method** is a renal radionuclide flow scan with captopril (showing high rennin and aldosterone). (3) **Confirmation** is done by angiography or by renal vein renin ratio (RVRR).

Treatment: (1) For atherosclerotic RAS: 1) Medical therapy first for most unilateral and bilateral RAS; 2) If hypertension still cannot be controlled, percutaneous angioplasty with stenting is recommended. Renal artery revascularization is reserved for those with complex anatomic lesions or failed stenting procedures. (2) For fibromuscular dysplasia: percutaneous angioplasty with stent is usually curative. (3) ACE-I can be a drug adjunct in elder patients for one-side stenosis, but contraindicated in bilateral renal stenosis because it can accelerate high-renin and renal failure by preferential vessel-dilation of the efferent artery.

4. **Primary hyperaldosteronism**: Characterized by hyper-aldosterone and hyper-Na, hypo-renin and hypo-K.

(1) **Conn syndrome**: 70% unilateral, mostly from an adrenal adenoma.

(2) **Cushing syndrome**: with above features, along with decreased glucose intolerance, central obesity, hirsutism, striae, "buffalo hump" (**Image 38**).

(3) Iatrogenesis: Usually due to chronic steroid use.

2° HTN

5. **Pheochromocytoma**: Triad—episodic hypertension, headache, and diaphoresis. Other features include young age, paroxysmal symptoms, and history of endocrine tumors (MEN IIA & IIB syndrome).

Diagnosis: By elevated 24-hour urinary catecholamines or VMA. CT or MRI is also helpful in diagnosis.

Treatment: Use both alpha- and beta-R blockers followed by surgical resection.

6. **PKD** (Polycystic kidney disease): Hypertension along with a family history of PKD, flank mass, and enlarged kidneys.

Treatment: Symptomatic and conservative.

Brachial- femoral Pulse delay. L-interscapular or continuous murmur   systolic

7. **Coarctation of the aorta**: Hypertension with upper limbs only; right arm BP > left arm BP, with lower limb muscle hypotrophy. Treatment options depend on conditions of the patient (age, severity, etc).

– LVH on EKG. TX surgery

ENDOCARDIAL AND VALVULAR HEART DISEASES

Endocarditis

It mostly refers to infectious endocarditis (IE), defined as an infection and inflammation of the endocardial surface of the heart (mainly a heart valve), usually secondary to bacterial or other infections. **Risk factors include** history of rheumatic or valvular heart diseases (mitral or aorta valve), **IV drug use** (tricuspid valve is the No.1 affected), immunosuppression, recent dental or surgical procedure, indwelling intravenous catheter, and use of prosthetic heart valve.

PEARLS—Table 2-7: Summary of Important Etiologies of Endocarditis

Classification / Causes
Acute endocarditis: IV drug use—#1 by Staph-aureus; others: Pneumococcus, Gonococcus.
Subacute endocarditis: Dental procedures, valve damage, kids: #1 by Strep-mutans (viridans); prosthetic heart valve: #1 by Staph-epidermidis; others: Enterococcus, Fungi.
Culture-negative infection: H. parainfluenza, Cardiobacterium, Actinobacillus, Eikenella, Kingella.
Autoimmune: Rheumatic fever; SLE—Libman-Sacks: autoantibody to valve causing warty vegetations.
Drug-induced & toxic: Cytotoxics (doxorubicin), emetine, catecholamines, etc.; causing inflammation & necrosis.
Marantic: Carcinoma—Metastasis seeds valves, causing emboli and infarcts; poor prognosis.

Essentials of diagnosis

1. Variable systemic symptoms: **High fever** with shaking chills (for acute cases) or low-grade fever (for the subacute); cough, dyspnea, anorexia, general weakness, and weight loss.

2. **P/E results and complications**: Include **murmur** (new or changed), joint tenderness, **Osler's nodes** (tender nodules on finger and toe pads, **Image 39**), **Janeway's spots** (small peripheral hemorrhages, **splinter hemorrhages** (subungual petechiae, **Images 40**), and **Roth's spots** (retinal hemorrhages, **Image 147**).

3. **Lab diagnosis**:

(1) Culture and sensitivity (**C/S**) use is the **best means of diagnosis (> 95% sensitivity) —three sets of blood cultures** separated in time (> 1 hour) and location, usually showing multiple positive same pathogens. **ALWAYS take blood for culture/sensitivity before use of antibiotics!** ESR is increased.

(2) **Echocardiogram: Positive finding of vegetations is confirmative**, but negative result does not rule it out. In general, transthoracic echocardiography (TTE) is the first diagnostic test for suspected patients. Transesophageal echocardiography (TEE) has higher sensitivity than TTE and is better for detection of cardiac complications such as abscess, leaflet perforation, and pseudoaneurysm. CXR may reveal septic emboli in right-sided endocarditis.

Other complications for diagnostic consideration

Conjunctival petechiae; brain lesion (mycotic aneurysm); renal lesions (hematuria, glomerulonephritis); splenomegaly; septic emboli to the lungs.

Treatment

1. Empiric **long-term antibiotic therapy** for 28 days, initially covering Gram$^+$ bacteria then adjusted by the culture/sensitivity results. **For Staph-aureus**: 14-day regimen of **nafcillin or vancomycin**; if > 60 y/a, add ampicillin (for Listeria). Choose **ceftriaxone (4 weeks) for pneumococcus or Strep-viridians/bovis, ampicillin + gentamicin for Enterococci, and choose amphotericin and valve replacement for fungal endocarditis.**

2. For **culture-negative/difficult endocarditis**, possible organisms include Hemophilus aphrophilus or parainfluenza, Actinobacillus, Cardiobacterium, Eikenella, and Kingella. **Ceftriaxone** is the drug of choice for this group of organisms.

3. Always monitor for relapse, add an aminoglycoside, and extend the duration of antibiotics. Perform **valve replacement** for recurrent Gram$^-$ or fungus infections, worsening valvular function (especially aorta or mitral stenosis), systemic emboli or conduction disturbances. For endocardial abscess or vegetation, perform immediate debridement. If valve replacement is intolerable, valvulotomy is used.

4. **Indications for antibiotic prophylaxis**:

(1) **High-risk procedures** (dental procedures, bronchoscopy with biopsy, GI or GU procedures with ongoing infection, procedures on infected skin or musculoskeletal tissue, or intracardiac procedures) **with high risk diseases** (unrepaired valvular diseases, cyanotic diseases, history of previous infectious endocarditis, and severe rheumatic heart diseases).

(2) **High-risk procedures (as above) with moderate-risk diseases:** ASD, PDA, VSD, bicuspid aorta, aorta coarctation, rheumatic valvular diseases, MVP, myxoma, hypertrophic cardiomyopathy.

Endocarditis

5. **Selection of preventive antibiotics:**

(1) **For oral, respiratory, esophageal procedures**: the first choice of medicines is amoxicillin, ampicillin or erythromycin (if not available, choose clindamycin, azithromycin, clarithromycin).

(2) **For GU, GI procedures**: choose ampicillin + gentamycin; if not available, choose vancomycin $\pm$ gentamycin.

Note: Low-moderate risks that do not need antibiotics:

GI-endoscopy, esophageal intubation (but needed for esophageal dilation), vaginal delivery, hysterectomy, and valvular diseases with arterial catheterization.

Rheumatic Fever

Rasi 294

It is a systemic nonsuppurative immune process following a pharyngeal streptococcal (Strep) infection. Most cases of acute rheumatic fever occur in children 5 to 15 years of age, more common in developing countries. Rheumatic fever may result in valvular heart disease, with mitral stenosis as the most common one. Other valvular lesions may also occur.

Major criteria for diagnosis:

1. Migratory arthritis (multiple large joints); 2. Carditis and valvulitis; 3. CNS involvement (eg, Sydenham chorea); 4. Erythema marginatum; 5. Subcutaneous nodules.

Minor criteria:

Fever, polyarthralgias, increased ESR, prolonged PR interval in ECG, prior history of rheumatic fever, preceding Strep infection, or ASO (+).

Diagnosis of acute rheumatic fever—Jones Criteria:

Two major criteria, or one major plus two minor criteria.

Differential diagnosis

Endocarditis, RA, SLE, osteomyelitis, SCD, and Lyme disease.

Treatment

1. Treat acute rheumatic fever with bed rest and **NSAIDs**—aspirin has been replaced by the stronger **naproxen** with less adverse effects. Treat streptococcal pharyngitis with **long-acting penicillin G benzathine** or erythromycin. **Antibiotics help prevent cardiac complications from Strep infection, but not post-Strep nephropathy**.

2. Treat the valvular pathology of rheumatic heart disease.

3. **Indications for antibiotic prophylaxis**: During dental, GI, or genitourinary procedures. Long-acting benzathine penicillin G is used as the secondary prevention of recurrent rheumatic fever.

VALVULAR HEART DISEASES

Mitral Stenosis (MS)   *more blood, more murmur*

MS is the most common cardiac lesion caused by rheumatic fever, consisting of thickened mitral valve leaflets, fused commissures, and chordae tendineae. It can lead to left-to-right ventricular failure. It affects more women than man.

Pathogenesis

Mitral valve stenosis impairs left ventricle filling. Increased left atrial pressure causes pulmonary   *↑ pulm pressures* congestion. Forward cardiac output is reduced, secondary pulmonary vasoconstriction occurs, and eventually right ventricular failure results.   *dyspnea, orthopnea, PND, hemoptysis*

Essentials of diagnosis   *↑ LA pressure → ↑ LA enlargement that predisposes to dev. of afib → ↑risk of LA thrombus formation & systemic thromboembolism complications, like stroke*

1. Most patients present with **gradual left-heart-failure symptoms**: Exertional dyspnea, orthopnea, PND (paroxysmal nocturnal dyspnea), fatigue, wasting, and hemoptysis. Later on with progression, systemic embolism, hoarseness (due to enlarged left atrium), and right-heart-failure signs (hepatomegaly, ascites, and peripheral edema). **History of pregnancy or immigration associated cardiomyopathy may be a precipitator and clue of diagnosis.**

2. **P/E** usually finds typical **low-pitched apical diastolic rumble**, loud S1, opening snap following S2, decreased pulse pressure, pulmonary rales (edema), and sternal lift. Murmurs are increased by squatting or leg lifting, and decreased by standing or Valsalva maneuver.

3. **Lab diagnosis:**

(1) **Echocardiography/Doppler confirms the diagnosis**: It usually shows thickening of mitral valve leaflets, a reduction in the excursion and area of the valve leaflets, and increased left atrial size.

(2) **ECG**: May show signs of RV hypertrophy, left and right atrial abnormalities, and atrial fibrillation.

(3) **CXR**: May show a large left atrium (early), straightening of the left heart border, elevation of the left main-stem bronchus, and **signs of pulmonary hypertension** (Kerley's B lines, increased vascular markings, and a large pulmonary artery; <u>Image 14</u>).

Treatment

1. Medical therapy: Diuretics and salt-restricted diet for pulmonary congestion and edema; digitalis (to control the ventricle rate) and long-term oral anticoagulants in patients with atrial fibrillation. For **rheumatic MS**, percutaneous mitral balloon valvotomy (**PMBV**) is preferred to surgery.

2. **Surgery:** For most congenital MS and cases with persistent symptomatic despite above treatment, **commissurotomy, balloon valvuloplasty, or valve replacement (more severe)** usually produces good results. Open mitral commissurotomy or valve replacement is often indicated for patients with contraindications for valvuloplasty. **Pulmonary hypertension is not a contraindication for the surgery.**

more blood more murmur

Mitral Regurgitation (MR)

It is insufficiency of the mitral valve that causes backflow of blood from the left ventricle (LV) into the left atrium. It may remain asymptomatic for many years (or for life) or cause left-sided heart failure.

Etiology

Common causes are rheumatic fever and dilation of the left ventricle, which lead to abnormalities of the mitral leaflets, annulus, and chordae tendineae. Male > female.

1. **Acute MR**: #1 cause is **post-MI papillary muscle dysfunction**. Others include chordae tendinae rupture, papillary muscle rupture, endocarditis, and trauma.

2. **Chronic MR**: #1 cause is **mitral valve prolapse**. Others include rheumatic heart disease (scarring and retraction of valve and leaflets), papillary muscle dysfunction, endocarditis, calcification of the mitral valve annulus, hypertrophic cardiomyopathy, congenital endocardial cushion defect, and severe left ventricle (LV) dilatation.

Pathogenesis

A portion of the left ventricular stroke volume is pumped backward into the left atrium resulting in increased left atrial pressure and decreased forward cardiac output. There are also overloaded volume, increased preload, and decreased afterload involved, which help compensate for the regurgitation by increasing ejection fraction. Nevertheless, prolonged compensation leads to left ventricular dysfunction.

Essentials of diagnosis

1. Rapid LV failure signs are common: Dyspnea, orthopnea, PND, fatigue, hemoptysis, etc. With severe MR, right-heart failure signs can co-exist (pulmonary hypertension, edema, and ascites).

2. **P/E:** Hyperdynamic and displaced (downward and to the left) LV impulse. Carotid upstroke is decreased and brisky. **There is a holosystolic apical murmur radiating to the axilla**, often with a thrill, S_3 with a soft S_1 and widely **split S_2**, and JVD. Murmurs are increased by squatting or leg lifting, and decreased by standing or Valsalva maneuver.

3. **Lab diagnosis:**

(1) **Echocardiography/Doppler confirms** the diagnosis (and helps decide when to operate): Will show abnormal movement of the mitral valve, and left atrial and ventricular enlargement if chronic.

(2) Others: ECG will show signs of LV hypertrophy and left atrial enlargement. CXR may show Cardiac enlargement, vascular congestion if with CHF. Catheterization may show a large "v" wave (due to volume overload on the left atrium).

Differential diagnosis

Mitral valve prolapse: See below.

Aortic stenosis:

Systolic ejection murmur radiating to the carotid/aorta area; delayed carotid upstroke; soft, single or absent S_2; echocardiogram features of aortic stenosis and calcification of the aortic valve.

Mitral Regurg

Hypertrophic obstructive cardiomyopathy (HOC):

It is also called **idiopathic hypertrophic subaortic stenosis**. (1) Typical systolic outflow murmur, increased with standing, Valsalva maneuver, or amyl nitrite, and decreased with squatting, leg raising, or hand grip. The mechanisms are similar with other types of valvular heart diseases. (2) Typical echocardiogram features of HOC.

Papillary muscle rupture with acute MR:

It occurs in about 1% of MI, mostly 3-5 days after infarction, more frequent in inferior-posterior infarcts (posterior papillary more frequent). Murmur is usually loud and **holosystolic radiating to the aorta area**. Echocardiogram usually shows flair or prolapsing leaflet. Doppler shows systolic regurgitant jet into left atrium.

Ventricular septal rupture:

It occurs in 1-2% of all infarcts; peak incidence is 3-5 days after infarction, more frequent in **anterior infarcts**. Murmur is loud and **holosystolic with widespread radiation** and 50% have palpable precordial thrill. Echocardiogram shows the septum defect. Doppler can show the transseptal left-to-right shunt.

Ventricular septal defect (VSD):

L→R shunt: plm overcirc, pulm HTN, growth failure, ↑S₂ bc ↑R↓ pressure diaphoresis, fatigability, CHF. from ↑ L-R flow ⇒ ↑ pressure on closing pulm valve

There is a holosystolic shrill murmur over lower left sternal border, with strong and **split S2.** Radionuclide studies or Doppler will confirm left-to-right shunt. Cardiac catheterization reveals oxygen jump from right atrium to ventricle.   *Eisenmenger: cyanosis from R-L shunting.*

Treatment

1. Medications for chronic MR: Use digitalis, diuretics, artery dilators (ACE-I), and warfarin to relieve symptoms by increasing forward cardiac output and reducing afterload and pulmonary venous hypertension.

2. **Surgery: Mitral valve repair (EF<30%) or replacement (>30%)** is the choice. Indications include persistent symptoms with severe MR despite optimal medications. The surgery carries more risk for patients with chronic heart failure and should be avoided if the heart failure is severe enough. With mild symptoms, surgery should be deferred because the condition may remain stable for years.

Aortic Stenosis (AS)

more blood more murmur

— stiff aortic valve doesn't wanna open, la blood gets thru aortic valve
— LV dilation, big loose floppy heart

Etiology and pathogenesis

atherosclerosis

The No.1 cause is calcification and fibrosis of a normally aged aortic valve (elderly patients) **or congenitally bicuspid aortic valve**. Rheumatic valvular diseases may affect both the mitral valve and aortic valve. The stroke volume is normal until late stages, with elevated LV end-diastolic pressure and gradual pulmonary congestion. LV hypertrophy and high intramyocardial wall tension will increase the oxygen demands and decrease diastolic coronary blood flow, resulting in the onset of angina.

Essentials of diagnosis

Aortic Stenosis

1. Most patients are asymptomatic until middle or old age. Typical manifestations include angina, syncope, and dyspnea from CHF; **harsh systolic ejection murmur radiating to the carotid or aorta** area; delayed carotid upstroke; S4 gallop, decreased A2, and aortic ejection click. Murmurs are increased by squatting or leg lifting, and decreased by standing or Valsalva maneuver.

2. **Lab diagnosis**:

(1) **Echocardiography/Doppler is the best means of diagnosis** and shows thick aortic valve leaflets with decreased excursion and LV hypertrophy.

(2) CXR may present with calcification, cardiomegaly, and pulmonary congestion.

Differential diagnosis

HOC, MR: See above.

Elderly aortic valve sclerosis (without stenosis):

Systolic murmur does not peak late; carotids do not have delayed upstrokes; no LV hypertrophy by ECG; no significant results by cardiac catheterization. Echocardiogram may show normal or reduced aortic valve leaflets.

Pulmonary stenosis: See below.

Treatment

1. Patients should be given antibiotic prophylaxis for endocarditis.

2. **Surgery** is indicated for symptoms and asymptomatic patients with severe aortic stenosis.

(1) **Valve replacement** is the **mainstay of surgery** for most AS cases when the valve area is ≤ **1.0 cm²**. Surgery can also improve the symptoms if angina, syncope, and left ventricle dysfunction are present, although the operative mortality is higher.

(2) **Balloon valvuloplasty** is preferred if the valve stenosis is very severe (usually the area is ≥**1.0 cm²**) without calcification, in selected children, or if the patient is too weak (with high risk) to tolerate surgery.

more blood more murmur

Aortic Regurgitation (AR) – _Aortic valve is weak & floppy, allowing back flow during diastole_
– big dilated floppy heart, eventual HF

Etiology and pathogenesis
– cardiogenic shock, ↓ forward flow, flash pulm edema

Acute AR: Causes include **endocarditis, aortic dissection**, traumatic leaflet rupture, hypertension, rupture of a congenitally fenestrated cusp, iatrogenic valve injury during surgery, and prosthetic aortic valve thrombosis or disk escape.

CHF
Chronic AR: Rheumatic fever is the #1 cause, with the mitral valve frequently affected together. Others include aortic root dilation, congenital bicuspid aortic valve, calcific valve disease, hypertension, and Marfan syndrome.

Aortic Regurg Insufficiency

AR results in a volume overload of the left ventricle (LV), which compensates by increasing its end-diastolic volume (Frank-Starling law). The LV over-dilation causes overstretch of the myofibrils and decreased contractility. In chronic AR the pulse, pressure and systolic pressure are increased, and the diastolic pressure is decreased due to the AR and large stroke volume.

Essentials of diagnosis

1. Severe acute AR commonly presents with sudden cardiovascular collapse and pulmonary edema.

2. Chronic AR is usually asymptomatic until middle age to present with graduate left-sided heart failure. History of dyspnea, **typical diastolic decrescendo murmur at the cardiac apex**, with systolic flow murmur; Austin-Flint murmur (a mid-diastolic rumbling murmur at the apex); S3 in early LV decompensation; systolic and diastolic thrill/murmur heard over the femoral artery. Murmurs are increased by squatting or leg lifting, and decreased by standing or Valsalva maneuver.

3. Chronic AR is staged as "A, B, and C" according to valve anatomy and hemodynamics, hemodynamic consequences, and symptoms.

2. **Lab diagnosis**:

(1) **Echocardiogram is diagnostic** by showing a dilated LV and aorta, volume overload, and fluttering of anterior mitral valve leaflet.

(2) Others: ECG may show LV hypertrophy, often with narrow deep Q-waves in left precordial leads. CXR may show LV and aortic dilation.

Differential diagnosis

Mitral stenosis and **aortic stenosis**: See above.

Pulmonic regurgitation:

Typical diastolic murmur, usually with pulmonary hypertension due to mitral stenosis or with right-to-left cardiac shunt; compensated RV enlargement; no peripheral manifestations of AR.

Patent ductus arteriosus:

Typical continued systole and diastole murmur with peak at S2, whereas systolic ejection murmur with AR usually peaks in midsystole. Angiography or cardiac catheterisation shows L-to-R shunt.

Treatment

1. **For acute AR: Emergent aortic valve replacement or repair** is performed. If there is any delay in surgery, temporary stabilization is attempted in ICU using IV vasodilators (nitroprusside) to reduce afterload, and possibly adding inotropic agents (dobutamine, digitalis) to lower LV end-diastolic pressure.

2. Medical treatment for chronic AR: Reduction in preload and afterload—Valsalva maneuver, salt restriction, diuresis; nitroglycerin, vasodilators.

3. **For severe chronic AR: Aortic valve replacement** is indicated when symptoms worsen or ejection fraction (EF) is decreased, and endocarditis prophylaxis is needed.

Tricuspid Stenosis (TS)

Tricuspid stenosis is characterized by right-sided heart failure. It is usually rheumatic in origin but carcinoid syndrome and tricuspid surgery are the more common causes in the US. Female has the predominance. TS rarely occurs as an isolated lesion; it is often accompanied by tricuspid regurgitation and associated with mitral valve disease or/and the aortic valve.

Essentials of diagnosis
1. **History** of rheumatic fever, carcinoid disease, or cardiac surgery.

2. Typical **manifestations of right heart failure**: JVD, hepatomegaly, ascites, and dependent edema; giant a wave in the JVP (pressure); **typical diastolic rumble** along the lower left sternal border (mimicking mitral stenosis)

3. Lab tests: ECG reveals RA enlargement without atrial fibrillation. CXR shows marked cardiomegaly with a normal PA size. **Echocardiography/Doppler** confirms diagnosis. Mean valve gradient > 5 mm Hg by echocardiography indicates severe stenosis.

Treatment
1. Diuretics are the main treatment to reduce symptoms associated with the fluid congestion.

2. When the stenosis progresses causing right heart failure, the most effective and definitive treatment is **tricuspid valve repair/replacement** (by a bioprosthetic valve) or balloon valvotomy. The tricuspid valve replacement is often combined with mitral valve replacement if it's also with stenosis.

Tricuspid Regurgitation (TR)

TR frequently occurs in patients with pulmonary or cardiac disease with pressure or volume overload on the right ventricle (**RV dilation**). Thus TR is usually a functional disorder.

Etiology includes pulmonary hypertension, MI, endocarditis, left heart failure, RV dysplasia, sarcoidosis, Ebstein anomaly, and tricuspid valve prolapse or injury. These can all result in RV dilation and TR, which in turn worsens the severity of the regurgitation.

Essentials of diagnosis
1. **History** of a pulmonary or cardiac disease/lesion (as above) associated with RV dilation.

2. Similar **manifestations of right heart failure** as in tricuspid stenosis: JVD, hepatomegaly, ascites, and dependent edema; **holosystolic TR murmur** may be audible along left sternal border, which increases with inspiration.

3. **Lab tests**: CXR may show an enlarged RA and pleural effusion. **Echocardiography** confirms the diagnosis with severity of the TR (low- or high-pressure TR), the RV size and RV function.

Treatment
1. Mild TR is common and usually well tolerated, and can be managed with diuretics (to reduce the fluid congestion).

Tricuspid Regurg

2. **Surgery**: When feasible, tricuspid valve repair is generally preferred to valve replacement. However, repair is associated with significant risk of recurrent TR. Definitive treatment requires elimination of the cause of the TR. With progressive right heart failure, tricuspid valve replacement is indicated.

Pulmonary Stenosis (PS)

It is the stenosis of the pulmonary valve or RV infundibulum, which increases the resistance to RV outflow and RV pressure, and decrease pulmonary blood flow. It is often congenital and associated with other cardiac lesions.

Essentials of diagnosis

1. **Asymptomatic** until the lesion is at least moderate. Severe cases may present with right-sided heart failure.

2. **There is a high-pitched systolic ejection murmur** maximal in the second left interspace and radiating to the shoulder. P2 is delayed and soft or absent. Ejection click often exists and decreases with inspiration –the only right heart auscultatory sign with this condition (all other ejection clicks increase with inspiration).

3. CXR and ECG may reveal enlarged right ventricle. 2-D **echocardiogram confirms diagnosis** by visualization of the valve stenosis.

4. Patients with peak pulmonic valve gradients > 60 mmHg or mean of 40 mmHg by echocardiography or Doppler should undergo intervention regardless of symptoms.

Treatment

A domed pulmonary valve stenosis (most cases) can be treated by balloon valvuloplasty, whereas a dysplastic pulmonary valve (with severe stenosis) usually requires surgery. Dynamic RV outflow obstruction may occur after surgical or percutaneous treatment and tends to regress with time.

Pulmonic Regurgitation (PR)

It is pulmonary valve regurgitation. Most cases are due to pulmonary hypertension (high-pressure PR) or surgical injury for treating RV outflow obstruction (low-pressure PR). Other "low-pressure" causes include a dilated pulmonary annulus, congenital bicuspid/dysplastic pulmonary valve, or carcinoid plaque.

Essentials of diagnosis

1. In high-pressure PR, the pulmonary diastolic murmur is readily audible, which is increased with inspiration and diminishes with the Valsalva maneuver. In low-pressure PR, there are rarely murmur and abnormal echocardiography/Doppler findings.

2. **Echocardiography** is definitive in diagnosis of high-pressure PR but may be less definitive in low-pressure PR.

Treatment

Pulmonar Regurgitation

1. In high-pressure PR: Target primary cause—pulmonary hypertension because it's poorly tolerated by the patient.

2. Low-pressure PR is usually tolerated by the patient and rarely requires treatment. Exercise and pregnancy are not interdicted.

3. **Pulmonary valve replacement is indicated with** (1) symptomatic, severe PR; (2) right ventricular enlargement and/or dysfunction; (3) PR plus progressive tricuspid valve regurgitation.

Untreated severe PR will result in right ventricular enlargement, systolic dysfunction, arrhythmia, and death.

CONGENITAL HEART DISEASES

The prevalence is less than 1% among live births. Most diagnoses can usually be made in early life, although initial murmurs and symptoms may not be noticeable. Etiology is unknown. Intrauterine **risk factors** include teratogens (maternal alcohol and drug use), congenital infections (rubella, etc.), and genetic diseases (Down syndrome, Marfan syndrome, etc.).

Classification

1. **By shunting:**

(1) **Right to left—cyanotic (mnemonics: "4T-blue baby"):** **T**etralogy of Fallot, **T**ransposition of the great arteries (TGA), **T**ricuspid atresia, and **T**runcus arteriosus (mixing shunts). Deoxygenated blood is shunted into the systemic circulation, causing serious cyanosis.

(2) **Left to right—noncyanotic (Memo: "Late blue child"; "VAP"):** **V**entricular septal defect, **A**trial septal defect, and **P**atent ductus. Oxygenated blood from the lungs is shunted back into the pulmonary circulation, with late and mild cyanosis.

2. **By stenosis:** Aortic stenosis, pulmonic stenosis, and coarctation.

Mitral valve prolapse (MVP) *more blood less murmur*

MVP (syndrome) is the most common congenital valvular abnormality, or is considered a normal anatomic variant occurring in 2-5% of the population and more commonly in young females and associated with connective tissue diseases (e.g., Marfan syndrome, Ehlers-Danlos syndrome, skeletal abnormalities, or idiopathic).

Essentials of diagnosis

Usually it remains asymptomatic but may show **non-anginal chest pain** (**#1 symptom**, due to arrhythmias), palpitations, exercise intolerance, dizziness, syncope, and panic and anxiety disorders. Auscultation typically finds **middle-to-late systolic click and a late systolic murmur** at the cardiac apex, worse with standing/Valsalva and improving with squatting or leg lifting.

Lab diagnosis: **Echocardiography** is the best method to confirm marked displacement of the mitral leaflets in systole into the left atrial side of the annulus. **Difference from MR**: there is only moderate systolic displacement of the leaflets with MR.

Treatment

1. Most cases are asymptomatic and not in need of treatment. Lifestyle modification is beneficial, including avoidance of stimulants (caffeine) and alcohol, reduction in stress, and moderate exercise. Beta blockers are used with symptoms.

2. Valve repairs can be performed with a catheter by placing clip to tighten up the valve, while surgery is rarely necessary. Neither is for endocarditis prophylaxis (even with a MR murmur).

Ventricular Septal Defect (VSD)

It's the congenital opening between the ventricles leading to left-to-right shunting, **the most common congenital heart disease**. It is often **associated with Down syndrome, fetal alcohol syndrome**, cri-du-chat syndrome, Apert syndrome (cranial deformities, finger/toe fusion), and trisomies 13/18.

Essentials of diagnosis

1. **Small defects** are often asymptomatic but with a harsh **holosystolic murmur** at the lower left border, usually **louder than with larger defects**.

2. Large defects can show dyspnea, frequent respiratory infections, failure to thrive, pulmonary hypertension, and CHF. The **holosystolic murmur is softer**, blowing and with a thrill, louder S2 and middle-diastolic murmur.

3. **Diagnosis:** Echocardiography or Doppler confirms diagnosis by showing blood flow between the ventricles. ECG and CXR may show LVH, RVH, and increased pulmonary vessel markings (CXR).

Treatment

1. Newborns are closely followed in the first weeks of life. If it's complicated with heart failure, a diuretic, inotropic, or ACE-I is used. Most small VSDs **close spontaneously,** and only need echocardiography monitoring.

2. For symptomatic VSD that fails medical treatment or has pulmonary hypertension, surgical repair is indicated.

3. **Antibiotic prophylaxis** should be given **to all VSD patients** before dental, oropharyngeal, or GU procedures to prevent bacterial endocarditis.

Atrial Septal Defect (ASD)

It's the congenital opening between the atria leading to **left-right shunting**. It's also associated with **Down syndrome and fetal alcohol syndrome**, etc.

Essentials of diagnosis

ASD

1. Mostly patients are asymptomatic and discovered on routine P/E. With a large defective size, patient can present with fatigability and frequent respiratory infections. P/E finds RV lift, a **wide, split S2 and systolic ejection murmur** at the upper left sternal border (from increased right ventricular blood).

2. **Lab tests: Echocardiography/Doppler** is diagnostic by showing blood flow between the atria. ECG reveals right-axis deviation and RVH. CXR shows enlarged heart size and pulmonary-vessel markings.

3. A **patent foramen ovale** is present in 25% of the population but can lead to paradoxic emboli and stroke. Patient with a history of cryotogenic stroke before age 50 should be highly suspected of it.

Treatment

1. Most small ASDs **close spontaneously**. If there is any evidence of an RV volume overload, a percutaneous device or surgery should be done to close it. Surgery is usually required for closure of primum ASDs, sinus venosus defects, and coronary sinus defects.

2. **Antibiotic** prophylaxis is required for **ostium primum defect** prior to dental procedures.

Patent Ductus Arteriosus (PDA)

It's the congenital failure of the arterial ductus to close in the first few days of life, causing a **left-right shunt** from the aorta to the pulmonary artery. **Risk factors** include maternal **rubella** infection (1ˢᵗ trimester), female gender, and prematurity.

Essentials of diagnosis

1. It's usually asymptomatic until middle age or larger ductal size. Patient with a large defect may present with recurrent respiratory infection, lower extremity clubbing, and CHF.

2. Typical P/E results include: A widened pulse pressure, load S2, "**continuous machinery murmur**" at the 2ⁿᵈ left intercostal space by the sternum, and bounding peripheral pulse.

3. **Lab tests:** A color-Doppler ultrasonography (U/S) is helpful in showing blood flow from the aorta into the pulmonary artery, but the lesion is best visualized by MRI, CT, or contrast angiography. With larger PDAs, echocardiography, ECG and CXR may all show left atrial/ventricular enlargement.

Treatment

1. **For premature infants, indomethacin is used to close the PDA,** unless the PDA is needed for survival (as in great artery transposition, Fallot tetralogy, severe aorta-coarctation, and hypoplastic left heart).

2. For **most infants > 6-8 months of age** (including indomethacin failure), **percutaneous PDA closure** (catheter occlusion and surgical ligation) is necessary.

Coarctation of the Aorta (CA)

It's the constriction of an aorta portion leading to decreased flow below or distal to it and increased flow above or proximal to it. Most cases are below the left subclavian artery. It's often associated with **Turner syndrome, Berry aneurysm**, bicuspid aorta valve, and male gender.

Essentials of diagnosis

1. Patient usually has a history of asymptomatic hypertension in childhood, and may presents with dyspnea on exertion, syncope, headache, claudication, and epistaxis.

2. **Typical P/E signs**: Systolic **BP is higher in the arms than in the lower limbs; right arm BP is higher than the left arm** (determined by the coarctation location); weak or absent femoral pulse; a late, short systolic murmur in the left axilla; forceful apical impulses.

3. **Lab tests**: Echocardiography/Doppler confirms the diagnosis (a gradient > 20 mm Hg). In older children, ECG may reveal LVH and CXR may show **"reverse 3" sign** (due to pre-/post-dilation of the coarctation), cardiomegaly, pulmonary congestion, and **"rib notching"** (due to collateral circulation through the intercostal artery).

4. 50% of cases are associated with bicuspid aortic valve; some with webbed neck (Turner syndrome).

Treatment

1. With severe infant coarctation, PDA needs be kept open with PGE_1 for survival.

2. Surgical correction or balloon angioplasty may be effective treatment. Early repair may lower risks of CHF and CAD.

3. It's important to have continuous prevention for endocarditis and monitoring for re-stenosis, aortic dissection, and aneurysm development.

Tetralogy of Fallot (Fallot Tetralogy)

It consists of "VPOR"—VSD, Pulmonary artery stenosis, overriding aorta, and RVH. It's the **most common cyanotic congenital heart disease in children > 24 hours of life**. Early cyanosis results from **right-to-left** shunting across the VSD, and may be milder in the initial 1-2 weeks because of the pressure decrease in the right ventricle after birth. The cyanosis can be worse over time if the pulmonary artery stenosis is severe to keep a high right-ventricle pressure. **Risk factors: Down syndrome,** cri-du-chat syndrome, maternal PKU, trisomy 13/18.

Essentials of diagnosis

1. Gradual cyanosis, fatigability, and dyspnea during infancy (> 24 hours after birth). Patients often squat (to increase systemic artery pressure) for symptomatic relief during hypoxemic episodes.

2. Hypoxemia may cause secondary failure to thrive, mental status changes or CHF.

Tetralogy of Fallot

3. **P/E** usually reveals a systolic ejection murmur at the left upper sternal border (pulmonary artery stenosis), RV lift and a single S_2, as well as signs of CHF.

4. **Lab tests: Echocardiography/Doppler and catheterisation are diagnostic.** Be wary if the RV is enlarged because the Echo/Doppler may underestimate significant pulmonic regurgitation. **CXR** shows a "**boot-shaped**" heart with decreased pulmonary-vessel markings (opposite to "single VSD"). ECG reveals RVH and right-axis deviation. Arrhythmias are common and period Holter monitoring is recommended. Patient may be risky of sudden death if the QRS width is > 180 msec.

Differential diagnosis

TGA, large VSD, PDA, tricuspid or pulmonary artery stenosis, hypoplastic left ventricle.

Treatment

1. Administer **PGE1 to keep the PDA open followed by surgical correction** (intracardiac repair by patch closure of the ventricular septal defect) to relieve severe pulmonary artery stenosis. An artificial shunt (balloon atrial septostomy) can be a temporary palliation.

2. Treat cyanosis with O_2, knee-chest position, alpha-agonist, beta-R blocker, morphine, and fluid.

Prognosis

It mostly depends on the degree of pulmonary artery stenosis. Arrhythmia may occur even after surgical repairs.

Transposition of the Great Arteries (TGA)

It's a congenital condition in which the pulmonary and systemic circulations exist in parallel—the aorta is connected to the right ventricle and the pulmonary artery to the left ventricle. It's the **#1 common cyanotic** congenital heart disease **in the newborn at birth. It's fatal without a PDA or VSD, and requires immediate correction.**

Risk factors: Down syndrome, cri-du-chat syndrome, Apert syndrome, trisomy 13/18, and diabetic mothers.

Essentials of diagnosis

1. A severely ill, weak newborn with cyanosis immediately after birth. Reverse cyanosis may be present if aorta stenosis or coarctation coexists.

2. P/E finds cyanosis, tachypnea, a single S2, progressive respiratory failure, or signs of CHF.

3. **Diagnosis** is confirmed by **echocardiogram**. CXR may show narrow heart base and absence of the main pulmonary artery segment ("egg-shaped silhouette"), and increased pulmonary vessel markings.

Differential diagnosis

Fallot tetralogy, large VSD, aortic coarctation, hypoplastic left heart syndrome.

Treatment

Transposition of the Great Vessels

1. It's necessary to administer IV **PGE1 to keep the PDA open followed by immediate surgical correction** (arterial or atrial switch).

2. If immediate surgery is not possible, a fast balloon atrial septostomy (creating an ASD) can be done for the first few days of life.

Persistent Truncus Arteriosus (PTA)

It's the congenital separation failure of the great vessels that causes **one single great vessel supplying both the systemic and pulmonary artery** beds with a mixture of oxygenated and deoxygenated blood.

Essentials of diagnosis

1. Cyanosis shortly after birth, followed by gradual dyspnea, easy fatigability, failure to thrive, and CHF signs.

2. P/E finds a harsh systolic murmur at the lower left sternal border, with a loud S_1/S_2 and systolic ejection click, cardiomegaly, CHF signs, and pounding pulses.

3. **Lab tests**: Angiocardiography is diagnostic. ECG often shows normal axis and evidence of LVH and RVH. CXR may reveal "boot-shaped heart", absent main pulmonary artery, and a large aorta arching to the right.

Differential diagnosis

Fallot tetralogy, large ASD or VSD, etc.

Treatment

Surgical repair is necessary.

Tricuspid Atresia (TA)

It's a congenital condition in which the **tricuspid heart valve is missing** or abnormally developed.

Clinical features and diagnosis

Early cyanosis exists at birth, 90% with VSD, and 30% with TGA. P/E shows **L2-sternal border systolic murmur and single S2**. ECG reveals left axis deviation and CXR shows **decreased pulmonary vessel** markings.

Treatment

Initially give oxygen and IV PGE1 to keep ASD, VSD, or the arterial duct open to allow survival, followed by 3-stage surgical palliation.

Hypoplastic Left Heart Syndrome

It's a congenital syndrome with left heart chamber defect, small left ventricle, stenosis of the aorta and mitral valves, ASD, pulmonary congestion, increased right-ventricle pressure, pre-cordial hyperactivity, and loud S2, but no murmur. Patient usually presents with cyanosis and heart failure in the 1st week of life.

Diagnosis

Echocardiography.

Treatment

Initially give oxygen and mechanical ventilation and IV PGE1 to keep the arterial duct open to allow survival, followed by 3-stage surgical palliation.

Kartagener Syndrome (KS) or Primary Ciliary Dyskinesia (PCD)

KS is also known as **immotile ciliary syndrome,** a rare, ciliopathic, autosomal recessive genetic disorder that causes a defect in the action of the cilia lining the respiratory tract (lower and upper, sinuses, Eustachian tube, and middle ear) and fallopian tube.

<u>Typical triad</u>: **Dextrocardia, recurrent sinusitis, and bronchiectasis**.

Treatment

It includes daily chest physiotherapy, antibiotics with good coverage on Pseudomonas, and supportive pulmonary care. Heart-lung transplantation may be the therapeutic choice for end-stage disease.

MYOCARDIAL DISEASES

Myocarditis

It's defined as the infection or inflammation of the myocardial cells, leading to reduced cardiac contractility and output. It can be acute, subacute, or chronic, and there may be either focal or diffuse involvement of the myocardium and a cause of heart failure (HF).

Etiology

It's mostly caused by **viruses—coxsachie B as #1,** then adenovirus, CMV, EBV, HSV, hepatitis C, etc. Other causes include **bacteria** (post-Strep-A rheumatic fever, Lyme disease), **autoimmune or autoreactive diseases** (SLE, giant cell myocarditis, eosinophilic myocarditis, sarcoidosis), rickettsia (Rocky Mountain spotted fever), protozoa (Chagas disease in South America), medications (sulphonamides), and irradiation, etc.

Clinical features and diagnosis

[Handwritten margin notes:]

Viral Myocarditis
- viral prodrome.
- HF: respiratory distress, murmur, hepatomegaly

dx: CXR = cardiomegaly
    & pulm edema
ekg: sinus tachy
echo: ↓ EJ fraction
Bx: gold. inflamm, necrosis

TX: supportive
    IV Ig

myocarditis

1. Most patients have non-specific symptoms such as fatigue, weakness, and fever (after an infection); some may have precordial pain, arrhythmias, and signs of heart failure.

2. Diagnosis is based on clinical manifestations and abnormal results from ECG (ST-T wave changes and deficient conduct), cardiac enzymes, and ESR. **Endomyocardial biopsy** confirms diagnosis, which may be indicated when patient shows unexplained new-onset heart failure of less than two week's duration associated with hemodynamic compromise or new ventricular arrhythmias.

Treatment

1. **Supportive and symptomatic therapy is the mainstay** of treatment is the choice for most cases. Because of the high risk of arrhythmias and cardiac shock, at-risk patients should be cared in ICU. IVIG is recommended. Anti-pathogen and anti-arrhythmia therapy should be started if indicated, but be cautious with antiarrhythmic drugs with negative inotropic activity. If heart failure develops, digitalis, ICEI or diuretics may be needed. Immunosuppressive therapy (including steroids) is suggested for giant cell myocarditis, sarcoidosis, noninfectious eosinophilic myocarditis, and autoreactive myocarditis.

2. Patients should **avoid NSAIDs,** heavy alcohol consumption, and exercise, and should receive routine follow-up with serial echocardiography. Most patients recover well.

Cardiomyopathies

Cardiomyopathies refer to diseases of the heart muscle itself that lead to cardiac dysfunctions. Current major definitions of cardiomyopathy exclude heart disease secondary to cardiovascular causes (such as hypertension, ischemic heart disease, or valvular disease). According to morphologic and hemodynamic features, they can be **classified as dilated (#1 common), hypertrophic, restrictive, arrhythmogenic right ventricular, and unclassified cardiomyopathies.**

I. Dilated (Congestive) Cardiomyopathy

It is the cardiac weakening and enlargement due to decreased systolic function (mainly LV).

Etiology

No.1—idiopathic; No.2—toxic: alcohol. Others: myocarditis (virus, parasite, mycobacteria, or Ricketts), peripartum, neuromuscular diseases (muscular dystrophy, myotonic dystrophy), chemotherapy toxicity (doxorubicin, cyclophosphamide, vincristine), Vit-B$_1$ deficiency, connective tissue diseases (rheumatoid arthritis, SLE, polyarteritis), glycogen storage diseases, toxins (cobalt, lead, arsenic), metabolic diseases (thyroid disease, pheochromocytoma, chronic Hypo-P$_2$, Hypo-K, Hypo-Ca, uremia).

Essentials of diagnosis

1. Symptoms and signs of left and right ventricular failure (due to decreased myocardial contractility, EF, and cardiac output); S$_3$, S$_4$ and murmur of mitral or tricuspid regurgitation may be present.

2. **Lab diagnosis:**

dilated congestive cardiomyopathy

(1) **Echocardiogram is the #1 diagnostic means**, showing dilated left ventricle, decreased wall motion, mitral valve regurgitation, and increased biventricular chamber size.

(2) CXR: Cardiomegaly with pulmonary congestion.

(3) ECG: Sinus tachycardia, arrhythmias, and conduction disturbances.

(4) Catheterization: Dilated hypocontractile ventricle; MR may also exist.

Differential diagnosis

Acute infectious myocarditis; valvular heart diseases; CAD; hypertensive heart diseases.

Treatment

1. **Same medications as for CHF:** digoxin, diuretics (spironolactone), Beta1 blockers, vasodilators (ACE-I, angiotensin-II-R blockers), and/or antiarrhythmic drugs. Most of these medications **can lower its mortality**. If the QRS is wide, a biventricular pacemaker can be placed to improve both symptoms and survival.

2. Remove the offending agent if possible. Preventive warfarin is recommended due to the high risk of pulmonary and systemic embolism.

3. Dilated cardiomyopathy is the No.1 reason for heart transplantation if other therapies fail.

Peripartum Cardiomyopathy (PPCM)

PPCM is a rare form of dilated cardiomyopathy, usually presenting between the last month of pregnancy and up to five months postpartum. PPCM also involves a decrease in the LV ejection fraction (EF), which is often limited and reversible. Some patients develop heart failure.

The etiology is unknown but may be associated with viruses, autoimmunity (by antibodies against myocardium), and toxins.

Essentials of diagnosis

1. Manifestations may be caused by gradual CHF and pulmonary edema: Orthopnea, dyspnea, pitting edema, cough, palpitations, chest pain, frequent night-time urination, and excessive weight gain during the last month of pregnancy.

2. PPCM is a diagnosis of exclusion—no prior history of heart disease and no other known causes of heart failure. Echocardiogram is used to both diagnose and monitor the effectiveness of treatment. Medications of treatment are the same as for dilated cardiomyopathy.

Treatment

1. Medications of treatment are the same as for dilated cardiomyopathy.

2. Prognosis is mostly good if treated in time. Repeat pregnancy in a patient with PPCM will provoke significant antibody production against the myocardium, with worse prognosis.

II. Hypertrophic Cardiomyopathy (HCM)

Etiology and pathogenesis

HCM   more blood less murmur

It's an **autosomal dominant** hereditary disease with **abnormal chromosome 14**. Pathologically it's characteristic by marked myocardial hypertrophy (mostly left ventricle) and disproportionate thickening of the inter-ventr septum. There are normal or increased chamber size, cardiac output and stroke volume, increased ejection fraction and decreased diastolic compliance. Obstruction may develop between inter-ventr septum and septal leaflet of mitral valve, causing hypertrophic obstructive cardiomyopathy (**HOCM**). MR may be present.

Essentials of diagnosis

1. **Family history** of the disease or of "sudden death" (especially HOCM).

2. Clinical manifestations include palpitations, dyspnea, angina, presyncope, and syncope; bifid carotid pulse, palpable/loud S_4 gallop, systolic ejection murmur and thrill, possible MR murmur, and large jugular "a" wave. Sudden death may occur without other symptoms, particularly among athletes.

3. **HOCM has more severe symptoms** (dyspnea, angina, and syncope), which are **worsened by factors causing increased heart rate** (exercise, dehydration, and diuretics) **and decreased LV chamber size** (ACE-I, ARBs, digoxin, hydralazine, Valsalva, suddenly standing, etc.).

4. **Lab diagnosis**:

(1) **Echocardiogram is the #1 means of diagnosis**, showing hypertrophy, systolic anterior motion of mitral valve and midsystolic closure of aortic valve.

(2) CXR: Shows left-Ventr predominance and dilated left atrium. ECG is usually normal.

(3) Catheterization: Shows hypertrophy with vigorous systolic function and cavity obliteration.

Treatment

1. All patients should avoid strenuous exercise. Symptomatic patients are **best treated with beta-blockers,** which help reduce myocardial contractility and improve diastolic filling and symptoms. A Ca-blocker or disopyramide may help improve symptoms if patient is unresponsive to beta-blockers. Implantable defibrillator is used in HOCM patient with syncope. **Diuretics may be helpful in HCM but are contraindicated in HOCM.**

2. Surgery: Septal ablation, myomectomy, or mitral valve replacement can be a good therapy for severe cases.

III. Restrictive Cardiomyopathy

Etiology and pathogenesis

It's less common. It is the infiltration of the myocardium results in rigid ventricular walls, reduced ventricular compliance, normal to decreased cardiac output and stroke volume, and decreased diastolic compliance. The ventricular pressure tracing resembles those as recorded in constrictive pericarditis, with an early diastolic dip-and-plateau pattern.

Causes and subtypes

1. **Infiltrative**: Sarcoidosis, amyloidosis, hemochromatosis, or neoplasia.

Restrictive CM

2. **Endocardial fibroelastosis**: Cardiac dilatation with diffuse endocardial hyperplasia.

3. **Endomyocardial fibrosis**: Fibrous endocardial lesions of the ventricular inflow portion.

4. **Loffler endocarditis**: Dense endocardial fibrosis with overlying thrombosis.

5. **Becker disease**: Cardiac dilatation with fibrosis of the papillary muscles and subendocardium associated with necrosis and mural thrombosis. It has been mostly found in South Africa.

Essentials of diagnosis

1. Weakness, dyspnea, exercise intolerance; JVD, edema, hepatomegaly, ascites, S4 and S3 gallop, and Kussmaul sign.

2. **Lab diagnosis**:

(1) **Echocardiogram** may show characteristic myocardial texture in amyloidosis with thickened pericardium, and increased left and right atrium sizes.

(2) CXR: Mild cardiomegaly and pulmonary congestion.

(3) ECG: Low voltage, conduction abnormalities, and Q-waves.

(4) Catheterization: Typical "square root sign"; M-shaped atrial wave form, elevated left- or right-sided filling pressures.

Treatment

There is no effective treatment but symptomatic and supportive care. Try to treat underlying disorders (amyloidosis, sarcoidosis, hemochromatosis, etc.). It will eventually result in death from CHF or arrhythmias. Heart transplantation may be the last resort.

IV. Arrhythmogenic Right Ventricular Cardiomyopathy (ARVC)

This is a genetically determined myocardial disease **characterized by ventricular arrhythmias, fibrous cardiomyopathy, and RV dysfunctions. Gene mutations** may be involved in the pathology.

Treatment

Recommended management includes antiarrhythmic medicines and implanted cardioverter-defibrillator (ICD) for secondary prevention of sudden cardiac death in patients with sustained ventricular tachycardia (VT) or ventricular fibrillation (VF) and for primary prevention in selected high-risk patients.

V. Unclassified Cardiomyopathies

These include cardiomyopathies that do not readily fit into any of the above phenotypic categories, such as LV noncompaction, stress-induced (takotsubo) cardiomyopathy, and cirrhotic cardiomyopathy.

Left ventricular noncompaction

Also called **isolated ventricular noncompaction**, it is a rare cardiomyopathy with an altered myocardial wall due to intrauterine arrest of compaction of the loose interwoven meshwork. When the LV

Cardio myopathies

noncompaction is severe, it may cause ventricular arrhythmias, heart failure, and thromboembolism. Treatment varies with the clinical manifestations.

Stress-induced cardiomyopathy

Also called apical ballooning syndrome, broken heart syndrome, and takotsubo cardiomyopathy, it is characterized by transient systolic dysfunction of the apical and/or mid segments of the LV that is often provoked by stress. This disorder is generally transient and only in need of supportive therapy.

Cirrhotic cardiomyopathy

While alcoholic cardiomyopathy is one cause of heart disease in patients with cirrhosis, cirrhosis is found to be associated with myocardial dysfunction independent of alcohol exposure. The pathophysiology remains unclear. Treatment is focused on supportive care of the cardiomyopathy and cirrhosis, and their complications.

PERICARDIAL DISEASES

Acute Pericarditis

It's the inflammation of the pericardial lining around the heart.

Etiology

1. Idiopathic (**Dressler syndrome**, postviral infections, etc.).

2. Infection (viruses, bacteria, fungi, toxoplasmosis), connective tissue and autoimmune diseases (vasculitis, SLE, rheumatoid arthritis, scleroderma, sarcoidosis), metabolic diseases, neoplasm, trauma, and drug reactions (lupus syndrome), radiation, etc.

Essentials of diagnosis

1. Patient typically has **positional, substernal chest pain** that is worsened by lying down, coughing and deep inspiration, and relieved by sitting up and leaning forward. Fever and nonproductive cough may be present.

2. Characteristic **pericardial friction rub (diagnostic of pericarditis)**—a high-pitched, scratchy sound, usually transient and best heard as the patient sits forward at forced-end expiration. The ventricular systole sound is present more consistently.

3. **ECG**: It's helpful in diagnosis, usually revealing a **diffuse ST-elevation** with upright T waves and PR depression at the onset of chest pain, but **no Q-wave (different from MI).** Echocardiogram is often normal but abnormal if pericarditis with effusion is present.

Treatment

For most acute idiopathic or viral pericarditis, **colchicine plus ibuprofen** is recommended. For post-MI and most pericarditis, **aspirin plus colchicine** is the mainstay of therapy. Treat underlying cause if known (including drainage of a pericardial effusion). Most cases are self-limited, resolving in 2-6 weeks.

Pericardial Effusion

Etiology and pathogenesis

Fluid may accumulate in the pericardial cavity in pericarditis and other forms of pericardial diseases.

1. A transudate indicates pericardial injury, and an exudate reflects inflammation.

2. Serosanguineous pericardial fluid is typically from TB or neoplasm.

3. Hemopericardium may be from aortic aneurysm rupture, aortic dissection, post-MI Ventr-rupture, severe chest trauma, or bleeding by coagulopathy. When fluid accumulates rapidly, it compresses the heart and inhibits cardiac filling, resulting in life-threatening cardiac tamponade.

Lab diagnosis

1. **Echocardiography** is the most sensitive and specific means of diagnosis, which can display > 20 mL of fluid).

2. CXR can show a "water-bottle" configuration of the cardiac silhouette (> 250 mL of fluid).

Treatment

1. If the effusion is small and clinically insignificant, a repeated echocardiography in 1-2 weeks is appropriate following etiologic therapies.

2. Patients with a significant pericardial effusion and evidence of hemodynamic compromise (E.g., cardiac tamponade) should undergo urgent drainage of the effusion.

Cardiac Tamponade

It's a life-threatening condition in which a pericardial effusion has developed so rapidly and largely that it compresses the heart, leading to decreased ventricular filling and cardiac output.

Etiology: It's mostly the same as for acute pericarditis and pericardial effusion.

Essentials of diagnosis

1. Patient typically has dyspnea, orthopnea, pulsus paradoxus (marked weakening pulses during inspiration), hypotension, JVD with clear lung, and decreased heart sounds. Paradoxical pulse is not diagnostic of cardiac tamponade and can occur in severe CHF, chronic pulmonary disease, acute asthma, and certain hypovolemic shock.

2. Echocardiography (must be performed) and cardiac catheterisation will confirm tamponade and equal pressure of the left and right atrium.

Treatment

Perform emergent pericardiocentesis and drainage to save life! If symptoms persist, perform subxiphoid surgical drainage.

Constrictive Pericarditis

Etiology and pathogenesis

Constrictive Pericarditis is **diffuse fibrous scarring and thickening of the pericardium** in reaction to prior inflammation, leading to obliteration of the pericardial cavity and reduced distensibility of the cardiac chambers and diastolic filling. Cardiac output is limited and filling pressures are increased to match the external constrictive force placed on the heart by the pericardium. The heart size is usually normal. The cause in most cases is **idiopathic**. Others include viruses, TB, chronic pericardial effusion, uremia, connective tissue diseases, heart surgery, and thoracic radiation.

Essentials of diagnosis

1. Most patients appear very ill. Initial manifestations are secondary to increased systemic venous pressure—edema, ascites, hepatomegaly, JVD, and Kussmaul sign. Later, patients usually have dyspnea on exertion and orthopnea. P/E usually finds distant heart sounds and "pericardial knock", which can be confused with an S3 gallop.

2. **Lab diagnosis**:

(1) ECG: Low-voltage and non-specific T-wave changes. Atrial fibrillation may occur in some patients.

(2) Chest CT or MRI scan: May show thickened pericardium, and pericardial calcifications (TB).

(3) Cardiac catheterization: A marked 'y' descent with the right atrial pressure tracing. Left and right ventricular pressure tracings may show a typical "square root" sign. The end-diastolic pressures in all four chambers and the pulmonary arteries are about the same.

Differential diagnosis

Restrictive and constrictive cardiomyopathy:

Left ventricular ejection fraction is more likely to be decreased in patients with restrictive cardiomyopathy. CT can effectively demonstrate the thickened pericardium. Differentiation can be difficult sometimes.

Treatment

Most newly diagnosed cases are initially treated conservatively with Na-restriction, mild diuretics, NSAIDs, steroids, or/and antibiotics, etc. Pericardiectomy or resection may be performed in chronic, severe cases as the definitive therapy. However, the mortality rate is high.

VASCULAR DISEASES

Aortic Dissection

It's a transverse tear in the intima of the aorta, leading blood into the media and creating a false lumen and a hematoma that propagates longitudinally. **Longstanding hypertension** is the major risk factor.

Other predisposing factors include trauma, connective tissue diseases (Marfan and Ehlers-Danlos syndrome), bicuspid aortic valve, coarctation of the aorta, etc. The most common site of origin is above the aortic valve and distal to the left subclavian artery. It's more common in 50-60 y/o men.

Essentials of diagnosis

1. **Sudden, severe, tearing pain** in the anterior chest (in ascending aorta dissection) or interscapular back pain (descending aorta dissection), accompanied with diaphoresis.

2. **P/E results** are usually **asymmetric pulses and BP (difference > 20 mmHg)** between the left and right arm. BP is mostly hypertensive. If it is hypotensive, pericardial tamponade (with pulsus paradoxus, decreased heart sound and JVD), acute MI from coronary ischemia (see "MI" for the symptoms), or hypovolemic shock from blood loss should be suspected. If the aorta valve is involved, signs and murmur of aorta regurgitation may exist. Neurologic signs may exist if carotid artery is obstructed.

3. **Lab diagnosis**:

(1) **CXR shows widened mediastinum** (usually >8 mm), cardiomegaly, or new pleural effusion.

(2) CT angiography is the most accurate means of diagnosis to show details of the dissection, if the patient is stable and confirmation is required.

(3) TEE is also sensitive and specific, showing details of the thoracic aorta, coronary arteries, aortic valve, and possible pericardial effusion. Serum biomarker **D-dimer** (increase) indicates recent or ongoing intravascular blood coagulation and possible acute aortic dissection.

4. There are **two classification systems**:

(1) **Stanford system**: Ascending aorta dissection is Type A, and all others are Type B.

(2) **DeBakey system**: Type I—dissection involving both the ascending and descending aorta; Type II—confined to the ascending aorta; Type III—confined to the descending aorta.

Differential diagnosis

Myocardial ischemia, pericarditis, pulmonary embolus, aortic regurgitation/aneurysm without dissection, musculoskeletal pain, pleuritis, and digestive disorders.

Treatment

1. For the life-threatening **ascending aorta dissection, an emergent surgical repair** is indicated.

2. For descending aorta dissection, BP and heart rate monitoring and control are needed. IV beta-blockers are given to reduce cardiac rate and force, and nitroprusside-Na to lower BP below 120 mmHg.

Aortic Aneurisms (AA)

AA is a localized dilation of the aorta, and **the most common one is abdominal AA (AAA)** secondary to atherosclerosis or hypertension, which causes local aorta wall weakness and dilation. Other causes include high cholesterol, family history, smoking, trauma, infection (No.1 is syphilis), congenital weakness (Marfan syndrome), or elder men. Most AAAs occur between the renal arteries and iliac bifurcation. The incidence increases with age and more common in men.

Essentials of diagnosis

1. It's usually asymptomatic and discovered incidentally on P/E or radiologic imaging.

2. It can be symptomatic, with "sense of fullness", severe or boring low back pain or flank pain radiating into the testis or leg. It may be confused with other back/flank pain. **P/E mostly reveals a pulsatile abdominal mass or abdominal bruit** +/- tenderness. Symptoms suggest expansion and impending rupture.

3. **Ruptured AA**: Acute, severe chest or abdominal pain, hypotension, shock, or MI. For an AAA rupture, **Grey Turner's sign** (ecchymoses on back and flanks, **Image 41**) and **Cullen's sign** (ecchymoses around umbilicus) may be seen.

4. **Lab diagnosis**:

(1) **Ultrasound** is usually the initial diagnostic tool.

(2) **CT or aortography** with contrast is the most **accurate** and confirmative means of diagnosis.

(3) Plain X-ray often picks up an AA accidentally with aortic wall calcification.

Treatment

1. Symptomatic patients should be hospitalized and prepared for surgical fixing. Ruptured AA or impending rupture requires IV fluid and packed RBC followed by an emergent operation to save life.

2. Asymptomatic, < 5 cm AA may be monitored for size changes and BP control (using beta blockers) as an outpatient; > 5 cm (ascending) or > 6 cm (descending) AA should be electively repaired (by surgical resection with grafting). CVS status evaluation is required prior to surgery.

Peripheral Vascular Diseases (PVD)

It refers to reduction or occlusion of the blood supply to the extremities caused by **atherosclerotic plaques (#1)**, thrombosis, embolism, or trauma. Chronic, insufficient blood supply to the affected area leads to ischemic pain and mostly affects the lower extremity, which is called **intermittent claudication**. Acute ischemic symptoms are usually caused by embolism from the heart. Symptoms depend on the vessel and extent involved.

Essentials of diagnosis

1. Most patients have **risk factors and history of atherosclerosis** (hyperlipidemia, hypertension, smoking, diabetes, lack of exercise), CAD, and intermittent claudication. The claudication can be relieved by exercise cessation or worsened by obstruction, leading to rest pain.

2. P/E are typically **"5Ps"—"Pain, Pallor, Pulseless, Paresthesia, Paralysis"**. Others are cool skin and hair loss. ABI (ankle-brachial index) measures the ankle-brachial systolic BP and provides objective evidence of obstruction. When ABI is < 0.4, ischemia is severe enough to cause rest pain.

3. Two common types:

(1) **Femoropopliteal obstruction**: With calf claudication but no pulses below the femoral artery.

(2) **Aortoiliac obstruction**: Associated with **Leriche syndrome**—decreased femoral pulses, buttock claudication, and male impotence.

4. **Lab diagnosis**:

(1) Initial ultrasound may show decreased blood flow due to the obstruction.

(2) **The best diagnostic means is angiography**, which will demonstrate the area and severity of stenosis necessary for surgical consideration.

Treatment

1. Most patients with claudication will improve with **smoking cessation** (highly important), diet modification, and gradual exercise program (mainly targeting lipid reduction), as well as control of the underlying disease. **Aspirin/clopidogrel** and thromboxane inhibitor also help reduce incidences.

2. **Surgical treatment**: Indications include rest pain, ischemic ulcerations (tissue necrosis), and severe symptoms refractory to conservative therapies that affect quality of life or work. Usually angioplasty (with patient's saphenous vein), stenting, or bypass grafting can be chosen. If the limb cannot be saved by angioplasty, amputation is the last option.

Deep Venous Thrombosis (DVT)

See "RESPIRATORY DISEASES: PE-DVT".

Virchow's triad factors for venous thrombosis:

Stasis, endothelial injury, and hypercoagulable states. See **Images 42 for DVT**.

Eisenmenger Syndrome (ES)

ES is a disorder of gradual right-to-left shunt, the triad of systemic-to-pulmonary shunt, pulmonary hypertension, and cyanosis. It usually develops in a patient with a ventricular septal defect and significant left-to-right shunting that eventually leads to pulmonary hypertension. Severe pulmonary hypertension eventually reverses the shunting to "right-to-left".

Diagnosis: P/E generally finds central cyanosis, digital clubbing, RV impulse, and a load/palpable P_2 sound. The prognosis is better than those with pulmonary hypertension who have similar hemodynamics. **Echocardiography** is confirmative.

Management: Most evaluations and treatment of ES should be performed in a center with expertise in managing cardiac catheterization, the congenital heart disease, and pulmonary hypertension. Heart or/and lung transplantation may be the last treatment option for severe ES.

VASCULITIS SYNDROMES

See Chapter 8: Diseases of the Musculoskeletal System and Connective Tissue.

Chapter 2: High-yield Questions (HYQ)

1. A 50 y/o man presents with chest pain, shortness of breath (SOB), palpitations, and ankle edema for the past month (mo), with worsening of symptoms over 2 days. Physical examination (P/E) finds tachycardia, normal BP, JVD, and lower limb edema. ECG (EKG) reveals an atrial rate of 380/min, irregular QRS, and no clear P-wave with baseline. What's the most appropriate next step of treatment (Tx)?

A. Aspirin

B. Warfarin for 3 weeks

C. Metoprolol

D. Digoxin

E. Electric cardioversion (50-100j)

2. A week later, the above patient complains of seeing flying objects and feeling extreme weak. Lab tests reveal hypo-K and hypo-Mg. ECG reveals atrial tachycardia and A-V block, with a ventricular rate of 50/min. The best immediate Tx is

A. atropine

B. KCl and MgCl2

C. electric pacing

D. anti-digitalis fragment

E. digoxin cessation

3-9: Match the following clinical scenarios with the best initial treatment.

A. Amiodarone

B. Atropine

C. Lidocaine

D. Verapamil

E. Propranolol

F. Procainamide

G. Digoxin

H. Aspirin

I. Synchronized cardioversion

J. Ventr-pacemaker

K. Unsynchronized cardioversion

L. t-PA

M. Metoprolol

N. Heparin

O. Warfarin

P. Morphine

3. A 55 y/o man complains of periodic palpitations and lightheadedness after an acute myocardial infarction (MI) two weeks ago. P/E finds stable vital signs. ECG reveals wide QRS and inverted T waves in V5-6 leads. Other findings are unremarkable.

4. A 55 y/o man with chronic heart disease complains of occasional palpitations, lightheadedness, and syncope. P/E finds a fast pulse with stable vital signs. ECG reveals an atrial rate of 300/min and a ventricular (Ventr) rate of 150/min. QRS waves are regular and P-waves are in a "sawtooth" pattern.

5. A 55 y/o man complains of frequent palpitations, lightheadedness, and syncope after an acute myocardial infarction 2 weeks ago. He is brought to the ER after a syncopal episode. P/E results: HR = 120/min; BP = 90/50 mmHg. ECG reveals a ventricular rate of 130/min, wide bizarre QRS with regular rhythms and A-V dissociation.

6. A 50 y/o female complains of frequent palpitations, lightheadedness, and syncope for the past 3 days. She has a 5-year history of chronic cardiomyopathy. P/E finds HR = 130/min, BP = 90/60 mmHg. ECG reveals ventricular rate = 150/min, short PR intervals and wide, slurred QRS (delta wave).

7. A 35 y/o female complains of frequent palpitations, dizziness, and syncope for the past 3 days. She has a congenital hearing deficit. P/E finds HR = 120/min, BP = 90/60 mmHg. Serum K and Mg levels are low. ECG reveals ventricular rate = 130/min, QRS rotations, and prolonged QT.

8. A 50 y/o man with SOB and crushing chest pain for 3 hours is brought to the ER. He has a history of hypertension (HTN), smoking, and alcohol use for the past 10 years. P/E finds a weak pulse of 120/min, labored

breathing at 24/min, BP of 90/60 mmHg, and an S3 gallop. ECG shows ST-elevation in leads II, III, and aVF. Lab tests show normal CBC, CK-MB, troponin, LDH, and CXR.

9. The above patient's symptoms were relieved within one week of Tx. One month later he presents with milder chest pain. P/E finds normal vital signs except a transient high-pitched, scratchy sound over the heart. ECG reveals a diffuse ST-elevation without Q-waves.

10. A 50 y/o man with a 10-year history of smoking comes to the physician for a health exam. He has no history of CAD or other diseases except chronic bronchitis with productive cough and sputum. P/E finds rough respiratory sound and normal vital signs. CXR shows increased tracks in both lungs. CBC is normal. His random total cholesterol (Chol) is 220, HDL is 40, and LDL is 140 (mg/dL). The best next step is

A. 3-mo diet and exercise plan   B. giving lovastatin   C. smoking cessation

D. giving gemfibrozil   E. lipid re-testing in a month

11. A 60 y/o man with a 3-month history of dyspnea on exertion and ankle edema complains of orthopnea and coughing up pink sputum for 1 hour. He has a history of smoking, hypertension and diabetes for the past 2 years and is on "intermittent oral drugs" for hypertension and diabetes. P/E finds HR =110/min, BP =150/100 mmHg, with an S3 gallop and JVD. CXR reveals pulmonary congestion, cardiac enlargement, and Kerley's B lines. Echo-cardiography reveals EF = 45%. Serum glucose is 150 mg/dL. What's the most appropriate medicine to use now?

A. Metoprolol   B. Thiazides   C. altace (ramipril)

D. Diltiazem   E. Doxazosin

12. The above patient obtains general relief of symptoms and stable BP of 145/95 mmHg after taking ramipril for 5 days, but now has oliguria, persistent dry cough and a skin rash. P/E finds a smoothly enlarged prostate and urinary bladder. Urine analysis reveals mild proteinuria without WBC. 300 mL of urine is drained out through a catheter. What's the best next drug for replacement?

A. Metoprolol   B. Thiazides   C. Valsartan

D. Diltiazem   E. Doxazosin

13. A 30 y/o man has his BP checked in your clinic for the first time and it is 150/95 mmHg. He denies any history of alcohol or drug use, or chronic diseases. What's the best next step of diagnosis (Dx)?

A. Abdominal ultrasound   B. Abdominal CT   C. Blood renin and aldosterone level

D. Angiography   E. BP re-testing in 2 weeks

14. The above patient comes back 2 weeks later and the BP is 145/95 mmHg. He has no other symptoms except for a periodic headache and sweating. P/E only finds a tachycardia. What's the most appropriate next step now?

A. Abdominal ultrasound   B. Abdominal CT   C. Blood renin and aldosterone test

D. 24-hr urinary VMA test   E. Alpha and beta R blocker use

15. A 65 y/o female complains of low-grade fever, short of breath, cough, joint pain, and generalized weakness for the past 3 days. She had a dental procedure performed a week ago. P/E finds rough systolic murmur at the apex, tender nodules on fingers, and subungual petechiae. ESR is increased. CXR shows increased vessel markings in the lungs. Echocardiography and ECG results are unremarkable. Blood samples are taken for culture and sensitivity (C/S). The best empirical antibiotics to start on this patient is

A. vancomycin   B. nafcillin + gentamicin   C. vancomycin + gentamicin

D. vancomycin + ampicillin   E. nafcillin + gentamicin + ampicillin

16. Ten days later, the above patient is found with (+) culture for S. aureus and a Gram⁻ rod, persistent fever, increased BUN and creatinine, and signs of progressive heart failure (HF). What's the strongest indication for valve replacement surgery for this patient?

A. S. aureus culture (+) after antibiotic Tx   B. Persistent fever after antibiotic Tx

C. Gram- rod culture (+) after antibiotic Tx   D. Progressive HF

E. Increased BUN and creatinine

17-22: Match the following clinical scenarios with the best treatment.

A. Conservative Tx   B. Valve commissurotomy   C. Valve replacement

D. Valvuloplasty   E. Diuretic   F. Surgical repair

G. Beta-R blockers   H. Antibiotic   I. Warfarin

J. Digitalis   K. Vascular dilator

17. A 65 y/o man complains of mild chest pain, dyspnea on exertion, and fatigability for the past month. P/E finds normal vital signs, and a harsh systolic murmur at the apex radiating to the aorta area without late peak and carotid upstrokes. ECG and CXR results are normal. Echocardiography reveals reduced aortic valve leaflets.

18. A 60 y/o female presents with an abrupt worsening of her chest pain and dyspnea 5 days after being treated for an acute MI. P/E finds tachypnea, tachycardia, hypotension, and diffuse pulmonary rales. A loud holosystolic murmur is heard at the apex radiating to the left axilla. CXR shows an enlarged left atrium and increased pulmonary infiltrates. Echocardiography shows prolapsing leaflet.

19. A 30 y/o female complains of lightheadedness, palpitations, and mild chest pain for the past 2 days. P/E finds normal vital signs, and a thin woman with long limbs. Auscultation reveals mid-systolic click and a late systolic murmur at the cardiac apex, getting worse with Valsalva and improving with squatting. Echocardiography confirms the diagnosis.

20. A 30 y/o man presents with fatigue, periodic chest pain, and dyspnea on exertion for the past 3 days. P/E finds a systolic murmur on the left sternal border between the 3-4th rib without radiation, increased with Valsalva maneuver, and decreased with squatting and handgrip. Echocardiography confirms the diagnosis.

21. A 55 y/o man has been treated for an acute MI (anterior infarct) for the past 3 days, and has an abrupt worsening of chest pain. P/E finds tachypnea, tachycardia, hypotension, and a loud holosystolic murmur at the cardiac apex with widespread radiation. Echocardiography confirms the diagnosis.

22. A 40 y/o female has fever, skin rash and migrant polyarthritis for a week followed by gradual dyspnea, orthopnea, and fatigability. P/E shows mild tachycardia and fever, normal BP, erythematous skin nodules, and a low-pitched apical diastolic rumble with loud S1. CXR shows mild increase in pulmonary vessel markings. CXR shows mild increase in pulmonary vessel markings. CBC is normal. ESR is increased. Aspirin has been used. She is scheduled for an echocardiography and arterial catheterization for diagnosis.

23. A 25 y/o man comes for a health check-up due to prolonged palpitations, chest pain, and dyspnea after an exercise program. P/E finds a man who generally looks in good health with normal vital signs, bifid carotid pulse, and a systolic murmur with thrill at the cardiac apex. What's the most important next step for diagnosis?

A. Echocardiography   B. ECG   C. CXR

D. Cardiac catheterization   E. Obtaining detailed history

24. A 50 y/o female presents with progressive weakness, dyspnea, and exercise intolerance for the past 3 days. P/E finds normal BP, JVD, S4 and S3 gallop, and ankle edema. ECG reveals low voltage, A-V block, and Q-waves. Echocardiography reveals thickened pericardium. CXR shows mild cardiomegaly and pulmonary congestion. Among the following causes, which one is the LEAST likely?

A. Alcohol and lipids   B. Hemochromatosis   C. Sarcoidosis

D. Endomyocardial fibrosis   E. Becker disease

25. A 60 y/o man presents with boring low back pain radiating down to the legs for the past 2 days. He has a 3-year history of hyperlipidemia and is on lovastatin. P/E finds normal vital signs and a pulsatile abdominal mass with bruits without tenderness. Blood tests reveal mild hyperlipidemia. Urine analysis (U/A) is normal. What's the most appropriate next step?

A. Abdominal ultrasound   B. Abdominal CT   C. Angiography

D. Abdominal X-ray   E. Abdominal MRI

26. A 50 y/o man presents with 1-month history of exercise intolerance and leg pain after more than 30 min walking. Symptoms are alleviated with rest. He has no history of alcohol use, smoking, drug use, or recent health evaluation. His wife complains of "too little sexual life." His family life is otherwise fine. P/E finds normal vital signs, pale and hairless legs, and weak femoral and ankle pulses. Ultrasound of the lower body is unremarkable. What's the most likely cause of his sexual problem?

A. Psycho-social factors   B. Atherosclerosis   C. Thrombosis

D. Embolism   E. Trauma

27. A 25 y/o man is brought to the ER by his friend for pressing chest pain and short of breath for a few hours after a fight. He denies any history of smoking, alcohol, drug use, and medical problems. He briefly mentions that both his parents have "heart disease." P/E results: pale, dyspneic, and diaphoretic; BP = 180/100 mmHg, HR = 120/min. He is irritable and aggressive, with dilated pupils. ABG is normal on room air. ECG shows acute ST-segment elevations in the anterolateral leads. What's the most likely cause for his conditions?

A. Alcoholic cardiomyopathy   B. Cardiac contusion   C. Pheochromocytoma

D. MI   E. Drug overdose

28. A 60 y/o man is brought to the ER with nausea and crushing chest pain radiating down the left arm after a big meal an hr ago. He feels an "impending doom" to come. He has a history of smoking, alcohol drinking, GERD, hypertension, and high cholesterol for several yrs. P/E results: Alert, pale, RR = 27/min, HR = 105/min, BP = 77/55 mmHg on both arms, T = 37.5°C, and ABG = 96% on room air. Neck shows JVD and lungs are (-) on auscultation. ECG reveals ST-elevations in the leads II, III, and aVF. CK-MB and troponin are (+). What's the best explanation for these findings?

A. Acute GERD   B. Diastolic heart failure   C. Acute mitral regurgitation

D. Left-ventr infarction   E. Right-ventr infarction   F. Acute aorta dissection

29. A 60 y/o man has progressive, unstable angina that is resistant to regular medical treatment. His uncle died of heart attacks before the age of 50. He has a 10-year history of moderate smoking, alcohol drinking, and

hyperlipidemia. Cardiac catheterization demonstrates about 70% occlusion of three coronary arteries. His left ventricular EF (ejection fraction) is 50%. Which of the following is the best therapy for this man?

A. Triple coronary bypass surgery using vessel grafts

B. Angioplasty and stenting of all three arteries

C. Intensive medical treatment until EF < 40%

D. Intensive medical treatment until his artery occlusion > 80% for surgical revascularization

E. Bypass surgery for the two main coronary arteries now

30. A 60 y/o man with prolonged hypertension presents with progressive short of breath at rest and at night in bed, and bilateral ankle swelling. P/E results are: RR = 22/min, HR = 85/min, BP = 120/80 mmHg; JVD (+), bilateral ankle edema (+), cardiac S3 gallop (+), bilateral lung crackles (+). CXR reveals an enlarged heart image and bilateral pulmonary edema. Among the following medicines used in this patient, which one does NOT show decrease in the mortality rate?

A. Aspirin	B. Digoxin	C. Captopril
D. Valsartan	E. Spironolactone	F. Hydralazine

31. A 30 y/o female is brought to the ER with sharp, shearing chest pain radiating to her mid back. It started 30 min ago and is still continuing. She is tall, thin, and generally healthy except for "occasional hypertension." P/E results: RR = 25/min, HR = 102/min, BP = 180/105 mmHg in the right arm and 140/95 in the left arm. Cardiac exam shows a blowing diastolic murmur best heard at the right upper sternal border. ECG reveals sinus tachycardia and normal QRS-ST waves. CXR, CT scan, and angiography all seem normal. What's the best diagnostic test next?

A. Cardiac enzymes	B. Transesophageal echocardiogram (TEE)
C. Repeat chest CT	D. Repeat angiography E. Chest MRI

32. A 30 y/o female comes to you for an evaluation before planning a pregnancy. She is generally active and healthy without any personal or family history of heart disease. She exercises often and feels well. P/E finds P = 85/min, normal BP, S1, and S2, a mid-diastolic rumbling murmur; the lungs are (-). CXR is normal. Echocardiogram reveals mild mitral stenosis and the left atrium enlargement; the left-ventr cavity size and systolic function are normal. Her blood glucose level is normal. Based on this information, what's your best advice to the patient?

A. She should avoid pregnancy because of her risky heart conditions

B. She can start pregnancy now

C. She should start a beta-R blocker before pregnancy

D. She needs an exercise stress test to evaluate the risk

E. She needs a prophylactic mitral balloon valvotomy before pregnancy

33. You are asked to review and decide antimicrobial prophylaxis for multiple cases of infective endocarditis. Which of the following cases is most likely to benefit from antimicrobial prophylaxis?

A. A 65 y/o man with aortic stenosis that is scheduled for a cardiac catheterization

B. A 45 y/o man with mitral stenosis that is scheduled for an esophageal dilatation

C. A 65 y/o man with mitral regurgitation that is scheduled for an esophageal endoscopy

D. A 45 y/o man with mitral stenosis that is scheduled for a TEE

E. A 35 y/o woman with mitral regurgitation that is scheduled for a hysterectomy

34. A 40 y/o man comes from the poor countryside presenting with progressive dyspnea on exertion, chronic cough, and chest pain for the past month. He denies any history of chronic diseases and present medication ingestion, except for a 4-kg weight loss over the past 2 months. P/E results: normal vital signs, low fever, and a cachectic appearance; the lungs are (-); JVD is (+) and alleviated with deep inspiration; S1 and S2 heart sounds are distant, with an early S3; the liver is enlarged. ECG shows low voltages without ST-elevation. CXR reveals an enlarged heart. What's the most likely diagnosis?

A. Tamponade

B. Congestive cardiomyopathy

C. Constrictive pericarditis

D. Restrictive cardiomyopathy

E. Right ventricular infarction

35. A 50 y/o administrative man comes to you for a health evaluation. He has a 5-year history of heavy smoking (1 pack/day) and alcohol drinking (> 5 cups/day). He also has a family history of hypertension and diabetes. He rarely goes to a physician for health examinations. P/E finds BP = 144/94 mmHg at rest, body weight = 70 kg, height = 1.65 meters. There are no other abnormal findings. What's your best advice for him to reduce the high BP?

A. Cut down alcohol drinking

B. Stop smoking

C. Reduce weight

D. Do regular exercise

E. Reduce work stress

36. A 65 y/o man complains of "crushing chest pain" radiating to the left arm and is brought to the emergency room. He also has anxiety, sweating, and nausea. His vital signs are stable. He has a history of diabetes mellitus. In the P/E, the physician will most likely find

A. a displaced point of maximal impulse (PMI)

B. S4 gallops

C. continuous "machinery" murmurs

D. triphasic scratchy sounds

E. increased jugular venous pressure on inhalation

37-38. 37. A 60 y/o woman presents with dyspnea, cough with pink sputum, and pressure-like chest pain for the past 3 months. P/E finds cyanosis, RR = 36/min, HR = 110/min, BP = 180/118 mmHg, PMI shift to the left, wet rales, and S3 gallops over the apex at auscultation. CXR and ECG confirm the diagnosis. The best immediate Tx is

A. metoprolol

B. nitroprusside

C. furosemide

D. valsartan

E. digoxin

F. nifedipine

38. The most likely cause of death for the above patient will be

A. myocardial infarction

B. myocardial rupture

C. pulmonary edema

D. pulmonary emboli

E. cardiac emboli

F. cardiac arrhythmia

39-42: Match the following clinical scenarios with the most likely Dx.

A. Ventricular septal Defect (VSD)   B. Atrial septal Defect (ASD)
C. Patent ductus arteriosus (PDA)   D. Coarctation of the aorta (CA)
E. Tetralogy of Fallot (TF)   F. Kartagener syndrome (KS)
G. Persistent truncus arteriosus (PTA)   H. Tricuspid atresia (TA)
I. Hypoplastic left heart syndrome   J. Transposition of the great arteries (TGA)

39. A 3 y/o boy is brought in for fatigue and frequent respiratory infections. The mother has a 5-year history of alcohol use and smoking before the pregnancy. P/E finds a weak, alert boy without cyanosis. A wide, split S2 and systolic ejection murmur is heard at the upper left sternal border. ECG reveals RVH. Echocardiography is ordered.

40. A 13 y/o girl is brought to the clinic for delayed development, fatigue, headache, and periodic syncope. P/E finds a pale girl with a short stature and tachycardia; no cyanosis. Systolic BP is higher in the right arm than in the left. ECG reveals LVH. CXR shows a "reverse 3" sign and pulmonary congestion.

41. A 1-month infant is found with a blue face, dyspnea, and weakness. The mother has a 5-year history of alcohol use and smoking before pregnancy at age 37. P/E finds a flat face and cyanosis. A systolic ejection murmur is heard at the upper left sternal border with a single S2. ECG reveals left axis deviation. CXR shows mildly reduced pulmonary vascular markings.

42. A 1-month infant is found with a blue face, dyspnea, and fatigability for the past week. The mother has a 5-year history of alcohol use and smoking for before pregnancy at age 37. P/E finds a weak infant with cyanosis and a flat facial profile. A systolic ejection murmur is heard at the upper left sternal border with a single S2. ECG reveals RVH. CXR shows a "boot-shaped" heart with decreased pulmonary vascular markings.

Answers and Explanations

1. (D). Digoxin is the best initial treatment (Tx) for this patient with CHF + atrial fibrillation. Warfarin (to prolong PT) +/- aspirin should be added for 3 weeks before cardioversion and be continued until normal (Nl) sinus rhythm has been maintained for at least 4 weeks, to prevent embolism. "C" is good for acute Atrial-fib rate control, but should be used cautiously with heart failure. "E" is indicated if the patient is unstable.

2. (A). It's a case of digitalis intoxication. A-V block must be first corrected with atropine; if the ventricular (Ventr) rate is still < 50 bpm after atropine administration, e-pacing is performed. Meanwhile, supply K + Mg and check digitalis levels; if it's > 10mg/L, stop it and add anti-digitalis fragment.

3. (J). This is a case of LBBB (left bundle branch block) and requires a Ventr-pacemaker. If the ECG signs are in leads V1-2, it's RBBB and only needs observation.

4. (D). This is typical atrial flutter and best treated with a Ca-blocker. If it's unstable, e-cardioversion is done.

5. (K). This is an unstable sustained monomorphic V-tachycardia requiring immediate unsynchronized e-cardioversion (defibrillation, "K"). If it's stable, amiodarone or lidocaine is the initial therapy for cardioversion. Common indications for synchronized cardioversion are unstable atrial fibrillation, atrial flutter, atrial tachycardia, and supraventricular tachycardias. Synchronization avoids the delivery of a LOW ENERGY shock during cardiac repolarization (t-wave), which may precipitate V-fibrillation.

6. (F). Wolff-Parkinson-White syndrome (WPW); procainamide is the choice of drug. Radiofrequency ablation is the definitive Tx. Beta-R blockers, Ca-channel blockers and digitalis are contraindicated.

7. (M). Most likely, it's a case of Torsade de Pointes or long Q-T syndrome, often associated with recurrent Ventr-tachycardia or Ventr-fibrillation. The best initial Tx is a beta1-R blocker plus correction of hypo-K/Mg. If unstable, e-cardioversion is needed.

8. (M). Most likely, an acute inferior MI, and best treated initially with "ABC" and a beta1-R blocker, followed by morphine, aspirin, t-PA, etc. Cardiac enzymes usually won't increase until 4-6 hours after MI.

9. (H). It's most likely a case of post-MI pericarditis (Dressler syndrome), and aspirin is the best Tx.

10. (E). The best strategy for this man with 2-3 risk factors for CAD is to confirm the hyperlipidemia first, then stop smoking, and "A" if the next LDL is < 160 mg/dL, or "A + B" if the LDL > 160.

11. (C). This is a complicated case of diabetes, hypertension, and HF. Diuretics should be first chosen with hypertension + HF, but contraindicated with hyperglycemia. Thus an ACE-I is best here. A beta1-R blocker is good with MI, but not with diabetes (DM) and hypoglycemia.

12. (E). Alpha-R-blocker is the best for this patient with mild hypertension + BPH (benign prostate hyperplasia). Otherwise, valsartan (an angiotensin-II-R blocker) is also a good replacement for ICE-I sensitivity.

13. (E). No special Dx or Tx is needed if the BP recheck is < 135/85 mmHg. If it's still > 140/90 mmHg, it's most likely secondary hypertension. Suspect renal artery stenosis, Conn's syndrome, Cushing's syndrome, or adrenal tumors.

14. (D). Most likely, a pheochromocytoma (clinical triad—episodic hypertension, headache, and diaphoresis), and "D" is the best Dx test to confirm it. "B" also helps locate the tumor. After the Dx is confirmed, Tx is an alpha and beta R blocker followed by surgical resection. If there are other manifestations, "A and C" help distinguish renal artery stenosis or Conn/Cushing syndrome. Polycystic kidney disease and coarctation of the aorta are other differential Dx.

15. (E). This is most likely subacute endocarditis caused by Strep or Listeria (> 60 y/a) after a dental procedure, and thus 'E' is the best choice. Vancomycin is usually saved for PCNase-resistant Staph-aureus and other life-threatening Gram⁺ infections; not as the initial trial.

16. (D). Absolute indications include progressive HF despite Tx, fungal endocarditis, valve ring abscess, and failure to clear infection after a long course of antibiotic Tx.

17. (A). It's a case of elderly aortic valve sclerosis without stenosis. Aortic stenosis has similar murmurs but also has a late peak and delayed carotid upstroke, with a soft or absent S2. Echocardiogram usually shows aortic stenosis and calcification of the aortic valve.

18. (C). Papillary muscle rupture with acute MR (mitral regurgitation) after acute MI: stabilize vital signs and perform an urgent valve replacement.

19. (A). Mitral valve prolapse: No.1 common congenital valvular abnormality, usually seen in young female and associated with Marfan syndrome, etc.; presenting with signs of chronic MR. Acute MR: M > F; No.1 cause is post-MI papillary muscle dysfunction; rapid Left-Ventr failure signs are common; holosystolic apical murmur radiating to the axilla, often with a thrill, S3, and widely split S2; treated with "E, F".

20. (G). A typical case of hypertrophic obstructive cardiomyopathy, distinguishable from aortic stenosis.

21. (F). A typical ventricular septal rupture that requires emergent supportive Tx and surgical repair.

22. (E). This patient has rheumatic fever with mitral stenosis, and should be treated with aspirin, diuretics and salt-restricted diet. If failed, mitral commissurotomy is indicated. Valvular diseases with arterial catheterization, GI-endoscopy, and esophageal intubation are low-moderate risks that do not need preventive antibiotics.

23. (E). This patient should be highly suspected of HOC for his age and P/E results, and detailed family history is the most important initial step of Dx. Because HOC is an autosomal dominant genetic disease, every generation of the family should have a similar patient or "sudden death". If the family history is positive, then "A" can be the first Dx test, and "D" is confirmative.

24. (A). It's a case of restrictive cardiomyopathy with HF due to rigid Ventr-walls and reduced Ventr-compliance and cardiac output. Heart transplants may be the only cure. Alcohol usually causes dilated cardiomyopathy, and high lipids (LDL) mostly cause CAD.

25. (A). Ultrasound is the proper initial Dx step for abdominal aortic aneurisms (AAA). CT or aortography with contrast supplies more accurate and confirmative Dx. Plain X-ray can pick up a calcified AA accidentally.

26. (B). This patient has intermittent claudication and impotence most likely caused by atherosclerosis and aortoiliac obstruction (Leriche syndrome). Other causes are less possible for this case. The best diagnostic tool is angiography.

27. (E). In a healthy young person with similar presentations of myocardial ischemia, drug abuse (especially with cocaine or amphetamine overdose) should be highly suspected, although patient usually denies it. Most myocardial ischemia by similar drug overdose is secondary to coronary vasospasm. Other differential Dx for ST-segment elevations on the ECG include: MI, cardiac contusion, Ventr-aneurysm, pericarditis, and normal variants. "A" usually causes dilated cardiomyopathy and heart failure. "B" usually requires a heavy blunt trauma as in a traffic accident. "C" is characterized by periodic hypertension, headache, profuse sweating, palpitations, and apprehension. MI usually occurs in a patient > age 45 with risk factors, low BP and ABG, and abnormal QRS-ST waves on the ECG.

28. (E). Patient has a typical right-sided MI, with the classic P/E triad of hypotension, JVD, and clear lungs on auscultation. ECG indicates infarction in an inferior and a posterior distribution. Since instances of isolated posterior wall MI is rare, isolated right-Ventr MI is the most likely Dx. "A or F" is also possible but less typical. "B" is mostly associated with a hypertrophied heart, as with long-standing hypertension or infiltrative cardiomyopathy, and mainly presenting with left-sided failure. "C" can occur during a large anterior wall MI secondary to papillary muscle dysfunction, causing left-sided failure. "D" is typically associated with ST-segment elevation in leads V1-4 in ECG and left-sided failure.

29. (A). For this patient with progressive angina, 70% major artery occlusion, and multiple risk factors, there is a clear indication for aggressive surgery. Coronary bypass surgery is better than angioplasty for multiple artery occlusions≥70%. The critical graft is usually done with the best available internal mammary artery. Angioplasty and stenting ("B") is better suited for isolated vessels rather than multiple ones. 70% occlusion is already an indication for surgery, not delayed until EF<40% ("C") or occlusion>80% ("D"). "E" is inadequate in this case.

30. (B). All the listed medicines, ACE-I, angiotensin-II-R blockers, vascular dilators, diuretics, aspirin, and beta-R blockers have documented evidence of reducing mortality in patients with heart failure except digitalis.

31. (B). Most likely it's an aortic dissection. Major risk factors include hypertension, blunt chest trauma, and connective tissue diseases (as Marfan syndrome probably in this case). Visualization is necessary to guide Dx and Tx. Although CT or angiography is usually the first test done, it misses about 10% of the cases. Thus TEE is the most sensitive test for aortic dissections. Cardiac enzymes a few hours after the onset may help exclude MI, but MI is less likely with the present presentations and normal ECG. Repeating previously (-) tests ("C and D") is unlikely to provide more information immediately. MRI for aortic dissection is not as sensitive and convenient as echocardiogram.

32. (C). Most patients with mild asymptomatic mitral stenosis with active daily activities can tolerate pregnancy without any complications. Thus she only needs a beta-R blocker to improve the cardiac function (without affecting the blood glucose level) before pregnancy rather than stress test or mitral valve procedures.

33. (B). Antimicrobial prophylaxis for infective endocarditis is mainly determined by two factors: the preexisting risk of the patient, and the risk of the procedure or surgery. All the above cases are with low to moderate risk of diseases (valvular diseases) and procedures except esophageal dilation, which is a high-risk traumatic procedure that induces bacterial translocation and microtrauma and thus requires antibiotics.

34. (C). Constrictive pericarditis usually results from the healing of a prior pericarditis, or destruction of pericardial cavity, and presents with diastolic dysfunction and low ECG voltages, etc. It's mostly idiopathic and may also follow infectious causes. Tamponade ("A") will typically show pulsus paradoxus and a significant decrease in the inspiratory systolic BP. "B" is dilated cardiomyopathy with systolic dysfunction, mostly caused by alcoholism, myocarditis, etc. Echocardiography shows an enlarged heart and ECG reveals arrhythmias. "D" usually results from infiltrative or connective tissue disease, typically showing apical beats, left-ventr hypertrophy, S3, diastolic dysfunction, and LBBB. "E" is less likely without acute crushing chest pain and abnormal QRS-ST in the ECG.

35. (A). Excessive alcohol intake (> 5 drinks/day) has been clearly associated with hypertension, cardiomyopathy, and liver disease, whereas mild alcohol intake (< 1 drink/day) may reduce the risk of CVD. Smoking significantly increases the risk of CVD but not hypertension directly. Weight reduction can reduce the risk of CVD but not hypertension. Reduction of work stress can help reduce hypertension but alcoholism is the major concern for this man.

36. (B). This is an acute coronary syndrome with cardiac ischemia, which leads to noncompliance of the left ventricle and S4 gallops. A displaced PMI towards the left is typical of left ventricular hypertrophy and dilated cardiomyopathy. Continuous "machinery" murmurs are characteristic of patent ductus arteriosus. Triphasic scratchy sounds are typical of chronic pericarditis. Kussmaul sign (E) is mostly associated with constrictive pericarditis.

37. (C). This is a case of hypertensive heart failure with pulmonary edema. The best treatment is IV furosemide to remove a large volume of fluid followed by nitroprusside to immediately reduce both preload and afterload of the heart. Metoprolol and valsartan can be added in the maintenance treatment of hypertension with HF, but the beta1 blocker should be watchfully used. Digoxin should be avoided with HTN and nifedipine is contraindicated in HF.

38. (F). This is a typical case of congestive heart failure (CHF) and the most common cause of death is from ventricular arrhythmia provoked by cardiac ischemia, not from direct pulmonary edema, dyspnea, emboli, or myocardial infarction or rupture. A diuretic and vasodilator are first-line therapies (especially with hypertension) to reduce preload, afterload, and mortality.

39. (B). Presentations are characteristic of ASD, which is associated with alcoholism, Down syndrome, etc. Echocardiography confirms Dx. Most small ASDs close spontaneously.

40. (D). CA is often associated with Turner syndrome and Berry aneurysm. It's diagnosed by echocardiogram and treated with surgery.

41. (H). This is a case of "TA + VSD + Down syndrome". TA is associated with early cyanosis at birth, 90% with VSD. VSD here has partially compensated for the reduced R-ventr and pulmonary artery blood flow from TA. Tx: Administer PGE1 to keep ASD and VSD open for survival.

42. (E). Fallot tetralogy is associated with Down syndrome and with gradual cyanosis and HF. Administer PGE1 followed by surgery to correct it.

Chapter 3

DISEASES OF THE RESPIRATORY SYSTEM

PULMONARY FUNCTION TESTS (PFTs)

Main applications

1. Categorization of different types of lung diseases—restrictive versus obstructive (Table 3-1).

2. Evaluation of disease severity—for surgery and prognosis.

3. Post-treatment evaluation of pulmonary function.

Commonly used PFTs

1. **Static lung volumes**: Total lung capacity (**TLC**) and residual volume (**RV**). Decreases indicate restrictive lung disease. Increases indicate obstructive lung disease.

2. **Airflow**: It is mostly measured by expiratory flow rate—**FEV_1/FVC** (ratio of forced expiratory volume in 1 sec to forced vital capacity). In an obstructive lung disease (asthma, emphysema, or chronic bronchitis), peak flow is diminished, FEV_1/FVC is decreased, and residual volume and TLC are increased.

3. **Alveolar membrane permeability—Diffusing capacity (DC):** Measured by the diffusing capacity of a gas in the lung, usually the one with carbon monoxide (**DLCO**). DC decrease exists in all interstitial lung diseases, most restrictive diseases, and some obstructive diseases (such as emphysema).

4. **Methacholine challenge** test: It can be used to evaluate bronchial hyperreactivity.

5. **Evaluation criteria:** < 80% of any predicted lung volume or flow rate is considered abnormal, whereas > 110% of the predicted values is considered air trapping.

PEARLS—Table 3-1: Obstructive Versus Restrictive Lung Diseases by PFTs

Measurement	Obstructive	Restrictive
FEV1	Low	Normal or slightly low
FEV1/FVC	**Low**	**Normal or high**
Peak expiratory flow rate	Low	Normal
Residual volume	High	Various
Total lung capacity	**High**	**Low**
Vital capacity	Low	Low

RESPIRATORY TRACT INFECTIONS

See "Chapter 1 INFECTIOUS DISEASES".

GAS EXCHANGE DISORDERS AND RESPIRATORY FAILURE

The cardiac output, hemoglobin (Hb) levels and the O_2-saturation, and the **arterial oxygen tension** (PaO_2) are the most important factors to deliver maximum O_2 to the needed organs. There will be minimal changes in O_2 delivery even if the PaO_2 is increased from 60 to 100 mmHg by giving patient 100% O_2.

The alveolar-arterial gradient (PAO_2-PaO_2 gradient) is useful in the assessment of oxygenation.

PAO_2-PaO_2 gradient $= 150 - 1.25 \times PCO_2 - PaO_2 = 5\sim15$ (Normal, Nl).

If the gradient is >15 after 100% O_2 inhalation, suspect "shunt" —**V/Q mismatch** due to:

(1) Atelectasis;

(2) Pulmonary edema or fibrosis;

(3) Vascular shunt within the lungs: pulmonary artery embolism (PE);

(4) Intra-cardiac shunt (right-left): VSD, ASD.

FiO_2 means inspired O_2 fraction (0.21 = room air), also used for the assessment of oxygenation.

Atelectasis

It's a collapse of part or the entire lung, commonly occurring < 24 hours after a surgery and due to poor inspiration or lack of coughing during this period of time. A mucous plug, tumor or foreign body can also lead to atelectasis. Thus atelectasis can be classified as obstructive (resorptive) or nonobstructive (pleural disease, parenchymal compression, surfactant dysfunction, scarring or infiltrative disease of the lung, etc.).

Essentials of diagnosis

1. Acute disease usually presents with tachycardia, dyspnea, fever, and hypoxemia.
2. Chronic cases may be asymptomatic, with only abnormal X-ray results.

3. On CXR, the atelectatic lobe appears densely consolidated and smaller than the normal lobe. Upper lobe atelectasis can appear as tracheal deviation to the affected side (secondary to volume loss from atelectasis). Lower lobe atelectasis may cause an elevation of the corresponding part of the diaphragm. Massive atelectasis may lead to a mediastinal shift to the involved side.

Treatment

1. Treat underlying cause. In the postoperative phase, it is important to help patients move early, induce deep breathing, and stimulate coughing. Incentive spirometry and pulmonary flushing are effective.

Atelectasis

2. For patients without abundant secretions, continuous positive airway pressure may be beneficial. For patients with abundant secretions, chest physiotherapy and suctioning are recommended. Bronchoscopy with subsequent removal of mucous plugs is the treatment of choice for spontaneous atelectasis (with secretions).

Acute Respiratory Distress Syndrome (ARDS) *FA5(P. 62(*

ARDS is characterized by increased permeability of the alveolar-capillary membrane and pulmonary edema, which eventually lead to severe hypoxemia, decreased pulmonary compliance, non-cardiogenic pulmonary edema, and acute respiratory failure. The general mortality is 30%−40%. It is also considered a restrictive lung disease.

Causes include trauma, pneumonia, sepsis, shock, pancreatitis, DIC, burns, drug overdose, inhaled toxins, Goodpasture syndrome, multiple transfusions, SLE, drowning, bypass surgery, etc. ARDS mostly develops within the first 24 hours of the initial attack. *diffuse alveolar dmg*

Essentials of diagnosis

1. History of the above causes, along with dyspnea, tachypnea, tachycardia, cyanosis, labored breathing, and diffuse rales and rhonchi on auscultation.

2. Recognize that ARDS can be developed in **4 phases**.
<1 week
Phase 1: Acute injury period, with normal P/E +/- respiratory alkalosis.

Phase 2: 6-48 hour period, with respiratory distress and increased A-a PO_2 gradient.

Phase 3: With typical signs of respiratory failure.

Phase 4: Life-threatening period, with severe hypoxemia and respiratory-metabolic acidosis unresponsive to most treatments.

3. **Lab diagnosis:**
Bilateral   *noncardiogenic pulm edema*
(1) CXR usually shows diffuse interstitial or alveolar infiltrates/opacities (Phase 3).

(2) ABG reveals decreased PaO_2 (< 100 on a supplemental oxygen fraction of 50%) and increased or normal $PaCO_2$ (Phase 2-3).

(3) Swan-Ganz catheter will reveal normal cardiac output and normal capillary wedge pressure (≤18 mmHg) but increased pulmonary artery pressure.

4. **Diagnostic criteria**

(1) Acute onset of respiratory distress without evidence of cardiac origin (capillary wedge pressure ≤ 8 mmHg).

(2) No evidence of left atrial hypertension: PaO_2/FiO_2 ratio ≤200 mmHg.

(3) Bilateral pulmonary infiltrates on CXR.
opacities
Treatment

Diffuse alv. hemorrhage:
- caused by DAD
- drugs, rheum conditions
- cough, fever, hemoptysis,
↓ in hemoglobin.

ARDS

1. Treat underlying disorders and precipitating conditions. Be cautious about using sedatives and neuromuscular blockers.

$\uparrow$PPEER $\downarrow$TV, $\uparrow FiO_2$

2. Maintain adequate perfusion and O_2 delivery to the organs. Mechanical support with increased positive end-expiratory pressure (PEEP) will help achieve adequate oxygenation ($PaO_2 > 60$ mmHg or $SaO_2 > 90\%$). PEEP is monitored by the cardiac output. Low tidal volumes are usually maintained to minimize injuries from mechanical ventilation. Conservative fluid therapy should aim at CVP < 4 mmHg. Corticosteroids may be helpful when given within the first 2 weeks after the onset of ARDS. If the patient has very severe gas exchange abnormalities (E.g., $PaO_2/FiO_2 \leqslant 120$ mmHg), it might be best for him/her to be treated with up to 48 hours of neuromuscular blockade while further investigation is under way.

Acute Respiratory Failure (ARF)

ARF or **acute hypercapnic respiratory failure** is a pathologic status when pulmonary function decreases to cause $PaCO_2 > 45$ mmHg, PaO_2 **under 60,** and respiratory acidosis (pH < 7.35). Mortality rate can be as high as $60\%-70\%$.

Causes are mostly similar to those of hypoxemia and ARDS, including hypoventilation (asthma, obstruction, pulmonary edema, etc.), right-to-left intracardiac shunt, V/Q mismatch (pulmonary embolism), diffusion impairment, and low O_2 content. Triggering factors include bronchitis, pneumonia, sepsis, trauma, pulmonary embolism (**PE**), toxins, etc.

Essentials of diagnosis

1. Hypoxemic manifestations: Tachypnea, short of breath (SOB), cyanosis, restlessness, pleuritic chest pain, confusion, and delirium.

2. **Lab tests**: Arterial blood gas (ABG) usually shows $PaCO_2 > 45$ mmHg, $PaO_2 < 60$, and abnormal $PAO_2 - PaO_2$ gradient (> 15 suggests "shunt"). Pulse oximetry demonstrates decreased HbO_2 saturation.

3. CXR: It can help demonstrate or rule out ARDS, atelectasis, pneumonia, trauma, and PE, etc.

Treatment

1. Start O_2 inhalation first. Place the patient on a ventilator to increase O_2 saturation by increasing FiO_2, I/E ratio, or positive end-expiratory pressure (PEEP, especially with COPD) to maintain the tidal volume $\geqslant 10$ mL/breath/kg.wt. (E.g., 70 kg.wt is $\geqslant 700$ mL/breath). Increase minute ventilation for hyper-CO_2 patients. Target arterial Hb saturation of $\geqslant 90\%$ ($PaO_2 \geqslant 60$ mmHg). Treat underlying causes.

2. Tracheal intubation—indications: (1) Upper airway obstruction (including retained secretions); (2) hypoxia or respiratory acidosis despite supplemental oxygen; (3) progressive tachypnea, dyspnea, or mental status deterioration; (4) apnea.

OBSTRUCTIVE LUNG DISEASES

Asthma

It's an obstructive lung disease characterized by inflammatory hyperreactivity of the respiratory tree to various stimuli, resulting in **reversible airway obstruction**. A combination of mucosal inflammation, bronchial constriction, and excessive, viscous, mucous plugs produces bronchial obstruction. It is mostly seen in young patients and the prevalence is decreased by adulthood.

Etiology and pathogenesis

[handwritten: Cold air causes mastcell degranulation => broncho constriction]

1. **Intrinsic or idiosyncratic asthma** occurs in 50% of non-allergic asthmatics. A bronchial reaction occurs secondary to non-immunologic stimuli, such as infections, irritating inhalants, cold air, exercise, and emotional upset. The intrinsic asthma attacks are more severe, and prognosis is less favorable.

2. **Extrinsic (allergic, atopic) asthma** results from sensitization. Specific IgE level is elevated. Family usually has a history of allergic disease. Extrinsic asthma is precipitated by allergens and accounts for about 20% of asthmatics, with better prognosis. Many cases have features of both types.

3. **Exacerbating factors**:

(1) Respiratory **infections—No.1 common** stimuli, RSV in young children and rhinoviruses in adults;

(2) Medicine (aspirin, beta-blockers, tartrazine, etc.).

4. **Pathogenesis**: During the attack, large and small airways become narrowed due to hypertrophy and spasm of bronchial smooth muscle, edema and inflammation of the bronchial mucosa, and production of viscous mucus. The mediators for those reactions are released by the mast cells, lymphocytes, and eosinophils, and include histamine, bradykinin, leukotrienes C, D, and E, and PG E_2, F_{2a}, and D_2.

Essentials of diagnosis

1. Mild attack: General tachypnea, tachycardia, SOB, prolonged expirations, and moderate diffuse wheezing, chest tightness, and cough. It usually occurs within 30 min of exposure to triggers.

2. **Acute severe asthma attack— "Status asthmaticus"**: Accessory muscle respiration, diminished breath sounds, loud wheezing, hyperresonance, and intercostal retraction.

3. **Spirometry or PFTs**: Typically showing an obstructive pattern (Peak flow is diminished, decreased FEV_1/FVC, increased residual volume and TLC), which mostly **reverses with bronchodilation** (by a beta2-agonist). Sometimes the PFTs may be normal during the reversible period. In this case, a methacholine or cold air challenge test should be done, which will show decreased FEV_1/FVC.

4. **ABG**: In the acute phase—a decrease in $PaCO_2$, increase in pH, and normal or low PaO_2. In severe asthma attack—a decreased PaO_2, increased $PaCO_2$, and decreased pH (HCO_3^- usually only increases in COPD). **A normal $PaCO_2$ with an asthmatic patient may indicate respiratory failure during a severe asthma attack!**

5. **CXR** (**Image 13**): Normal in mild cases; hyperinflation in severe asthma. It may help rule out pneumonia, pneumothorax, pneumomediastinum, etc.

[handwritten notes at bottom:]
Severe Life threatening Asthma: acute asthma exacerbation with impending resp failure (sob, access muscles).
Vital sign instability (pulse >120, respirations >30, hypoxia O_2 sat <90%)
RFs: previous intubation
- prev. ICU admission
- poorly ctrl asthma (↑ sx, ↑ albuterol use)

Asthma

6. Variants of asthma: Include nocturnal cough and exercise-induced asthma. The typical **aspirin sensitivity—nasal polyposis syndrome** affects adults with perennial vasomotor rhinitis and then asthma following minimal ingestion of aspirin. There is significant cross-reactivity between aspirin and other NSAIDs (ibuprofen, etc.). Leukotriene inhibitors can be the effective therapy.

Treatment

1. **Immediate relief (aided with supplemental O$_2$):**

(1) **Beta$_2$-R agonist inhalers**: Saligenins (**albuterol/salbutamol**) and the resorcinols (terbutaline, metaproterenol) are the **major therapies** in acute and chronic asthma, ending about 70% of attacks. Inhaled (metered-dose inhalers) beta$_2$-R agonists are the preferred route for maximal bronchodilation with minimal adverse effects. **The most common S/E is tremor. Salmeterol is a long-acting** (12 hours) type of albuterol that is effective in nocturnal cough variant and exercise-induced asthma. Beta-R agonists must be used with caution in patients who have coexisting CAD, hypothyroidism, diabetes, or hypertension.

(2) Anticholinergic drugs (ipratropium bromide): They have particular benefit in patients with heart disease and patients who have risks with the use of beta-R agonists and theophylline. Major disadvantages: They are too slow to achieve the maximal effect (90 min) and only of medium potency.

(3) Aminophylline and theophylline are modest bronchodilators, sometimes of benefit in chronic patients with nocturnal cough by improving contractility of the diaphragm and other respiratory muscles.

2. **Long-term control:**

(1) **Corticosteroids:** First-generation—beclomethasone, prednisone; second-generation with more specific receptor binding in the lungs—fluticasone, budesonide. Inhibit the synthesis of all cytokines and TNF-alpha (by inhibition of NF-kB). They are indicated as the No.1 long-term therapy with more than two asthma attacks per week, showing the optimal effects by inhalation. They are the **main therapy for chronic asthma** in adults and are very effective in reducing airway inflammation. **For severe or persistent chronic asthma, high-dose inhaled steroids along with long-acting beta$_2$-R agonists (inhaled salmeterol) are the most effective treatment**. Systemic IV steroids are used acutely and shortly, and are the last resort for chronic, persistent asthma.

Adverse effects (S/E) of long, systemic use of steroids include oral candidiasis, weight gain, diabetes, hypertension, glaucoma, cataracts, muscle weakness, and osteoporosis.

(2) **Mast cell stabilizers**: **Cromolyn-Na and nedocromil**, slowly inhibiting the release of mediators and used only for prophylaxis in exercise and allergic asthma. They are the first-line chronic **treatment in children**, demonstrating better effects compared to adults. **Anti-IgE agent omalizumab** may be considered with evidence of sensitivity to a perennial allergen. *Pretty much only useful in exercise induced asthma*

(3) **Anti-leukotrienes: Zileuton**—it inhibits 5-lipoxygenase and then reduces leukotriene production (LT-C$_4$, D$_4$, and E$_4$), or competitively antagonizes the main LTD$_4$.

Zafirlukast and montelukast are **LTD$_4$-R antagonists**, spared for severe asthma that is resistant to maximal doses of inhaled steroids, and as a last resort before chronic use of systemic steroids.

(4) **Prevention**: Avoid allergens and any potential exacerbating factors.

Chronic Obstructive Pulmonary Disease (COPD)

COPD is a preventable and treatable disease characterized by nonreversible airflow obstruction and decreased lung function. The airflow limitation is usually progressive and associated with an enhanced chronic inflammatory response in the airways and the lung to noxious particles or gases. Substantial overlap exists between COPD and other disorders with airflow limitation—chronic bronchitis, emphysema, asthma, bronchiectasis, and bronchiolitis. Thus, COPD may be divided into 4-5 stages and forms based on its severity.

Etiology and pathogenesis

Smoking is a major cause of COPD, and 80-90% of COPD are cigarette smokers. Numbers of pack-years of smoking correlates closely to the FEV1 decrease. Airway infections, pollution, and allergies can also lead to bronchitis and COPD.

1. **Chronic bronchitis**: It is considered a common form of COPD. Patients have chronic inflammatory and productive cough for at least 3 months per year for over two consecutive years. Smoking is a major cause and increased airway resistance is the hallmark. Inflammatory mucus plugs in lumens (blocking exodus of CO_2) is the basic pathogenesis.

2. **Emphysema**: Another common form of COPD. Patients have abnormal permanent dilation of air spaces distal to the destructed terminal bronchioles. Decreased pulmonary elastic recoil is the major pathologic mark, but mass exodus of CO_2 is not affected by partial damage of the distal terminal bronchioles. The pathognomonic difference on PFTs for asthma is that the airflow obstruction is reversible. Centrilobular emphysema is mainly associated with smoking, and panlobular emphysema is associated with alpha1-**antitrypsin deficiency** (a rare hereditary autosomal recessive disease associated with liver disease).

3. **Cor pulmonale:** It is considered a late complication of COPD, and occurs with symptoms and signs of right heart failure (RHF) secondary to chronic pulmonary hypertension without any left heart disease. Other causes include pulmonary embolism (PE), asthma, interstitial lung diseases (ILD), cystic fibrosis (CF), sleep apnea, and pneumoconiosis.

Essentials of diagnosis and differentiation   *EKG: right axis deviation 2° to RVH from pulm HTN*

1. **Chronic bronchitis ("The blue bloater"):** Recurrent productive cough with sputum, **cyanosis,** mild dyspnea, rhonchi, wheezes, clubbing, and barrel chest. **PaCO2 is mostly increased**. CXR usually shows increased pulmonary markings (**"dirty lungs"**, **Image 11**). The course is usually longer than 3 months lasting at least 2 years to be diagnosed.

2. **Emphysema ("The pink puffer"):** Dyspnea, **pursed lip breathing**, distant breath sounds, barrel chest, and **minimal cyanosis and cough**. **CXR** (**Image 13**) shows hyperinflation of bilateral lung fields with diaphragm flattening, small heart size, and increase in retrosternal space. **PaCO2 is mostly normal**.

3. **The diagnosis of COPD** should be considered and spirometry performed in all patients who have any combination of dyspnea, chronic cough, or chronic sputum production, especially if there is a history of exposure to triggers of COPD (tobacco smoke, occupational dust) or a family history of chronic lung disease. The physical exam and CXR may vary with the severity of the COPD. **COPD is confirmed by**

COPD

PFTs showing a post-bronchodilator decrease in FEV1/FVC (< 0.7), increased RV, and TLC in COPD. **DLCO is decreased in emphysema but normal in chronic bronchitis**. ABG may show hypoxemia and respiratory acidosis (decreased PaO2, increased PaCO2). **Sputum Gram staining and culture**, blood culture, and sensitivity are done for patients with productive cough and fever.

4. Cor pulmonale: Dyspnea, cyanosis, digital clubbing, and signs of right heart failure (JVD, edema, hepatomegaly). CXR shows enlarged RA, RV, and pulmonary arteries. Echocardiogram reveals right ventricular dilation but normal left ventricular size and function. Give etiologic and symptomatic treatment.

Complications

Hypoxemia, secondary erythrocytosis, chronic respiratory failure, pulmonary hypertension, cor pulmonale, and gradual RHF (right heart failure).

Treatment

1. **Acute COPD exacerbation:**

(1) **Airway and O2**: Give O2 when the PaO2 is acutely < 60 mmHg or with desaturation, to maintain a PaO2 > 60 mmHg, or SaO2 ≥ 90%. Perform PPMV for severe cases and intubation for impending respiratory failure.

(2) **First-line medications**: Inhaled **short-acting bronchodilators are the mainstay of therapy—a beta2-R agonist** (albuterol or terbutaline) or/and an **anticholinergic** (ipratropium or atrovent) for **synergism**, plus IV steroids for best effects. Systemic steroids should be slowly tapered within 2 weeks.

(3) **Antibiotics**: Should be used empirically to cover both Pneumococcus and H. Inf (Hib).

2. **Chronic COPD treatment:**

(1) **Smoking cessation**: the most important, definite intervention to slow the progression—it prolongs the survival rate but does not reduce it to the level of a non-smoker.

(2) Inhaled long-acting beta2-agonists and anticholinergics +/- steroids. If it's still persistent, adding the **phosphodiesterase-4 inhibitor roflumilast** or chronic azithromycin may reduce the frequency of exacerbations.

(3) **Supplemental home oxygen**: It should be started when resting PaO2 is ≤ 55 mmHg or SaO2 is ≤ 88%, and PaO2 is ≤ 60 mmHg for cor pulmonale.

Complication

Acute exacerbations, secondary polycythemia, pulmonary hypertension, and cor pulmonale (after long-standing COPD).

Prognosis and vaccination

Post-bronchodilator FEV1 is the best predictor of survival—the higher the better; the faster the FEV1 declines, the worse the survival rate will be. Despite all the above treatments, **only smoking cessation and supplemental home oxygen can reduce the mortality of COPD. Vaccinations against pneumococcus (every 5 years) and influenza virus (every year) are highly important**.

Bronchiectasis

Bronchiectasis is a syndrome of chronic cough and viscid sputum production associated with **permanent dilation and wall-thickening of small- and medium-sized bronchi** that result from destruction of bronchial elastic and muscular elements. It can occur as focal bronchiectasis secondary to repeated pulmonary infections (such as TB, fungal infections, lung abscess, and pneumonia), or as diffuse bronchiectasis in cystic fibrosis and immotile cilia syndrome (50% of this may have Kartagener syndrome). Exacerbations are usually caused by acute bacterial infections. The disease is less common now probably due to timely antibiotic treatment for infections.

Essentials of diagnosis

1. Chronic/persistent cough, copious foul-smelling purulent sputum production, wheezes, crackles, hemoptysis (various), and dyspnea.

2. Significant history of recurrent pulmonary infections (mostly Gram⁻ bacteria), sinusitis, and immunodeficient disorders. Hypoxemia and secondary polycythemia may occur.

3. **Lab diagnosis: CXR (Image 13)** may be normal or with streaking shadowing in early stage, and later will show 1-2cm cysts, wall thickening, and crowding of the bronchi (**tram-tracking**). High-resolution **CT scan of the chest is the best** noninvasive test. PFTs reveal an obstructive pattern.

Treatment

1. **Antibiotics: Antibiotics:** (1) **For out-patients** with mild-moderate symptoms: Amoxicillin, **amoxicillin plus clavulanate** (beta-lactamase producing bacteria), doxycycline, or a fluoroquinolone (multiple bacteria) should be used. (2) **For in-patients (severe or with pneumonia): IV antibiotics for >10 days that cover Gram- bacteria (Hib, Pseudomonas, etc.) —antipseudomonal (ceftazidime or cefepime) or antipseudomonal penicillins in combination with a beta-lactamase inhibitor (piperacillin-tazobactam or ticarcillin-clavulanate).** Rotating antibiotics is helpful to diminish resistance by microorganisms.

2. Bronchodilators (albuterol), chest physical therapy, and postural drainage are used to control and improve drainage of bronchial secretions. Bronchial hygiene is very important.

3. Indications for surgery: Recurrent bronchiectasis with failure of medical treatment, massive hemoptysis, or with a lung abscess.

4. **Vaccinations**: All patients with bronchiectasis require pneumococcal and influenza vaccines.

Complications

Massive hemoptysis, amyloidosis, cor pulmonale, and visceral abscesses.

Cystic Fibrosis (CF)

CF is an autosomal recessive disease predominantly affecting young Caucasians (white) people. The defect in chloride-channel protein due to the CFTR gene mutation on chromosome 7, causing impaired chloride and water transport, which leads to widespread exocrine gland dysfunctions with excessively

Cystic Fibrosis

thick, viscous secretions in the respiratory tract, exocrine pancreas, sweat glands, intestines, and genitourinary tract. CF is traditionally considered a pediatric disorder but now the median survival age is over 30 years.

Essentials of diagnosis *Prenatal screen - meconium ileus - H2O enema - recurrent pulm inf xns   mom: kid tastes salty*

1. CF typically results in obstructive lung disease pattern, presenting with chronic cough, sputum production, dyspnea, wheezing, cyanosis, hemoptysis, bronchiectasis, chronic sinusitis, or digital clubbing, accompanied with recurrent, aggressive respiratory infections with Pseudomonas, Hib, or S. aureus. *→ failure to thrive*

2. Pancreatic insufficiency, recurrent pancreatitis, nutritional deficiencies, steatorrhea, biliary cirrhosis, gallstones, distal intestinal obstruction, and male genital abnormalities, etc.

3. **Diagnosis is confirmed by sweat chloride test—concentration above 60 mEq/L on two occasions.** If chloride testing is intermediate, cystic fibrosis transmembrane conductance regulator **(CFTR) gene analysis** should be done to confirm. CFTR genotyping is also necessary for most patients to determine if they carry one of the mutations approved for ivacaftor use.

Treatment *1) screen 2) confirm sweat chloride test*

1. Respiratory system: Long-term antibiotics (oral azithromycin for age > 6), inhaled bronchodilators (beta2-agonists) or steroids, high-dose ibuprofen (if the lung function is good), chest physical therapy and DNase I are recommended. For all ≥ 2-y/o patients being positive for ivacaftor-approved mutations, **ivacaftor** is used. *Pulm toilet, Also Pseudomonas*

2. Digestive system: pancreatic enzymes and fat-soluble Vit (A, D, E, K) for malabsorption.

3. Lung or pancreas transplantation may be the only definitive treatment for advanced CF.
genetic counseling - ① don't procreate → pass this disease. ② you're infertile bro absence of sperm canal

RESTRICTIVE AND INTERSTITIAL LUNG DISEASES

Restrictive lung diseases and interstitial lung diseases associated with hypersensitivity, environmental exposure, and granulomas have been included in this category.

Hypersensitivity Pneumonitis (HP)

It's also known as **extrinsic allergic alveolitis**, defined as hypersensitive reactions of the lungs after environmental exposure to antigens. Chronic exposure may lead to alveolar thickening, granulomas, and restrictive lung disease.

Etiology

1. Spores of actinomycetes can cause "Farmer's lung", "Air conditioner lung", "Mushroom worker's lung", or "Bagassosis" (from dust of sugarcane processing).

2. Antigens from bird's feathers and excreta can cause "Bird fancier's lung".

3. Spores of Aspergillus can cause "Malt worker's lung".

4. Grain weevil (an insect) dust may cause "Miller's/Grain handler's lung".

Essentials of diagnosis

1. Acute HP: Symptoms usually start 4-6 hours after exposure to provocative antigens -- dyspnea, cough, fever, shivering, and malaise.

2. Chronic HP: Patient mostly presents with progressive dyspnea, P/E reveals bilateral rales.

3. Lab tests: CXR is usually normal, or shows military nodular infiltrate in acute disease and upper-lobe fibrosis in chronic disease. Bronchoalveolar lavage shows lymphocytosis; positive inhalation challenge testing; histology with noncaseating granulomas or a mononuclear cell infiltrate.

Treatment

1. The cornerstone of prevention and treatment is **environmental controls to reduce or eliminate exposure to the agricultural dusts, bioaerosols, and chemicals that cause HP.**

2. All patients with HP should be strongly encouraged to avoid or minimize ongoing exposure. In patients with mild or moderate HP, avoidance may be adequate to resolve the clinical manifestations.

3. **Glucocorticoids should be used in severely symptomatic patients**, especially if there is physiologic and radiographic evidence of progression of disease.

4. Advanced chronic HP may be best treated with lung transplantation.

Eosinophilic Pulmonary Syndrome

It is a diverse group of interstitial lung diseases with hypersensitivity, characterized by **eosinophilic pulmonary infiltration (CXR) and blood eosinophilia**. This group of diseases can be acute or chronic and includes allergic broncho-pulmonary Aspergillosis, acute eosinophilic pneumonia, and Loeffler syndrome.

Etiology

1. Helminth infections: Ascaris, hookworms, Strongyloides, Paragonimus lung flukes or cestodes, Trichinella, and Schistosomia.

2. Nonhelminthic infections: Coccidioidomycosis and Mycobacterium tuberculosis (less common).

Essentials of diagnosis

1. Symptoms of dyspnea, cough, and fever after exposure to allergic agents or parasites.

2. CBC shows peripheral eosinophilia. CXR reveals peripheral pulmonary infiltrates.

Differential diagnosis

Churg-Strauss syndrome:

It's a granulomatous vasculitis characterized by asthma, pulmonary infiltrates, rash, muscle pain, and significant eosinophilia. Perinuclear antineutrophilic cytoplasmic antibody (+) helps confirm diagnosis.

Treatment

Treat underlying cause. **Glucocorticoids** can effectively control inflammation. Avoid re-exposure to known antigens.

Idiopathic Pulmonary Fibrosis (IPF, Usual Interstitial Pneumonia)

IPF is an inflammatory lung disease of unknown origin that causes lung fibrosis and restrictive lung disease without extra-pulmonary manifestations except clubbing. It mostly occurs in the 50's of life after possible occupational exposure of < 5 years, and more often in men and smokers. The mean survival is only 3-7 years after the initial diagnosis is made.

Essentials of diagnosis

1. Chronic, progressive exercise intolerance and dyspnea are most common, with coarse dry crackles on auscultation.

2. **PFTs** demonstrate obvious **restrictive** intrapulmonary process.

3. **CXR** may show reticular, nodular lesions (**diffuse fibrosis**). **CT** scan usually reveals "**ground-glass or honeycombing**" appearance without calcification. Bronchoalveolar lavage may show nonspecific increase in macrophages.

Treatment

1. There is generally no effective treatment except for supportive care (supplemental oxygen, pulmonary rehabilitation, and pneumococcal and influenza vaccinations).

2. For patients with mild-to-moderate IPF, **pirfenidone or nintedanib** may be helpful. Corticosteroids and cytotoxic agents (azathioprine, cyclophosphamide) should not be routinely used due to limited benefits. The rest of patients may progress to advanced lung fibrosis and gradual respiratory failure, which may require lung transplantation. The best prognostic indicator may be the response to steroids, which is assessed by PFTs.

Environmental Lung Disease — Pneumoconiosis

It is an occupational lung disease in which inhalation of certain fibers generates a chronic, inflammatory process leading to progressive pulmonary fibrosis. Usually it occurs after more than 15-year constant exposure to offending chemicals (metal mining of gold, silver, lead, copper) but can develop in less than 10 years when dust contents of those agents are extremely high.

Pathogenesis

Alveolar macrophages engulf offending agents, causing inflammation and fibrosis of the lung parenchyma in pneumoconiosis. Respiratory insufficiency is the ultimate consequence of silicosis and the other pneumoconioses. Treatment is mainly supportive care plus O_2 supply.

Essentials of diagnosis

1. **History of occupational exposure for > 10 years** is very important for the diagnosis.

2. Non-specific symptoms and signs of exertional dyspnea, shortness of breath, cough with sputum, clubbing, and cor pulmonale.

3. **PFTs** demonstrate a **restrictive pattern** with a decreased DLCO. Hypoxemia is evident with an increased PA_{O2}-Pa_{O2} gradient.

4. **CXR** (**Image 15**) mostly shows multiple small irregular opacities, interstitial densities, and **"ground glass"** or **"honeycombing"** appearance.

Specific types

I. Coal Miner's Lung (Coal worker's Pneumoconiosis)

(1) Depending on the amount and time of coal dust (containing carbon and silica) exposure, most patients will have simple coal worker's pneumoconiosis (exertional dyspnea) without significant respiratory dysfunction, whereas some may develop complicated fibrosis and restrictive lung disease.

(2) Lab: CXR usually shows small round, **nodular densities** usually in the upper lung zones. Large densities with **massive fibrosis** can be seen in severe progressive disease. Lab testing may show immunologic abnormalities—IgA, IgG, C_3, ANA, and rheumatoid factor may increase.

(3) **Diagnosis** is mainly based on the exposure history, CXR, and exclusion.

(4) **Differential diagnosis—Caplan syndrome:** Coal miner's lung plus rheumatoid arthritis plus rheumatoid nodules in the pulmonary periphery.

(5) **Treatment:** Symptomatic and supportive care. Lung transplantation is the last option.

II. Asbestosis

(1) It's caused by inhalation of asbestos fiber dust, mostly from mining, milling, foundry work, ship-yards, or the application of asbestos products to pipes, brake linings, insulation, and boilers.

(2) Most patients are asymptomatic until 20 years later, with progressive dyspnea with exertion.

(3) **Lab: CXR** shows **hazy infiltration with bilateral linear opacities,** effusions, pleural thickening, plaques, and calcification in the **lower lobes**. A **lung biopsy**, which shows barbell-shaped asbestos fiber, is usually necessary for the diagnosis.

(4) **Treatment**: No specific therapy is available except for supportive care (avoidance of exposure, supplemental oxygen, pneumococcal and influenza vaccinations). Death mostly comes from eventual respiratory failure. It is highly important to stop smoking with asbestosis because the **risk of developing bronchogenic carcinoma** (synergistic effects) is 70 times that of the normal population, and less commonly, the risk of peritoneal **malignant mesotheliomas.**

III. Silicosis

(1) Caused by inhalation of silica dust from glass and pottery making, stone-cutting, tunneling, etc.

(2) Acute silicosis (silicoproteinosis) develops a few weeks to a few years after exposure to high concentrations of respirable crystalline silica and results in symptoms—cough, weight loss, fatigue, and pleuritic pain. **CXR** usually shows **a bilateral patchy alveolar filling pattern**.

(3) Chronic silicosis (includes simple and massive fibrosis) has multiple, rounded nodules (<10mm). It typically appears 10 to 30 years after exposure, mainly with progressive dyspnea with exertion. Accelerated silicosis develops within 10 years of the initial exposure and is associated with high levels of exposure. **CXR** typically shows **localized nodular hyaline opacities with calcification—the pathologic mark,** which is most prominent in the **upper lobe zones**. **Eggshell calcification** is typical but rare. In progressive massive fibrosis, densities look like large masses (>10 mm).

(4) **Diagnosis**: Based upon the exposure history, typical CXR, and exclusion. A bronchoalveolar lavage (BAL) showing milky and lipoproteinaceous effluent is helpful.

(5) **Treatment**: No specific therapy is available except for supportive care. Death occurs usually due to respiratory failure. Silicosis is highly associated with pulmonary TB; therefore, the patient should have yearly PPD tuberculin testing. Patient with positive PPD (> 10 mm) should get isoniazid (INH) prophylaxis for 9 months. Lung transplantation may be the last resort for advanced disease.

IV. Berylliosis

It is a chronic lung inflammation caused by inhaling dust or fumes that contain beryllium (metal or alloy) and is characterized **by noncaseating granulomas in the lungs**. It shares many clinical and histopathological features with pulmonary sarcoidosis, and differs from other occupational lung diseases in that lung inflammation occurs only **in people sensitive to beryllium**, even at low levels of exposure.

(1) Diagnosis is based on the exposure history—**high-tech fields** (electronics, nuclear power, telecommunications and aerospace), foundries, ceramics, plating, dental materials, and dyes; a positive beryllium lymphocyte proliferation test (BeLPT); **CXR** showing **diffuse infiltration and hilar adenopathy**; and the presence of noncaseating granulomas (if biopsy is possible).

(2) **Treatment**: **Steroid (prednisone) therapy** is recommended for both acute and chronic disease to slow progression, as well as symptomatic treatment.

Systemic Sarcoidosis

Sarcoidosis is a multisystem disease of unknown etiology, characterized by nonspecific **noncaseating granulomas in the lung (mostly) and other organs** such as the eyes, skin, heart, GIT, and the joints. It's more common among 30-40 y/o patients and Blacks.

Essentials of diagnosis

1. Most of the sarcoidosis is found in an asymptomatic patient, usually in the form of **bilateral hilar adenopathy on a CXR (90% of cases; Image 16)**. Common symptoms include cough, dyspnea, chest pain, eye lesions, and/or skin lesions.

2. There are two distinct acute sarcoid syndromes:

(1) **Lofgren syndrome**: Erythema nodosum, arthritis, eosinophilia in the blood, and hilar adenopathy by CXR.

(2) **Heerfordt-Waldenstrom syndrome**: Fever, parotid enlargement, uveitis, and facial palsy.

3. **Lab tests**:

(1) **Hyper-Ca or hypercalcuria**, caused by high Vit-D (produced by macrophages).

(2) Nonspecific **increase in ACE** in 60% of patients; used for the follow-up of the disease.

(3) Abnormal liver function tests may exist in 30% patients with hepatic lesion and symptoms.

4. Other findings: Skin anergy, and normal or restrictive PFTs. Ophthalmologic exam is always necessary to check uveitis.

5. **Definitive diagnosis is biopsy** of suspected tissues, which shows noncaseating granulomas.

Treatment

1. An initial trial of **topical steroids** can be used in skin lesions.

2. For more severe sarcoidosis, **systemic glucocorticoids (prednisone) is the main treatment.** Methotrexate or doxycycline may be used to reduce the organ impairment. Mandatory indications of steroid use include uveitis, CNS-sarcoidosis, and hypercalcemia. If the above therapy fails, a trial of anti-TNF therapy (infliximab, adalimumab, or thalidomide) may be considered. However, most of the treatment may not change the course of the disease.

Prognosis

80% of patients remain stable or resolved and 20% progress into end-organ complications.

ALVEOLAR FILLING DISEASES

Anti-GBM Antibody (Goodpasture) Disease

Anti-glomerular basement membrane (anti-GBM) antibody disease is a rare **autoimmune disease (type II) caused by IgG antibody against GBM and alveolar basement membranes.** It's also considered a nephritic syndrome (see Chapter 7). Patients usually present with rapidly progressive glomerulonephritis, and with pulmonary involvement (alveolar hemorrhage) in 50-60% of cases.

Essentials of diagnosis

1. Typical manifestations include **hemorrhagic pneumonitis (hemoptysis, dyspnea) and rapidly progressive glomerulonephritis (hematuria, acute renal injury,** nephritic urine sediment, and non-nephrotic proteinuria). Systemic symptoms are usually absent unless vasculitis in involved.

Anti GBM antibody dz Good pasture

2. **Diagnosis is usually made by positive anti-GBM IgG in serology**. Kidney biopsy showing linear deposits of IgG in the specimen is diagnostic, and activity of renal involvement may help guide therapy. If tissue biopsy is not available, Western blot testing may be added.

3. Note that 40% of patients with anti-GBM antibody disease also test positive for ANCA at the time of diagnosis and may have a systemic vasculitis, which may alter treatment decisions and indicate worse prognosis.

Treatment

Early diagnosis and treatment are critical for achieving the best response to therapy with minimal crescents formed in the kidney. The treatment of choice is **plasmapheresis in conjunction with immunosuppression—prednisone and cyclophosphamide for 2-3 months**. Plasmapheresis removes circulating anti-GBM antibodies and other mediators of inflammation, such as complement, and the immunosuppressive agents minimize new antibody formation. Prognosis varies. If left untreated, this disease usually progresses rapidly to end-stage renal failure. Recovery of kidney function is rare if dialysis is required at initiation of treatment.

Pulmonary Alveolar Proteinosis (Phospholipoproteinosis) (PAP)

It's a rare condition caused by diffuse accumulation of **surfactant-like, lipoproteinaceous and phospholipid material in the alveoli. There are three main categories of PAP: (1) Autoimmune and hereditary PAP**—disruption of granulocyte-macrophage colony-stimulating factor signaling; **(2) Congenital PAP—disorders of surfactant production; (3) Secondary PAP**—develops in adulthood associated with high level dust exposures (silica, aluminum, titanium, or indium-tin oxide), hematologic dyscrasias, etc.

Essentials of diagnosis

1. Patient usually presents with dry cough, dyspnea, hypoxia, and rales.

2. **Lab**: Typical **BAL fluid has an opaque or milky appearance** and cytology reveals alveolar macrophages engorged with **PAS-positive** material. Suspected adult patients should have serologic testing for antibodies to granulocyte macrophage-colony stimulating factor (**GM-CSF**). **CXR typically shows a ground-glass appearance with bilateral alveolar infiltrates resembling a bat shape.**

3. **Definitive diagnosis** is made by **lung biopsy** (filling with flocculent, granular lipoproteinaceous material that stains pink with PAS stain).

Treatment

For asymptomatic or mild cases despite extensive radiographic abnormalities, observation is recommended. For patients with severe dyspnea and hypoxemia, whole lung lavage via a double-lumen endotracheal tube is recommended. **Rituximab and therapeutic plasma exchange** may be helpful. Steroids are not beneficial to patients and may cause more infections. Generally, no effective therapies have been confirmed presently.

Cryptogenic Organizing Pneumonia (COP)

Cryptogenic (or bronchiolitis obliterans) organizing pneumonia (**COP**) is one of the idiopathic interstitial pneumonias. Etiology is unknown. When organizing pneumonia is seen in association with other processes, such as connective tissue diseases, certain drugs, or malignancy, it is called secondary organizing pneumonia.

Essentials of diagnosis

1. Common manifestations include cough, dyspnea, and flu-like symptoms.

2. CXR often shows bilateral ground-glass patchy infiltrates. BAL is frequently used to evaluate for infection, hemorrhage, and malignancy. Biopsy as the means of confirmation usually shows excessive proliferation or "plugs" of granulation tissue within alveolar ducts and alveoli.

Treatment

For patients with moderate to severe symptoms, **corticosteroids can be used, with over 60% of cases alleviated**. If steroids fail, immunosuppressive agents (cyclophosphamide or azathioprine) may be tried. Antibiotics are generally not effective. Relapses may occur after cessation of steroids.

DISEASES OF THE PULMONARY VASCULATURE

Pulmonary Embolism (PE)

PE is a blockage of one or more pulmonary arteries by an embolus, a serious and potentially fatal pathologic condition and a common complication of deep venous thrombosis (**DVT**, about 70%) mostly from the lower body. **Virchow's triad** for venous thrombosis is stasis, endothelial damage, and hypercoagulable state. A small proportion of cases are due to the embolization of air, fat, talc in drugs of IV drug abusers or amniotic fluid. The obstruction of the blood flow through the lungs and the resultant pressure on the right ventricle of the heart lead to the symptoms and signs of PE. Efficient clinical evaluation and testing is necessary before anticoagulation therapy to reduce mortality.

Etiology

PEARLS: Typical PE patients—pregnant/postpartum, oral contraceptive users, smokers, long-distance travellers (in cars, planes, etc.). _Prophylactic dose anticoag does not elim. risk_

High-risk factors include venous stasis (surgery, long-term immobility, pregnancy), > 40 y/a with history of DVT or PE, OCP use, cancer, and hypercoagulable state or thrombophilias (Factor V Leiden, antithrombin III deficiency, protein C or S deficiency, and antiphospholipid syndrome). Factor V Leiden is the #1 cause of thrombophilia among European patients, in which the protein C level is normal but non-functional.

Essentials of diagnosis

Pulm Embolism

dx:

dyspnea, hypoxemia

1. **Sudden onset of dyspnea along with tachypnea, tachycardia, and chest pain** is the most common symptom. Syncope may occur with massive PE, accompanied with fever, diaphoresis, cough, and hemoptysis. However, many patients have mild or nonspecific symptoms.

2. **CT pulmonary angiography** has essentially supplanted V/Q scanning as **the preferred** imaging modality. The demonstration of a filling defect in any branch of the pulmonary artery (main, lobar, segmental, subsegmental) by contrast enhancement is diagnostic of PE. It's the gold-standard testing for confirmation of PE but is invasive (with certain mortality).

3. **Ventilation-perfusion lung scanning (V/Q scan):** A high-probability V/Q scan (showing a defect on perfusion) is sufficient to diagnose PE, whereas a normal scan is sufficient to exclude clinically significant PE. All other patterns (low or intermediate probability) are nondiagnostic. V/Q scanning is sensitive but not highly specific because abnormally matched V/Q defects may also be seen with pneumonia, pleural effusion, or asthma. *for pts w renal insuff or allergy*

4. **Contrast-enhanced or magnetic resonance pulmonary angiography:** The demonstration of a filling defect or abrupt cutoff of a vessel on either of these modalities is diagnostic of an embolus. However, nondiagnostic scans are reported when the filling defect is not clearly visualized.

5. **Venous thrombosis studies: Doppler ultrasound (U/S)** may be good to initially diagnose suspected lower limb DVTs before angiography. **Contrast venography** is the gold-standard test for lower DVTs. **MRI** has similar sensitivity and specificity as contrast venography.

6. **Others:** (1) **ABG** is sensitive and helpful in showing **low PO_2, low PCO_2, a widened alveolar-arterial PO_2 difference**, and mild respiratory alkalosis (hyperventilation). Negative ABG results may exclude PE. (2) **CXR** is necessary to exclude other common lung diseases and aid in V/Q scan, but it does not establish the diagnosis by itself. It may be normal or sometimes show platelike atelectasis (Kerley B lines), wedge-shaped infarct (Hampton hump), or oligemia (Westermark's sign). (3) **ECG** usually shows sinus tachycardia without changes in ST segment, which helps exclude MI.

Treatment

1. **Anticoagulation: It is the mainstay of therapy and a form of secondary prevention for most stable patients.**

(1) **Standard regimen of heparin (including LMWH) followed by 6 months of oral warfarin results in > 80% reduction in the risk of both recurrent venous thrombosis and death from PE.**

 Heparin should be continued for at least 5 days to prolong the PTT to 1.5-2x of the normal value; loading dose plus constant infusion. **Adverse effects of heparin**: Thrombocytopenia occurs in 4% of patients owing to antiplatelet antibodies (7-10 days after the treatment is started). LMWH does not protect against antiplatelet antibodies. Bleeding occurs in 5-10% of patients taking heparin. The antidote to heparin toxicity is protamine sulfate (with hypotensive effect).

(2) **Warfarin: Long-term therapy** is started on day1 and given at a dose to prolong PT (prothrombin time) to 1.3-1.5x baselines for 6 months. Follow INR (International Normalized Ratio) goal of 2-3.

(3) **Coumadin:** It's a Vit-K antagonist that blocks clotting factors 2, 7, 9, and 10. It requires 2-3 days to reach effective levels and 5 days to reach maximal anticoagulation effect. Thus, even though the PT is prolonged after 2-3 days on coumadin treatment, heparin should be continued for more than 5 days.

Tx

Coumadin also inhibits the Vit-K-dependent synthesis of protein C. **Adverse effects of coumadin**: (1) Bleeding and skin necrosis (more common in protein C-deficient patients), because of the initial and transient hypercoagulable effect from the decreased protein C. (2) Teratogenic effects and CNS toxicity: contraindicated in 6-12 weeks of gestation.

2. **Thrombolytics**: Usually not indicated in suspected mild PE due to the fibrinolytic feature of the lung. In patients with established PE, thrombolytic therapy accelerates resolution of emboli within the first 24 hours compared with standard heparin therapy. It is thus **recommended in PE patients at high risk for death (hemodynamically unstable patients or patients with MI)**, which may be lifesaving. **Main contraindications** include uncontrolled hypertension, recent surgery and trauma within the past 6 weeks.

3. **Embolectomy**: It's the therapy in an unstable patient for whom thrombolysis is contraindicated.

4. **DVT prophylaxis:**

Preventive means: Elastic stockings, pneumatic compression stockings, low-dose oral anticoagulants, and heparin SC.

(1) Placement of a Greenfield vena cava filter for patients with a contraindication or with recurrent PE despite adequate anticoagulant therapy.

(2) Administration of heparin SC, LMWH (low molecular weight heparin), intermittent pneumatic compression of the lower limbs for bed-ridden patients with high-risk stasis, and early ambulation with the best effects.

5. **Pregnancy** with PE or DVT: Administration of LMWH for 6 months is required.

Pulmonary Hypertension (PH)

PH is a state of elevated pulmonary vascular resistance (PVR) and pulmonary circulation pressure. **Pulmonary artery hypertension (PAH) is a major type of PH and defined as pulmonary artery pressure $\geq$ 25 mmHg at rest.** It is classified by etiology as primary (idiopathic) and secondary pulmonary hypertension.

Etiology

1. **Idiopathic PH**: Absence of other disease of the lungs or heart. Etiology is unknown but may be associated with genetics. It's more common in young and middle-aged women.

2. **Secondary PH**:

(1) Increased pulmonary venous pressure from mitral valve disease or left-side heart failure.

(2) Increased pulmonary blood flow from congenital heart disease with left-right shunt.

(3) Hypoxic vasoconstriction from COPD; thromboembolic disease; interstitial lung disease.

Essentials of diagnosis

1. Idiopathic PH usually starts early without diseases of the heart or lungs.

2. Secondary PH mostly follows a history of heart disease, PE, COPD, emphysema, or interstitial lung disease.

3. Main manifestations include dyspnea on exertion, chest pain, syncope with exertion, lethargy, fatigue, and signs of right-sided CHF (JVD, lower limb edema, abdominal distention, etc.).

4. P/E will show a loud, split, palpable S_2, a systolic ejection murmur (from tricuspid or pulmonary valve insufficiency), or an S_4.

5. **Lab diagnosis**:

(1) **Echocardiography** as the main tool usually demonstrates RA and RV hypertrophy and suggests PH. If echocardiography is not suggestive of PH but the suspicion is still high, right heart catheterization should be performed. Confirmative diagnosis of PH requires that RHC shows pulmonary artery pressure ≥25 mmHg at rest and mean pulmonary capillary wedge pressure < 15 mmHg.

(2) Others: CXR mostly displays enlarged central pulmonary arteries and narrowing of distal vessels. ECG may reveal RA and RV hypertrophy. CBC may show polycythemia from chronic hypoxia. Helical CT or V/Q scanning may identify chronic PE as the cause of the chronic PH.

Treatment

1. Secondary PH: Treat underlying cause.

2. Idiopathic PH:

(1) Initial supplemental **oxygen and vasodilators** (Ca blockers—diltiazem, prostacyclins) can help reduce pulmonary vascular resistance and symptoms.

(2) If ineffective, either phosphodiesterase inhibitors (sildenafil, tadalafil) or endothelin receptor blockers (bosentan) are recommended.

(3) **Long-term anticoagulation with warfarin** is usually recommended (keeping INR around 2.0) due to venous stasis, physical inactivity, and hypercoagulable states. Diuretics are helpful with right heart failure and edema.

(4) In severe or late-stage PH, pregnancy should be avoided and lung transplantation is recommended.

Complication

Cor pulmonale, etc. Most patients die of right-ventricle failure.

PLEURAL DISEASES

Pleural Effusions

It's the accumulation of transudative or exudative fluid in the pleural cavity.

Types and etiology

1. **Transudative effusions:** Caused by **systemic, mechanical factors**—either increased capillary hydrostatic pressure (as in CHF) or decreased plasma oncotic pressure (as in hypoalbuminemia caused by nephrotic syndrome or cirrhosis). They usually cause bilateral effusions and only need treatment of the primary disease.

2. **Exudative effusions**: Caused by **local, inflammatory factors**—commonly seen in pneumonia, cancer, TB, pancreatitis, trauma, and collagen disease. They are mostly unilateral and in need of further evaluation. Tests of suspected fluid usually include glucose, pH, amylase, triglycerides, differential cell count, microbiology, and cytology.

Pulmonary embolism (**PE**) can cause either a transudate or exudate. If a patient has a transudative effusion but no apparent cause, consider PE.

Parapneumonic effusions: Caused by bacterial pneumonias, and should be demonstrated by a positive Gram stain or culture, or a pH < 7.2, or a glucose level < 60 mg/dL. A thoracentesis is required to rule out a complicated parapneumonic effusion—empyema, which requires drainage.

Differential diagnosis

Transudative: LDH < 200; LDH: effusion/serum < 0.6; protein: effusion/serum < 0.5.

Exudative: LDH > 200; LDH: effusion/serum > 0.6; protein: effusion/serum > 0.5.

All the above three values in the effusion must be "less than" that in the serum to be transudative (< **200, 0.6, and 0.5**), otherwise the effusion is exudative.

Treatment

Treatment is targeting underlying causes. Complicated parapneumonic effusions and empyema need antibiotics and chest-tube drainage together (chemical pleurodesis talc plus doxycycline is a good option).

Pneumothorax

See "Chapter 15 SURGERY".

NEOPLASMS OF THE RESPIRATORY TRACT

Pulmonary Nodules

It's common to find a pulmonary nodule on an incidental CXR. About 1/3 of all solitary nodules are malignant.

PEARLS: Differential diagnosis and management of pulmonary nodules

1. **Low risk or benign nodule:**

Patient's age < 35 y/a, non-smokers, with a < 2cm calcified nodule, smooth distinct margins, popcorn calcification (caused by hamartomas), bull-eye calcification (caused by granulomas), and stable size in comparison with an old CXR film.

Treatment: CXR follow-up every 3 months for 2 years. Follow-up can be stopped if there is no growth in 2 years.

2. **High risk or malignant nodule:**

A patient > 50 y/a, with a smoking history, and a nodule > 2cm with obscure margins, is more likely to have bronchogenic cancer. The best diagnostic means is chest CT scan followed by a FNA or open-lung biopsy. The best **diagnostic treatment** procedure is to remove the nodule with an open-lung biopsy. Bronchoscopy will not reach peripheral lesions and is only helpful for central tumors.

Lung Cancer--Bronchogenic Carcinoma

Bronchogenic Carcinoma is the most common cause of cancer mortality worldwide for both men and women. The two most common types are adenocarcinoma and squamous cell carcinoma. Small cell lung cancer (SCLC) is less common but more aggressive. The overall 5-year survival rate for SCLC is less than 5% and for non-small cell lung cancer (NSCLC) is less than 10%. There is no efficient screening test for lung cancer so far, and thus early diagnosis is difficult.

Etiology and risk factors

1. **The No.1 risk factor is smoking. 90% of cases are strongly associated with smoking** (only bronchoalveolar cancer is weakly associated). Smoking increases the risk by more than 10 times and is the major cause of lung cancer. If heavy smoking begins from early age, lifetime risk is 15%. Second-hand smoke exposure is more harmful than 1st-hand and has a relative risk of 1.3%.

2. Other risk factors include gender (male > female), age, occupation (exposure to asbestos, arsenic beryllium, hydrocarbons, or nickel), air pollution, and radiation. **Asbestos** exposure increases the risk by more than 70 times.

Pathologic types and features

1. **Adenocarcinoma**: This is **the most common type**, mostly a **peripheral** tumor and metastasized distantly by blood circulation. **Bronchioalveolar** carcinoma is a subtype of adenocarcinoma, a **low-grade** cancer that can occur in single, or multiple nodules, more common in non-smokers (2/3 of cases) and women. **Asbestos** exposure can be an underlying cause with a latent period of 30 years. Adenocarcinoma is usually associated with pleural effusions that have **high hyaluronidase** levels. **Thoracotomy with pleural biopsy** is the most helpful means of diagnosis.

2. **Squamous cell carcinoma (SCC)**: It's **centrally** located, associated with **cavitary** lesions, and **hyper-Ca** (from PTH-like substance). It mostly metastasizes by **direct extension** into the hilar node and mediastinum.

3. **Adenosquamous carcinoma**: With mixed features of the above two types.

4. **Large cell or neuroendocrine carcinoma**: Least common and peripherally located; associated with **cavitation and gynecomastia**. It can metastasize distantly late with poor prognosis.

5. **Small cell lung cancer (SCLC)**: Centrally located; rapidly growing with early distant metastases by blood to liver, adrenal glands, brain, and bone. It's **of neuroendocrine origin and often associated with paraneoplastic syndrome (Cushing syndrome, SIADH, myasthenia or Lambert-Eaton syndrome)**. It is also the **No.1** cause of superior vena cava (**SVC**) syndrome. Prognosis is poor, and not improved by early diagnosis.

Essentials of diagnosis

1. **Perform CXR screening first** for patients with risk factors and any symptom of cough, fatigue, dyspnea, chest pain, hemoptysis, or weight loss. Consider other coexisting conditions such as repeated pneumonia, hematopathy, and dermatomyositis.

2. Suspect **SCLC or Pancoast tumor** if patient has Horner syndrome (miosis, ptosis, anhidrosis), paraneoplastic syndrome, or hypertrophic pulmonary osteoarthropathy. See **Image 17** for SCLC.

3. **Lab diagnosis:**

(1) **Sputum cytology** may have high yield for **squamous cell cancer** (>80% because it is centrally located).

(2) **Bronchoscopy** with biopsy is highly sensitive for the "**central cancer**", and helpful in staging.

(3) **CT scan** of the chest and upper abdomen is required for most suspected patients. **CT**-guided fine needle aspiration (**FNA**) is more sensitive for **peripheral** nodules. New technology **PET** may be better used in operable patients with CT stage IB to IIIA lung cancer.

(4) Thoracoscopic biopsy with open thoracotomy for suspected cancer may supply an effective diagnosis and treatment. Mediastinoscopy is useful in diagnosing and staging mediastinal tumors.

Treatment

1. Stage I and II non-small cell lung cancer (NSCLC): For patients with adequate pulmonary function and without serious medical comorbidity, **surgical lobectomy** is the best initial treatment, followed by adjuvant cisplatin-based chemotherapy for stage II NSCLC, and postoperative radiotherapy for patients with positive surgical resection margins. Video-assisted thoracoscopy (**VATS**) is helpful with decreased operative morbidity and a faster recovery. If the tumor involves the mediastinal lymph nodes in the final surgical specimen, it is stage III disease and treated with combined surgery, radiation, and chemotherapy. Stereotactic body radiation therapy (**SBRT**) is an alternative that has comparable outcomes in selected stage I patients.

2. Nonsurgical cases: (1) For patients with small primary tumors (< 5 cm), impaired pulmonary function (tidal volume < 800 ml), or severe medical conditions that preclude surgical resection, and for those who refuse surgery, **stereotactic body radiation therapy** (SBRT) is recommended.

(2) For **most patients** with **unresectable cancer (SCLC)** or **unresectable signs**—involvement of mediastinal organs or lymph nodes (**N2 or N3**), bilateral tumors, hoarseness, malignant pleural effusion, atelectasis (suggesting central airway obstruction), bone pain or other extrathoracic metastasis, or CNS

symptoms, widely used regimens are combined chemotherapy of **cisplatin and etoposide, in conjunction with radiotherapy.** Superior vena cava (**SVC**) **syndrome** requires urgent radiotherapy.

3. Targeted therapy—targeting the epidermal growth factor receptor (**EGFR**) pathway: **Cetuximab, erlotinib, or crizotinib** is in clinical trial with hope, particularly for late-stage cancer.

Prevention

Smoking avoidance is highly important and CXR screening for risky patients is helpful.

Nasopharyngeal carcinoma (NPC)

NPC is a relatively rare cancer, originating in the nasopharynx and arising from the mucosal epithelium of the nasopharynx. It is more common in male individuals and in certain regions of Southeast Asia (e.g., Guangdong Province, China) and North Africa.

WHO classifies NPC in three types. Type 1 is squamous cell carcinoma. Type 2a (II) is undifferentiated, keratinizing carcinoma. **Type 2b (III) is undifferentiated, nonkeratinizing carcinoma, which is the most common form and associated with EBV** infection. Other possible causes include smoking, genetic susceptibility, and particular foods (such as salted fish) containing carcinogenic volatile nitrosamines.

Essentials of diagnosis

1. Patient may present with **nasal regurgitation, bleeding**, obstruction, a "nasal twang", **headache, and a lump/swelling in the neck** (lymph node metastasis). **The clinical triad** of a neck mass, nasal obstruction with epistaxis, and serous otitis media occurs infrequently. Late signs include hearing loss, trismus, bone pain, and cranial nerve palsies, etc.

2. Lab tests: Cervical lymph node biopsy is performed for diagnosis in many cases (mostly at stage III-IV). For the primary NPC, endoscopy plus biopsy is the definite means of diagnosis. Staging is clinical. Testing of EBV DNA levels is recommended for the treatment monitoring and prognostic significance.

Treatment

(1) **Stage I** (early stage): **Radiotherapy** is the mainstay of treatment.
(2) **Stage II** or higher: **Radiotherapy plus chemotherapy** (gemcitabine-cisplatinc-fluorouracil) reduce the rate of distant metastasis and overall mortality. Surgery is rarely used presently.

Juvenile Nasopharyngeal Angiofibroma (JNA)

JNA is an uncommon benign tumor in the nasopharynx that tends to bleed and usually occurs in adolescent boys.

Diagnostic Triad

1. Easy, recurrent epistaxis.
2. Nasal obstruction (stuffy nose and nasal discharge).

3. Nasopharyngeal mass. Decreased hearing may co-exist.

Treatment

Most episodes of epistaxis respond to simple compression. Treatment with surgery or radiotherapy is only required if the angiofibroma is growing larger, blocking the airways, or causing repeated nosebleeds. However, surgery is difficult.

Differential diagnosis

Nasal polyps:

It's characterized by recurrent rhinitis, chronic nasal obstruction, decreased sense of smell and taste, and persistent postnasal drip. It may be associated with asthma. Treatment can be oral steroids or surgery, but either therapy may have a high incidence of recurrence.

MISCELLANEOUS DISEASES

Allergic Rhinitis   *vs nonallergic Rhinitis: Allergic has predominant eye sx, itching, sneezing, ? identifiable trigger*

It's an allergic inflammation of the nasal airways introduced by IgE, usually seasonal. It occurs when an allergen (such as pollen, dust, or animal dander) is inhaled by an individual with preformed IgE, which causes mast cells and basophils to release histamine. Plant pollens cause **pollinosis**, and grass pollens cause **hay fever.** *Nasal congestion, rhinorrhea, sneezing, nasal itch, cough 2° to post-nasal drip, ocular itching ? tearing.*

Essentials of diagnosis

1. Recurrent, seasonal episodes of watery, itchy eyes and nose, and sneezing **without fever**. P/E *can have low-grade fever* usually finds inflamed, boggy nasal mucosa, and pale turbinates and nasal polyps. *Pharyngeal cobblestoning*

2. Diagnosis is usually based on history and clinical presentations. Skin testing and increased specific IgE levels can be helpful.

Treatment

1. Glucocorticoid nasal spray is most effective and adequate for mild to moderate symptoms. If more severe, an antihistamine nasal spray (azelastine, olopatadine) or oral antihistamine (second-generation cetirizine, levocetirizine) can be used. Cromolyn nasal spray is safer for children.

2. Prevention: Avoidance of the precipitating allergen—use of air purifiers, dust filters, and mattress/pillow covers; use of air conditioner (with windows closed); removal of pets that patient is allergic to; desensitization to allergens that patient cannot avoid.

Sleep Apnea

See Chapter 16: Sleep-Wake Disorders.

Chapter 3: High-yield Questions (HYQ)

1. A 60 y/o man with COPD is brought to the emergency room (ER) with tachypnea, shortness of breath (SOB), cyanosis, pleuritic chest pain, and altered mental status. After O_2 supplementation and mechanical ventilation, his PaO2 is 50 and PaCO2 is 35 mmHg. What's the most appropriate next step?
A. Continuous O_2 inhalation and close monitoring   B. Immediate intubation
C. Administer a respiratory center stimulant   D. Treat underlying cause
E. Increase the ventilation pressure

2. A 60 y/o man is dyspneic 24 hours after a general abdominal surgery. Physical examination (P/E) reveals that his HR = 100/min, T = 38.5°C, respiratory rate (RR) = 22/min with decreased breath sounds in the left lower lobe, and mild redness and tenderness around the surgical cut. WBC is 18,000/uL. What's the most appropriate next step?
A. IV antibiotics   B. O_2 inhalation
C. Anti-inflammation drugs   D. Help patient increase activity level and coughing
E. Explore the surgical cut

3. A 40-y-old man is found to have a 2-cm calcified nodule in the right lower lung on routine CXR. He has never had a previous CXR or history of smoking, and generally feels well. P/E results are unremarkable. What's the most appropriate next step for the nodule?
A. CXR follow-up in 3 months   B. Chest CT scan
C. CT-guided FNA (biopsy)   D. Surgical removal and biopsy
E. TB test

4. A 60 y/o smoker has headache, blurry vision, hypertrophic osteoarthritis, synovitis, and clubbing. P/E shows JVD and deformed joints in the hands and feet. Lab tests reveal anemia and hyper-Ca. The most appropriate next step is
A. CXR   B. Chest CT with FNA
C. Sputum cytology   D. Bronchoscopy with biopsy
E. Joint fluid analysis

5. A 30 y/o female who has a recent history of asthma with fever and cough comes to the hospital again with progressive wheezing and shortness of breath for the past week. P/E shows T = 37.5°C, P = 108/min, and RR = 27/min with diffuse wheezing throughout both lungs without crackles. She has taken inhaled albuterol for the past week and has no history of CVD. What's the most appropriate next treatment?
A. Higher albuterol dosage   B. Inhaled steroids + salmeterol
C. IV steroids   D. Zafirlukast (LTD4-R antagonist)
E. Ipratropium (anticholinergic)

6. The above patient has completed a 2-week's course of high-dose inhaled steroids and salmeterol but still has persistent asthma symptoms. What's the most appropriate next treatment now?
A. Higher albuterol dose   B. Higher doses of inhaled steroids and salmeterol

C. Chronic IV steroids   D. Zafirlukast

E. High-dose ipratropium

7. A 30 y/o female is brought to the ER with acute onset of SOB and pleuritic chest pain that occurred while standing from a seated position. She has never been sick before and takes no drugs except oral contraceptives (OCP). Her RR is 26/min and pulse is 107/min. Auscultation and other P/E results are unremarkable. CXR is normal. Her ABG shows $PO_2 = 70$ and $PCO_2 = 35$ mmHg on room air. What's the most appropriate next step?

A. Close observation and supportive care   B. OCP cessation and exercise program

C. Spiral CT on the chest   D. Continuous heparin and warfarin

E. Thrombolytics

8. A 55 y/o man who has worked for 15 years as a shipyard worker complains of fatigue, exertional dyspnea, shortness of breath, cough with sputum, and clubbing. He has smoked for 20 years. CXR shows hazy infiltration with calcification and effusions. PFTs demonstrate a restrictive pattern. What's the most appropriate next step?

A. Lung biopsy at the opacity site   B. Chest CT scan

C. Bronchoscopy   D. Advice on patient's change in occupation

E. Advice on patient's cessation of smoking

9. Continued from Q8: What's the most likely type of pulmonary carcinoma that may be accompanied with this patient?

A. Adenocarcinoma   B. Mesotheliomas

C. Squamous cell carcinoma   D. Small cell lung cancer

E. Large cell carcinoma

10. A 62 y/o man with recurrent and exacerbated COPD is hospitalized for evaluation for lung resection. He has a history of heavy smoking and alcoholism. His daily activities have been affected by the status of the disease. Which of the following is most useful in the evaluation for his surgery?

A. Result of exercise testing   B. Arterial PO_2 level

C. Arterial PCO_2 level   D. Predicted postoperative EFV1

E. PAO_2-PaO_2 gradient

11. A 55 y/o man comes to the clinic for fever, persistent cough, hemoptysis, foul-smelling purulent sputum and cyanosis for the past week. He had similar symptoms with sinusitis 2 months ago and has a 5-year history of smoking. P/E shows low-grade fever, and wheezes and crackles in both lungs. CXR reveals a 2-cm cyst on each side of the lungs. What's the most like diagnosis?

A. Chronic bronchitis   B. Bronchiectasis

C. Acute bronchitis   D. Lung cancer with infection

E. Lung abscesses

12. For the same patient in Q11, what's the most appropriate next step?

A. Sputum cytology   B. Sputum culture and sensitivity

C. PO ceftazidime +/- quinolones   D. IV ceftazidime +/- quinolones

E. CT scan

13. A 35 y/o female comes to the physician with dyspnea on exertion, chest pain, lethargy, fatigue, and lower limb edema for the past month. She has had an occasional cough for the past month and takes no medicine except an OCP. P/E shows a loud split S_2 and a systolic ejection murmur. CXR shows enlarged central pulmonary arteries. ECG and arterial blood gas (ABG) are ordered. Her RR is 25/min and pulse is 105/min. What's the most likely diagnosis?

A. Pulmonary embolism   B. CAD with right heart failure   C. COPD

D. Primary pulmonary hypertension   E. Secondary pulmonary hypertension

14. For Q13, all the following therapies are indicated EXCEPT:

A. O_2 supply   B. Vasodilators   C. Anticoagulants

D. Diuretics   E. IV fluid

15. A 40 y/o man has mild fever, non-productive cough, weak vision, painful joints, and nodular erythema on multiple sites for the past 2 weeks. He has a 5-year history of smoking and reports general good health before this episode. PFTs show a restrictive pattern. Lab tests reveal blood eosinophilia, Hyper-Ca, and hypercalcuria. CXR shows bilateral hilar adenopathy. What's the most likely diagnosis?

A. Small-cell lung cancer   B. SCC of the lung   C. Sarcoidosis

D. Hyperparathyroidism   E. Gout

16. A 50 y/o man has quit his job as a miner after 2 years of employment because of progressive activity intolerance and dyspnea. P/E finds finger clubbing and coarse dry crackles on auscultation. PFTs show an obvious restrictive intrapulmonary process. CXR reveals reticular, nodular lesions (diffuse fibrosis). Chest CT scan shows a "ground-glass" image. What's the most likely diagnosis?

A. Coal-miner's lung   B. Asbestosis   C. Idiopathic pulmonary fibrosis (IPF)

D. Silicosis   E. Berylliosis

17. A 55 y/o man comes to the physician because of progressive activity intolerance and dyspnea. He has worked in a glass and pottery factory for the past 10 years. P/E finds finger clubbing and coarse dry crackles in the upper lobes on auscultation. PFTs show a restrictive intrapulmonary process. CXR reveals hyaline nodules with calcification. What's the most likely diagnosis?

A. Coal-miner's lung   B. Asbestosis   C. Idiopathic pulmonary fibrosis (IPF)

D. Silicosis   E. Berylliosis

18. A 30 y/o female at 30 week's gestation is brought to the ER with acute onset of dyspnea and pleuritic chest pain that occurred while she was sitting in the sofa. She has never been sick before. Her respiratory rate is 26/min and HR is 107/min. Auscultation and other P/E results are unremarkable. CXR is normal. Her ABG shows $PO_2 = 75$ and $PCO_2 = 35$ mmHg. This patient needs:

A. O_2 supply and mechanical ventilation   B. O_2 supply and LMWH for 6 months

C. Spiral CT on the chest   D. Heparin and warfarin for 6 months

E. Thrombolytics

19. A 50 y/o female undergoes a 6-hour abdominal surgery. On the 3rd day, she develops tachypnea, dyspnea, and chest pain. P/E of the heart and lungs is unremarkable except for rough respiratory sounds. T = 37.5°C. CXR

shows bilateral hazy infiltrates. WBC is 9500/uL with 1.5% bands. Sputum culture is (-). Mechanical ventilation is used for 8 hours and ABG shows PO_2 = 60, PCO_2=46 mmHg. What's the most likely diagnosis?

A. Pneumothorax   B. Atelectasis   C. pulmonary embolism

D. ARDS   E. Pneumonia

20. A 35 y/o man comes to the ER complaining of cough with sputum and blood for the past 3 days. He has a 5-year history of smoking and alcohol use, and had a "cold" 2 weeks ago. P/E shows that he is cyanotic, with bilateral wheezing on auscultation. Heart exam and PFTs are normal. Urine analysis (U/A) reveals WBC (-), RBC (+), protein (+), cast (+). Serum creatinine is 3 mg/dL. What's the most likely diagnosis?

A. Lung cancer   B. Rapidly progressive glomerulonephritis

C. Granulomatosis with polyangiitis   D. Acute glomerulonephritis

E. Goodpasture syndrome

21. A 12 y/o boy with poor living conditions presents with fever, headache, sore throat, and weakness for the past 5 days, and a cough with sputum and threads of blood for a day. P/E shows T=38.5°C, erythematous throat, and stable vital signs. CXR reveals bilateral pulmonary infiltrates of lymph nodes. Urine analysis shows RBC (+) and protein (+). Blood tests show increased lymphocytes. TB skin testing is (+/-). What's the most likely diagnosis?

A. Acute pulmonary TB   B. Granulomatosis with polyangiitis   C. Allergic interstitial nephritis

D. Goodpasture syndrome   E. Atypical pneumonia

22-25: Match the following clinical scenarios with the most appropriate next step in diagnosis.

A. Serum Ca level test   B. Sputum cytology   C. CT with FNA

D. Bronchoscopy with biopsy   E. Hyaluronidase level test   F. Endocrine tests

G. Thoracoscopic biopsy with open thoracotomy   H. Biopsy of the lymph node

I. Diagnostic antibiotics   J. Specific immunologic test

22. A 50 y/o man with a 15-year history of smoking and cough presents with increased fatigue and cough with sputum and threads of blood for the past month. CXR reveals multiple infiltrates with cavitary lesions near the bronchi. There are no other abnormal findings.

23. A 55 y/o man with a 10-year history of smoking and asbestos exposure presents with progressive fatigue and cough with sputum and threads of blood for the past month. CXR reveals multiple infiltrates in the lungs. There are no other abnormal findings.

24. A 58 y/o man with a 12-year history of smoking and cough presents with fatigue, low fever, throat and nasal discomfort, and right ear and neck pain for the past 2 months. P/E finds T = 38°C, cloudy red eardrum, and a swollen, tender lymph node on the right side. CXR reveals increased reveals multiple infiltrates in the lungs.

25. A 30 y/o woman presents with tachypnea, tachycardia, short of breath, cough with threads of blood wheezing, prolonged expirations, and multiple painful erythematous lesions on the limbs for the past month. Blood testing shows eosinophilia. CXR reveals bilateral pulmonary infiltrates of lymph nodes.

Answers and Explanations

1. (B). Severe hypoxemia with normal P_{CO2} in a COPD or asthmatic patient indicates imminent respiratory failure, and requires immediate intubation. All other options are less helpful.

2. (D). This patient has atelectasis commonly seen a day after a major surgery, and initially only requires choice 'D.' If the fever and high WBC continue > 3 days, infection should be suspected.

3. (A). It's a low-risk lung nodule and only CXR follow-up every 3 months (mo) for 2 years is needed; no more CXR if there is no growth. If he has higher cancer risk factors (> 50y, smoking, etc), "B, C, and D" may be needed.

4. (A). This patient most likely has SCC of the lung with hyper-Ca, hypertrophic osteoarthritis, and metastasis. Bronchoscopy with biopsy is best for centrally located cancer (SCC), and "C" also has a high (+) rate, but initial CXR is still the basic means to obtain a general picture of lung cancer. "B" is the best Dx for peripheral lung cancer.

5. (B). Albuterol (beta2-agonist) is the major initial treatment (Tx) for asthma. For severe or persistent chronic asthma, high-dose inhaled steroids and long-acting beta2-agonists (inhaled salmeterol) are the most effective Tx. Anticholinergics have special benefit in patients with heart disease and in those at high risk for negative effects of beta-agonists and theophylline. Major disadvantages are slow action and only medium potency. Systemic IV steroids are used acutely and briefly as a last resort for chronic, persistent asthma.

6. (D). LTD4-R antagonists (zafirlukast and montelukast) are reserved for severe asthma resistant to maximal doses of inhaled steroids and as a last resort before using chronic systemic steroids.

7. (D). This is a typical case of PE with initial Dx by ABG. Tx is continuous heparin for > 5 days along with warfarin for 6 months. "A" is for spontaneous plain pneumothorax. "B" should follow "D". "C" is only sensitive for a proximal PE, which may not be the case here. "E" is indicated for severe PE +/- CAD.

8. (B). It's typical of asbestosis with high risk of lung cancer. A chest CT with FNA is the best to exclude cancer. "A" can only confirm the Dx of asbestosis. "C" is good for a suspected "central" cancer, which is less likely here.

9. (A). "A" (Adenocarcinoma) is #1 common and "B" may be the 2nd common for this patient with a long history of asbestos exposure and smoking.

10. (D). PFT-predicted postoperative EFV1 is the most useful means to evaluate the benefit from lung resection. ABG is not of much value for this purpose.

11. (B). This is bronchiectasis with typical symptoms, signs of recurrent pulmonary infection (mostly Gram⁻), sinusitis, and immunodeficiency. "A" —Productive cough with sputum, cyanosis with mild dyspnea, rhonchi and wheezes, clubbing, and barrel chest; usually > 3 months of course. CXR shows increased pulmonary markings.

12. (B). This patient is mostly complicated with severe Gram⁻ pulmonary infection, and should be given IV aminoglycosides, ceftazidime, or/and quinolones after the sputum culture/sensitivity (C/S) is started. "A" is for suspected lung cancer, which is less likely since CXR didn't show any mass.

13. (D). This patient has manifestations of pulmonary hypertension but no history of related causes. CXR demonstrates enlarged central pulmonary arteries. ECG and echocardiography will demonstrate R-ventricular hypertrophy and signs of R-Ventr overload. PE usually occurs suddenly with similar symptoms and may not show R-Ventr hypertrophy and failure so early. CAD is less likely because the patient has low-risk for her age and history.

14. (E). IV fluid is good for right heart failure caused by R-Ventr MI, but not by pulmonary hypertension. All other Tx is helpful for pulmonary hypertension.

15. (C). Systemic sarcoidosis involves multiple organs in a short period of time in a 30's y/o patient. Definitive Dx is biopsy of suspected tissues, which mostly show noncaseating granulomas. Other diagnoses are only partially represented here. Lung cancer is less likely for his low risk factors of age, history, symptoms, and CXR result.

16. (C). IPF usually has occupational exposure of < 5 years, progressive manifestations mainly within the lungs, and diffuse fibrosis without calcification on CXR.

17. (D). It's a typical case of silicosis. "A": > 5-10 years of coal exposure + progressive respiratory dysfunction + diffuse fibrosis on CXR. "B": > 5-10 years of asbestos exposure in mining/shipyards + progressive respiratory dysfunction + hazy infiltration and pleural thickening on CXR +/- lung cancer. "E": < 5 years of exposure to high-tech materials + progressive respiratory dysfunction + diffuse infiltration and hilar adenopathy on CXR.

18. (B). It's another case of pulmonary embolism (PE), initially diagnosed by symptoms and ABG. Only low molecular weight heparin (B) is safe for PE with pregnancy, and warfarin is contraindicated. "A" is for respiratory obstruction or failure. "C" is only sensitive for a proximal PE, which may not be proper here. "E" is indicated for severe PE +/- CAD.

19. (D). This patient has respiratory symptoms following a long operation, and needs to be evaluated for PE, MI, pneumonia, and ARDS. Her presentations are most consistent with ARDS.

20. (E). GPS involves both lungs and kidneys with the typical presentation seen in this patient. Granulomatosis with polyangiitis (Wegener granulomatosis) is a major differential diagnosis (Dx), typically with necrotizing granulomatous vasculitis of the upper and lower respiratory tracts (cough with blood), and focal necrotizing glomerulonephritis (hematuria may be present). Asthma or wheezing is usually absent. "A" is a low possibility here. "B and D" should not have these severe respiratory symptoms.

21. (B). It's more typical of granulomatosis with polyangiitis, with pulmonary and renal abnormalities following an URI. Acute pulmonary TB is usually associated with non-productive cough and night sweats, but not hematuria. GPS has more diffuse pulmonary infiltrates and signs of renal failure; BP may be increased. "C" is typically accompanied by increased IgE and eosinophils in the blood. "E" usually does not have signs of renal dysfunction.

22. (B). It could be chronic bronchitis, but more likely SCC of the lung, which is centrally located and associated with cavitary lesions and hyper-Ca. Sputum cytology is 80% sensitive for initial detection of cancer cells. "D" is the most sensitive and definite means of Dx and tumor staging. "A" is not specific.

23. (C). According to the age, history and presentations, this could be chronic bronchitis but bronchioalveolar carcinoma (adenocarcinoma) is more likely ("C"). It's the #1 common lung cancer and is mostly peripherally located. CT scan with biopsy is the most sensitive means of Dx. "E" may be increased but not specific. "F" is helpful in diagnosing SCLC and large cell carcinoma. "G" after "C" can be an effective way of both Dx and Tx for a located tumor.

24. (H). Among other possibilities, this is most likely a nasopharyngeal carcinoma (NPC) with lymphatic metastasis and otitis media. NPC can be asymptomatic or with late presentations of nasal regurgitation, bleeding, obstruction, enlarged cervical lymph node, otitis media, hearing loss, bone pain, etc. Biopsy of the cervical lymph node is the best initial test. Other associated tests should be done later to exclude possible lung cancer.

25. (J). This is most likely a Churg-Strauss syndrome, a granulomatous vasculitis characterized by asthma, pulmonary infiltrates, rash, muscle pain, and significant eosinophilia. Positive p-ANCA (perinuclear antineutrophilic cytoplasmic antibody, 70-80%) helps confirm diagnosis and exclude other diseases such as eosinophilic pulmonary syndrome (no skin lesions from vasculitis), hypersensitivity pneumonitis, systemic sarcoidosis, etc.

Chapter 4

DIGESTIVE AND NUTRITIONAL DISEASES

DISEASES OF THE ESOPHAGUS

The upper esophageal sphincter (UES) and lower esophageal sphincter (LES) have the functions of preventing regurgitation of food upon swallowing. Any disruption in peristalsis, LES, UES, or esophageal (Esoph) anatomy can cause dysphagia or odynophagia.

Dysphagia refers to difficult swallowing, usually present in esophageal diseases.

Odynophagia refers to painful swallowing, most often associated with esophagitis.

In-time differential diagnosis and management are highly important.

PEARLS—Differential Diagnosis of Dysphagia (Table 4-1)

Oropharyngeal dysphagia
Causes include thyroid disease, Zenker diverticulum (bad breath + neck mass), tumor (progressive), neurologic disease (cranial nerve or bulbar lesion), muscular disease, sphincter dysfunction, and post-surgery/radiation dysphagia. **Diagnosis of choice: Cine-esophagram (videofluoroscopic swallowing exam)** + esophageal manometry (motility study). Treat underlying cause.
Esophageal dysphagia
(1) **Mechanical obstruction**: Mostly partial obstruction and for solid foods, includes Schatzki ring (lower esophageal webs with periodic dysphagia), peptic stricture (progress + chronic heart-burn), cancer (progress + smoking + drinking). **Diagnosis of choice: Barium (Ba) X-ray** followed by endoscopy with biopsy. (2) **Motility disorder**: Mostly near-full obstruction for solid and liquid foods—achalasia (progressive LES pressure increase), diffuse esophageal spasm (intermittent), scleroderma (chronic heart-burn + Raynaud or CREST syndrome). **Diagnosis of choice: Manometry.** Treat underlying cause.
Odynophagia
Causes include neuromuscular disease, candida infection (HIV history + diffuse ulcers), CMV (large shallow ulcers), HSV (small deep ulcers), chemicals (lye or pill ingestion + atypical ulcer). **Diagnosis of choice:** Ba X-Ray, Cine-esophagram, or endoscopy. Treat underlying cause.
Diagnostic treatment (Tx) with nitrates and Ca-blockers
Treatment can lower the pressure in the LES and improve achalasia and diffuse esophageal spasm, but worsen GERD.

Gastroesophageal Reflux Disease (GERD)

GERD is a functional disorder of transient gastroesophageal reflux due to incompetence of the LES. Causes of decreased LES tone include: Pregnancy (by increased progesterone), hiatal hernia, foods (chocolate, pepper, caffeine, ethanol, and fatty foods), smoking, smooth muscle relaxants (beta-R agonists, nitrates, and Ca-blockers).

Essentials of diagnosis

1. Based mainly on history and diagnostic treatment:

The most common symptom is substernal burning ("heartburn"), usually an hour after a meal, alleviated by antacids, standing or sitting but not by nitroglycerin, and worsened with reclining. It's the **most common noncardiac chest pain**. It may also have nonproductive cough, hoarseness, and asthma-like symptoms.

2. The best diagnostic test: **24-hour pH monitoring**, usually done in refractory cases. Esophageal manometry can also help. **EGD**—esophagogastroduodenoscopy with biopsy may be needed for unresponsive and suspected cases.

3. If it's a simple GERD (with recurrent antiacid use and without dysphagia or cancer risks), EGD can be done first for Barrett esophagus or peptic ulcer.

Differential diagnosis

Achalasia, esophageal spasm, esophagitis, gastritis, PUD, CAD, and pericarditis.

Complications

Esophagitis, peptic esophageal stricture/ulcer, **Barrett esophagus**, and bleeding.

Treatment

1. Lifestyle modification is the best initial therapy: Weight reduction, small meals and last meal 3 hours before bedtime, sleep with elevated head, smoking cessation, and avoidance of fatty meals or sweets at bedtime.

2. Medical treatment:

(1) Initial drugs for mild and moderate cases: Antacids (aluminium hydroxide), H2-blockers (cimetidine, ranitidine).

(2) Severe cases: Proton pump inhibitors (**PPI**, -azole) heal 80% of GERD patients with esophagitis, better than H2-blockers. It's usually more effective with a PPI plus amoxicillin and clarithromycin against H. pylori.

(3) Prokinetic drugs (metoclopramide): Ingestion 30 min before meals may improve esophageal and gastric emptying and raise LES pressure, but not heal esophagitis.

3. Surgery: Nissen's fundoplication is reserved for cases refractory to all the above medical therapies.

Achalasia

It's a smooth muscle motor disorder with esophageal dilatation, decreased peristalsis, and increased LES tone. It's mostly idiopathic in etiology. Secondary causes include Chagas disease (cardiomyopathy, megacolon, and achalasia), gastric carcinoma, or lymphoma that infiltrates the lower esophagus, and scleroderma.

Essentials of diagnosis

1. Dysphagia to both liquids and solids and regurgitation of foods usually in a young patient.

2. **Ba X-ray should be done first** to show typical **"bird beak sign"**—dilated esophagus and tapered narrowing at gastroesophageal junction, or "air/fluid."

3. **Manometry accurately** demonstrates increased LES tone and abnormal peristalsis.

4. **Endoscopy is eventually needed in all patients** (especially with risk factors) to rule out achalasia caused by gastric carcinoma or lymphoma.

Differential diagnosis

Scleroderma (Image 43):

It's a chronic multisystem disease characterized by **thickening of the skin** (including **sclerodactyly**) **and fibrosis of visceral organs** causing GI dysmotility, pulmonary fibrosis, and renal hypertension with renal failure. GI symptoms include **progressive dysphagia** to solids and liquids, **GERD** symptoms due to decreased LES tone, and poor absorption. **Diagnosis is confirmed by anti-centromere and/or Scl-70 antibody (+). Treatment** is symptomatic.

Treatment

1. **Ca-blockers** and nitrates: With temporary relief of symptoms.
2. Pneumatic dilation of LES: Conditional because perforation risk is 5%.
3. Botulinum toxin injection in LES: Blocking cholinergic nerves with about 65% effect; used in patients not suitable for pneumatic dilation or surgery.
4. Surgical **myotomy**: Circular muscle incision is the definitive therapy for refractory cases.

Diffuse Esophageal Spasm

It refers to non-peristaltic, uncoordinated, spontaneous contractions from the degeneration of nerve processes.

Essentials of diagnosis

1. **Crushing chest pain and dysphagia** (for solids and liquids) are common, usually alleviated by nitrates or Ca-blockers.
2. **Ba X-Ray:** Shows typical wobbly shape **"corkscrew esophagus"** (**Image 44**).
3. **Manometry:** Accurately shows **nonperistaltic** uncoordinated contractions.

Differential diagnosis

Nutcracker esophagus:

It refers to increased excitatory activity that results in **high-amplitude all-esophageal contractions**. **Diagnosis:** 1. Clinical features are the same as diffuse esophageal spasm. 2. **Manometry:** Will show **high-amplitude peristaltic contractions**. **Treatment** is the same as for diffuse esophageal spasm.

Treatment

Ca-blockers (diltiazem) and nitrates are the mostly effective therapies. If it's refractory, anxiolytics or antidepressants (imipramine) may be helpful.

The Schatzki Ring

It's the **most common** mechanical obstruction of the esophagus—a weblike mucosal ring located at the squamocolumnar junction or proximal to LES (supra-sphincter ring). Schatzki rings are further subdivided into A rings (above the esophagus-stomach junction) and B rings (below the squamocolumnar junction). It's usually seen in young patients with episodic dysphagia to solids and sometimes liquids.

Essentials of diagnosis

1. Episodic dysphagia with solid foods, or a sensation that the food "sticks" when the patient swallows. About 10% cases are asymptomatic.

2. Ba X-ray or endoscopy confirms diagnosis by showing a narrowing near the stomach (**Image 45**).

Treatment

Asymptomatic Schatzki rings seldom worsen over time and need no treatment. Symptomatic Schatzki rings may be treated with dilatation of the esophageal stricture using bougie or balloon dilators. For refractory rings, intralesional steroid injection prior to dilation or endoscopic electrosurgical incision may be considered.

Plummer-Vinson Syndrome (PVS)

PVS, also called Paterson–Brown–Kelly syndrome or sideropenic dysphagia, is a hypopharyngeal-cervical web associated with glossitis and iron deficiency anemia. It's more common in middle-aged and post-menopausal women, with increased risk of squamous cell carcinoma (SCC).

Essentials of diagnosis

1. **Triad** in a middle-aged or post-menopausal female: Intermittent dysphagia, glossitis (a burning sensation with the tongue and oral mucosa), and iron deficiency anemia.

2. Ba-X-Ray can diagnose both PVS and the Schatzki ring. Endoscopy can be both diagnostic and therapeutic.

Treatment

1. Treatment is primarily aimed at correcting the iron-deficiency anemia. Patients should receive iron supplementation in their diet. This may improve dysphagia and pain.

2. If the symptoms persist, the web can be dilated by pneumatic dilation during upper endoscopy to allow normal swallowing, followed by long-term PPI. Surgical incision is reserved for refractory cases.

Esophagitis

It is acute or chronic inflammation of the esophagus. Acute esophagitis can be catarrhal or phlegmonous, whereas chronic esophagitis may be hypertrophic or atrophic.

Etiology

1. **Infection: most common cause**, usually by Candida (No.1 with AIDS) or viruses (HSV, CMV, varicella-zoster virus, or HIV) and mainly in immunodeficient patients.

2. Drug-induced esophagitis: Oral medicines with inadequate water—alendronate, doxycycline, anti-inflammatory drugs (NSAIDs), Fe-sulfate, and quinidine.

3. Corrosive esophagitis: Ingestion of strong acids or alkali. This type of esophagitis is severe and complicated by stricture formation, especially with alkali (the effect is slow and long).

Clinical feature

Odynophagia following an irritating factor.

Diagnosis and treatment

—Based on history and diagnostic therapy.

1. Erosive (GERD) esophagitis: PPIs are more effective than H_2-R blockers in healing.

2. Drug-induced esophagitis: Best prevented with hydration and drug ingestion in an upright position.

3. Immunosuppressive and HIV esophagitis: Empirical trial of antifungals first (fluconazole, amphotericin); if there is no response, antiviral agents (acyclovir for HSV and VZV; ganciclovir for CMV) are recommended.

4. EGD—Esophagogastroduodenoscopy: Reserved for non-responded cases from above or corrosive esophagitis.

Barrett Esophagus

It refers to transformation of squamous esophageal epithelium to columnar epithelium due to chronic reflux. It occurs in 10-20% of GERD patients and carries a high incidence of **adenocarcinoma**, especially if the size is > 8 cm, with dysplasia and smoking history.

Essentials of diagnosis

Patients usually show chronic reflux symptoms. Suspects should be examined by EGD and biopsies, which may show columnar metaplasia.

Treatment

Similar anti-reflux medications as for GERD.

PEARLS—EGD surveillance—depending on the grade of dysplasia.

(1) No dysplasia: surveillance (repeat) every 3-5 years;

(2) Low-grade dysplasia: endoscopic eradication therapy or surveillance every 6-12 months with biopsies;

(3) High-grade dysplasia: endoscopic eradication therapy (if no submucosal invasion) or esophageal resection (if adenocarcinoma is suspected).

Zenker Diverticulum

Also known as **pharyngoesophageal/hypopharyngeal diverticulum** or pharyngeal pouch, it is a diverticulum of the mucosa of the pharynx, just above the cricopharyngeal muscle. It is a false diverticulum caused by a weak posterior hypopharyngeal wall. It mainly affects older patients.

Essentials of diagnosis

1. An elderly patient has bad breath and dysphagia at initial swallowing, and regurgitation of old food with a gurgling sense and neck mass. It may be complicated with aspirated pneumonia.

2. A Ba X-ray (showing an **outpouching of mucosa, Image 46**) followed by an **EGD is diagnostic**. Avoid nasogastric intubation for risk of perforation.

Treatment

If it's small and asymptomatic, no treatment is necessary. Symptomatic cases can be treated by surgical cricopharyngeal myotomy or diverticulectomy (especially if the patient is < 50 y/a).

Mallory-Weiss Syndrome

It's also known as **gastro-esophageal laceration syndrome**, a partial longitudinal mucosal tear in the mucosa at the squamo-columnar junction of the stomach and esophagus, usually caused by severe alcoholism, forceful retching, coughing, or vomiting.

Essentials of diagnosis

1. Hematemesis after an episode of violent nonbloody emesis or retching. Patient may also show old blood in the stool (melena). In most cases, the bleeding stops spontaneously in 24 hours.

2. EGD usually confirms the diagnosis.

Treatment

1. Most cases are self-limited and only need observation for 24-48 hours in hospital and conservative treatment. **All patients should receive PPI therapy**.

2. Patients with active bleeding at endoscopy should be treated with endoscopic hemostasis. Angiographic embolization or vasopressin may be considered in refractory cases.

Boerhaave Syndrome

Also known as **effort rupture of the esophagus**, it is full-thickness rupture of the distal esophagus adjoining the stomach that results from a sudden increase in intraesophageal pressure combined with negative intrathoracic pressure, particularly from straining or forceful vomiting. Common esophageal rupture or perforation is rupture of the esophageal wall and 60% of cases are iatrogenic (by instrumentation or surgery).

Essentials of diagnosis

1. Patient mostly presents with sudden severe chest pain with swallowing or inspiration, mostly after severe vomiting and bulimia, accompanied by crepitus (pneumomediastina).

2. Diagnosis is suggested on the plain **CXR (displaying mediastinal or peritoneal air) and confirmed by contrast esophagram or chest CT scan**, which usually shows esophageal wall thickening, extraesophageal air and fluid, and mediastinal widening, etc.

Treatment

1. All patients with an esophageal perforation require the following: (1) Avoidance of all oral intake; (2) Parenteral nutritional support; (3) IV broad spectrum antibiotics (e.g., ticarcillin-clavulanate) to prevent mediastinitis and sepsis; (4) IV PPIs; (5) Drainage of fluid collections/debridement of infected and necrotic tissue if present.

2. Most patients require **urgent surgical repair to save life**. The death rate is high if delayed.

Esophageal Carcinoma

It is the malignancy arising from the esophagus. There are two major types—squamous cell carcinoma, which is more common in the developing world, and adenocarcinoma, which is more common in the developed world.

Etiology and pathogenesis

1. **Squamous cell carcinoma (SCC)**: It accounts for approximately 50% of cases and mostly occurs in the proximal 2/3 esophagus. It's highly associated with **alcohol** and **smoking**; other risk factors include achalasia, Plummer-Vinson syndrome, a diet high in nitrates and pickled vegetables, hot foods, and Asian or Black males.

2. **Adenocarcinoma (ACC)**: Accounts for the other 50% of cases; mostly in the distal 1/3 esophagus and associated with **Barrett esophagus**. The incidence is rising, and more common in White males.

Essentials of diagnosis

1. **Elder patient, with history of alcohol drinking, smoking,** or **Barrett esophagus,** presents with **progressive dysphagia** for solids and later liquids (if with 60% obstruction). Weight loss, malnutrition, cough, nausea/vomiting, and chest/back pain are late symptoms.

2. **Lab diagnosis**: Ba X-ray (<u>Image 47</u>) is usually done **first** as a map, showing uneven ulcerated edges. Then **EGD** with biopsy is followed **to confirm the diagnosis**. Hyper-Ca may co-exist with SCC.

Diagnostic laparoscopy is optional for patients without evidence of metastasis and for tumor located at the EGJ. Preoperative bronchoscopy with biopsy and brush cytology is indicated for patients with locally advanced tumors located at or above the level of the carina.

Differential diagnosis

See "Differential Diagnosis of Esophageal Dysphagia" above.

Treatment

1. **Thoracic esophageal cancer**

(1) T1N0 cancer or EGJ adenocarcinoma or SCC: Endoscopic surgery alone is preferred.

(2) T3N0 stage I: Chemoradiotherapy (weekly carboplatin plus paclitaxel preferred) followed by surgery provides the best survival rate.

2. **EGJ cancers**: Chemoradiotherapy followed by surgery is recommended.

3. **Cervical esophageal cancer**: Chemoradiotherapy is preferred over surgery.

4. For most metastatic cancers: Chemotherapy with paclitaxel plus carboplatin/cisplatin +/- 5-fluorouracil plus radiation.

Prognosis

Prognosis is generally poor, with < 5% 5-year survival rate for M1 stage (distal metastasis), because early screening and diagnosis are difficult; with about 20% rate for T4N1 (regional) stage.

DISEASES OF THE STOMACH AND DUODENUM

Gastritis

Gastric inflammatory disease can be broadly categorized into gastritides and gastropathies. Gastritis is an inflammatory process of the lining of the stomach while gastropathy denotes gastric mucosal pathology with minimal to no inflammation. Gastritis can be classified into two basic types—acute (erosive) and chronic (nonerosive) gastritis. There is no universal classification so far in the world.

I. **Acute (erosive) gastritis** is usually caused by alcohol, NSAIDs, or severe physiologic stress (in very sick patients).

II. **Chronic gastritis:** Previously further classified into "Type A (Atrophic)" and "Type B (Antrum)" subtypes; mostly caused by H. pylori infection.

Essentials of diagnosis

1. **Most chronic gastritis (about 80% cases) is associated with H. pylori infection and located in the antrum-body** of the stomach, leading to increased gastric acid secretion. Patient usually presents with abdominal pain, early satiety, nausea and vomiting, and GI bleeding. H. pylori infection is also associated with GERD and duodenal ulcer disease.

2. **With disease progression and other etiology such as** autoimmune processes involved, atrophic gastritis, pernicious anemia and achlorhydria occur. It involves antibodies that destroy parietal cells and intrinsic factor, which eventually leads to low gastric acid levels. **Atrophic gastritis is closely associated with Vit B12 deficiency and increased risk of gastric adenocarcinoma.**

3. **Lab tests:** (1) Stomach-specific serum pepsinogens (PGs) have been used to screen patients for gastric atrophy.

(2) Serology (**ELISA for IgG)** is both sensitive and specific for confirming or ruling out H. pylori infection. Gastroscopy plus biopsy is the most accurate testing for gastritis.

(3) **Urease tests** (95% sensitive and specific): They include the Campylobacter-like organism test and urea breath test (radiolabeled urea). The breath test has a relatively high false (-) rate after PPI use, and is usually used after negative ELISA, and best for the therapeutic follow-up.

(4) In most patients with dyspepsia (gastritis/PUD) with low risk of cancer and < 45 y/a: First perform ELISA or urea breath test for H. pylori. If (+), treat with antibiotics; if (-), use H2-blockers or PPI.

(5) If > 45 y/a and with risk factors of cancer (bleeding, anemia, weight loss): Perform both H. pylori testing and Ba-study/endoscopy. If no tumor is found but H. pylori is (+), use antibiotics.

Treatment

1. **Erosive gastritis:** Treated with H2-blockers or PPIs +/- misoprostol (similar to "PUD" below).

2. **Atrophic gastritis:** It requires lifelong use of Vit-B12 for pernicious anemia.

3. **H. pylori gastritis:** It requires **antibiotics to cure the H. pylori infection.** New standard therapy is (1) PPI + clarithromycin + amoxicillin ± metronidazole; or (2) PPI + bismuth subcitrate, or bismuth subcitrate + metronidazole + tetracycline, for 10-14 days.

Peptic Ulcer Disease (PUD)

It's the disruption of the mucosal integrity in the stomach or duodenum. **The two major causes are H. pylori and NSAID, and the two major types are gastric and duodenal ulcers (different).**

Etiology

1. **H. pylori** is associated with 70-80% cases of PUD and almost 100% **duodenal** ulcer. H. pylori-associated PUD is usually accompanied by antral gastritis or duodenitis.

2. **NSAID-induced PUD**: 20-30% cases, due to direct toxicity to the gastric mucosa. Others causes include ethanol, corrosive substances (strong acids or alkali), stress (**Curling ulcer**, due to mucosal injury

and ischemia), **Cushing ulcer** (due to intracranial injuries, mechanical ventilation, sepsis, or coagulopathy).

Essentials of diagnosis

I. Gastric ulcer

1. Epigastric pain occurs or worsens shortly after food intake and not relieved by antacids and H_2-R blockers, and accompanied by nausea, vomiting, and weight loss.

2. Low gastric acid and high H. pylori levels. It may be associated with stomach cancer and significant bleeding (25% cases), with higher morbidity and mortality than duodenal ulcers.

3. Confirmed by Ba-study or **EGD** (gold standard) after H. pylori test (No.1 specific test is ELISA).

II. Duodenal ulcer

1. Epigastric pain usually occurs at hunger or midnight, relieved by food, antacids, and H_2-R blockers. Vomiting is rare and may indicate complications.

2. High gastric acid and high H. pylori levels. Cancer is rarely associated. Pyloric stenosis or posterior penetration may be an infrequent complication.

3. Confirmed by Ba-study or **EGD** (gold standard) after H. pylori test.

Differential diagnosis

Non-ulcer dyspepsia:

It is **functional dyspepsia** that carries similar ulcer-like symptoms (epigastric pain and bloating) but is not with ulcer disease. Etiology is unclear but may be associated with abnormal gastric or small intestine motility. Results of gastric acid secretion, EGD or Ba-study are all normal. Diagnosis can only be confirmed by endoscopy. **Treatment is empiric PPIs if < age 45, and endoscopy if > age 55 or symptoms persist (to exclude malignancy).**

Gastroparesis (Delayed gastric emptying):

Early satiety and postprandial nausea/vomiting are the most common symptoms. Treatment is metoclopramide to promote gastric emptying.

Treatment of PUD

1. **H. pylori eradication if the test is positive**:
(1) Initial **triple therapy**: A PPI (-azole) plus clarithromycin plus amoxicillin (metronidazole if amoxicillin-allergic) for 10-14 days.
(2) **Quadruple therapy**: Recommended when it's resistant to the triple therapy—a PPI plus bismuth salt, metronidazole, and tetracycline (or doxycycline) for 10-14 days.
The combination of two antibiotics plus a PPI (omeprazole), H_2 blocker (cimetidine), or bismuth salts have similar success rates. **PPI** is the most potent gastric acid inhibitor, and the second is H_2-R blockers. **Octreotide** is also helpful by decreasing GI blood flow and gastric acid secretion.
Adverse effects: Cimetidine has weak anti-androgenic effects causing gynecomastia and impotence at high doses, and can inhibit cytochrome-P450 (increasing toxicity of warfarin, theophylline, and phenytoin).

2. **Antisecretory therapy: H2-blockers or PPIs** should be used. Misoprostol is a PG-E1 derivative which helps maintain mucosal integrity and repair. NSAIDs should be avoided. Maintenance antisecretory therapy should be limited to high-risk subgroups of PUD including refractory or giant (> 2cm) peptic ulcer and age > 50 years, etc.

3. **H. pylori can also cause MALT** (mucosa-associated lymphoid tissue) lymphomas and stomach cancer. H. Pylori should be treated before the lymphoma. Surveillance endoscopy (with biopsies of the ulcer) should be performed after 3 months of antisecretory therapy in patients with persistent symptoms, gastric ulcers, or risk factors for gastric cancer.

4. Surgical management (selective vagotomy) for refractory/recurrent PUD: It is rarely required and is reserved for the gastric ulcers (> 5mm) that fail to heal after twice-daily antisecretory therapy with a PPI for 24 weeks in whom other correctable factors (e.g., medication noncompliance, NSAID use, and H. pylori infection) have been addressed.

Complications

1. PUD: May cause hemorrhage and perforation.

2. Long-term H. pylori infection: Chronic superficial gastritis, PUD, MALT, and chronic atrophic gastritis.

Zollinger-Ellison Syndrome (ZES)

It's a syndrome caused by a gastrin-producing tumor (**gastrinoma**), which results in severe and refractory peptic ulcer disease, diarrhea, and mild malabsorption.

Gastrinomas: Mostly found in the duodenum and the head of the pancreas. 60% cases are malignant with metastatic potentials, 25% are associated with **MEN-I ("3 Ps"**: parathyroid, pituitary, and pancreatic tumors) and hyper-Ca.

Essentials of diagnosis

1. History of recurrent PUD (especially after surgery), with diarrhea and mild malabsorption. Multiple peptic ulcers found on EGD.

2. Elevated gastrin levels (> 200 ng/L) and an abnormal IV secretin test confirm the diagnosis.

Treatment

1. A **high-dose PPI** (omeprazole, esomeprazole, etc.) should be started with or without metastasis. 30-50% of cases may have metastases at diagnosis and require further investigation and surgical resection of the metastases along with the primary tumor. Other therapeutic options for unresectable metastases include embolization, chemoembolization, radiation, somatostatin analogs, and cryoablation.

2. If there is no metastatic evidence, **exploratory laparotomy with total gastrectomy** is the effective therapy to decrease mortality, since metastatic gastrinoma is the most common cause of mortality in patients with ZES.

Dumping Syndrome

It refers to postprandial vasomotor symptoms after a major gastroduodenal surgery, caused by distention of the small intestine and shift of fluids that result from the rapid emptying of gastric contents into the small intestine. Dumping is a phenomenon caused by the destruction or bypass of the pyloric sphincter.

Essentials of diagnosis

History of a gastroduodenal surgery followed by diaphoresis, lightheadedness, palpitations, nausea, and vomiting, usually 0.5-1 hour after having meals rich in carbohydrates (#1 inducing content is sucrose). Diagnosis is confirmed by upper gastrointestinal series, upper endoscopy, or/and gastric emptying study.

Treatment

Once diagnosed by upper gastrointestinal series, upper endoscopy, and gastric emptying study, dietary and medications (prokinetic agents) are initiated. Dietary modification is helpful—restriction of sweets and liquid intake with meals; frequent, small meals. Intractable patients require completion near or total gastrectomy. Note that nutritional deficiencies may develop following partial gastrectomy, including malabsorption of vitamins or minerals. Patients with a **previous partial gastrectomy for benign diseases are at an increased risk for developing gastric cancer after 15 to 20 years.**

Gastric Carcinoma

It's a common GIT malignancy in Japan and other Asian countries, but uncommon in the West. The majority are adenocarcinomas.

Etiology and risk factors

1. H. pylori infection or pernicious anemia: With more than threefold higher risk;

2. Severe atrophic gastritis, chronic atrophic gastritis, gastric ulcer/dysplasia, adenomatous gastric polyps, intestinal metaplasia;

3. High intake of preserved foods (high salt, nitrates, nitrites—smoked meat);

4. Others: Blood type A, Menetrier disease (10%), postantrectomy, etc.

Pathology

1. Ulcerative carcinoma: ulcer through all layers.
2. Polypoid carcinoma: solid mass projecting into stomach lumen.
3. Superficial spreading: most favorable prognosis.
4. Linitis Plastica—"leather bottle": tendency of early infiltration through all layers, causing the stomach wall thick and rigid; with poor prognosis.

Essentials of diagnosis

1. History of one or more of the above risk factors.

2. Reduced appetite and weight, anorexia, dyspepsia, early satiety, abdominal pain, nausea, vomiting, anemia, and melena are common symptoms.

3. **Lab diagnosis**: FOBT is usually (+). CBC may show anemia. **Endoscopy with multiple biopsies** is now the initial and most accurate diagnostic test. Upper GI series **Ba X-ray (Image 48)** can be used as a complement test for complicated cases (such as with linitis plastica). Abdominal CT scan is for staging and detecting presence of metastases.

Treatment (Based on TNM staging)

1. **Early stage**: (1) No lymph node (LN) metastases—gastrectomy +/- adjuvant chemotherapy is preferred; (2) With suspected local LN metastases—gastrectomy with removal of perigastric lymph nodes plus adjuvant chemotherapy. The **FLOT chemotherapy** regimen docetaxel plus oxaliplatin, leucovorin and short-term infusional fluorouracil) is recommended for patients with N_1 tumor, before or/and after surgery. **5-year survival rate for early stage gastric cancer is over 90%.**

2. For most patients with unresectable and metastatic esophageal or gastric cancer, palliative treatment with cytotoxic chemotherapy or chemoradiotherapy can improve symptoms, quality of life, and prolong survival.

DISEASES OF THE PANCREAS

The pancreas secretes up to 3 liters of alkaline fluid daily with suitable pH and major enzymes for the digestion. Secretin, cholecystokinin, and bile salts stimulate pancreatic secretion. Disorders of the pancreas and gallbladder will affect both digestion and metabolism.

Acute Pancreatitis

It's the acute pancreatic inflammation caused by autodigestion by proteolytic enzymes. **Ethanol is the No.1 cause and gallstones the No.2.** Other causes include hyper-TG (>1,000 mg/dL), hyper-Ca, and medications (anti-AIDS medicines, Bactrim, pentamidine, oral hypoglycemics, diuretics). According to the Atlanta classification, acute pancreatitis can be divided into two broad categories: (1) Interstitial edematous acute pancreatitis, which is characterized by acute inflammation of the pancreatic parenchyma and peripancreatic tissues, but without recognizable tissue necrosis. (2) Necrotizing acute pancreatitis, which is characterized by inflammation associated with pancreatic parenchymal and/or peripancreatic necrosis, and carries 10% mortality rate. According to the severity, acute pancreatitis is divided into mild, moderately severe, and severe acute pancreatitis.

Essentials of diagnosis

1. Sharp epigastric pain radiating to the back, usually after a big meal; with nausea, vomiting, fever, or shock.

Acute Pancreatitis

2. P/E may show decreased bowel sounds and palpable pseudocyst. Severe, necrotizing pancreatitis can present with **Cullen's sign** (blue umbilical discoloration secondary to hemoperitineum) and **Grey-Turner's sign** (blue discoloration in the flank area, **Image 41**).

3. **Lab tests**: Elevated serum lipase and amylase. **The lipase is more sensitive and specific** than the amylase for acute pancreatitis.

4. **Abdominal CT scan is indicated for suspected complications only (not as a routine on the first day)**:

Phlegmon (inflamed, edematous pancreas by 48 hours in 85% of cases); pancreatic necrosis (by 2 weeks); pseudocyst (1-4 weeks); abscess (4-6 weeks); splenic vein-thrombosis (with gastric varices).

Prognosis

—**Ranson's criteria:**

1. On admission: **(1) Age > 55 years; (2) WBC > 16,000/uL; (3) LDH > 350 IU/L; (4) glucose > 200 mg/dL; (5) AST > 250 IU/L.**

2. At 48 hours: (1) PO_2 < 60 mmHg; (2) Ca < 8 mg/dL; (3) BUN > 5 mg/dL; (4) decrease in hematocrit by 10%; (5) serum albumin < 3.2 g/dl; (6) fluid deficit > 4L.

Note: More than 2-3 criteria indicate high mortality; More than 7-8 criteria almost mean 100% death.

Treatment

1. 90% of cases are self-limited and in basic need of bowel rest, nothing PO (NPO), supportive care, IV fluid, and analgesics (morphine or fentanyl). For severe type (hemorrhagic or necrotic), apply nasojejunal tube nutrition and add antiacid drugs to prevent stressful gastric erosion.

2. Diagnosis and treatment by ERCP are indicated if coexisting stones in common bile duct are suspected.

3. Surgical pancreatic debridement plus antibiotics is used for pancreatic necrosis.

4. Severe cases: Daily CT scans can help find and treat bleeding and infection early to reduce mortality.

5. For a walled-off pancreatic fluid collection, abscess or pseudocyst (usually "mature", > 6 weeks): surgical drainage, endoscopic drainage, and/or percutaneous drainage under CT guide is indicated.

Chronic Pancreatitis

It's the result of chronic inflammation of the pancreas. 70-90% is caused by chronic alcohol use and the rest is idiopathic. Pediatric cases are mostly associated with cystic fibrosis.

Essentials of diagnosis

1. **The primary manefestations of chronic pancreatitis are persistent epigastric pain, steatorrhea, and malabsorption (Vit. A, D, E, and K deficiencies).** Some patients may have diabetic status if with 80% of pancreas dysfunction.

2. Abdominal X-ray or **CT** may be normal or show pancreas calcifications, mild ileus, and pseudocyst **(Image 49)**.

3. **Serum amylase and lipase are commonly normal**, although they may be slightly increased occasionally. If the image studies are also normal and no steatorrhea, secretin stimulation test (most sensitive) or endoscopic ultrasound should be performed for suspected cases.

4. For recurrent pancreatitis without a clear cause, obtain ERCP to search pancreatic duct dilation and branch narrowing "chains of lakes".

Treatment

1. Stop alcohol and tobacco use and eat small meals that are low in fat. Give acid suppression, pancreatic enzyme and vitamin supplements, medium-chain triglycerides in diet (independent digestion), and analgesics.
2. Treat diabetes. Avoid over-control of glucose level due to the tendency towards hypoglycemia.
3. For refractory pain or complications, surgery (such as lateral pancreatico-jejunotomy) may be considered. Watch for increased risk for pancreatic adenocarcinoma.

Pancreatic Carcinoma

It mostly refers to a ductal adenocarcinoma that originates from the exocrine pancreas and occurs in the pancreatic head. Thus it is also called exocrine pancreatic cancer. It's usually highly malignant with a poor prognosis.

Risk factors

Etiology is unknown. No.1 risk factor is **smoking**. Others include family history, high-fat diet, obesity, low-fiber diet, diabetes, > 60 y/o men, chronic pancreatitis (other than direct alcoholism or cholelithiasis), and blacks.

Essentials of diagnosis

1. Usually asymptomatic until past early stage, with progressive epigastric pain (radiating to the back), nausea, vomiting, fatigue, and weight loss.

2. **Courvoisier's sign**—palpable, nontender gallbladder with jaundice (**Image 51**); **Trousseau's sign**--migratory thrombophlebitis, only 10% cases.

3. **Lab tests**: AKP and direct bilirubin are usually increased. Serum biomarker cancer antigen **(CA)**19-9 has limited sensitivity and specificity and should not be a diagnostic means.

4. **PEARLS: Important diagnostic steps for progressive jaundice, RUQ pain, or mass:**

(1) First obtain an ultrasound, which is cost-effective for stones, abscess, and mass. If stones or mass are positive, perform an ERCP. Ultrasound is not preferred if no jaundice or obstruction is present.

(2) If stones are negative by ultrasound, obtain a CT/MRI scan with better sensitivity, which usually shows the tumor (**Image 50**).

(3) If CT/MRI is negative, perform ERCP with biopsy to identify a small mass. ERCP is both diagnostic and therapeutic in most cases.

Differential diagnosis

<u>Duodenoampullary cancer</u>:

Similar to features of pancreatic cancer (RUQ pain, progressive jaundice, nausea, vomiting, etc.), FOBT (+), and LFTs are normal. The best diagnostic means is EGD with biopsy.

Treatment

1. **Potentially resectable cancer:** (1) **Tumors in the head or uncinate process**, the standard operation is pancreaticoduodenectomy (Whipple procedure). (2) **Tumors of the tail/body**: distal pancreatectomy, usually combined with splenectomy. Adjuvant chemotherapy may be considered.

2. **Locally advanced, unresectable cancer:** Suggested therapies are combination chemotherapy regimens—(gemcitabine +/- capecitabine or leucovorin-modulated fluorouracil (FU).

3. For tumors with **known BRCA mutation**, a **platinum-based chemotherapy** regimen is preferred.

4. **Posttreatment surveillance—For a locally advanced or borderline resectable pancreatic cancer:** Testing for tumor markers **(CA)19-9** (if initially elevated) and CT scanning at least every 3-4 months during the first two years, and then every six months once the disease is in stabilized stage.

Prognosis: 80% of pancreatic cancers have metastases at diagnosis and the prognosis is very poor (only 6 months of mean survival rate after diagnosis).

DISEASES OF THE GALLBLADDER

Gallstones

Cholelithiasis involves the presence of gallstones in the gallbladder. Choledocholithiasis refers to the presence of gallstones in the common bile duct (CBD). Gallstones is a common disease more prevalent in middle-aged women and increasing with age.

Etiology and pathogenesis

<u>Gallstones carry the "5-F risk factor features"—"female, fat, forty, fertile and flatulent."</u> Other risk factors include estrogen use, pregnancy, Crohn disease, hyper-triglyceride, large-scale small bowel resection, total parenteral nutrition, etc. Pigmented stones are associated with alcohol abuse, chronic hemolysis, and cirrhosis.

The most common type is **mixed stones** (bilirubinate-Ca and pigmented stones) originated from cholesterol in the gallbladder. Symptoms are caused by transient cystic duct blockage from impacted stones, often complicated with acute cholecystitis, ascending cholangitis, or pancreatitis.

Essentials of diagnosis

1. **Most patients with choledocholithiasis are symptomatic (typically biliary colic)**—RUQ and epigastric pain after meals and lasting about 30 min; with fever and leukocytosis in cholecystitis; **Charcot triad** (fever, jaundice, and RUQ pain)—with ascending cholangitis.

2. **Ultrasonography is 90% sensitive** and the best means of diagnosis.

3. **ERCP** is for both diagnosis and treatment and preferred for common bile duct (CBD) stones.

Treatment

1. Asymptomatic cases: Watchful waiting. Treatment is only needed with porcelain gallbladder (cancer-risky), Sickle cell anemia, or salmonella infection.

2. Symptomatic cases: (1) Patients with high risk: ERCP with stone removal, followed by elective cholecystectomy. (2) Low risk: ERCP with cholecystectomy (or with sphincterotomy for common bile duct stones). Cholecystectomy followed by manual gallstone extraction is reserved for patients with acute recurrent symptoms and complicated gallstone disease who cannot undergo surgery.

3. Oral bile acids (ursodeoxycholic acid) are for surgery-intolerant cases and effective in noncalcified cholesterol stones < 5 mm.

Complications

Usually late onset—empyema, gangrene, perforation, sepsis, abscess or fistula formation, post-cholecystectomy pain, and gallbladder cancer.

PEARLS——**Common causes of post-cholecystectomy RUQ pain**

(1) Oddi's sphincter dysfunctioning: ERCP sphinctectomy should be performed if the pressure is increased.

(2) CBD stones: Imaging tests are abnormal.

(3) Functional pain: Ultrasonography and hepatic enzyme tests are normal.

Acute Cholecystitis

It's caused by **prolonged blockage of the cystic duct**, mostly from an impacted stone, resulting in post-obstructive distention, inflammation, infection, or gangrene of the gallbladder.

Essentials of diagnosis

1. History of **RUQ pain/tenderness and nausea/vomiting similar to but more severe and longer than biliary colic. Murphy's sign** is usually (+); may also have low fever, abdominal guarding or rebound tenderness.

2. **Lab tests**:
(1) Increased WBC and amylase; LFTs may be high or normal.

(2) **Ultrasonography:** The best initial tool to demonstrate stones, pericholecystic fluid, a thickened gallbladder wall, or gas inside.

(3) If the ultrasonography is equivocal, **cholescintigraphy (HIDA scan)** is the best to visualize and confirm cystic duct obstruction and cholecystitis. **Morphine cholescintigraphy** is particularly useful in critically ill patients.

(4) If the gallbladder is enlarged with jaundice but without stones, CT is obtained for possible tumor.

(5) **ERCP vs HIDA:** Most effective in showing intra-/extra-hepatic biliary trees and also therapeutic for the stony obstruction, but not so as HIDA for the cystic duct obstruction.

Differential diagnosis

Acalculous cholecystitis:

It is mostly in a chronic debilitated patient in a hospital, with severe trauma, burns, prolonged TPN, or mechanical ventilation. It's diagnosed by ultrasound first, then by CT or HIDA with more sensitivity.

Other differential diagnosis: Biliary colic, cholangitis, PUD, acute pancreatitis, GERD, MI, hepatitis, STD perihepatitis, renal colic, etc.

Treatment

1. Hospitalize the patient and administer IV fluid, electrolytes, and antibiotics.

Antibiotics: (1) For community-acquired cholecystitis of mild-to-moderate severity: cefazolin, cefuroxime, or ceftriaxone. (2) For acute cholecystitis of severe state, advanced age, or immune-suppression: imipenem-cilastatin, piperacillin-tazobactam, or ciprofloxacin/cefepime plus metronidazole. Vancomycin is added to each regimen for healthcare-associated biliary infection of any severity.

2. Perform **early cholecystectomy** (< 72 hours); obtain a **cholangiogram** during the surgery to rule out CBD stones. If the conditions are serious (as with diabetes), first perform a cholecystostomy to remove stones (faster), and remove the gallbladder later when the patient is stable. If surgery is not tolerable, ursodeoxycholic acid can be used.

Complications

Empyema, abscess, gangrene, perforation, fistula, sepsis, and chronic post-surgery pain, etc.

Acute Cholangitis

It's an inflammation or infection of the biliary tree, usually after obstruction from gallstones or cancer. The commonest pathogens are Gram⁻ rods—E coli, Enterobacter, and pseudomonas.

Essentials of diagnosis

1. Usually presents with **Charcot triad** (RUQ pain, jaundice and fever/chills), or if severe, **Reynold pentad** (Charcot triad plus shock and altered mental status), mostly in acute suppurative cholangitis.

2. **Increased WBC, direct bilirubin, and AKP.** Obtain blood for **culture and sensitivity.**

3. **ERCP is the best diagnostic means and fast initial therapy.**

Differential diagnosis

Hepatitis, cholecystitis, pancreatitis, sclerosing cholangitis, cholangiocarcinoma, pancreatic cancer, and primary biliary cirrhosis.

Treatment

1. Because it's a life-threatening disease, patient should be first in ICU with monitoring, supportive care, aggressive IV fluid, and **empiric antibiotic coverage for colonic bacteria**—ciprofloxacin, ampicillin-sulbactam, piperacillin-tazobactam, ticarcillin-clavulanate, or ceftazidime plus metronidazole. Anti-sepsis therapies may be needed.

2. Perform **emergent bile duct decompression** via endoscopic sphincterotomy, percutaneous transhepatic drainage, or operative decompression. If possible, ERCP should be done early after patient is stable to locate the obstruction, remove the stones, and place the stent.

ERCP complications

Pancreatitis, perforation, peritonitis, sepsis, hemorrhage, and biliary-enteric fistula (after sphincterotomy).

Gallbladder Cancer

It's an uncommon but **highly malignant tumor, mostly as adenocarcinoma**. Related **risk factors** include female gender (2 times more than male), ages 50-60, obesity, chronic cholecystitis and cholelithiasis, porcelain gallbladder, gallbladder polyps, and congenital biliary cysts. The incidence is alarmingly increasing in China and India.

Essentials of diagnosis

1. Most cases are asymptomatic and found incidentally. Early symptoms mimic gallbladder inflammation due to gallstones—steady pain in the upper right abdomen (URQ), nausea, loss of appetite, weakness, etc.

2. Later manifestations may be weight loss and jaundice and vomiting due to biliary and stomach obstruction.

3. **Courvoisier's sign** (palpable, nontender gallbladder with jaundice, **Image 51**) is a late indication of the gallbladder or pancreas cancer.

4. Early diagnosis is rare. Transabdominal ultrasonography, CT scan, endoscopic ultrasound, MRI, and magnetic resonance cholangiopancreatography (MRCP) can be used for accurate diagnosis. A biopsy confirms the diagnosis.

Treatment

1. If it is diagnosed in early stage (T_1, < 10% cases), the cancer can be treated effectively by surgical removal of the gallbladder, part of the liver and associated lymph nodes.

2. Most often it is found with late symptoms and treated with new systemic chemotherapy—gemcitabine plus cisplatin, or leucovorin-modulated FU regimen. The prognosis is poor—the 5-year survival rate is generally < 10%.

DISORDERS OF THE LIVER

The liver has an abundant dual blood supply and enzymes that allows it to remove toxins from the circulation. It breaks down exogenous (drugs) and endogenous (bilirubin) toxins via enzymatic oxidation, reduction, and conjugation reactions. Enzymatic **P450 system** is mostly involved in hepatic metabolism. Degradation of amino acids is done via the transaminases—ALT (GPT) and AST (GOT). Liver disease can be divided into different patterns based on liver function tests (LFTs):

1. **Hepatocyte integrity destruction or injury:** Elevated **ALT** (more specific than AST) and **AKP** (alkaline phosphatase, more sensitive) +/- GGT and bilirubin.

2. **Cholestasis:** Elevated **AKP, GGT, and bilirubin**, +/- ALT and AST.

3. **Isolated hyperbilirubinemia:** Elevated **bilirubin;** normal AKP and aminotransferases.

In hepatic injury, prolonged **PT is most prognostic** (normal: 11-14 sec); then it is low albumin. **Jaundice** is the most common symptom in liver-gallbladder disease. It can be secondary to hepatocellular disease, intrahepatic obstruction (causing cholestasis) or extrahepatic biliary obstruction.

Liver Injury and Hepatitis

Hepatitis is acute or chronic liver inflammation caused by various agents. The most common types are **alcoholic hepatitis and viral hepatitis.** Viral hepatitis is caused by systemic **viral** infections (mostly RNA viruses, except hepatitis B by a DNA virus). It mainly affects the hepatocytes and causes an increase in transaminases (**ALT:AST > 2, opposite to alcoholic hepatitis**). Cirrhosis can develop secondary to chronic hepatitis from either viral hepatitis (B and C) or alcohol. Fulminant hepatitis and hepatic failure is rare but can occur with acetaminophen and viral hepatitis.

PEARLS—**Table 4-2: Summary of Liver Injury and Hepatitis**

Cause / Clinical features, diagnosis, and treatment
Viral Hepatitis: See "Chapter 1: INFECTIOUS DISEASE".
Fatty Liver
It refers to hepatic ballooning and fat degeneration, mainly associated with hyperlipidemia, obesity, alcoholism, mostly **reversible** after alcohol cessation. Related drugs are amiodarone, tetracycline, valproic acid, and anti-HIV medicines. **Tx:** For nonalcoholic fatty liver, only weight loss is effective. For alcoholic fatty liver, only alcohol abstinence is effective. Vitamin E may be helpful. **Hepatic steatosis: Late stage of fatty liver,** with PMN infiltration, necrosis, and high ALT and AKP. Prevention of cirrhosis is necessary.
Alcoholic Hepatitis

Alcohol in any amount is toxic to the liver and can cause acute and chronic injury and hepatitis. After years of alcohol intake, **fatty liver** and acute or chronic hepatitis may occur with various severities. **Typical presentations include AST:ALT > 2**, ALT < AST < 300 IU/L. **Tx:** Alcohol abstinence, prednisone or pentoxifylline, treatment of alcohol withdrawal, and supportive care. **Prognosis: Women are more vulnerable than men for alcohol hepatic injury. For alcoholic and HCV hepatitis, men usually have faster progression towards cirrhosis** than women regardless of age.

Drug-induced Liver Injury

It's associated with halothane, INH, phenytoin, alpha-methyldopa, CCl4, etc. Acetaminophen may cause fulminant hepatitis with a rare incidence. **Dx:** History of the above drug ingestion, GI symptoms, along with elevated liver function tests—ALT) is more than three times the upper limit of normal, serum alkaline phosphatase and the total bilirubin > two folds. **Tx:** Cessation of associated drugs and supportive care. **Prognosis:** Most patients will recover fully. **Cholestasis:** Associated with chlorpromazine (CPZ), nitrofurantoin, erythromycin, or steroid use. Female with OCP use or pregnancy may have it, but it's self-limited. **AKP, GGT and bilirubin are elevated.**

Autoimmune Hepatitis

Previously known as autoimmune chronic active hepatitis, it is a chronic hepatitis **characterized by autoimmunologic features** including the presence of circulating autoantibodies and a high serum globulin concentration. **Diagnosis:** (1) History of autoimmune disease (ITP, etc.) but no symptoms of liver disease. (2) Enlarged liver-spleen, increased serum LFTs, AKP and proteins but decreased albumin. ANA and anti-smith are (+). **Tx: Immunosuppression:** Prednisone +/- azathioprine (not methotrexate). This disease is usually more severe in children and should be treated promptly with prednisone first. **Prognosis:** Most patients will recover fully with treatment.

Granulomatous Hepatitis and Hepatic Granulomas

Both may be caused by drugs (allopurinone and –butazones), sarcoidosis, primary biliary cirrhosis, TB or fungal infection, etc. The difference is that hepatic **granulomas does not imply hepatocellular inflammation**. **Dx:** Liver biopsy. **Tx: Immunosuppression** (prednisone +/- methotrexate) +/- antibiotics for suspected infections (e.g., anti-TB therapy should start before immunosuppression). Prognosis varies.

Hereditary liver diseases: Hemochromatosis, Wilson disease, alpha-antitrypsin deficiency, etc.

Alpha1-antitrypsin deficiency: It's a rare autosomal recessive disease with alpha1-antitrypsin deficiency, leading to chronic hepatitis, cirrhosis, and emphysema in early adulthood. It accounts for 20% of liver diseases among neonates. **Dx:** (1) Asymptomatic transaminase increase in a young patient with emphysema; (2) Absence of alpha-antitrypsin in electrophoresis and low serum alpha1-antitrypsin. **Tx:** (1) Asymptomatic: regular follow-up with pulmonary function test every 3 months; (2) Symptomatic: alpha-antitrypsin supplements plus supportive care.

Lactulose: ↓ serum albumin = poor itout

Cirrhosis

It's defined as irreversible chronic injury of the hepatic parenchyma with significant fibrosis, a complication of liver disease. **Alcohol is the #1 cause of cirrhosis.** Other common causes include chronic hepatitis B or C, primary biliary cirrhosis, primary sclerosing cholangitis, drugs, toxins, hemochromatosis, Wilson disease, and alpha₁-antitrypsin deficiency.

Clinical manifestations depend on the extent of liver damage rather than the cause. Fibrosis and vascular distortion in the liver lead to portal hypertension, ascites, and varices. Loss of most of the hepatic mass (usually > 70%) causes signs and symptoms of hepatic decompensation (jaundice, pruritus, signs of upper gastrointestinal bleeding, edema, spontaneous bacterial peritonitis, and confusion due to hepatic encephalopathy). Physical examination findings may include jaundice, spider angiomata, gynecomastia, ascites, splenomegaly, palmar erythema, digital clubbing, and asterixis. Laboratory abnormalities may include elevated serum bilirubin, abnormal aminotransferases, elevated alkaline phosphatase/gamma-glutamyl transpeptidase, a prolonged prothrombin time/elevated international normalized ratio (INR) (coagulopathy), hyponatremia, and thrombocytopenia.

Diagnosis is mostly based on clinical manifestations, although a liver biopsy is required for confirmation.

Treatment of cirrhosis includes prevention and treatment of potential complications (usually in late stage): variceal hemorrhage, ascites, spontaneous bacterial peritonitis, hepatic encephalopathy, hepatorenal syndrome, hepatopulmonary syndrome, portal vein thrombosis, cardiomyopathy, and hepatocellular carcinoma.

Portal Hypertension

It's a pathologic condition or complication rather than a disease. A variety of pathologic processes can cause the portal vein pressure (PVP) > 5 mmHg above the inferior vena cava (IVC) pressure, resulting in **ascites, bacterial peritonitis, esophageal varices, splenomegaly, hepatorenal syndrome, and hepatic encephalopathy.** Evaluation should include LFTs (ALT, AST, AKP, bilirubin, PT/PTT, and albumin) to assess the liver functions. **Common causes:**

1. Pre-sinusoidal—portal or splenic vein thrombosis, granulomatosis, or schistosomiasis;

2. Sinusoidal—cirrhosis or granulomatosis;

3. Post-sinusoidal—RHF, constrictive pericarditis, or hepatic vein thrombosis;

4. Budd-Chiari syndrome—Hepatic vein or IVC thrombosis secondary to hypercoagulation status. It requires treatment with thrombolytics or liver transplantation, with a high mortality.

PEARLS—**Table 4-3: Complications of Portal Hypertension**

Complication / Clinical features, diagnosis (Dx), and treatment (Tx)
Ascites
It's mostly the result of portal hypertension and heart failure (serum-ascites albumin gradient >1.1); also in nephritic syndrome, TB-peritonitis and peritoneal cancer without portal hypertension (serum-ascites albumin gradient <1). Thus, etiologic Tx is important. **Tx**: 1. Na-restriction and diuretics (K-saving spironolactone plus furosemide is preferred). **Avoid anti-HTN agents (propranolol, ACE-I) because low BP may increase mortality with refractory ascites.** 2. If it's severe: Large volume of paracentesis (tapping) along with IV albumin (if no peripheral edema) is effective. 3. Perivenous shunt: (1) Portal-caval shunt: With long effect and most usage; ascites and esophageal varices decrease but risk of hepatic encephalopathy increases. (2) TIPS—Transjugular intrahepatic portosystemic shunt: Indicated for refractory ascites and hydrothorax, with low mortality but short effects; useful before liver transplantation. (3) Distal splenorenal shunt: Portal hypertension decreases but ascites increases.
Spontaneous Bacterial Peritonitis (SBP)
It is indolent infection of the ascetic fluid and may be a complication of chronic liver diseases or portal hypertension (as the history). **Dx**: Fever and abdominal pain; ascitic fluid neutrophils >250/mm³/uL (or >500/uL in asymptomatic patient). Bacterial culture is mostly negative. **Tx**: IV antibiotics (usually a 3rd-generation cephalosporin such as cefotaxime) to cover both Gram⁻ bacteria (**E coli #1**, Klebsiella) and Gram⁺ bacteria (Enterococcus) until the pathogen is identified.
Esophageal Varices
Usually it occurs when portal pressure >12 mmHg. **Tx**: 1. Monitor for GI bleeding. 2. A beta-blocker (Prop) is the best prophylaxis after the first bleeding and re-bleeding. 3. For severe acute bleeding: two IV lines with octreotide (decreased GI motility, secretion and bleeding) infusion. 4. If not stopped: Endoscopic banding ligation or sclerotherapy is the effective Tx. 5. If still refractory: Venous shunt (TIPS) and liver transplantation.
Hepatorenal Syndrome
It's **a syndrome of acute kidney injury and renal dysfunctioning caused by acute or chronic liver disease, resulting in renal azotemia, oliguria, and urine Na <10 mEq/L (very low rate of sodium excretion).** Affected patients usually have portal hypertension due to cirrhosis, severe alcoholic hepatitis, or metastatic tumors. **Dx**: By hepatic history and excluding other causes of acute kidney injury (including prerenal azotemia and tubular necrosis). **Tx**: The ideal therapy is treatment of original liver disease, improvement of hepatic functions, or **liver transplantation (cure).** Supportive care, **diuretic cessation (terlipressin plus albumin)** and dialysis are helpful.
Hepatic Encephalopathy
It's a **reversible impairment of neuropsychiatric function associated with impaired hepatic function. Increased serum ammonia** concentration may be an important role for inhibitory neurotransmission **through GABA** receptors in the CNS and changes in central neurotransmitters and circulating amino acids. **Precipitating factors:** SBP, low-K alkalosis, azotemia, GI bleeding, and sedative use. **Typical hepatic and neuropsychological presentations:** Cognitive impairments in attention, reaction, and memory; diurnal sleep pattern (insomnia and hypersomnia); neuromuscular impairments (bradykinesia, hyperreflexia, rigidity, myoclonus, and asterixis); hepatic coma. **Tx:** 1. Identification and **correction of precipitating causes**. Measures to lower the blood NH3 concentration and **decrease protein intake--#1 important**. **Lactulose** (#1) or rifaximin +/- neomycin to decrease NH3 absorption in the bowel, with fast and short effects. 2. Perivenous shunt and liver transplantation as the cure.

Hemochromatosis

It's an autosomal recessive disease of **iron malabsorption**. Excess iron is absorbed and deposited in tissues and organs-predominantly in the liver, pancreas, heart, pituitary, testes, adrenals and kidneys, causing fibrosis, diabetes and heart failure (CHF), etc. It's more common in men due to lack of female menstruations, and associated with about 30% incidence of liver cancer.

Essentials of diagnosis

1. Most patients are asymptomatic until after middle ages, with skin pigmentation and hepatomegaly (90% cases). Other associated disorders include cirrhosis, diabetes, arthropathy, gout, restrictive heart failure, and hypogonadism or impotence (not relieved by sildenafil).

2. Lab tests: Increased iron, transferrin, and **ferritin** (**>1000** ng/mL or ug/L); ALT, AKP and glucose may also increase.

3. DNA test (revealing HFE gene mutation) or liver biopsy confirms diagnosis.

Treatment

1. Patient should avoid foods rich in iron (such as red meat, raw shellfish), alcohol, Vit C, etc.

2. **Phlebotomy**: It's the **most effective and simple therapy** to remove excess iron; used weekly or biweekly.

3. **Iron-chelating agents: Deferoxamine is effective for acute intoxication**, but less effective, more expensive and rarely necessary for hemochromatosis after phlebotomy.

Complications

Most patients die of cirrhosis or heart failure. Other complications include diabetes, liver cancer, impotence, arthropathy, and hypopituitarism.

Wilson Disease

It's an autosomal recessive disease with impaired hepatic secretion of copper (Cu), causing excessive Cu accumulation and deposit in the liver, brain, and cornea. Basal ganglia dysfunction can occur with CNS deposit. It occurs mostly in adolescent ages.

Essentials of diagnosis

1. **Neuropsychiatric disturbances are early signs**: tremor, chorea, dysarthria; bizarre behavior, psychosis; **Kayser-Fleischer rings in the cornea** (**Image 155**, pathognomonic sign); acute hepatitis or cirrhosis (showing jaundice, hepatomegaly and elevated LFTs).

2. Low serum ceruloplasmin and high urine Cu (serum-Cu may be high or normal).

3. Liver biopsy with high Cu confirms the diagnosis.

Treatment

1. Restrict diet Cu along with lifetime use of the first-line drug—**D-penicillamine** (a Cu-chelator, plus Vit-B6). Adverse effects include sensitivity reactions, nephrotic syndrome, etc. Trientine is the second-line medicine with fewer side effects.

2. Oral zinc is a maintenance therapy to increase fecal Cu excretion.

3. Liver transplantation: Curative treatment for late-stage Wilson disease and hemochromatosis.

Primary Biliary Cholangitis

Previously known as **primary biliary cirrhosis**, it is an **autoimmune disease of chronic cholestasis** (decreased bile acid flow) that leads to destruction of intrahepatic bile ducts and eventual cirrhosis and liver failure. It is **characterized by accumulation in serum of cholesterol, bilirubin, and bile acids**, which are normally secreted in bile. It's predominant in females and associated with other autoimmune diseases (Sjogren syndrome, rheumatoid arthritis, Hashimoto thyroiditis, scleroderma, etc.).

Essentials of diagnosis

1. Usually a middle-aged female presents with fatigue (#1 symptom), pruritus, and obstructive jaundice (later stages). About 30% patients are asymptomatic. Complications include metabolic bone disease, hypercholesterolemia, malabsorption, vitamin deficiency, hypothyroidism, and anemia.

2. **Lab tests**: Elevated AKP, GGT, bilirubin, Chol, and AST or ALT (mildly). Anti-mitochondria antibodies are positive. Ultrasonography usually shows normal extrahepatic bile ducts. **Liver biopsy** confirms diagnosis by showing destruction of intrahepatic bile ducts.

Treatment

1. **Ursodeoxycholic acid (UDCA)** is the best therapy to improve hepative functions and symptoms.

2. **Liver transplantation** may be the only curable way of treatment in the end stage of the disease.

Primary Sclerosing Cholangitis

It's usually a disease in a middle-aged man, with focal cholestasis leading to progressive destruction of both intra-/extra-hepatic bile ducts. Bile ducts have a characteristic pearl-like appearance, caused by strictures and dilations of the bile ducts secondary to fibrosis and inflammation. The disease ultimately progresses to cirrhosis. 80% of cases are associated with ulcerative colitis, and 15% with cholangiocarcinoma. It's also associated with hepatocellular carcinoma and colon cancer. Other complications are similar to those of primary biliary cholangitis.

Essentials of diagnosis

1. Usually a middle-aged man presents with fatigue first, then pruritus, and obstructive jaundice later.

2. **Lab tests**: Elevated AKP, GGT, direct bilirubin, and AST or ALT (mildly); anti-centromere (+).

ERCP: Typical irregular intra-/extra-hepatic bile ducts with stricturing and beading.

Liver biopsy: Confirms diagnosis by showing inflammation and fibrosis of hepatic ducts.

Treatment

1. Patients with this disease should undergo **screening for gallbladder carcinoma, cholangiocarcinoma, colon cancer, and hepatocellular carcinoma** due to the increased risk.

2. **Ursodeoxycholic acid** is the best available therapy to improve the liver functions and symptoms. Immunosuppressive therapy has limited effects.

3. **Liver transplantation** may be the only curable therapy in the end stage of the disease. Median survival without transplantation is 10-12 years.

Hepatocellular Carcinoma (HCC)

It's a common aggressive cancer in the digestive system with a poor prognosis. **Risk factors** include **cirrhosis and HCV** (more common in the West), **HBV and aflatoxins** (more in developing countries). Median survival following diagnosis is approximately 6-20 months.

Essentials of diagnosis

1. Most patients are asymptomatic until late stage. Initial presentations are commonly chronic abdominal distension and RUQ tenderness; later with jaundice, easy bruisability (coagulopathy), fatigability, and cachexia (wasting and weight loss). P/E may find an enlarged, tender liver.

2. **Lab tests**: Elevated LFTs and **marked AFP increase** are often seen. Initial abdominal MRI may find < 1cm mass in suspected patient. If it's negative, follow-up ultrasound (may show a mass) is suggested every 3 months. Larger lesions require further evaluation with CT or MRI. Liver biopsy confirms the diagnosis.

Treatment

1. If a small, solitary tumor is diagnosed early, aggressive major liver resection with the tumor can be the effective treatment, with a good 5-year survival.

2. For tumors that are not surgically resectable, liver transplantation is the only potentially curative option. For late-stage cancer (unresectable tumor +/- metastasis) that cannot go through liver transplantation, suggested therapies include radiofrequency ablation (shrinking) +/- transarterial chemoembolization +/- percutaneous ethanol injection +/- surgical resection. Standard chemotherapy alone is not effective; clinical trial showed sorafenib plus doxorubicin is better than doxorubicin alone.

3. **AFP is used to monitor tumor recurrence**. Avoidance of exposure to hepatic carcinogens and alcohol, and vaccination against HBV together have recorded decreases in morbidity.

GENETIC BILIRUBINEMIA

It's a group of uncommon diseases and summarized in the table below.

Table 4-4: Summary of Genetic Bilirubinemia

Disease / Clinical features, diagnosis, and treatment
Gilbert syndrome (disease)
It's the most common genetic cause of indirect bilirubinemia, a benign autosomal recessive or dominant disease due to a mild **deficiency of glucuronosyltransferase**. The jaundice fluctuates and is exacerbated by physical stress, infection, fasting, fever, surgery, or ethanol, and **alleviated by barbital use**. Elevated bilirubin is mostly < 5 mg/dL. Patient usually has no other abnormalities and requires no special treatment.
Crigler-Najjar syndrome
It's an autosomal recessive disease, with **more severe deficiency in glucuronosyltransferase than Gilbert syndrome**, causing a significant indirect bilirubinemia (20-40 mg/dL), which is not alleviated by barbital use. **Tx**: Most patients present with kernicterus in infancy and thus require phototherapy, etc.
Dubin-Johnson syndrome
It's a benign, autosomal recessive disease with **defects in biliary excretion**. Patient is usually asymptomatic except for jaundice, increased direct bilirubin and GGT, and occasional abdominal pain and hepatomegaly, with **black granules** in hepatocytes. The jaundice is exacerbated by infections, pregnancy, or OCP use. No special Tx.
Rotor syndrome
It's similar to DJS but there are **no pigmented granules** in hepatocytes. Decreased secretion of bilirubin causes direct bilirubin to increase (> 50% total bilirubin). GGT is increased. Most patients have no symptoms and no need for Tx.

DISORDERS OF THE INTESTINE

Diarrhea

It's defined as increase in stool weight or frequency. **Acute:** < 14 days; **Chronic:** > 2-3 weeks. Types by pathogenesis include infectious, secretory, and osmotic diarrhea.

Etiology

1. **Acute: GI infection (No.1 cause)**, food poisoning, systemic infection, or prolonged antibiotic use.

2. **Chronic: Lactase deficiency (No.1 cause)**, milk or soy intolerance, indigestion, celiac disease, cystic fibrosis, IBS, IBD, Giardiasis, or laxative abuse.

I. Infectious diarrhea (for details, refer to "Chapter 1 INFECTIOUS DISEASES")

Table 4-5: A Brief Summary of Infectious Diarrhea by Etiology

Causes / Clinical features
Virus: **#1** cause of infectious diarrhea; in schools or child-care center—**#1 rotavirus**, then adenovirus, Norwalk virus.
Campylobacter: **#1 cause of bacterial diarrhea** by contaminated foods. It can be watery or bloody diarrhea and can be associated with reactive arthritis.
Enterotoxigenic E. coli: #1 common when travelling in underdeveloped areas ("Traveller's diarrhea"). It mostly causes watery diarrhea.
Enteroinvasive E. coli O157:H7: Often in undercooked beef, hamburgers or milk, and causes bloody diarrhea, fever, and even hemolytic uremic syndrome (HUS) and thrombotic thrombocytopenic purpura (TTP).
Shigella: Transmitted by contaminated food or water; causes local invasion and bloody diarrhea.
Salmonella: A movable bacterium, often in raw eggs or dairy products; diarrhea + systemic symptoms.
Yersinia: Diarrhea + RLQ pain + joint pain + rash + fever. **Appendicitis is a differential diagnosis**.
C. difficile: With a history of recent hospitalization or antibiotic use.
Bacillus: Often in undercooked, leftover rice.
Giardia: Often from mountain water or camping.
M. Avium, cryptosporidia, isospora: Mostly in immunocompromised patients.

II. Secretory diarrhea

It's a large volume of diarrhea, usually > 1L, usually hormone mediated (carcinoid syndrome, Z-E-S, or VIPoma). Laxative use such as phenolphthalein can also cause it.

III. Osmotic diarrhea

It's caused by undigested solute pulling fluid in intestinal lumen by the osmotic pressure. Common solutes are lactate, fructose, and sorbitol.

Lactase Deficiency (Lactose intolerance)

It's the #1 cause of osmotic diarrhea and more common in Asian and Black populations.

Diagnosis: 1. Abdominal cramps, bloating, foul-smelling loose stool after ingestion of milk products. Occurs after milk-meals (bloating + diarrhea) and improves with fasting.

2. Hydrogen breath test (+), clinitest of stool for reducing substances (+), increased osmotic gap.

Treatment: Avoid milk product and supply lactase.

Diagnosis of diarrhea

1. Fecal leukocytes: in IBD and all enteroinvasive diarrheas (except Giardia and Cryptosporidia).

2. Stool culture, ova, and parasite. String test and stool giardia antigen are performed if Giardia is suspected.

3. Fecal Na(OH) test: Turns red in phenolphthalein use.

4. Colonoscopy or biopsy may be done for complicated cases.

Treatment of diarrhea

Most infectious diarrhea is self-limited. IV fluid plus antibiotics can be used in severe, invasive diarrheas: TMP-SMX (Bactrim) or ciprofloxacin is the first-line drug. Metronidazole is the best choice for Giardia.

Antibiotic-associated Colitis (Pseudomembranous Colitis)

It's caused by Clostridium difficile overgrowth (thus also called "**fulminant C. difficile colitis**") in the colon and toxin production usually after prolonged (several weeks) use of any antibiotic, with cephalosporins as the most common one.

Essentials of diagnosis

1. History of antibiotic use, fever, abdominal cramps, diarrhea without blood or mucus, and increase WBC.

2. **No.1 test—stool toxin assay for C. difficile**: Most assays are positive with three stool tests.

3. If complicated, colonoscopy can be done to demonstrate the pseudomembranes, plaques, and exudates.

Treatment

The first step of management is cessation of the inciting antibiotic. **The drug of choice is oral vancomycin** (also covering metronidazole-resistant cases). IV metronidazole is added in patients with fulminant or refractory disease. If it recurs (about 10%), this therapy is repeated. **Note that IV vancomycin is not effective.**

Malabsorption Syndromes

It refers to disruption in absorption of dietary nutrients across the intestinal wall, mostly accompanied with steatorrhea and fat-soluble Vit (A, D, E, K) deficiencies (by pancreatic insufficiency, cystic fibrosis or celiac sprue). Clinical types may include:

I. Celiac sprue

It's an autoimmune disorder of the small intestine with atrophy. It is associated with **gluten sensitivity** and intolerance (protein in wheat, cereal, pasta, etc.), **anti-endomysial and anti-gliadin antibodies**, and dermatitis herpetiformis. It's more common in females and the Caucasian (White) population.

II. Tropical sprue

It's an acquired malabsorption disease in tropics without clear causes, marked with abnormal flattening of the villi and inflammation of the lining of the small intestine. It may be secondary to an infectious pathogen or toxin. It differs significantly from celiac sprue.

III. Lactase deficiency

It's congenital lactase deficiency with the inability to digest lactose, causing milk product intolerance.

Essentials of diagnosis

1. Sprues typically have steatorrhea (> 14g/dL fecal fat) that is determined by 48-72 hour stool collection for Sudan staining. Patients may also have presentations of deficiencies of iron, folate, and fat-soluble vitamins (A, D, E, K), abdominal bloating, growth retardation, weight loss, osteoporosis, lactose or B_{12} deficiency (in tropical sprue).

2. **Differential diagnosis**: **D-Xylose test** is normal in pancreatic insufficiency and cystic fibrosis, and abnormal in small bowel diseases. Small **bowel biopsy** can confirm and distinguish diseases of the small bowel (celiac, tropical sprue, etc.), from decreased trypsin and secretin levels (chronic pancreatitis).

(1) <u>Celiac sprue</u>: (a) Steatorrhea improvement after gluten removal from the diet. (b) Abnormal small bowel biopsy ("flattening" of the villi). B_{12} deficiency is more common than tropical sprue.

(2) <u>Tropical sprue</u>: Symptoms are similar to those of celiac sprue but not improved with gluten-free diet.

(3) <u>Lactase deficiency</u>: Abdominal bloating and cramps, flatulence, diarrhea, nausea, or vomiting after consuming significant amounts of lactose. Dairy product challenge tests may help with diagnosis.

Treatment--Based on specific etiology.

1. Celiac sprue: Gluten-free diet, vitamin (A, D, E, K, B_{12}, folic acid) supplements and psyllium seed husks are recommended.

2. Tropical sprue: Tetracycline (more effective than TMP-SMX) plus folic acid for 3-6 months are recommended.

3. Bacterial overgrowth: Empiric antibiotics.

4. Pancreatic insufficiency: Pancreatic enzymes and vitamin supplements are needed.

5. Lactase deficiency: No treatment is necessary. Foods containing lactose should be avoided.

Complication

Celiac sprue: Intestinal lymphoma is common.

Whipple Disease

It's a rare GI infection and disorder caused by Tropheryma whippleii (a Gram$^+$, non-acid-fast, PAS-positive rod) infection, leading to intestinal lymphatic obstruction. Symptoms are similar to other malabsorption syndromes (abdominal bloating and cramps, flatulence, diarrhea/steatorrhea, vitamin deficiencies), except with characteristic extraintestinal manifestations—arthralgia and CNS symptoms (dementia, ophthalmoplegia, etc.).

Whipple dz

Essentials of diagnosis

Diagnosis is based on the above manifestations, upper endoscopy and biopsies of the small intestine for T. whipplei testing—showing **foamy macrophages (acid-Schiff stain)**. **Xylose test** (GI mucosa defects) is mostly positive.

Treatment

The recommended therapies include supportive care plus **penicillin or ceftriaxone** for 2-4 weeks followed by maintenance therapy with oral **TMP-SMX** (Bactrim) or doxycycline for 12 months.

Irritable Bowel Syndrome (IBS)

IBS is defined as recurrent abdominal pain or discomfort at least three days per month in the last three months with two or more of the following: improvement with defecation, onset associated with a change in frequency of stool (diarrhea or constipation), onset associated with a change in form of stool. It's a common, idiopathic functional GID and more common in young patients with stress, anxiety, or depression.

Essentials of diagnosis

1. > 3-month recurrent abdominal distention and pain relieved by defecation with altered bowel habits (diarrhea or constipation +/- mucus in stool). Weight is usually normal.

2. Rule out lactose intolerance, inflammatory bowel disease, and hypo- or hyperthyroidism.

3. If > 40 y/a, always rule out colorectal tumors by a sigmoidoscopy (or colonoscopy if patient has the family history).

Treatment

1. Reassurance and modification of life style and diet (stress reduction, exclusion of gas-producing foods, fiber supplements).

2. Symptomatic treatment: Antispasmodic agents (hyoscyamine, dicyclomine); antimotility agents (loperamide for diarrhea); promoting bowel movement (psyllium, polyethylene glycol, or lubiprostone); antidepressants.

INFLAMMATORY BOWEL DISEASES (IBD)

Ulcerative Colitis (UC)

It's a common chronic IBD characterized by continuous, superficial, ulcerative lesions in the lining of the rectum (most common) and colon. There is a risk of colorectal cancer, especially with pancolitis.

Essentials of diagnosis

1. Local: LLQ abdominal cramps and bloody diarrhea with mucus or pus in most patients.

Ulcerative Colitis

2. Systemic: Mild fever, weight loss, arthritis, iritis or uveitis, erythema nodosum, and pyoderma gangrenosum.

3. Lab tests: Evidence of iron deficient anemia and elevated ESR. Vit-B12 deficiency is rare.

4. Sigmoidoscopy/colonoscopy: Shows **diffuse and continuous inflammation and superficial ulcers** and pseudopolyps without granulomas, mostly involving the rectum. Biopsy is indicated if the case is complicated.

Treatment

1. Acute, mild-moderate cases: Topical (enema) anti-inflammative agent 5-aminosalicylic acid (5-ASA) +/- topical steroids +/- antibiotics (such as sulfonamide). Other NSAIDs may not be very effective for small bowel inflammation.

2. Resistant cases: Combined oral and topical 5-ASA plus steroids (prednisone) are recommended. Immunosuppressants (6-MP, azathioprine, infliximab) may be reserved for more refractory cases. If all the above treatment fails, colectomy is curative.

Complications

They include severe bleeding, toxic megacolon, perforation, strictures, primary sclerosing cholangitis, and the development of dysplasia and colorectal cancer. Toxic megacolon is a severe, fulminant stage of UC, usually leading to dilation and microperforation of the bowel, hypotension, and sepsis, *and, peritonitis*

Crohn Disease (CD)

Also known as **regional enteritis,** it is an **IBD** mostly involving all layers of the bowel wall, particularly the ileocecal region. It may affect any part of the gastrointestinal tract and lead to a wide variety of symptoms. This disease may be caused by interactions between environmental, immunological and bacterial factors in genetically susceptible individuals.

Essentials of diagnosis

1. Local: RLQ abdominal pain or mass, nonbloody diarrhea +/- mucus.

ant. uveitis: painful redness photophobia, tearing. ↓ visual acuity
episcleritis: red eye, tearing, no pain or ↓ visual acuity

2. Systemic: Mild fever, nausea/vomiting, weight loss, arthritis, iritis or uveitis, episcleritis, erythema nodosum, and pyoderma gangrenosum.

3. Lab tests: Evidence of iron-deficient anemia, Vit B12 deficiency, and elevated ESR.

4. Colono/sigmoido-scopy: Aphthoid or linear ulcers, strictures, **"cobblestoning and skip lesion."** **Non-caseating granuloma**(s) is the pathologic mark.

PEARLS — Differential points between CD and UC

CD commonly has skin lesions, regional transmural granulomas, fistulas, abscesses, masses, obstruction, perianal disease, and Vit B12 deficiency. UC usually has none of those, but lesions on the superficial mucosa, with more risk of colorectal cancer, and the cure by colectomy.

Treatment

1. Sulfasalazine or mesalamine (5-ASA) +/- sulfonamide is usually effective.

Inflamm bowel dz tx

2. Prednisone +/- immunosuppressants +/- antibiotics (ciprofloxacin or metronidazole): Reserved for refractory cases. Metronidazole is good for patients with fistulas.

3. Surgical resection: Indicated for severe complications (such as perforation), with a relatively high recurrent rate.

Complications

Fistula formation, obstruction, and urinary oxalate stones. *Ant. uveitis.*

Acute Mesenteric Ischemia

sudden abd pn followed by rectal bleeding.
/ due to inadequate perfusion of watershed colon 'splenic flexure'

Acute mesenteric Thrombosis:
- Abd pn out of proportion to PE, N/V, s.
bloody diarrhea due to mucosal sloughing.
- numerous atherosclerotic RFs

Acute mesenteric ischemia (AMI) is a syndrome or **ischemic colitis** caused by inadequate blood flow through the mesenteric vessels, resulting in ischemia and eventual gangrene of the bowel wall. Although relatively rare, it is a potentially **life-threatening** condition.

I. Superior mesenteric artery (SMA) ischemia

SMA is mostly due to low blood flow (CHF or hypotension), **occlusion** (atrial fibrillation embolus, thrombus), or vessel spasm (as by digitalis).

Clinical features and diagnosis

(1) Abdominal pain 0.5-1 hour after meals, constant and out of proportion to exam.

(2) Lab tests: Elevated WBC and K^+, with acidosis; serum amylase may also increase.

(3) **Imaging: CT angiography without contrast is the initial test with a high degree of accuracy for diagnosing AMI**. CT can also confirm possible mechanical bowel obstruction. **Early arteriography** may be necessary and important in a suspected patient. AXR may show "**fingerprinting**" sign. Colonoscopy or sigmoidoscopy is used to confirm colonic ischemia.

Treatment

1. For occlusive ischemia—to restore intestinal blood flow as rapidly as possible: Early embolectomy (< 12 hours) plus artery dilation (stent placement) are critical to reduce mortality. Other therapies may include revascularization, resection of infarcted bowel, intra-artery infusion of a thrombolytic agent or a vasodilator, systemic anticoagulation, and empiric broad-spectrum antibiotics.

2. For nonocclusive ischemia: Infusion of a vasodilator (usually papaverine-HCl) into the SMA. Long-term management is aimed at preventing future embolic events with anticoagulation, and cardiovascular risk reduction strategies.

Differentiation

Superior mesenteric artery (SMA) syndrome:

It is a is a gastro-vascular disorder in which the third and final portion of the duodenum is compressed between the abdominal aorta (AA) and the overlying SMA due to the loss of mesenteric fat between the SMA and aorta resulting in compression of the third portion of the duodenum. Patients

SMA ischemia

present with symptoms consistent with a proximal small bowel obstruction. The diagnosis is based on clinical features indicating duodenal obstruction and CT/MRI showing an abnormal angle between the aorta and the SMA. Conventional arteriography may be needed for unconfirmed patients. **Treatment** may include gastric decompression, fluid resuscitation, correction of electrolyte abnormalities first, and then enteral or parenteral nutritional support. If conservative management is not effective, surgical options include mobilization of the ligament of Treitz, gastrojejunostomy, and duodenojejunostomy (best).

II. Inferior mesenteric Artery (IMA) ischemia

IMA is usually due to **low blood flow** caused by small vessel disease, myocardial infarction, aortic insufficiency, sepsis, cardiac arrhythmias, post-aneurysm-surgery damage, administration of digoxin or alpha-adrenergic agonists, cocaine, cardiopulmonary bypass, or dialysis.

Clinical features and diagnosis

(1) Painless bleeding or bloody diarrhea with LLQ pain.

(2) The commonest location is in **"watershed areas"**—splenic flexure & rectosigmoid. Angiogram is not as helpful as for occlusive ischemia. Diagnosis is mostly clinical.

Treatment

1. For acute nonocclusive ischemia: Infusion of a vasodilator (papaverine hydrochloride) is effective.

2. For chronic, isolated IMA occlusion: Treatment options include arterial embolectomy, arterial bypass, arterial stenting, and arterial or venous thrombolysis. Revascularization is the best therapy.

Diverticular Diseases of the Colon

I. Diverticulosis

Large-volume bleeding = frank, red blood
Low-moderate bleeding from Right colon will mix into stool → hematochezia.

It's the outpouching of colonic mucosa through the muscle layers; maybe due to an increased colonic intraluminal pressure caused by low fiber diet. It's most common in sigmoid colon and usually asymptomatic unless complicated by diverticulitis or hemorrhage. Incidence increases with age.

Essentials of diagnosis

1. LLQ colicky pain and relieved by defecation (painful diverticular syndrome). Patient may also have typical painless rectal bleeding or **hematochezia** (melena)—**No.1 common complication and cause of lower GI bleeding in patient > 40 y/a**.

2. Colonoscopy or barium enema confirms the diagnosis. A bleeding scan or angiography is indicated if the hemorrhage is severe.

Treatment

1. Non-bleeding disease: Symptomatic treatment and addition of fiber in the diet (metamucil).

Diverticulosis

2. **Diverticular bleeding:** It's mostly self-limited (75%). If the bleeding is severe, recurrent, or complicated, angiography with embolization or endoscopic surgery is indicated.

II. **Diverticulitis**

It's a complication of diverticulosis and is inflammation and microperforation caused by infection, obstruction, undigested food or fecalith trapped in the diverticula (mostly sigmoid). It is often associated with segmental colitis.

Essentials of diagnosis

1. LLQ pain, low fever, and a possibly palpable sigmoid mass but **no lower GI bleeding**.

2. WBC is increased and stool guaiac test is positive.

3. **CT** is the best means of diagnosis. Sigmoidoscopy and barium enema may increase the risk of perforation and are only indicated after the acute phase in patients > 50 y/a to rule out colon cancer.

Treatment

1. Bowel rest (no enteric foods) for a day, antibiotics (ciprofloxacin plus metronidazole for 10-14 days), and hydration. Approximately six weeks after recovery, a colonoscopy should be performed (if not done yet) to evaluate the extent of the diverticulosis and exclude colonic neoplasia.

2. If a surgical complication is suspected, such as septic colon, obstruction, or fistula, an operation may be necessary.

NEOPLASMS OF THE INTESTINE

Carcinoid Tumors and Carcinoid Syndrome

Tumors of neuroendocrine origin and may produce serotonin, tryptophan, or tachykinins (substance-P) and thus cause a set of typical clinical manifestations.

Location: Appendix (the most common local, nonsecreting carcinoid), ileum (the most common "systemic syndrome", secreting 5-HT), or bronchi (symptomatic).

Essentials of diagnosis

1. Classic syndrome with tumors of the ileum and bronchi (70% metastatic): intermittent diarrhea, facial flushing, wheezing, ethanol intolerance, tachycardia, and hypotension. Right heart abnormalities may be present.

2. 24-hour urine collection for 5-HIAA (5-hydroxyindolacetic acid) test confirms the diagnosis. Contrast-enhanced MRI of the abdomen and pelvis has high sensitivity for metastases.

Treatment

Surgical resection of the involved segment and small bowel mesentery with regional lymphadenectomy is recommended for most localized, nonmetastatic carcinoid tumors. **Octreotide**

(somatostatin analogue) can help improve symptoms for patients with the rare bronchial neuroendocrine tumors and metastatic tumors.

Colorectal Carcinoma (CRC)

The morbidity and mortality of CRC is the **third most common malignancy** for both male and female. Most colorectal carcinomas arise from adenomatous polyps > 2 cm and after 5-10 years.

There are four types of colon polyps:

(1) Tubular adenoma (adenomatous polyp, most common type);

(2) Villous or tubulovillous adenoma;

(3) Hyperplastic polyp;

(4) Inflammatory polyp (commonly seen in ulcerative colitis or Crohn disease; considered non-cancerous). Degree of cancer risk: Villous > tubular > hyperplastic polyps (low risk).

Risk factors

Family history of CRC (No.1 factor), familial polyposis syndrome and genetics (APC gene, p54), diet (high fat, high "red-meat" and low fiber), smoking, obesity, ulcerative colitis, alcohol consumption, chronic history of constipation, Strep-bovis infection, and high-income population. High fiber diet and aspirin may decrease risk.

Essentials of diagnosis

1. **Hematochezia** (melena, the most common symptom) and a change in bowel habits are relatively early symptoms. Later, pencil-thin stools, abdominal obstruction (left colon cancer), anemia (right colon cancer), abdominal pain, fatigue, and weight loss may be present. 20% of patients present with metastatic disease. The most common metastatic sites are the regional lymph nodes, liver, lungs, and peritoneum.

2. **Colonoscopy with biopsy is the most accurate means of diagnosis**. **Ba-enema followed by colonoscopy** is the most commonly used way of diagnosis. Ba-enema X-ray usually shows an **"apple-core" filling defect** (**Image 53**), or image of polyps.

3. **Anatomic staging by the TNM and Duke** system.

Stage I (Tis, T_1, T_2, N_0, M_0)—Duke A: mucosa and submucosa; >80% of 5-year survival rate.

Stage II (II_A, II_B, II_C; T_{3-4}, N_0, M_0)—Duke B: muscularis (B_1) into or through serosa (B_2); 60-80% of 5-year survival.

Stage III (III_A, III_B, III_C, N_{1-2}, M_0)—Duke C: regional lymph nodes—LN (+); 35-60% of 5-year survival.

Stage IV (any $T+N+M_1$; no Duke Class): distant metastasis (#1 common to the liver); 1-5% of 5-year survival.

Treatment

1. **For Stage I and II, lymph nodes (LN (-):** Surgical resection along with follow-ups by colonoscopy in 6-12 months, then 3-5 years.

2. **Stage III, LN (+):** Resection along with chemo/radio-therapy (oxaliplatin-based or 5-fluorouracil). Small to moderate metastases to liver or other organs are resected as much as possible, along with chemotherapy. Postoperative chemotherapy eradicates micrometastases, reduces the likelihood of disease recurrence, and increases cure rates. For non-surgical candidates, palliative chemotherapy is considered.

3. **Postsurgery follow-up**: Colonoscopy in 6 months and then 3 years are commonly used. Carcinoembryonic antigen (CEA) should be obtained before and after surgery and used to monitor recurrence at least for the first three years.

Important Prevention

Healthy life style: (1) Regular exercise and no smoking; (2) Reduction of fat in diet carries more benefits than high-fiber diet, though both are good.

PEARLS — Recommended CRC Screening

—**With benefits of early diagnosis and reduced mortality.**

1. **For most people with average risk:**

(1) **Annual FIT or iFOBT** (fecal immunochemical test) starts at age 50 and through age 75. If (+), colonoscopy is indicated and per 2-4 years.

(2) **Colonoscopy every 10 years** or CT colonography every 5 years through age 75 starts at age 50 (45 for the Black population).

2. **For patients at increased risk:**

(1) If a first-degree relative had CRC < 50 y/a, colonoscopy is started at age 40 or 10 years earlier than the age when the family member had CRC, and per 3-5 years.

(2) If the family CRC was diagnosed > 50 y/a, colonoscopy is started at age 50 and per 5 years.

(3) If patient has a personal history of CRC or adenomatous polyps, ulcerative colitis, or Crohn disease, colonoscopy and consultation are needed. Patient should have colonoscopy at 1 year after tumor resection, then at 3 years, then every 5 years. With family adenomatous polyposis (FAP), sigmoidoscopy is started at age 12 and every year. If the FAP or ulcerative colitis is present for 10 years, prophylactic colectomy is recommended.

(4) If multiple family members or 2-generations had CRC, or family with Lynch syndrome (HNPCC), colonoscopy is started at age 25 and every 1-2 years.

HEMORRHAGE OF THE DIGESTIVE TRACT

Upper GI Hemorrhage

It refers to GI tract bleeding proximal to the ligament of Treitz, which connects the fourth portion of the duodenum to the diaphragm near the splenic flexure of the colon. Sources include gastric erosions, PUD, esophageal varices, Mallory-Weiss tear, esophagitis, and gastric tumor.

Essentials of diagnosis

1. **History** of **hematemesis** (bright red if fresh or coffee-ground vomiting if not), **melena** (black stool, indicating > 60 ml blood loss), **orthostatic hypotension, occult bleeding, and iron-deficiency anemia** (in slower chronic bleeding). **BUN** may be elevated because of bacterial breakdown of blood.

2. **Nasogastric lavage**: Fast, blood (+) indicates an active bleed.

3. **EGD-scopy: Both diagnostic and therapeutic.** It's also prognostic. Erythromycin use is recommended prior to the examination.

Treatment

1. Adequate IV fluid is very important to save life in case of major bleeding. Emergent EGD is diagnostic and therapeutic—indicated for all patients—electrocoagulation, injection therapy, sclerotherapy, and band ligation for varices.

2. IV omeprazole (PPI) helps reduce risk of recurrent bleeding from PUD.

Lower GI Hemorrhage

It refers to GI tract bleeding distal to the ligament of Treitz and superior to the anus, mostly involving the colon.

Sources: Diverticulosis (No.1 common in the elderly), hemorrhoids (No.1 in the young), angiodysplasia, infectious colitis (E. coli O157:H7, Shigella, Salmonella, Campylobacter jejuni), IBD, cancer, mesenteric ischemia, Meckel diverticulum, and coagulopathy (a bleeding diathesis).

Essentials of diagnosis

1. Based on vital signs (hypovolemia), mental status, and patient history.

2. Laboratory tests: Decreased hemoglobin, hematocrit, and platelets are good evidence of hypovolemia or blood loss. aPTT may also be tested.

Treatment

Treat underlying cause. In most cases emergency hospital admission is required and the bleeding resolves spontaneously. Adequate IV fluid is very important to save life in case of major bleeding.

GI Angiodysplasia (Vascular ectasia)

It is a small vascular malformation of the bowel, the second common lower GI tract bleeding in the elderly and a common cause of otherwise unexplained GI bleeding and anemia. Lesions are often multiple, and frequently involve the cecum or ascending colon. It may also be part of hereditary **Osler-Rendu-Weber syndrome**—multiple angiodysplasias on nose, skin, mucosa, lung, brain, and GI tract.

Assoc. w vWF def, Aortic Stenosis (delayed carotid pulses)

Clinical features and diagnosis

R.colon

1. Painless lower GI bleeding in elder patients; cecum is the commonest site.
2. Perform colonoscopy first--for active bleeding; both diagnostic and therapeutic. If negative, labelled-RBC scan is confirmative.   *cautery*

Treatment

Endoscopic injection therapy is effective. Medication or occasional surgery may be needed. Adequate IV fluid is very important to save life in case of major bleeding. Angiogenesis inhibitors or octreotide may have some effects.

PEARLS—Indications for Diagnostic Tests for GI Bleeding

Labelled-RBC scan: Endoscopy unrevealing in a massive acute hemorrhage .

Angiography: Specific vessel or site of bleeding that needs to be identified before surgery or embolization of the vessel; use only in unresponsive, massive bleeding.

Capsule endoscopy: Small bowel bleeding; cause unidentified after upper and lower endoscopy.

CT or MRI: Not very helpful.

MISCELLANEOUS DISEASES

Hereditary (Familial) Colorectal Cancer Syndromes

These are **autosomal dominant polyposis syndromes** associated with malignancy and are mostly from adenomatous polyps (pre-cancerous disease). **Familial** adenomatous polyposis (FAP) and **Lynch syndrome** (hereditary nonpolyposis colorectal cancer [HNPCC]) are the most common of the familial colon cancer syndromes.

I. Familial adenomatous polyposis (FAP)

This is the most common familial polyposis syndrome. It's associated with an APC gene mutation in the adenomatous polyposis coli (APC) test. It is characterized by the early onset of hundreds to thousands of adenomatous polyps (and adenocarcinoma) throughout the colon. If left untreated, all patients (100%) with this syndrome develop colon cancer by age 35-40 years. In addition, an increased risk exists for the development of other malignancies.

Diagnosis: FAP should be suspected in patients with >10 cumulative colorectal adenomas or a history of adenomas in combination with extracolonic features associated with FAP. Germline mutations in the APC gene establish the diagnosis of FAP or attenuated FAP.

Treatment: Total colectomy is recommended.

Gardner syndrome

Also known as **brain tumor-polyposis syndrome, mismatch repair cancer syndrome** (MMRCS), it is a rare cancer syndrome associated with biallelic DNA mismatch repair mutations—colonic polyps along with CNS tumors (medulloblastomas and gliomas). It's an autosomal recessive disorder, perhaps a variant of FAP, and not curable.

Turcot syndrome

Also known as mismatch repair cancer syndrome (MMRCS), it is a rare cancer syndrome associated with biallelic DNA mismatch repair mutations—colonic polyps along with CNS tumors. It's an autosomal recessive disorder, perhaps a variant of FAP, and not curable.

II. Lynch Syndrome—Hereditary Nonpolyposis Colorectal Cancer (HNPCC)

It is an **autosomal dominant genetic cancer syndrome that carries a high risk of colorectal cancer (50-80% lifetime and earlier than 45 y/a), brain tumors** (astrocytoma or glioblastoma), and other malignancies including the endometrium, ovary, GIT, and skin cancers. The increased risk for these cancers is due to inherited multi-gene mutations that impair DNA mismatch repair. Family history is usually significant (first-degree relatives, more than two generations).

Diagnosis

Evaluation is warranted in patients with personal or familial history of any of the above cancers at young age. Diagnosis is suspected by tumor tissue immunohistochemical staining for mismatched proteins, and confirmed by genetic testing.

Management

1. Colonoscopy starting at age 25 years, or 10 years prior to earliest family diagnosis, whichever is earlier; then every 1-2 years.

2. Esophagogastroduodenoscopy (EGD) starting at age 30 years.

3. Urine cytology with or without urinalysis starting at age 30-35 years.

4. Consider endometrial sampling and/or concurrent transvaginal ultrasound.

5. Consider prophylactic hysterectomy and bilateral salpingo-oophorectomy if childbearing is completed.

Hamartomatous Polyposis Syndromes

It's a heterogeneous group of disorders that share an autosomal dominant pattern of inheritance. These are GI polyps with low malignant potential and they should stll be removed by colonoscopy followed by surveillance. Associated syndromes include:

I. Peutz-Jeghers syndrome

Multiple hamartomatous polyps are found in large and small intestines, and are associated with mucocutaneous pigmentation—melanotic spots on the lips and skin, and increased frequency of **breast, gonadal, and pancreatic cancers**.

II. Familial juvenile polyposis (syndrome)

It's also autosomal dominant and is characterized by multiple (>10) hamartomatous polyps in the colon. There is an increased risk of adenocarcinoma. Genetic testing (to reveal defects) is helpful in diagnosis.

III. PTEN multiple hamartoma (tumor) syndrome (Cowden disease)

It is characterized by hamartomatous polyps and lipomas throughout the GI tract with cerebellar lesions. There is an increased risk of malignancy in the thyroid, breast, and urogenital tract.

VITAMIN DEFICIENCIES

Clinical features and treatment of common vitamin (Vit) deficiencies are summarized below.

I. Thiamine (Vitamin B1) deficiency

1. Most common in patients with chronic alcoholism—poor dietary intakes and impaired absorption of B1; other causes—renal dialysis, high-dose glucose IV.

2. Early symptoms: anorexia, muscle cramps, paresthesias, irritability.

3. Advanced syndromes: high-output heart failure ("wet beriberi"), peripheral nerve disorders, and **Wernicke-Korsakoff syndrome** (WKS, "dry beriberi").

WKS Triad: (1) Encephalopathy (disorientation and confusion); **(2) ataxia** (polyneuropathy, cerebellar and vestibular dysfunction); **(3) ophthalmoplegia** (nystagmus, conjugate-gaze palsy, and lateral rectus palsy). **Korsakoff dementia: (1) Same clinical triad of WKS.** (2) Additional anterograde and retrograde amnesia, confabulation, and horizontal nystagmus, which are **irreversible**.

Treatment: Large doses of Vit-B1 IV (before glucose) can reverse symptoms rapidly.

II. Riboflavin (Vitamin B2) deficiency

1. Always coexists with other Vit deficiencies due to dietary inadequacy and interactions with alcoholism and some drugs.

2. Cheilosis, angular stomatitis, glossitis, seborrheic dermatitis, anemia, and corneal vascularization.

Treatment: 1. Foods rich in meat and dairy products. 2. Supplemental Vit-B2.

III. Niacin (Vitamin B3) Deficiency

1. More commonly due to alcoholism and nutrient-drug interactions.

2. Anorexia, stomatitis, and "**triad of pellagra--DDD**" (dermatitis, diarrhea, and dementia).

Treatment: Oral niacin is effective.

IV. Vitamin B6 Deficiency

1. #1 cause is interactions with medications—especially isoniazid, cycloserine, penicillamine, and oral contraceptives, or alcoholism.

2. Similar symptoms as Vit-B2 deficiency plus peripheral neuritis.

Treatment: Oral Vit-B6 supplement is effective.

V. Vitamin B12 deficiency

1. **Major pathology**: Pernicious anemia; degeneration of the posterior and lateral columns of the spinal cord.

2. **Risk factors**: Strict vegetarians and gastric or ileal resection.

3. **Clinical features**: Gradual, progressive, symmetric paresthesia, stocking/glove- sensory deficits, spasticity, paraplegia, leg stiffness, bowel and bladder dysfunction, and dementia.

Treatment: Vit-B12 IM or large-dose PO.

VI. Folate deficiency—pernicious anemia

1. **Risk factors**: Alcoholics; diet lack of green vegetables.

2. **Features**: Symptoms of anemia, irritability, and personality changes; no neuro-deficiency.

Treatment: Reversible with early supplemental folate in diet.

VII. Vitamin C deficiency

1. **Causes**: Mostly due to dietary inadequacy in the poor, the elderly, and chronic alcoholics.

2. **Typical "scurvy"**—perifollicular/splinter/gum hemorrhage, petechiae, purpura, anemia, delayed wound healing, etc.

Treatment: Oral Vit-C is effective.

VIII. Vitamin A deficiency

1. A common nutritional deficiency and cause of blindness in poor families.

2. Early presentations: night blindness, xerosis (dry conjunctiva), "**Bitot spots**" (conjunctival white patches); later: keratomalacia (corneal ulceration & necrosis), perforation, endophthalmitis, blindness, and skin hyperkeratinization.

Treatment: Oral Vit-A is effective.

Vit-A toxicity: Excess intake of beta-carotenes can cause toxic presentations of dry, scaly skin, hair loss, painful mouth and hyperostosis, anorexia, vomiting, and headache, etc. Withdrawal of Vit-A from the diet is the treatment.

IX. Vitamin **D deficiency**

See "Osteomalacia" in this chapter.

X. Vitamin **K deficiency**

See "Chapter 6: Hematology".

XI. Vitamin **E deficiency**

1. It can be caused by severe malabsorption and chronic diarrhea.

2. Presenting with areflexia, disturbances of gait, decreased proprioception and vibration, and ophthalmoplegia.

Treatment: Supplemental Vit-E is helpful. Large dose of Vit-E can improve neurologic complications.

PEARLS—Table 4-6: Summary of Vitamin Deficiencies and Manifestations

Vit-A: "**OD**" —Ocular lesions (xerosis, night blindness), dry scaly skin.
Vit-B1 (thiamine): **Beriberi ("HEN")** —Heart failure, encephalopathy (Wernicke-Korsakoff syndrome), neuritis.
Vit-B2 (riboflavin): "**ACC**" —Angular stomatitis, cheilosis, corneal vascularization.
Vit-B3 (niacin): **Pellagra ("DDD")** —Dermatitis, diarrhea, dementia.
Vit-B5 (pantothenate): Rare; dermatitis, enteritis, alopecia, adrenal insufficiency.
Vit-B6 (pyridoxine): "**DNA**" —Dermatitis, neuritis, anemia.
Vit B12 (cobalamin): "**ANG**" —Megaloblastic anemia, neuritis, glossitis.
Vit-C: **Scurvy** —Pseudoparalysis, scorbutic rosary, mucous membrane bleeding.
Vit-D: **Rickets** —Craniotabes, rachitic rosary, bowlegs; infantile tetany.
Vit-E: "**MAC**" —Muscle weakness, anemia, creatinuria.
Vit-K: "**HB**" —Hypoprothrombinemia, bleeding (prolonged PT and aPTT, normal BT).
Biotin ("Vit-H"): "**DE**" —Dermatitis, enteritis.
Folic Acid: Megaloblastic anemia without neurologic symptoms.
Selenium: Cardiomyopathy (e.g., **Keshan disease**).

Obesity

Definition: Obesity is a complex disorder involving excessive body fat that increases the risk of health problems. For adults, overweight and obesity ranges are determined by the body mass index (BMI), which is calculated by the body weight (kg) divided by height squared (meters). BMI closely correlates with the amount of body fat. BMI of 25-29.9 kg/m^2 is considered overweight; BMI > 30 kg/m^2 is obese. As children approach adulthood, the 85th and 95th percentiles for BMI are approximately 25 and 30 kg/m^2, the thresholds for overweight and obesity in adults, respectively.

Etiology

Obesity usually results from a combination of causes and contributing factors, including:

Genetics (not the decisive factor), family lifestyle (similar eating, lifestyle and activity habits), inactivity, unhealthy diet and eating habits (high in calories, lacking in fruits and vegetables, full of fast food, missing breakfast, etc), smoking cessation, pregnancy, lack of sleep (increasing the appetite), certain medications (antidepressants, anti-seizure drugs, diabetes medications, antipsychotics, steroids, and beta blockers), and rare disorders (Cushing syndrome, Prader-Willi syndrome).

PEARLS: Obesity-increased risk

1. Cardiovascular diseases (CVD): Heart disease (CAD, CHF, arrhythmia), hypertension, hyperlipidemia, stroke, etc.

2. Diabetes: Obesity increases insulin resistance, which can lead to type II diabetes.

3. Cancer: Endometrial cancer, breast cancer after menopause, colorectal cancer, gallbladder cancer, esophageal cancer, and kidney cancer.

4. Digestive disorders: Gallstones, fatty liver, cirrhosis, and gastroesophageal reflux disease (GERD).

5. Respiratory disorders: Sleep apnea, obesity hypoventilation syndrome (OHS), asthma, and Pickwickian syndrome (eventually causing heart disease).

6. Arthritis: Due to extra weight on the joints, especially knees, hips, and lower back.

7. Sex hormone disorders: Increased risk of infertility, irregular menstruation, and birth defects (especially neural tube defects).

Management

Generally, only about 20% of overweight people both eat fewer calories and engage in at least 150 min of physical activity each week. Thus, clinicians can play an important role in educating people regarding losing weight. The therapeutic goal is to prevent, reverse, or ameliorate the complications of obesity, and to achieve a realistic weight loss goal (5-7%). Treatment is based on initial risk assessment.

(1) BMI of 25-29.9 and no risk factors for CVD: At low risk. Individual should receive advice on dietary habits and physical activity.

(2) BMI of 25-29.9 and with one or more risk factors for CVD (diabetes, hypertension, dyslipidemia), or with a BMI of 30 to 34.9: At moderate risk. Patient is counseled about weight loss therapies (diet, physical activity, behavioral modification, and for some, medications).

(3) BMI of 35-40: At high risk. Patient should receive the most aggressive treatment (lifestyle intervention, pharmacologic therapy, and bariatric surgery).

1. Initial treatment: Comprehensive lifestyle intervention (a combination of diet, exercise, and behavioral modification) is the most important strategy for weight management. One example of a successful lifestyle intervention program is the Diabetes Prevention Program (DPP).

2. Drug therapy: Medications (such as orlistat or lorcaserin) may be a helpful therapy for those with a BMI around or > 30. However, the side effects and potential for abuse should be considered.

3. Surgery: Bariatric surgery is recommended for patients with (1) BMI ≥ 40 who have failed to lose weight with diet, exercise, and medication therapy; (2) BMI > 35 with obesity-related comorbidities (hypertension, diabetes, dyslipidemia, sleep apnea) who have failed other therapies.

Liposuction can significantly reduce fat mass and weight but not improve insulin sensitivity or risk factors for heart disease.

Chapter 4: High-yield Questions (YHQ)

1. A 30 y/o man presents with a 2-month history of progressive odynophagia, fatigue, cough, and weight loss. He has a history of repeated IV drug abuse and risky sexual behavior. He's currently taking an anti-inflammatory drug for the pain. Physical examination (P/E) finds a low-grade fever and low body weight. CXR and blood tests are ordered. Esophagoscopy finds diffuse shallow ulceration. What's the most likely esophageal complication in this patient?

A. Candida infection   B. CMV infection   C. HSV infection

D. Cancer   E. Drug lesion

2. A 50 y/o man comes to the physician for a 2-month history of progressive dysphagia, chest pain, cough, and fatigue. He has a 15-year history of smoking, alcohol use, and a sedentary lifestyle. P/E, CXR and CBC results are unremarkable. Serum Ca = 13.5 mg/dL. What's the most appropriate next step?

A. Endoscopy   B. Chest CT   C. Manometry

D. 24-hour pH monitoring   E. Ba-study

3. From the above patient (Q2), Ba-study and endoscopy reveal a mass with uneven ulcerated edges in the proximal 2/3 esophagus. Biopsy will most likely show which pathologic result?

A. ACC   B. SCC   C. ACC + Barrett esophagus

D. SCC + achalasia   E. Inflammatory mass

4—7: Match the following clinical scenarios with the most likely diagnosis.

A. Barrett esophagus   B. Zenker diverticulum   C. Mallory-Weiss syndrome

D. Achalasia   E. Diffuse esophageal spasm   F. Nutcracker esophagus

G. The Schatzki ring   H. Plummer-Vinson syndrome (P-V-S)

I. GERD   J. Boerhaave syndrome

4. A 55 y/o man complains of substernal burning after meals that is alleviated by standing/sitting and worsened with reclining. He has a 10-year history of alcohol drinking. At the doctor's office, he has an episode of bloody emesis. Endoscopy is scheduled.

5. A 60 y/o man is hospitalized for acute fever, shivering, and coughs with sputum. He has a 10-year history of alcohol use, and a month's history of difficulty in the initial stages of swallowing. P/E finds T = 39°C, tachypnea, bad breath, rough breath sound, and a mass in the upper neck. CXR reveals infiltrates in the right lung.

6. A 25 y/o woman complains of episodic dysphagia to solid foods. She occasionally drinks a small cup of wine and denies other abnormal symptoms. Endoscopy finds a lesion in the squamocolumnar junction near LES.

7. A 60 y/o woman presents with a 2-month history of progressive dysphagia, chest pain, cough, and fatigue. She has a 10-year history of smoking and alcohol use with recent difficulties in the initial stages of swallowing. P/E finds a pale patient with a low body weight. CXR is normal. CBC shows microcytic anemia. Ba-study reveals a hypopharyngeal fill defect with obscure margins.

8. A 46 y/o man complains of "dull stomach pain" 0.5-1 hour after meals, and occasional nausea/vomiting (N/V) and black stools for the past 2 months. He has a 5-year history of smoking and alcohol use. P/E finds a soft

abdominal with epigastric tenderness. CBC reveals microcytic anemia. FOBT (fecal occult blood test) is (+). What's the best next step?

A. H. pylori test   B. Ba X-ray   C. Endoscopy

D. Ba X-ray + endoscopy   E. H. pylori test + Ba X-ray

9. From the above patient, Ba X-ray reveals signs of antral gastritis without a mass, and ELISA for H. pylori is (+). Now what's the best next step?

A. Amoxicillin + bismuth salts   B. Metronidazole + Vit-B$_{12}$

C. Endoscopy + antral biopsy   D. Endoscopy + biopsy + surgery

E. Clarithromycin + metronidazole

10. A 55 y/o man presents with painless black stools and post-prandial abdominal pain for the past few days. He had surgery for an abdominal aneurysm 3 months ago but denies history of heart disease, alcohol abuse, or reflux. P/E reveals a soft abdomen with LLQ tenderness. CBC is normal and FOBT is (+). The best diagnostic step now is

A. Ultrasonography (U/S)   B. CT   C. angiogram

D. endoscopy   E. clinical basis

11. A 60 y/o woman comes to the clinic with upper abdominal cramp and nausea for 4 hours. She has no fever or other symptoms. P/E finds mild RUQ abdominal tenderness. CBC is normal. Ultrasound shows two small gallstones without bile duct dilation. What's the best next step?

A. Oral quinolones   B. ERCP   C. Surgical stone removal

D. Oral ampicillin   E. Symptomatic treatment and observation

12. A 50 y/o man is brought to the ER for constant, severe abdominal pain for 5 hours. He has a 2-month history of fatigue and itching after bathing. P/E finds a jaundiced patient with a smoothly enlarged and tender liver and spleen; no fever. Lab tests show elevated CBC, ALT, and AST. What's the most appropriate next abdominal exam?

A. CT   B. Ultrasonography   C. MRI

D. Arteriography   E. Venography

13. A 50 y/o man is brought to the ER for fever, sharp epigastric pain radiating to the back, and nausea for 4 hours after a big dinner. He also has a 6-mo history of chronic RUQ pain and periodic jaundice. P/E shows T = 39°C, HR = 100/min, BP = 90/70 mmHg; jaundiced skin, a soft abdomen, decreased bowel sounds, and a palpable mass with tenderness in the epigastric area. Lab tests show elevated serum lipase, amylase, AKP, and direct bilirubin; WBC = 15,000/uL, ALT and LDH both = 300 IU/L. IV fluid, analgesics and antibiotics are given. What's the best next step?

A. CT   B. Ultrasonography   C. MRI

D. ERCP   E. Surgical exploration

14. Continued with the above patient: two stones are seen by ERCP in the mildly swollen common bile duct and then removed. Ultrasound reveals a 5.5-cm pancreatic pseudocyst. Now what's the best next step?

A. CT + internal drainage   B. CT + external drainage   C. MRI

D. Symptomatic treatment   E. Surgical resection

15. A 50 y/o man complains of constant RUQ pain, fatigue, yellowing skin and weight loss for the past month. He has a 10-year history of smoking and alcohol use. P/E finds T = 37.5°C, jaundice, a soft abdomen, and a small mass in the RUQ with tenderness. Lab tests show FOBT (+) and elevated AKP and direct bilirubin. CBC is normal. What's the most appropriate next step?

A. CT   B. Ultrasonography   C. MRI

D. ERCP   E. CA 19-9 test

16—18: Match the following clinical scenarios with the most likely diagnosis.

A. Autoimmune hepatitis   C. Viral hepatitis   D. Rotor syndrome

E. Dubin-Johnson syndrome   F. Crigler-Najjar syndrome   G. Gilbert disease

H. Hemolytic anemia

16. A student just finished a final exam and comes to the clinic for yellowing eyes. He describes it as on and off for the past few days, and seemed alleviated after he took some "private sleeping pills." P/E finds mild jaundice of the sclera. Serum total bilirubin is 7 mg/dL (normal value < 1 mg/dL). CBC and platelet counts are normal.

17. A 40 y/o man complains of abdominal distension and yellowing skin for the past 3 days. He smokes and drinks a small cup of wine daily for the past 1-2 years. His uncle has a similar medical history. He denies chronic disease. P/E finds T = 37.5°C and jaundice of the skin and sclera. Ultrasound reveals an enlarged liver and spleen without a mass. Lab tests show direct bilirubin = 15 mg/dL (Nl value < 0.2mg); both ALT and AST are 300 IU/L; urine bilirubin is (+); CBC is normal. FNB of the liver shows black granules.

18. A 40 y/o man complains of abdominal distension and yellowing skin for the past 3 days. He smokes and drinks a small cup of wine occasionally for the past 1-2 years. His uncle had a similar history. He denies any chronic liver disease. P/E finds T = 37.7°C and jaundice of the skin and sclera. Ultrasound reveals an enlarged liver and spleen without a mass. Lab tests show total bilirubin = 8 mg/dL; both ALT and AST = 300 IU/L; platelets = 125,000/uL; ANA is (+); CBC is normal.

19. A 55 y/o man complains of progressive abdominal distension, yellowing skin, difficulty swallowing, foot swelling, shortness of breath, and weight loss for the past 2 months. Symptoms are not alleviated by daily use of spironolactone. He has a 10-year history of alcohol use and smoking. P/E finds tachycardia, jaundice, and lower limb edema. Lab tests: LFTs are increased; FOBT is (+). Ultrasound reveals a small liver with fluid in the abdomen. What's the most effective treatment to control the ascites without significant risk of hepatic encephalopathy?

A. Na-restriction + oral neomycin   B. Distal splenorenal shunt

C. Large volume of paracentesis + IV albumin   D. Portal-caval shunt

E. TIPS (transjugular intrahepatic portosystemic shunt)

20. The above patient (Q19) has decreased ascites after treatment, but new tests show his urine output = 300 ml/24 hrs, urine-Na = 10 mEq/L, urine-K = 0.8 mEq/L, serum K = 5.6 mEq/L, and creatinine = 2.5 mg/dL. What's your immediate next step?

A. Diuretic cessation   B. Dialysis   C. Preparation for liver transplantation

D. Stronger diuretics   E. IV saline

21—28: Match the following clinical scenarios with the best diagnostic test.

A. D-Xylose test   B. Stool toxin test   C. Hydrogen breath test

D. Schilling test   E. Stool culture, ova, and parasite

F. Stool antigen test   G. FOBT   H. Anti-endomysial antibody

I. Abdominal CT   J. Colonoscopy   K. Ba-enema

L. Urine 5-HIAA (5-Hydroxyindoleacetic acid)   M. Reassurance

21. A 30 y/o woman presents with fever, abdominal pain, and diarrhea with mucus and blood after a large meal in a local restaurant. She completes a 10-day course of ampicillin and the bloody diarrhea stops. A few days later, she again has fever, abdominal cramps, and diarrhea but no blood or mucus. In CBC, WBC is increased.

22. A 30 y/o woman presents with occasional abdominal cramps, bloating, and foul-smelling diarrhea for the past 2 months. She says it often occurs after drinking milk and improves with fasting. She has no fever and no mucus or blood in the stool.

23. A 40 y/o woman presents with periodic abdominal cramps, bloating, and oily, loose stools for the past 10 months, accompanied with fatigue and decreased touch sensation and ataxia. She has been taking digestive enzymes and gluten-free diet but symptoms persist. She denies fever and mucus or blood in the stool.

24. A 50 y/o woman presents with periodic abdominal cramps, bloating, oily, loose stools for the past 3 months, accompanied with fatigue, joint pain, and decreased vision and memory. Stool exam reveals WBC and Gram$^+$ bacillus.

25. A 35 y/o man presents with a 3-month history of recurrent abdominal distention and pain, which is relieved by defecation and accompanied by periodic diarrhea and constipation with sparse mucus in stool. He received a recent promotion at work and denies history of fever, alcohol use, "food allergy", or other abnormal symptoms. FOBT, stool WBC and clinitest are (-).

26. A 41 y/o man presents with occasional joint pain, eye pain, skin rash, mild fever, fatigue, LLQ abdominal pain and bloody diarrhea with mucus for the past month. He denies personal and family history of colon cancer or polyps. CBC reveals mild anemia, and stool exam shows RBC and WBC.

27. A 60 y/o man presents with 1-month history of mild fever and LLQ colicky pain relieved by defecation, which is loose with mucus but no blood. P/E finds T = 38°C and LLQ tenderness. Lab tests reveal increased WBC and ESR, and stool guaiac test is (+). His colonoscopy 6-month ago reported "inflammation".

28. A 40 y/o female presents with progressive cough, pounding heart, RLQ pain, diarrhea, facial flushing, and fatigue for the past 2 months. She denies history of smoking, alcohol use, fever, or black stools. P/E finds tachycardia, hypotension and RLQ tenderness. CXR reveals a bronchial infiltrate. FOBT is (-).

29. A 55 y/o female presents with a 3-month history of frequent black stools, changes in bowel habits (with both diarrhea and constipation), Wt loss, and fatigability. She admits that she likes to "eat lots of meat but few vegetables." P/E finds a pale patient with an enlarged liver and a RLQ mass. FOBT is (+). Hb = 9.5 mg/dL. Ba-enema X-ray shows a filling defect in the right colon. Colonoscopy and biopsy confirm the diagnosis. Which of the following lesions has the highest potential for transformation to this type of neoplasms?

A. Adenomatous polyp   B. Inflammatory polyp   C. Hyperplastic polyp

D. Villous adenoma   E. Tubulovillous adenoma

30. What's the most appropriate next step for this patient?

A. Tumor staging   B. CT scan   C. CEA test

D. Chemo/radio-therapy   E. Surgery along with Chemo/radio-therapy

<u>31—33</u>. Match the following clinical scenarios with the most likely diagnosis.

A. Acute ulcerative colitis   B. Acute appendicitis   C. Diverticulosis

D. Acute diverticulitis   E. Crohn disease   F. Acute pancreatitis

G. Cholecystitis   H. Ectopic pregnancy   I. Small bowel obstruction

31. A 65 y/o woman presents with severe left quadrant pain, fever, and anorexia for the past 10 hours. She has no significant history of chronic diseases or medication use. She often has constipations and takes stool softeners for it. P/E shows guarding and rigidity on the middle left abdomen. FOBT is (-). WBC count is 12×10^3/uL.

32. A 38 y/o obese woman presents with progressive upper abdomen pain after a big meal with some wine. The pain started as "gnawing" and now becomes "sharp" and radiates to the right shoulder. Her last menstruation was 4 weeks ago. P/E reveals a cessation of inspiration upon palpation of the RUQ, with rebound tenderness. Lab tests: WBC = 14×10^3/uL with a left shift. Further tests are scheduled.

33. A 41y/o woman presents with nausea, vomiting, and severe abdominal pain that has gradually been increasing in intensity. The patient has no bowel movement or passing gas for the past 3 days. She has a history of abdominal hysterectomy a year ago. Her last menstruation was 4 weeks ago. P/E results: T = 38.5°C; hyperactive, tinkling bowel sounds sound. Lab tests: WBC = 16×10^3/uL.

Answers and Explanations

1. (A). Patient most likely has AIDS plus esophageal (Esoph) candidiasis (with lung infection). Differential diagnosis (Dx): CMV infection (big shallow ulcer); HSV infection (small deep ulcer); chemicals (history of ingestion + atypical ulcer). After the Dx of AIDS is confirmed, anti-HIV and anti-fungal medicine can be started.

2. (E). This patient is at higher risk for Esoph-cancer than for lung cancer according to his symptoms and CXR results, and thus Ba-study is done first (as a map), followed by endoscopy and biopsy to confirm the Dx.

3. (B). About 50% of Esoph-cancers are SCC, typically occurring in the proximal 2/3 esophagus, and may be associated with hyper-Ca and achalasia (not showing in this case). The other 50% are ACC and occur in the distal 1/3 esophagus, mostly associated with Barrett esophagus (columnar metaplasia).

4. (C). Mallory-Weiss syndrome is a partial mucosal tear in the squamocolumnar junction due to chronic vomiting. It is mostly based on GERD and is self-limited. 'J' is a full-thickness rupture of the distal esophagus, mostly associated with alcoholism.

5. (B). Zenker diverticulum is an out-pouching located in the upper esophagus caused by a weak posterior hypopharyngeal wall, often complicated with aspiration pneumonia in the elderly. Dx is made by Ba-study first. Surgery may be needed.

6. (G). The Schatzki ring is a common mechanical esophageal obstruction in young patients—a web-like mucosal ring proximal to LES. Tx is dilation of the ring.

7. (H). Plummer-Vinson syndrome (P-V-S) is hypopharyngeal web associated with iron deficient anemia, more common in middle-aged female and with increased risk of SCC, as with this patient. Ba-study will diagnose both the Schatzki ring and P-V-S, confirmed by endoscopy.

8. (E). Most likely it's a case of type B chronic gastritis with risk factors of cancer, and thus 'E' is the best initial Dx step to confirm H. pylori infection and exclude cancer. Usually type A (atrophic) gastritis is associated with Vit-B12 deficiency and gastric ACC.

9. (E). Since Ba-study did not show tumor and H. pylori is (+) in a 46 y/o patient, it's best to use 'E' or 'A' + metronidazole for 2-4 weeks. If a tumor is positive, endoscopy + antral biopsy are done followed by surgery.

10. (E). This is most likely a case of inferior mesenteric artery (IMA) ischemia due to low-flow secondary to post-aneurysm-surgery damage (small vessels). The #1 location is the "watershed areas." Angiogram is not as helpful as for SMA occlusion, and thus Dx is mostly clinical. SMA ischemia usually presents with extensive upper abdominal pain, acidosis, and leukocytosis, and is best diagnosed by angiogram.

11. (E). This patient has uncomplicated cholecystitis without biliary duct obstruction or systemic infection, and conservative Tx is the best. With complications, antibiotics, ERCP and surgery are indicated.

12. (B). Ultrasonography is 80% sensitive for hepatic vein thrombosis—Budd-Chiari syndrome, a common complication of erythrocytosis vera with high mortality. Hepatovenography is the next best exam for confirmation.

13. (D). Most likely acute cholangitis (with "Charcot triad") and pancreatitis secondary to gallstone obstruction of the common bile duct, thus ERCP is the 'best' means of Dx and Tx to confirm and remove the stones. Ultrasound (U/S) is the initial diagnostic step for most gallstones and cholecystitis, but ERCP is the best here.

14. (B). CT-guided drainage of abscess or pseudocyst: external drainage if "immature" (size > 5 cm or persisting < 6 weeks); internal drainage if "mature" (> 6 weeks).

15. (B). There is high suspicion for pancreatic or duodenoampullary cancer in this patient with risk factors, constant abdominal pain without fever, FOBT (+), and Courvoisier's sign. Gallstones need to be excluded. Remember the important diagnostic steps for this kind of cases: (1) First obtain an ultrasonography: if stones are (+), perform ERCP; (2) if stones are (-), obtain CT (very sensitive for the tumor); (3) if CT is (-), perform ERCP + biopsy for small mass. CA19-9 is most specific for pancreatic cancer but not the 1st means of Dx. MRI is more expensive and only indicated when CT cannot distinguish well.

16. (G). Gilbert disease is the most common genetic jaundice with mild indirect bilirubinemia, precipitated by stress and alleviated by barbital use. 'F' (C-N-S) is more severe than Gilbert disease and has higher indirect bilirubinemia (20-40 mg/dL), often causing infant kernicterus. Rotor syndrome causes direct bilirubin increase (> 50% of total bilirubin).

17. (E). Dubin Johnson syndrome (D-J-S) causes direct bilirubin increase, an enlarged liver and spleen, and black pigmentation in hepatocytes. Rotor syndrome is similar to D-J-S but there are no black granules.

18. (A). 'A' has a history of autoimmune diseases (ITP), hepatosplenomegaly, and elevated LFTs. ANA and Anti-smith are (+). Tx is steroid +/- Azathioprine. 'B' takes yrs of alcohol intake to cause fatty liver; AST:ALT > 2.

19. (E). TIPS—Transjugular intrahepatic portosystemic shunt is good for refractory ascites, especially useful before liver transplant because of low mortality and short effect. 'A' can reduce risk of hepatic encephalopathy (but not ascites), whereas most other shunts increase it. IV albumin should be avoided with signs of CHF.

20. (A). Patient has developed hepatorenal syndrome, a difficult medical condition that should be treated first by supportive Tx and diuretic cessation (spironolactone). Dialysis is indicated if serum K > 6 mEq/L or creatinine > 3 mg/dL, but only liver transplantation is curative.

21. (B). It's most likely pseudomembranous colitis. Stool toxin test for C. diff is diagnostic and the drug of choice is metronidazole for 10 days.

22. (C). It's a typical case of lactose intolerance. Dx is made by hydrogen breath test or clinitest of stool. Tx is to avoid milk product and supply lactase.

23. (D). Most likely it's a case of tropical sprue with B12 deficiency, and thus Schilling test is highly specific. 'H' is specific for celiac sprue, in which B12 deficiency is rare.

24. (A). Most likely it's a case of Whipple disease caused by Tropheryma whippleii, with malabsorption syndrome along with extra-GI symptoms. D-Xylose test is (+) and distinguish it from pancreatic insufficiency (Nl Xylose test). Tx: Same as for tropical sprue—Bactrim for 3-6 months.

25. (M). IBS is the initial Dx since lactose intolerance; IBD and thyroid disease are mostly excluded. If the patient is > 40 y/a, always rule out colorectal tumors by a sigmoidoscopy (or colonoscopy with family history). Reassurance and life style and dietary modification are the best management.

26. (J). Ulcerative colitis is most likely and colonoscopy should be done since he's > 40 y/a. Crohn disease mostly shows RLQ abdominal pain and nonbloody diarrhea +/- mucus, B$_{12}$ deficiency, etc.

27. (I). Diverticulitis is mostly likely and CT is the best tool of Dx. Sigmoidoscopy and Ba-enema may incur a high risk of perforation and are only indicated after the acute phase and with risk of colon cancer, which was initially excluded by his colonoscopy 6 months ago.

28. (L). Carcinoid syndrome is most likely and 24-hour urine 5-HIAA test confirms the Dx. Location: Appendix (No.1 common local, nonsecreting carcinoid tumor), ileum (No.1 systemic carcinoid syndrome, secreting 5-HT), or bronchi (with 70% metastasis). Octreotide is the first Tx; surgical resection if it fails.

29. (D). Colorectal cancer is mostly from adenomatous polyps > 2 cm and after 5-10 years. Cancer risk order for polyp types are: villous > tubular > inflammatory polyp (as in UC or Crohn disease) and hyperplastic polyp.

30. (B). Since the pathologic nature has been diagnosed by biopsy, the best next step is to specify the tumor size and extent of the metastasis (liver, lymph nodes) with CT, to get an initial staging to guide the Tx ('E'; final staging is after surgery). Post-surgery monitoring: colonoscopy in 6 months followed by 3 years. Follow-ups of CEA levels help in monitoring for postsurgery recurrence, but not in Dx.

31. (D). Acute diverticulitis: acute onset of severe LLQ pain, fever; no lower GI bleeding; increased WBCs.

32. (G). It's a typical cholecystitis case in a mid-aged obese woman with RUQ pain, Murphy's sign (+), and leukocytosis. Ultrasonography shows pericholecystic fluid and a thickened gallbladder wall. Acute pancreatitis typically has sharp epigastric pain radiating to the back after a big meal. Serum lipase and amylase levels (increase) are necessary to differentiate and confirm Dx. Acute appendicitis usually presents with RLQ pain and an ectopic pregnancy with LLQ or RLQ pain following a menopause.

33. (I). Typical small bowel obstruction—no stool and flatus, along with nausea, vomiting, and abdominal pain with hyperactive bowel sounds. An abdominal surgery is a major risk for its cause.

Chapter 5

ENDOCRINE AND METABOLIC DISEASES

DISORDERS OF GLUCOSE AND FAT METABOLISM

Diabetes Mellitus (DM)

DM is a disorder of carbohydrate metabolism caused by absolute or relative deficiency of insulin, and characterized by hyperglycemia (fasting glucose > 125 mg/dL or 6.9 mmol/L on two separate occasions), metabolic disturbances, and end-organ complications, including nephropathy, neuropathy, retinopathy, and accelerated atherosclerosis.

Classification

Type 1 diabetes (IDDM, insulin-dependent or juvenile-onset DM):

Prevalence: It accounts for **10%-20%** of all DM, male (M) = female (F). The age of onset is usually < 30 y/a. **Genetic trend is less than type 2 DM**. 95% of type 1 DM is immune-mediated and called type IA. The main mechanisms are **autoimmune destruction** of the pancreatic beta cells, evidenced by increased autoimmune antibodies (Auto-Ab) to islet cells and other tissues. It's usually associated with viral infection and HLA-DR3/-DR4, etc. Patient has **more typical symptoms ("3-polys & 1-loss"** — polyuria, polydipsia, polyphagia, and weight loss), more risk of ketoacidosis and coma due to **insulin deficiency,** and always requires exogenous insulin therapy. About 5% of type I DM is idiopathic (no evidence of autoimmune destruction) and named type IB DM. The **No.1 cause of death with type 1 DM is renal failure.**

Type 2 diabetes (NIDDM, non-insulin-dependent or adult-onset DM):

Prevalence: Accounts for **80%-90%** of all DM, male > female, mostly in obese patients > 40 y/a. It's genetically associated with strong family history (**autosomal dominant trait**, 90%-100% occurrence in identical twins), but no autoimmune antibodies or HLA linkage. There are two clear pathologic defects— **abnormal insulin secretion and resistance to insulin** action in target tissues, and insulin levels may be high, normal (Nl), or low. Symptoms are more insidious and various, and most patients are found with hyperglycemia at asymptomatic screening. Complications such as hyperosmolar dehydration and coma may occur. The **No.1 cause of death with type 2 DM is a cardiovascular complication (MI, CVD).**

PEARLS—Important diagnostic criteria for diabetes

1. **Symptomatic patients**: Random plasma glucose ≥ **200 mg/dL (11.1 mmol/L) along with typical symptoms** (polyuria, polydipsia, polyphagia, and weight loss) **can be diagnostic (mostly for type 1 DM).**

2. **For asymptomatic patients**, any of the standards below met (mostly on two separate occasions):

(1) **Fasting plasma glucose: ≥ 126 mg/dL or 7 mmol/L** (Nl: < 100 mg/dL or 5.6 mmol/L; impaired glucose tolerance: 100-125 mg/dL or 5.6-6.9 mmol/L); for both type 1 and type 2 diabetes.

(2) **2 hours after 75g glucose load (75g GTT): > 200 mg/dL** or 11.1 mmol/L (Nl: <140 mg/dL or 7.8 mmol/L; impaired or prediabetic: ≥ 140-199 mg/dL or 7.8-11.0 mmol/L); **mostly for type 2 diabetes.**

(3) **HbA1c (%): ≥ 6.5%** (Nl: < 5.7; impaired: 5.7-6.4). **HbA1c** is usually used for follow-ups of the treatment compliance and glucose control in diabetic patients (**normal value is < 5.7%; therapeutic goal is ≤ 7% for most diabetic patients**). Higher levels indicate poor control of the diabetes or chronic state.

PEARLS—Important diagnostic steps for diabetes

1. Patient with random plasma glucose ≥ **200 mg/dL (11.1 mmol/L) along with typical symptoms** (polyuria, polydipsia, polyphagia, ketonuria, and weight loss) **can be diagnosed** (mostly type 1 DM) without further testing.

2. **Asymptomatic** patient with risk factors (> 35y/a, family history, hypertension, obesity, increased lipid, back pain) or increased plasma/urine glucose during screening will need 8-hour **fasting plasma glucose ≥126** mg/dL on two separate occasions to be diagnostic.

3. **75g** oral glucose tolerance test (**GTT**): usually required when the repeated fasting screening test is uncertain. GTT is diagnostic if the **2-hour plasma glucose is ≥ 200** mg/dL or **glycosylated HbA1c ≥ 6.5%** on two separate occasions.

Important screening and diagnosis of gestational diabetes

See Chapter 12: OBSTETRICS.

Treatment of type 1 diabetes

Insulin replacement is the main therapy. The goal is to control symptoms and prevent or restrict acute and long-term complications. Therapeutic effects of hyperglycemia and ketoacidosis are best monitored by AG (**anion gap, new normal AG = 3-10**). **Hypoglycemia** is the most common complication with insulin therapy. It may result from a meal delay, unusual exercise without supplemental calories or decrease in insulin dose, or combined use with sulfonylureas.

Table 5-1: Important Insulin Formulations*

Insulin Type	Onset of Action	Peak Action	Effective duration
Lispro, aspart, glulisine	5-15 min	1-1.5 hours	3-4 hours
Regular insulin	30-60 min	2 hours	6-8 hours
NPH (intermediate/long-acting)	2-4 hours	6-7 hours	10-20 hours
Detemir (long-acting)	1 hour	Flat	17 hours
Glargine (long-acting)	1.5 hours	Flat	18-24 hours

* Adapted from Current Medical Diagnosis and Treatment 2016.

Guidelines for insulin dosing:

(1) Morning: 2/3 of total daily dose; (2) afternoon: 1/3 of daily dose. It's better to use long- and short-acting mixture— "intermediate" (2/3 NPH + 1/3 Regular, or 70% NPH/30% Regular) to provide immediate and extended effects in the same injection. The goal is to keep plasma glucose level at 100-120 mg/dL, which should be measured before the meal and at bedtime.

PEARLS—Important conceptual differentiations

1. **The "Honeymoon" period**: In Type 1 DM, an initial episode of ketoacidosis followed by a symptom-free interval, presumably caused by stress-induced epinephrine release blocking insulin secretion. **No treatment** is needed.

2. **The Somogyi effect:** Blood glucose decreases at 3am and increases at 7am. **Rebound hyperglycemia** in the morning is due to counterregulatory hormone release after an episode of hypoglycemia in the middle of the night. **Treatment is decrease in the evening insulin dose**.

3. **The Dawn phenomenon:** An early **morning hyperglycemia**; insulin level is normal at 3am but low at dawn (7am hyperglycemia). **Treatment is increase in the evening insulin dose** to maintain euglycemia.

4. **Insulin dose waning:** Insulin level remains low; blood glucose increases at both 3am and 7am. **Treatment is maintenance of insulin doses**.

Treatment of type 2 diabetes

1. Initial nonmedical therapies include patient education, weight reduction, low-fat diet, exercise, and control of hypertension, which is very important to reduce diabetic complications.

2. **Oral hypoglycemic drugs**:

(1) **Metformin:** It inhibits hepatic gluconeogenesis and increases peripheral tissue sensitivity to insulin. **It should be the initial medicine for type 2 DM, particularly patients with obesity (BMI > 30)**, benefited by the adverse effect (S/E) of nausea/vomiting that causes weight loss, and by reducing insulin resistance and triglycerides. **Contraindication**: Elderly and patient with renal disease, due to the rare adverse effect of lactic acidosis.

(2) **Sulfonylureas** (#1 **glipizide**): Increase pancreatic insulin secretion and peripheral tissue sensitivity to insulin. It's the **#1 choice for patients with BMI < 30, asymptomatic or mild DM** with metformin contraindication or without pregnancy. Compared with metformin, they have the disadvantage of hypoglycemia and weight gain. If HbA1c > 7%, acarbose or thiazolidine (inhibiting GI absorption of glucose) or insulin should be added.

(3) Others: **Pioglitazone** can improve peripheral insulin resistance and lower glucose without causing hypoglycemia. Adverse effects include weight gain, fluid retention (**heart failure**), and potential of **bladder cancer**. **Alpha-glucosidase inhibitors** have modest glucose lowering effects with S/E of GI. The **GLP-1R agonists (exenatide and liraglutide)** promote weight loss and have a lower risk of hypoglycemia than the sulfonylureas.

3. Insulin is usually required when hyperglycemia is out of control (HbA1c > 9%), even with insulin resistance.

Acute complications of diabetes

1. **Diabetic ketoacidosis (DKA):**

It results from severe insulin insufficiency and hyperglycemia, predominantly in **type 1 DM**. It may be the initial presentation and can be precipitated by insufficient or interrupted insulin treatment, infection, stress, myocardial infarction, alcohol, and drugs (steroids, thiazides). The major concerns are metabolic acidosis and dehydration, patient presenting with nausea, vomiting, nonspecific abdominal pain, Kussmaul respiration (slow, deep breathing), "fruity" breath odor (acetone), signs of dehydration (dry skin and mucous membranes and poor skin turgor), and mental status changes.

Lab tests: Serum glucose usually > 250 mg/dL, HCO_3^- < 15 mEq/L, AG > 10 (anion gap metabolic acidosis), and increased ketones (acetoacetate, acetone, and hydroxybutyrate).

Treatment: IV moderate volume of normal saline (N.S.) with large dose of insulin. $NaHCO_3$ is only administered when pH ≤ 6.9. It's best to check AG for therapeutic effect.

2. **Hyperosmolar nonketotic coma (HONK):**

It's predominantly in **type 2 DM**, characterized by severe hyperglycemia in the absence of significant ketosis; precipitated by noncompliance in treatment, inadequate water intake, infections, drugs (diuretics, phenytoin, steroids), and strokes. This is common in elderly DM patients living in nursing homes. **The major problem is fatal dehydration resulting from hyperglycemic diuresis,** causing manifestations of weakness, polyuria, polydipsia, lethargy, confusion, convulsions, and coma.

Lab tests: High serum glucose (> 600 mg/dL), BUN, and plasma osmolality; mild metabolic nonketotic acidosis (HCO_3^- = 20-24 mEq/L and AG is normal).

Treatment: It's necessary to replace a **large volume of IV N.S. with a moderate dose of insulin.** Up to 10 L of N.S. along with ½ tension saline can be administered.

Chronic complications of diabetes

1. **Retinopathy:** *both DM1 & DM2*

It appears in 50% of cases after 5 years of DM, and the other 50% after 10 years of DM. It's the leading cause of blindness (whereas glaucoma is the No.1 cause of blindness for the Black population).

(1) **Most cases are non-proliferative (Image 148),** with microaneurysms, exudate, hemorrhages, and edema. **Treatment is control of glucose levels.** *Non prolif => background or simple retinopathy. Visual impairment occurs w development of macular edema*

(2) **Proliferative retinopathy (Image 149):** with scars and visual deficits. **Treatment** is panretinal *Argon* laser photocoagulation for neovascularization (also as prophylaxis). *cotton wool spots*

2. **Nephropathy:**

It affects about 30% of DM, characterized by glomerular hyper-infiltration or proliferation and mesangial thickening (diffuse or nodular—Kim-Wilson's) followed by microalbuminuria. End-stage renal failure can develop. Random or 24-hour **urine albumin > 30 mg** is the **#1 sensitive** test and **earliest marker** of DM nephropathy.

2. Diabetic Nephropathy

Treatment: Strict control of glucose and hypertension; early use of **ACE-I** or **angiotensin II receptor blockers (ARBs)** with microalbuminuria; in late stage, dialysis or renal transplantation.

3. Neuropathy:

It is **peripheral, symmetric and polyneuropathy**, with manifestations of "**stocking & glove**" **numbness**, refractory pain and dysfunctioning of the limbs ("**Charcot's joint**"), GI, UT, or CVS symptoms (difficult swallowing, urine retention, impotence, orthostatic hypotension, syncope). **P/E:** Absent reflexes and loss of vibratory sense, ulcers; peripheral **median nerve or CN3** are the most frequently affected (CN3 paralysis but with normal pupil reflex).

Treatment: (1) Glucose control. (2) **For painful diabetic neuropathy**, initial therapy using either **amitriptyline/venlafaxine or duloxetine/pregabalin** is recommended. Gabapentin or carbamazepine can be used if the pain persists. (3) For gastroparesis, metoclopramide or erythromycin can be used.

4. Macrovascular complications:

These include increased risk of strokes, myocardial infarction, and peripheral vascular diseases. Optimal control: BP < 135/85 mmHg, LDL < 130 mg/dL (LDL < 100, TG < 200 with history of CAD).

PEARLS—Differential diagnosis of diabetes

Glucagonoma:

It's a glucagon-producing tumor located in the pancreas. Clinical features include necrotizing migratory erythema (mostly below the waist), stomatitis, glossitis, mild diabetes, and hyperglycemia (with low amino acid levels and high glucagon levels). Efficient treatment is surgical resection.

Somatostatinoma:

It's a rare malignancy in the pancreas. Most cases are with metastasis at diagnosis and with poor prognosis. **Classical triad is diabetes, gallstones, and steatorrhea**.

VIPoma:

It's also known as **Verner-Morrison** or **w**atery **d**iarrhea, **h**ypokalemia and **a**chlorhydria **(WDHA) syndrome**, a rare pancreatic tumor (> 50% are malignant). Clinical features include watery diarrhea (causing dehydration, hypokalemia, acidosis), achlorhydria (due to VIP inhibiting gastric acid secretion), hyperglycemia, and hyper-Ca. Treatment is surgical resection.

Health maintenance for diabetic patients

1. Pneumococcal vaccination.

2. Annual examinations for the retinopathy, neuropathy, and ulcerations.

3. Antihypertensive agents (ACE-I or ARBs) are used if the BP is > 130/80 mmHg, or urine tests are positive for microalbumuria.

4. Aspirin is suggested for all > age 30; statins for those with LDL > 100 mg/dL.

Hypoglycemia

Etiology, clinical features, and diagnosis

Hypoglycemia is a state of abnormally low levels of glucose in the blood (generally < 70 mg/mL). Symptoms may not occur until blood glucose levels are $\leqslant$ 20 mg/dL, including sweating, tremor, tachycardia, anxiety, dizziness, headache, blurred vision, confusion, convulsions, and coma due to over-secretion of epinephrine and CNS dysfunction. Major causes and clinical features are summarized below:

1. **Fasting hypoglycemia:** It can result from hormone deficiency (panhypopituitarism, adrenal insufficiency, hyperinsulinism), enzyme deficiency, substrate deficiency (severe malnutrition, late pregnancy), chronic liver diseases, or drug use (sulfonylureas, alcohol, propranolol, salicylates, etc.).

2. **Factitious hyperinsulinism:** It's caused by self use of insulin or oral sulfonylureas, and more common than by insulinoma. Most patients are health workers or have access to these drugs. A **triad of hypoglycemia, suppressed C-peptide and high immunoreactivity of insulin** is the pathologic mark.

3. **Insulinoma** (pancreatic B cell tumor): 90% of cases are single and benign but can cause hypoglycemia. Clinical features are chronic hypoglycemia leading to neuroglycopenic symptoms (blurred vision, headache, slurred speech, and weakness) or acute sympathetic activation (palpitations, diaphoresis, tremors, high blood pressure, and anxiety). **Diagnosis is by high insulin level** (> 8 mg/mL) **and low glucose level** (< 40 mg/dL) in blood, particularly after fasting. CT scan or ultrasound can also support diagnosis. **Surgical resection** is the best treatment.

4. **Ethanol-induced hypoglycemia**: It can occur with (1) prolonged starvation after glycogen is depleted in 24 hours; (2) ethanol inhibition of gluconeogenesis. History is important in diagnosis.

Treatment

Treat underlying causes.

PITUITARY AND HYPOTHALAMIC DISEASES

The pituitary lies in the sella turcica near the hypothalamus and optic chiasm, and is divided into two lobes—anterior and posterior lobe.

Anterior lobe (80%): It secrets **ACTH** (adrenocorticotropic hormone), **LH** (luteinizing hormone), **FSH** (follicle-stimulating hormone), **GH** (growth hormone), prolactin, and **TSH** (thyroid stimulating hormone). Disorders of the anterior lobe will cause partial or complete deficiency of one or any combination of these hormones.

Posterior lobe: It's the storage site for **ADH** (antidiuretic hormone, produced by supraoptic nuclei) and **oxytocin** (produced by paraventricular nuclei in the hypothalamus). Disorders of the posterior lobe will result in deficiency of either ADH or oxytocin or both.

The hypothalamus regulates the anterior pituitary hormones by different releasing and inhibitive hormones (hypothalamic-pituitary axis). The released hormones are **CRH** (corticotropin-releasing hormone), **GnRH** (gonadotropin-releasing hormone), **GHRH** (growth hormone-releasing hormone), and **TRH** (thyrotropin-releasing hormone).

DISORDERS OF THE ANTERIOR PITUITARY LOBE

Hyperprolactinemia

It is a common disorder in female causing the galactorrhea-amenorrhea syndrome, due to secondary LH & FSH decrease. It can also occur in natural physiologic states such as pregnancy, early nursing, stress, sleep, and nipple stimulation. It is rarely seen in males.

Etiology

1. **Pituitary adenomas** (prolactinomas): The most common cause of pathologic hyperprolactinemia, usually presenting as microadenomas in female and macroadenomas in male.

2. Medications: Decreased inhibitory action of dopamine (DA). (1) DA synthesis blockers (phenothiazines, metoclopramide); (2) DA-depleting agents (alpha-methyldopa, reserpine).

3. Stimuli that overcome normal DA inhibition: primary hypothyroidism (increased TRH).

Essentials of diagnosis

1. First exclude conditions such as physiologic status, hypothyroidism, and medications before the work-up of hyperprolactinemia.

2. Look for manifestations of syndrome of galactorrhea-amenorrhea, with LH & FSH decrease and possible peripheral vision defects.

3. Prolactin > 100 ng/mL suggests potential pituitary adenoma. The concentration is proportional to the tumor size.

Differential diagnosis

Craniopharyngioma: See "Chapter 9 Neurologic Diseases" (Table 9-2).

Treatment

1. **Cabergoline,** a new long acting dopamine (DA) agonist is the initial option, which can effectively reduce prolactin levels in most patients. If it's ineffective, bromocriptine is considered.

2. Surgery and radiotherapy are reserved only for macroadenomas not responsive to medications or with significant compressive effects.

Acromegaly

Acromegaly is a disorder of excessive secretion of GH leading to bone and soft tissue overgrowth throughout the body. It's usually caused by a pituitary adenoma (macroadenoma). In children, it is called "gigantism". Acromegaly is an insidious, chronic debilitating disease associated with bone and soft tissue overgrowth, but rarely with ectopic neoplasms.

Essentials of diagnosis

1. 30-50 y/o patient, with **gradual skeletal and soft tissue growth over years: enlarged hands, feet, nose, tongue, mandible, coarsening of facial features, and thickened skin folds (Image 55)**. Hint: increased hat, glove/shoe size, ring, **body odor** (due to sweat gland hypertrophy), etc.

2. Enlarged internal organs (heart, lung, spleen, liver, and kidneys, with colon polyps) and soft tissues, with possible interstitial edema, osteoarthritis (arthralgia), signs of neurologic entrapment (due to carpal tunnel syndrome), deep voice, and obstructive sleep apnea.

3. Evidence of impaired glucose tolerance (80%), diabetes (15%), and hypertension (30-50%). Impotence may occur due to increased prolactin cosecreted with the pituitary adenoma. Headaches and visual field loss can also occur. Levels of somatomedin or insulin-like growth factor (IGF) positively correlate with the disease.

4. Screening test: It's positive if GH > 5 ng/mL after 100g of oral glucose. Normally a glucose load should suppress GH secretion.

5. CT or MRI usually confirms diagnosis and localizes the tumor after screening.

Treatment—To decrease GH level and tumor size

1. Medications:

(1) Dopamine agonist: **Cabergoline** is long acting and more effective in inhibiting GH release and better tolerated than bromocriptine as the initial therapy.

(2) **Octreotide or lanreotide**: A somatostatin analogue that can reduce GH release in 2/3 patients and tumor size in 1/3 patients.

(3) **Pegvisomant**: A GH receptor antagonist that inhibits IGF release from the liver.

2. **Transphenoidal surgery**: This provides the best therapy if patient does not respond to medications (surgery is effective in 70% of cases), but hypopituitarism can result in < 20% of patients.

3. Radiotherapy: It's only used in those who do not respond to medications or surgery.

Complications

Cardiac failure—the No.1 cause of death. Others include diabetes, cord compression, and visual field defects. Most complications are due to the tumor compression on the surrounding structures or rupture into the brain or sinuses.

Differential diagnosis

Empty sella syndrome:

Enlarged sella without bony erosion, caused by herniation of the suprasellar subarachnoid space through an incomplete diaphragm sella. Most patients are obese, multiparous females with headaches; hypertension and endocrine symptoms are less common. Management is reassurance and follow-ups.

Hypopituitarism

Definition and etiology

Hypopituitarism is the anterior function decrease or loss due to any lesion of the pituitary or hypothalamus, or their regulating functions. **FSH, LH, and GH levels are usually reduced earlier than TSH and ACTH. Common causes** include ischemic or hemorrhagic disorders, large pituitary **tumors** and hypothalamic tumors (craniopharyngiomas, meningiomas, gliomas), and inflammatory diseases (granulomatous disease and autoimmune disease).

Pituitary apoplexy is an emergent syndrome associated with acute hemorrhagic infarction of a pre-existing pituitary adenoma. Patient usually presents with severe headache, nausea and vomiting, and decreased cognitive and pituitary functions.

Sheehan syndrome (Postpartum pituitary necrosis) is a common cause due to pituitary ischemia secondary to heavy blood loss during delivering. **The early sign is unable to lactate after delivery**.

Essentials of diagnosis and treatment

The following hormone deficiencies will occur in order with hypopituitarism.

I. Gonadotropin deficiency—LH and FSH decrease first. In female, it leads to amenorrhea, genital atrophy, infertility, decreased libido, and loss of axillary and pubic hair. In male, it leads to impotence, testicular atrophy, infertility, decreased libido, and loss of axillary and pubic hair.
Lab tests: Low serum LH, FSH, and estrogen (in female) or testosterone (in male).

Treatment: Treat underlying causes and replace deficient hormones. In men, testosterone or gonadotropins/GnRH (for secondary cause) is indicated. In women, estradiol and progestin replacements and gonadotropin or pulsatile GnRH for induction of ovulation are indicated if fertility is pursued.

II. GH deficiency: It occurs the second and is not easily detectable in time in adults, with gradual decrease in muscle mass, bone density, serum glucose (increased sensitivity to insulin), and memory. In children, it may present with hypoglycemia, short stature, and growth failure.
Lab tests: The most reliable test for GH stimulation is **insulin-induced hypoglycemia**: GH < 10 mg/dL following insulin IM is diagnostic; GH > 10 mg/dL after insulin can exclude GH deficiency.
Treatment: Recombinant GH should be started at the youngest possible age to achieve the best growth response. Measure IGF-I approximately four weeks after starting the GH therapy or make a dose adjustment, and lower the GH dose if the level is above the normal range.

III. Thyrotropin (TSH) deficiency: It results in central hypothyroidism, presenting with fatigue, cold intolerance, and puffy skin without goiter.

Lab tests: Low serum T4 and T3, normal to low TSH.

Treatment: Synthetic T4 supplement, with the dose adjusted according to the patient's symptoms and serum free T4 levels.

IV. ACTH deficiency: This occurs last after pituitary disorders, and results in secondary adrenal insufficiency.

(1) Decreased cortisol showing fatigue, decreased appetite, weight, and skin pigmentation.

(2) Decreased response to stress, fever, hypotension, and hypo-Na with high mortality.

(3) Electrolytes: Mild hyper-K and hypo-Na are with secondary adrenal insufficiency because aldosterone is mainly maintained by the renin-angiotensin (which is normal).

(4) **Specific Lab tests:** Basal cortisol levels may be low to normal. **Insulin tolerance test (+) is diagnostic**—cortisol < 19 mg/dL after insulin IM. Cortisol increase (> 19 mg/dL) after insulin administration excludes ACTH deficiency.

Treatment: Administration of hydrocortisone or other glucocorticoid in an amount and timing to mimic the normal pattern of cortisol secretion.

DISORDERS OF THE POSTERIOR PITUITARY LOBE

Diabetes Insipidus (DI)

DI is a disorder of the neurohypophyseal system caused by a **deficiency of vasopressin (Central DI), or renal unresponsiveness to vasopressin (Renal DI)**. Both deficiencies result in excessive, dilute urine (not alleviated by reduced fluid intake) and increased thirst due to hyper-Na.

Subtypes by etiology

I. Central DI

1. Due to neoplastic or infiltrative lesions in the hypothalamus or pituitary (adenomas, craniopharyngiomas, leukemia, or sarcoidosis);

2. Pituitary or hypothalamic surgery, or radiotherapy; severe head injuries, hypertension, infection, or autoimmune disease;

3. Idiopathic DI: Accounts for 50% of cases and mostly starts in childhood;

4. Risk factors: This disorder occurs more often in young males.

II. Nephrogenic DI

This is caused by renal resistance to the action of vasopressin; it can be idiopathic or secondary to **hyper-Ca, hypo-K, drugs (lithium, demeclocycline, colchicine, chlorpromazine, anticholinergics, thioridazine)**, Sickle cell anemia, pyelonephritis, or sarcoidosis.

Essentials of diagnosis

1. Related history and hyper-Na symptoms: Polyuria, excessive thirst, polydipsia (> 15 L/day), severe dehydration, prostration, fever, and even coma and death.

2. **Lab tests**: Increased serum Na and osmolality, urine specific gravity < 1.010; increased levels of vasopressin and osmolality ratio of plasma to urine.

3. **Water deprivation test**:

(1) In central DI: Water deprivation with ADH challenge will normally decrease urine output and increase urine osmolality. MRI may show a pituitary or hypothalamic mass.

Diabetes Insipidus

(2) In nephrogenic DI: Water deprivation with ADH challenge cannot stop patient from secreting a high volume of dilute urine.

Differential diagnosis

Primary (Psychogenic) polydipsia:

(1) Polydipsia, polyuria with large volumes of dilute urine, and symptoms of **Hypo-Na** and low plasma osmolality.

(2) After long water deprivation, maximum plasma osmolality is low (around 290 mOsm/kg) and urine osmolality is high (around 690 mOsm/kg); after using an ADH analogue, urine osmolality increases little (about 710 mOsm/kg).

Treatment

I. Central DI: Three main effective therapies include (1) a low-solute (sodium and protein) diet, **(2) desmopressin (dDAVP, an ADH analog), (3)** and other drugs such as **thiazide** diuretics. Some medications can also be used to increase the secretion or release of vasopressin (chlorpropamide, clofibrate, or carbamazepine).

II. Nephrogenic DI:

1. Stop irritating medications, treat underlying disease, and restrict salt.

2. Increase water intake along with a **thiazide (highly effective). A thiazide** can effectively enhance the reabsorption of fluid from the proximal tubule (**paradoxical effect**). **Amiloride** is added if the urine output is insufficiently reduced. **Chlorthalidone** is also helpful. If polyuria persists, adding indomethacin is suggested.

Syndrome of Inappropriate Secretion of Vasopressin (SIADH)

It is abnormal secretion of ADH caused by non-osmotic stimulation or beyond physiologic conditions (such as dehydration, stress, injury, etc.), leading to water retention, hypervolemia, and concentrated urine with reduced volume.

Etiology

1. **Malignancies**: Small cell lung carcinoma (SCLC), pancreatic carcinoma, etc., producing ectopic vasopressin secretion.

2. Nonmalignant causes: CNS disorders—head injury, CVA, and infections; pulmonary diseases—infections and sarcoidosis; **drugs**—antipsychotics, antidepressants, and cytotoxics (chlorpropamide, clofibrate, vincristine, vinblastine, cyclophosphamide, and carbamazepine) can all induce SIADH.

Essentials of diagnosis

1. Manifestations of water retention, Hypo-Na and hypervolemia without edema or hypertension, owing to natriuresis: lethargy, muscle weakness, and oliguria; if severe acute hypo-Na (serum Na < 120 mEq/L) —signs of cerebral edema (irritability, confusion, seizures, and coma).

SIADH

2. **Lab tests**: **Hypo-Na and concentrated urine,** plasma Na < 130 mEq/L and osmolality < 270 mOsm/kg, urine osmolality > 300 mOsm/kg and Na > 20 mEq/L (abnormal natriuresis); suppressed renin-angiotensin system and no matching ANP; low BUN, creatinine, albumin, and uric acid.

Treatment—Targeting underlying causes.

1. Mild (serum Na$^+$ > 130 mEq/L): Water and fluid restriction, and treat the underlying disease. First restrict fluid to 800-1,000/day to recover serum Na level.

2. Moderate (serum Na$^+$ 120-130 mEq/L): Limited normal saline (N.S.) +/- hypertonic saline IV.

3. Severe (serum Na$^+$ < 120 mEq/L, or with seizure or coma): IV 3% saline (200-300 mL in a few hours) followed by furosemide.

4. Chronic or refractory SIADH: Hypertonic saline in combination with **desmopressin or demeclocycline** (potent ADH inhibitor) or lithium (anti-ADH) can help correct Hypo-Na slowly. The new vasopressin receptor antagonist conivaptan (IV) or tolvaptan (PO) produces a selective water diuresis without affecting sodium and potassium excretion.

DISEASES OF THE THYROID

Graves infiltrative ophthalmopathy:
- proptosis, impaired ocular movement, ocular irritation, redness - vision loss.

Thyroid diseases could be quantitative or qualitative changes in hormone secretion with or without thyroid enlargement. Deficient hormone secretion results in hypothyroidism, excess secretion in hyperthyroidism. Thyroid enlargement can be associated with neoplasms (focal, benign or malignant), hyper-/hypothyroidism, or normal functions depending on the nature and status of the disease.

PEARLS— **Important lab tests for thyroid disorders**

1. **The most sensitive test is the TSH**. If the TSH is normal, then the patient is euthyroid.

2. Total T4 and T3 do not always reflect actual thyroid function. E.g., increased thyroxine-binding globulin (TBG) levels are seen in pregnancy and OCP use, which will increase total T4 but the free/active T4 level is normal. Decreased TBG levels are seen in nephrotic syndrome and the use of androgens, which will decrease total T4 but the free or active T4 level is normal (patient is euthyroid).

3. Serum thyroglobulin concentration can be used to assess therapeutic effects and for the follow-ups of thyroid cancer.

FA87 p.321   - Sx: tachycardia, anxiety, wt loss.

Hyperthyroidism (Thyrotoxicosis)

Etiology and pathologic types

It's mainly due to abnormal thyroid stimulation or excess production of TSH (rare).

1. **Graves disease** or **toxic diffuse goiter**:

- Toxic adenoma, Toxic multinodular. MCC hyperthyroidism (after graves dz, usually caused by activating mutations in the TSH receptor. (221)

- TSH-independent thyroid hormone secretion, focal (TA) or multifocal follicular hyperplasia.

↑ hyperTh
- overproduction (graves, toxic nodular goiter),
↑ uptake
- release of preformed (painless thyroiditis, subacute thyroiditis),
↓ uptake

Hyper thyroid, Thyrotoxicosis

Hyperthyroidism + diffuse goiter + exophthalmos + pretibial myxedema.

This is **the most common** cause of **hyperthyroidism**. It is more common in > 40 y/o females and associated with Anti-TSH-R antibodies in thyroid cell membranes, which stimulates the gland to hyperthyroidism (thyroid-stimulating immunoglobulin). It may also be related to other systemic autoimmune diseases such as pernicious anemia, myasthenia gravis, and diabetes.

2. **Toxic multinodular goiter (Plummer disease):**

It's a hyperfunctioning, non-autoimmune disease of the elderly, commonly associated with arrhythmia and CHF. It can also follow a simple goiter. **There is no exophthalmos.**

3. **Transient hyperthyroidism:**

It usually results **from subacute thyroiditis (painful, virus) and lymphocytic thyroiditis (painless, postpartum).**

4. **Extrathyroid source of hormones:**

They include thyrotoxicosis factitia and ectopic thyroid tissue (struma ovarii, functioning follicular carcinoma).

Essentials of diagnosis

Thyrotoxic Myopathy: 1. Clinical features of a specific type; more neurologic symptoms in young patients and more CVS
- distal or proximal symptoms in older patients: emotional lability, sleeplessness, tremors, sweating, and heat intolerance,
weakness diarrhea, increased appetite but decreased weight and strength; dyspnea, palpitations, angina, or cardiac
- muscle atrophy failure in older patients; warm moist skin, silky hair and lid lag.

painless
Thyroid:
- Riedel, painless
subacute, silent
thyroiditis

2. **Lab tests**: High T4 & T3 and low TSH in primary hyperthyroidism and high TSH in secondary hyperthyroidism. I^{131} uptake is increased.

Differential diagnosis

Anxiety, neurosis, and mania, pheochromocytoma, acromegaly, cardiac disease, myasthenia gravis. It is important to distinguish primary hyperthyroidism from thyroiditis due to different treatment applied.

Treatment

1. **Acute or urgent: Atenolol or propranolol** is first administered to control adrenergic symptoms, then iodine to decrease T3/T4 release and shrink the thyroid for surgery.

2. **Antithyroid drugs** as the main therapy: **Methimazole** or **propylthiouracil (PTU, safe in** pregnancy); **thionamide.**   ↓thyroid hormone production

3. **Ablative therapy with I^{131}**: Good for **Graves or Plummer** disease but risky of hypothyroidism, in which T4 supplement may be needed.

4. **Subtotal thyroidectomy**: Reserved for patients in pregnancy (2nd trimester) and for children forbidden for radiation.

If left untreated.
- rapid bone loss → osteoporosis
from ↑ osteoclastic resorption
- hypercalcemia & hypercalciuria
from ↑ bone turnover
- tachycardia, systolic HTN, ↑
pulse pressure, tachy arrhythmias

fetal hyperthyroidism:
- mother w active Graves dz
TSH receptor antibodies cross
the placenta

Thyroid Storm

It is **an extreme and dangerous form of thyrotoxicosis**, precipitated by stress, surgery, or trauma. Manifestations include extreme irritability, delirium, coma, tachycardia, restlessness, vomiting, diarrhea, high fever, dehydration, and hypotension.

Treatment

1. Urgent supportive therapies with saline and glucose hydration, glucocorticoids, oxygen, and a cooling blanket. *Initial tx = beta blockade*

2. **Propranolol** is used for immediate symptom relief, and antithyroid agents (PTU every 2 hours) plus iodine to inhibit T3/T4 release. Methimazole is used for maintenance. *or methimazole* *or cool.*
definitive: sws, radioiodine ablation. for toxic adenoma

3. Finally glucocorticoids (dexamethasone) to inhibit hormone release and peripheral production of T3 from T4, and to strengthen adrenal functions. Cholestyramine may also be of benefit in severe cases to reduce enterohepatic recycling of thyroid hormones.

Hypothyroidism

The most common primary hypothyroidism is due to chronic thyroiditis—**Hashimoto** disease, which is goitrous and associated with **anti-microsomal** antibodies. Other causes include I^{131} therapy, surgery, iodine deficiency, inherent synthetic defects, and medicines (lithium, amiodarone, and ASA). Secondary hypothyroidism is mostly from hypopituitarism and tertiary hypothyroidism is hypothalamus-induced.

Essentials of diagnosis

1. In newborns and children: **Cretinism** and juvenile hypothyroidism are the major manifestations. At birth, persistent physiologic jaundice, hoarse cry, constipation, somnolence, and feeding problems. In later months, delayed milestones and dwarfism, coarse facial features, sparse hair, dry skin, protuberant abdomen (+/- hernia), intellectual disability, and delayed bone development.

2. In adults: Weakness, fatigue, cold intolerance, constipation, muscle cramping, carpal tunnel syndrome, and menorrhagia. In later stage, depression, decreased intelligence, movement, deep tender reflexes, and appetite; increased weight and lipid; dry skin, brittle hair, deeper voice, and myxoedema.

3. **Lab tests: Low T4, T3 and high TSH levels confirm the diagnosis.** Others results: low Hb and Na; hyperlipidemia.

Differential diagnosis

Iodine deficiency disorder and endemic goiter:

(1) It is common in regions with low-iodine diets. (2) It has a high rate of congenital hypothyroidism and cretinism. (3) There is usually an enlarged, multinodular goiter. (4) Most adults with endemic goiter are euthyroid while some are hypothyroid. (5) Treatment is supplemental iodine $\pm$ surgery (for goiter).

Treatment

1. T4 is administered and TSH/T3 levels are monitored—it takes weeks for the dosing to be stabilized.

Hyperthyroidism

2. Hydrocortisone is administered followed by T4 if supra-thyroid hypothyroidism (such as ACTH deficiency) is suspected. The goal is to restore metabolic state gradually in the elderly and patient with heart disease.

Complications

1. **Hyperlipidemia:** Mainly with high LDL or cholesterol (Chol). Fasting cholesterol testing for patients with hypothyroid symptoms is the best means of diagnosis.

2. **Myxoedema coma:** Usually caused by severe and long-time hypothyroidism without treatment; presenting with bradycardia (HR < 40/min), respiratory depression, hypothermic (T < 30°C), and fatal stuporous state. Precipitating factors include cold exposure, trauma, infections, and CNS depressants. **Treatment is IV high-dose T4 and T3.**

Thyroiditis

It is inflammation of the thyroid with different causes and clinical courses, and can affect individuals of both sexes and all ages. **It can be a euthyroid, thyrotoxic, or hypothyroid state**.

I. Subacute Thyroiditis

deQuervain

typically preceeded by URI

It's the most common form of thyroiditis, also called **subacute granulomatous thyroiditis** or **de Quervain thyroiditis**, usually associated with **viral infection, granulomatous diseases, and giant cell arteritis**. It mostly occurs in middle-aged women following an upper respiratory infection (URI).

Essentials of diagnosis

1. Patient usually starts with an URI, accompanied with fever, malaise, muscle aches, and a **painful, enlarged, and firm thyroid**. The pain radiates to the lower jaw, ears, or neck. Then **brief hyperthyroid symptoms** appear followed by hypothyroidism.

2. **Lab tests**: Increased TSH, ESR, decreased I^{131} uptake; **initially elevated T4 and T3 followed by decrease** (T4-T3 depletion and hypothyroidism).

Differential diagnosis: Graves disease.

Treatment

Thyroid pri if NSAIDs dont work

Anti-inflammatory or symptomatic treatment with aspirin/naproxen/ibuprofen, prednisone, and propranolol is effective. The disease eventually subsides and the functions recover over months. If symptomatic hypothyroidism persists, T4 can be administered.

II. Painless or Silent Thyroiditis

lymphocytic (Hashimoto)

Painless thyroiditis is considered a variant form of chronic autoimmune thyroiditis and also known as **postpartum thyroiditis.** Etiology is unclear. The typical changes in thyroid function is transient hyperthyroidism (anxiety, sweating, tremor, warm skin, tachycardia, etc.), followed by a self-limited phase of hypothyroidism (weakness, fatigue, cold intolerance, etc.), and then recovery. It is more common

similar to postpartum,

hypothyroid state may persist or return to euthyroid.

Painless Silent Thyroiditis

in postpartum women. The thyroid is usually nontender, firm, symmetrical, and mildly enlarged. **Lab tests vary**. Initially T4 and T3 may be high and I^{131} uptake and TSH low. ESR is mostly normal. Anti-thyroid peroxidase antibody titers are mildly high in 50% patients. Recurrence is possible.

Painless

Treatment

Mild cases may not need treatment. If severe, symptomatic hyperthyroidism is treated with propranolol and/or NSAIDs, and hypothyroidism is treated with propranolol.

causes adrenergic stim, like tremors & palpitations

Treatment

rarely, Levothyroxine

Mild postpartum thyroiditis may need no treatment. Symptomatic cases can be treated with propranolol and/or NSAIDs.

III. Chronic Autoimmune (Lymphocytic) Thyroiditis   *Hashimoto*

Also known as **Hashimoto thyroiditis,** it is a chronic **autoimmune** inflammatory disease of the thyroid with **lymphocytic (LC) infiltration**, in which the thyroid gland is attacked by a variety of cell- and antibody-mediated immune processes. It was the first disease to be recognized as an autoimmune disease. It's more common in middle-aged females, and is the **#1 common sporadic goiter in children**.

Essentials of diagnosis

1. **Painless**, rubber or firm, non-toxic goiter with **hypothyroidism** (with bouts of hyperthyroidism) -- myxoedematous psychosis, weight gain, depression, mania, sensitivity cold, paresthesia, chronic fatigue, bradycardia, muscle weakness, and hair loss.

2. **Lab tests**: T4 and T3 are initially normal and then decreased, and **TSH is increased**. Anti-thyroglobulin antibody is usually positive and anti-thyroid peroxidase antibody is strongly positive.

Treatment

T4 supplement daily is mostly necessary for the rest of the patient's life. Immunosuppressive therapies may be needed for severe cases.

IV. Fibrous (Riedel) Thyroiditis

It's an infiltrative thyroiditis with a state of hypothyroidism caused by idiopathic, intense **fibrosis** of the thyroid and surrounding structures (including mediastinal and retroperitoneal fibrosis). Patient mostly presents with a painless, non-toxic goiter with hypothyroid symptoms. T4 and TSH are mostly normal until hypothyroidism is present.

Treatment

Thyroid hormone may be supplied if hypothyroidism is present. Corticosteroid can be used to inhibit inflammation and the actions of fibrinogenic cytokines. Surgery may be necessary if complications occur.

PEARLS—Table 5-2: Comparison of Hyperthyroidism and Hypothyroidism

Hyperthyroidism	Hypothyroidism
Fever, heat intolerance	Hypothermia, cold intolerance, edema, hair loss
Tachycardia, palpitations, atrial fibrillation	Bradycardia
Diarrhea; weight loss	Constipation; weight gain
Anxiety, nervousness, restlessness; hyperreflexia	Fatigue, lethargy, coma; hyporeflexia
Graves disease: low TSH, high RAIU*, Ab (+); Tx: I^{131}	**Chronic antoimmune/lymphocytic thyroiditis**: normal to low T4 & T3, high TSH; Ab (+)
Exogenous T4 & T3 use: low TSH and RAIU; drug history (+), nonpalpable gland; Tx: Stop use	**Fibrous thyroiditis**: low T4 & T3, high TSH; Tx: T4.
Subacute thyroiditis: low TSH and RAIU; gland tenderness; Tx: Aspirin	
Silent thyroiditis: low TSH and RAIU; painless	
Pituitary adenoma: high TSH, MRI confirms; Tx: Resection.	

*RAIU: radioactive iodine (I^{131}) uptake.

NEOPLASMS OF THE THYROID

Thyroid Adenoma

It is a solitary benign neoplasm resulting from a genetic mutation in a single precursor cell. It may be nonfunctional ("cold" nodule) or hyperfunctional ("hot" nodule with hyperthyroid symptoms), slowly growing over years. FNB (fine needle biopsy) is the best means of confirmative diagnosis.

Sub-types

1. Follicular adenoma—the most common and a highly differentiated, autonomous nodule. It can be normofollicular (simple), microfollicular (fetal) with the potential for microinvasion, or macrofollicular (colloid) without the potential for microinvasion.

2. Atypical (embryonal) adenoma has the potential for microinvasion.

3. Hurthle-cell (oxyphil) adenoma has the potential for microinvasion.

4. Papillary adenoma: Rare.

Differential diagnosis

A **multinodular goiter** is considered to result from a hyperplastic response of the entire thyroid gland to a stimulus, such as iodine deficiency. Careful pathological examination may be necessary to distinguish a thyroid adenoma from a minimally invasive follicular thyroid carcinoma.

Treatment

1. Benign nodules (macrofollicular or adenomatoid/hyperplastic nodules, colloid adenomas, nodular goiter, and Hashimoto's thyroiditis) are usually followed without surgery.

2. Hyperfunctioning adenomas are treated with ablation by surgery or I^{131} radiation.

Thyroid Carcinoma

The incidence increases with age and the overall female: male ratio is 3:1.

Essentials of diagnosis

1. **History of radiation** therapy or exposure of the head/neck (especially in childhood and women).

2. A recent thyroid mass without tenderness or hoarseness, or a solitary nodule with high calcitonin level. I^{131} scan shows **"cold nodule"**.

3. Calcifications on x-rays such as psammoma bodies suggest papillary carcinoma; increased density suggests medullary carcinoma.

4. FNB (FNA) is the best means of diagnosis.

PEARLS—Important differential and managing steps for a solitary thyroid nodule

1. First perform thyroid function tests (TFTs; TSH, T4, and T3). If they are normal (a non-functional nodule) or of hypothyroidism, then proceed to a FNA for cytology, which is the most appropriate initial procedure for most patients. FNA has high sensitivity and moderate specificity.

2. If it's hyperthyroidism or uncertain, I^{131} scan is applied to determine if it's a "cold or hot" nodule. Functioning ("hot") nodules are rarely malignant.

3. If the FNA result is benign, treat with T4 to suppress TSH and shrink nodule, along with ultrasound follow-up.

4. If the FNA result is malignant, perform thyroidectomy along with I^{131} scan—it's both diagnostic and therapeutic, especially with follicular cancer and lymph node (LN) metastasis (do not resect LN).

5. If it's difficult to judge the "benign or malignant" nature, perform a lobectomy and wait for the biopsy report.

6. Ultrasound may help determine if the nodule is cystic or solid, but FNA is eventually required.

Pathologic types and treatment

I. Papillary carcinoma:

It's the most common type (accounting for 75-85% of thyroid carcinomas), and usually associated with history of **radiation** exposure. Females are more frequently affected, with a bi-modal distribution by age in 20-30's and elder age. The tumor grows slowly and **spreads via lymphatic channels** after many years. It may occur in women with familial adenomatous polyposis and in patients with Cowden syndrome.

Treatment: (1) Surgery for small and localized tumor (thyroid lobectomy and isthmusectomy for tumor < 1cm); (2) surgery plus radioiodine ablation for large tumor +/- metastases (regional lymph node dissection); (3) TSH suppression therapy is also helpful. General prognosis is good.

II. Follicular carcinoma:

It accounts for about 15% of all thyroid cancers. It is more common in the elderly females and more malignant than papillary carcinoma. It **spreads via blood** with distant metastasis (Met) to the lung and bone. It's occasionally seen in patients with Cowden syndrome.

Treatment requires near total thyroidectomy with postoperative I^{131} ablation.

III. Anaplastic carcinoma:

It accounts for about 10% of all thyroid cancers and occurs more in elderly females. It is the **most malignant** type with rapid and painful enlargement. 80% of patients die within 1 year of diagnosis.

IV. Medullary carcinoma:

It accounts for about 5%. It arises from **parafollicular cells** of the thyroid and is more malignant than follicular carcinoma, often **producing calcitonin and metastasis via lymph or blood** (mostly to the liver). It is often part of the two subtypes of multiple endocrine neoplasias 2 (**MEN-2**).

Treatment: The only effective **therapy** is thyroidectomy along with I^{131} radiation.

Follow-up

Patients with differentiated thyroid cancer usually require post-surgery T4 replacement and follow-up with physical examinations, biochemical tests (including serum Ca, TSH and thyroglobulin measurements), and ultrasonography.

Multiple Endocrine Neoplasias (MEN)

It's a group of endocrine neoplastic syndromes that carries **autosomal dominant inheritance** and encompasses several distinct neoplasms (tumors) of endocrine glands, each with its own characteristic pattern. Some of the tumors are malignant and some are benign. Gene testing allows a diagnosis before tumors or symptoms develop. Subtypes are:

MEN 1 (Wermer syndrome): Including **P**arathyroid (hyper-PTD, 95%), **P**ancreatic islet cell tumors (54%, including gastrinoma, insulinoma, glucagonoma, and VIPoma), **P**ituitary (42%), **F**acial angiofibroma and collagenases (85%), etc. **Mnemonic: "PPPFace".**

MEN 1 should be suspected in patients with an endocrinopathy of two of the three characteristic affected organs, or with an endocrinopathy of one of these organs plus a first-degree relative affected by MEN 1 syndrome. Many tumors in MEN 1 are **benign** and cause symptoms by overproduction of hormones (mostly **PTH plus gastrin**) and tumor effects, such as nephrolithiasis, amenorrhea, galactorrhea, erectile dysfunction, peptic ulcer disease, diarrhea, and neuroglycopenic or sympathoadrenal symptoms from hypoglycemia. The average age of death in patients with MEN 1 is 55 years for men and 47 years for women. Family history is significant. DNA testing for MEN 1 gene mutations can be used for specific diagnosis.

MEN 2A (Sipple syndrome, mostly malignant): Including **M**edullary thyroid carcinoma (**MTC**, >90%), **A**drenal pheochromocytoma (20-35%), and **P**arathyroid hyperplasia (20-50%). **Mnemonic: "MAP"**. In MEN 2A, **MTC represents the most frequent initial diagnosis**.

MEN 2B or MEN 3 (mostly malignant): Including **m**edullary thyroid carcinoma (85%), **A**drenal pheochromocytoma (60%), **M**ucosal neuromas (100%), and **M**arfanoid habitus (> 80%). **Mnemonic: "MAMM"**. In MEN 2B, MTC, mucosal neuromas, pheochromocytoma and Marfanoid features may manifest together, with characteristic musculoskeletal and/or lip and/or GI findings. If pheochromocytoma is found together, it should be removed prior to thyroidectomy. **If the initial testing for coexisting tumors is negative, it is important to evaluate the index patient for pheochromocytoma (MEN 2A and 2B) and hyperparathyroidism (MEN 2A) annually.**

DISORDERS OF THE PARATHYROID GLANDS

Pathophysiology

Parathyroid hormone (PTH) acts directly on the bone and kidney, and indirectly on intestine (by synthesis of $1, 25(OH)_2$-D_3 to increase serum Ca. **Ionized Ca** is the major regulating factor for Ca metabolism, which involves three tissues—the bone, kidney, and intestine, and three hormones: PTH, calcitonin, and activated vitamin D. Normal serum Ca is 8.5-10.5 mg/dL.

Hyper-Ca: It can be a sign of a serious disease, with symptoms when Ca > 11.5-12 mg/dL (**#1 cause is primary hyper-PTD),** or showing crisis with **cancer (Ca > 14** mg/dL) —mostly via PTH-related proteins [$1, 25(OH)_2$-D_3], IL, TNF, and osteoclastic-activating factor. Other causes are tertiary hyperparathyroidism, chronic renal failure, drugs (thiazides or lithium), sarcoidosis, thyrotoxicosis, familial hypocalciuric hyper-Ca, and immobilization.

Hyperparathyroidism and Hypercalcemia

Primary hyperparathyroidism (hyper-PTD) represents **90% of mild hyper-Ca (serum Ca 10.5-11.5** mg/dL), mostly due to one gland hyperplasia or adenoma and accidentally found in middle-aged women. Parathyroid adenoma is also part of **MEN-1 and MEN-2**.

Essentials of diagnosis

1. **Clinical features:** (1) Most patients are asymptomatic with mild hypercalcemia. When serum Ca is over 11.5 mg/dL, typical symptoms will appear as **"Bones** (pain and fractures with osteitis)**, Groans** (PUD, pancreatitis), **Stones** (nephrolithiasis), **and Psychic** overtones (anxiety, depression, irritability and sleep disturbances)."

(2) CVS: Hypertension and arrhythmias (short QT).

(3) UT: polyuria, polydipsia, and nephrocalcinosis with renal failure.

(4) GI: anorexia, weight loss, constipation, nausea/vomiting, thirst, abdominal pain.

(5) NS: Neuromuscular weakness, psychosis, or mental disturbances.

2. **Lab tests**: Serum Ca > 10.5 mg/dL and PO_4 < 2.5 mg/dL with elevated PTH can be diagnostic.

Differential diagnosis

High oral Ca-intake, secondary hyper-PTD, tertiary hyper-PTD, sarcoidosis, MEN syndrome, etc.

Secondary hyper-PTD:

[handwritten: — ↑ Phosphate = directly Stim parathyroid gland. — Vit·D def: causes 2° Hyper PTH. — ↓ to normal phos, — normal Ca²⁺]

The excessive secretion of PTH is **due to hypocalcemia** and associated hypertrophy of the parathyroid glands, most commonly seen in **chronic renal failure**. Manifestations include hypo-Ca, bone and joint pain, increased BUN:creatinine ratio, and neurologic or immunologic abnormalities. **Treatment** (with renal failure) includes dietary restriction of phosphorus, supplements with an active form of Vit-D such as calcitriol. If left untreated, the disease will progress to tertiary hyperparathyroidism.

[handwritten left margin: ↓ GFR → ↓ 1,25-(OH)₂ Vit·D ↓ ↓ intestinal Ca²⁺ abs ↓ ↓ serum Ca²⁺ ↓ PTH synth; Phosphate retention ↓ ↑ serum phosphate]

Tertiary hyper-PTD:

It's a state of excessive **secretion of PTH after a long period of secondary hyperparathyroidism and resulting in hypercalcemia**. It reflects development of **unregulated parathyroid** function following a period of persistent parathyroid stimulation. The basis of **treatment is still prevention in chronic renal failure**, starting medication and dietary restrictions long before dialysis treatment is initiated. **Cinacalcet** has greatly reduced needed surgery for surgery. If hyper-PTD persists despite medical treatment, **surgical removal** of most of the parathyroid glands is indicated.

Treatment

1. **Medications: pamidronate (P_2)** is used for asymptomatic patients with hyperparathyroidism, with serum Ca 10.5-11.5 mg/dL or with surgery contraindication. Diet Ca restriction to 400 mg/day and oral fluid 2-3 L/day are also effective. Estrogen may be indicated in hyper-PTD with menopause.

2. **Urgent treatment of severe hypercalcemia (Ca > 12 mg/dL):** This includes the simultaneous IV administration of **saline, calcitonin (effective < 48 hours), and a bisphosphonate**. Isotonic saline corrects possible volume depletion due to hypercalcemia-induced urinary salt wasting or vomiting. Hypovolemia exacerbates hypercalcemia by impairing the renal clearance of calcium.

3. **Primary hyperparathyroidism (symptomatic): Parathyroidectomy** is the effective therapy that cures the disease, decreases the risk of kidney stones, and improves bone mineral density. Surgical therapy is the effective cure for hypercalcemia caused by parathyroid neoplasms, but not applied to familial hypocalciuric hypercalcemia.

Complication

"Hungry bones syndrome": It refers to severe and prolonged hypocalcemia caused by surgical removal of a hyper-PTD gland normal or elevated PTH. The hypocalcemia may be treated with oral or IV calcium supplementation or by dialysis.

Hypoparathyroidism and Hypocalcemia

Hypocalcemia (serum Ca < 8.5 mg/dL) can be associated with low or high parathyroid hormone. Low PTH levels are seen in hereditary hypo-PTD, acquired hypo-PTD (**surgery is the #1 cause**), and hypo-Mg. High PTH levels are seen in CRF and low vitamin D, due to decreased diet intake or defective metabolism (secondary to anticonvulsant therapy or Vit-D-dependent rickets type 1). Ineffective vitamin D can also lead to high PTH levels, seen in GI malabsorption and vitamin D-dependent rickets type 2.

Essentials of diagnosis

1. **Neuromuscular irritability**: Tetany, laryngospasm, cramping, seizures, and amnesia. **Chvostek sign** (percussion of the facial nerve) and **Trousseau sign** (cuff on the arm) may be (+).

2. CVS: Prolonged QT, hypotension and refractory CHF may be seen. Chronic: possible cataracts and soft tissue calcifications.

3. **Lab tests: Serum calcium (Ca) is low**. It is important to measure ionized Ca, pH and albumin level and correct them accordingly, because the low Ca may be caused by low albumin or alkalosis. The serum total calcium concentration falls approximately 0.8 mg/dL for every 1 g/dL reduction in the serum albumin concentration.

Differential diagnosis

Hypo-Ca and hyper-P (PO_4): Can be due to **hypo-PTD**, pseudohypo-PTD, renal failure, and massive tissue destruction.

Hypo-Ca and hypo-PO_4: It's due to **vitamin D deficiency (with secondary hyper-PTD)**, whereas primary hyper-PTD may alleviate vitamin D deficiency.

Treatment

1. **Acute symptomatic hypo-Ca ($\leq$ 7.5 mg/dL or 1.9 mmol/L): $CaCl_2$ or Ca-gluconate IV**. Oral calcium and Vit-D supplement is for maintenance therapy or patients with mild symptoms (e.g., paresthesias) and hypocalcemia (corrected serum calcium >7.5 mg/dL).

2. **Chronic disease:** Treat original causes. If hyper-PO_4 coexists, diet restriction and phosphate binders (Ca-carbonate or aluminum hydroxide) are indicated.

Osteomalacia

It's defined as decreased bone mineralization and density while bone mass or volume is normal. Defective mineralization of the growing skeleton in children results in permanent bone deformities (rickets). Defective skeletal mineralization in adults causes osteomalacia. It can result from any condition causing inadequate Ca or phosphate mineralization of bone osteoid.

Etiology

1. **Vitamin D deficiency (#1 cause) and resistance:** Lower availability or nutritional supply of Vit D; insufficient sunlight exposure; malabsorption (including pancreatic disease); chronic kidney or liver disease; Vit D-dependent rickets type 1; medications (phenytoin, carbamazepine, or barbiturate therapy).

2. **Deficient Ca intake:** due to long-term nutrition-imbalanced diet.

3. **Phosphate deficiency: It results in rickets in childhood and osteomalacia in adults. Causes** include malnutrition or malabsorption, genetic disorder (high FGF_{23}, low P_2), mesenchymal tumors (high FGF_{23}, low P_2), and renal disease.

 4. **Aluminum toxicity or bisphosphonates:** Inhibition of mineralization.

 5. **Disorders of bone matrix:** hypophosphatemia; fibrogenesis imperfecta; axial osteomalacia.

Essentials of diagnosis

 1. **Painful proximal muscle weakness (particularly pelvic girdle); bone pain and tenderness.**

 2. **Decreased bone density** from defective mineralization.

 3. **Abnormal lab results: increased alkaline phosphatase; decreased 25-OH-D, Ca, and phosphate; secondary hyperparathyroidism.** Bone X-ray typically shows **"looser zones"**.

Treatment

Supplemental calcium plus phosphate plus vitamin D are more effective for nutritional osteomalacia than others. Underlying cause should be treated. Hereditary hypophosphatemic rickets is treated with a combination of phosphate supplementation and calcitriol.

DISORDERS OF THE ADRENAL GLAND

 The adrenal gland is divided into two areas, the cortex, and medulla. The cortex is divided into three areas: glomerulosa (aldosterone synthesis), fasciculate (cortisol synthesis) and reticularis (androgen synthesis). Hyperfunctional adrenal disorders include Cushing syndrome (primary hypercortisolism), hyperaldosteronism, and increased adrenal androgens (female-virilization). Hypofunctional adrenal disorders include Addison disease (Primary) and secondary adrenal hypofunction (due to pituitary gland hypofunction or resection).

Cushing Syndrome ~ ⊕ 24 hr urine free cortisol

 It's a group of clinical abnormalities caused by chronic or prolonged hypercortisolism. **The No.1 cause is excessive use of corticosteroids.** The No.2 cause is **ACTH hypersecretion** by the pituitary microadenoma (**Cushing disease, accounting for 70% of organic hypercortisolism**). Other causes include adrenal hyperplasia secondary to ACTH or CRH produced by non-endocrine cancers (small cell lung carcinoma, thymus tumor, pancreatic carcinoma, and bronchial adenoma) and adrenal adenoma or carcinoma.

Essentials of diagnosis

 1. **Classical manifestations (Image 38) of "moon face", interscapular, "buffalo hump", and truncal obesity** (caused by adipose deposition); glucose intolerance or hyperglycemia (20% with diabetes), hypo-K; hypertension, muscle weakness, and fatigability; osteoporosis (caused by increased bone catabolism); cutaneous striae and easy bruisability.

 2. Emotional lability, irritability, depression, or even psychosis can also occur. Female patient may have acne, hirsutism, and oligomenorrhea or amenorrhea resulting from the higher levels of adrenal androgen.

Cushing syndrome

— dexamethasone suppresses pituitary ACTH release, which subsequently reduces adrenal cortisol production.

3. Confirmative steps of lab tests:

(1) **The first test is low-dose dexamethasone** suppression: if suppression is positive (cortisol reduction the next morning), it indicates the adrenal gland may or may not be normal, then 24-hour free urinary cortisol collection is done (this can also be done first as a screening test).

(2) If persistent cortisol elevation exists after the low-dose inhibition test, a high-dose dexamethasone suppression test is done: pituitary tumors will be suppressed but ectopic cancers will not (e.g., small cell lung cancer).

(3) CT (adrenal) or MRI (sphenoid) can further localize the lesion.

Treatment

1. ACTH-secreting pituitary or ectopic tumor or cortisol-secreting adrenal tumors: Surgical resection is the best therapy. Cabergoline may be added after surgery if hyper-ACTH persists.

2. Medicines: Ketoconazole, metyrapone, cabergoline, pasireotide or octreotide can be used to inhibit cortisol secretion in adrenal cancer or small cell lung carcinoma.

Hyperaldosteronism

It's a syndrome associated with hypersecretion of the major adrenal mineralocorticoid—aldosterone. By etiology, it can be divided into primary and secondary aldosteronism.

I. Primary Aldosteronism

Most cases (70%) result from a unilateral adrenal tumor (Conn syndrome); 30% from bilateral adrenocortical hyperplasia.

Essentials of diagnosis

1. Typical manifestations include Hyper-Na, hypertension, headache, hypo-K, muscle weakness, metabolic alkalosis, and polyuria (hypo-K causing secondary decreased ADH sensitivity).

2. With above manifestations, first obtain plasma aldosterone and renin levels. Increased aldosterone and decreased renin level is specific for the diagnosis, which is confirmed by salt loading test. If aldosterone is NOT suppressed after salt loading ("positive"), then primary aldosteronism is confirmed.

3. Next, abdominal CT or MRI is performed to locate the adrenal tumor.

4. If extra-adrenal tumors are suspected: NP-59 scan (iodine-scintillation) is done for chest or abdominal tumors.

5. In patients with low K^+, low aldosterone and high renin: 24-hour urine K^+ secretion is tested (which should be low) for suspected secret vomiting ("Bulimia disorder").

Treatment

1. **Conn syndrome**: Laparoscopic or open adrenalectomy is the therapy of choice.

2. **Bilateral hyperplasia**: Aldosterone-R antagonist—spironolactone (#1) or eplerenone (#2).

II. Bartter Syndrome

Bartter syndrome and Gitelman syndrome (milder form) are rare autosomal recessive disorders (except Bartter's type V as dominant) characterized by **hypo-Cl, hypokalemia, metabolic alkalosis, secondary hyperreninemia and hyperaldosteronism**, and normal to low blood pressure and Mg (no edema). There is a **defect in renal reabsorption of NaCl** (especially Cl$^-$) and juxtaglomerular hyperplasia. **Most cases are neonatal and classical types and diagnosed by clinical exclusion.**

Treatment

Lifelong administration of **spironolactone** (to block distal tubule Na$^+$-K$^+$ exchange) plus KCl, NaCl, and magnesium supplements are usually required. Additional NSAIDs may be helpful.

Syndrome of Adrenal Androgen Excess

It's a disorder or syndrome due to excessive production of dehydroepiandrosterone (**DHEA**), sulfated analogue (**DHEAS**), and **androstenedione**. Some of them are converted into various estrogenic and androgenic compounds in peripheral tissues, mainly resulting in androgenic effects.

Etiology

The adrenal glands produce all of the body's DHEAS and 80% of the DHEA. Thus most of the causes include congenital adrenal hyperplasia, adrenal carcinomas, adrenal adenomas (rare), and polycystic ovary syndrome.

Clinical features

Acne, female hirsutism, oligomenorrhea, and virilization.

Treatment

Target etiologic and surgical therapies.

Congenital Adrenal Hyperplasia

It's a syndrome associated with adrenal androgen or estrogen production due to congenital enzymatic defects for cortisol synthesis, mostly from autosomal recessive mutations. It's the commonest adrenal disorder of infancy and childhood. Family history and short stature are common.

Etiology & clinical features

1. **21-hydroxylase deficiency**: **No.1 common** type (95%, early onset), associated with decreased cortisol and aldosterone, increased 17-OH progesterone, DHEA, and ACTH, causing congenital **masculine (virilization)** signs (ambiguous female genitalia—**Image 56**) or male macrogenitosomia), **hypo-Na, hyper-K, dehydration, and hypotension.**

2. **11-hydroxylase deficiency**: Late onset, impaired conversion of 11-deoxycorticosterone to corticosterone causing (1) increased 11-deoxycorticosterone (a potent mineralocorticoid), presenting with

hypertension, hyper-Na, and hypo-K; (2) increased **17-OH progesterone** (markedly) and DHEA (mildly), presenting with irregular menses (anovulation), **hirsutism** (without much virilization**)**, and **precocious puberty** (<u>Image 57</u>).

3. **17-hydroxylase deficiency: Both androgen and estrogen are decreased** and aldosterone is increased, causing hypertension with low K, high Na, **hypogonadism, and feminism.**

4. **3-beta-hydroxylase deficiency**: Rare, it causes **decrease in all three adrenal cortical steroids** (mineralocorticoids, glucocorticoids, and sex steroids), resulting in decreased BP, glucose, and sexual development (this **resembles 17-hydroxylase deficiency**).

Essentials of diagnosis

1. Suspected infants usually present with failure to thrive, episodes of adrenal insufficiency, salt wasting, hypertension, or/and abnormal genitalia.

2. The above enzyme products and serum chemistry should be tested to specify the deficiency.

Treatment

Long-term glucocorticoid replacement is usually required and adequate. It may also cease the androgenic signs and restore ovulatory cycles in women. Mineralocorticoid may be added if necessary.

Adrenal Insufficiency   *Loss of Cortisol, loss of aldosterone*

FAS1 315

Primary—Addison disease: chronic adrenal insufficiency. *loss of cortisol, ACTH maintained*
Secondary—ACTH insufficiency; **Adrenal crisis—**Acute adrenal insufficiency: *→ NO ACTH created*

1. Weakness, abdominal pain, fever, confusion (mental changes), nausea, vomiting, and diarrhea

2. Low BP, dehydration; +/- skin pigmentation . *Not N*

3. Serum K$^+$ is high, Na$^+$ is low, and BUN is high.

4. ACTH 1-24 is unable to increase serum cortisol to $\geq$ 20 ug/dL

Addison Disease

It's a primary adrenal insufficiency following acute or chronic destruction of the gland, mostly through **idiopathic or autoimmune destruction**. Other causes are congenital enzyme deficiencies, surgery, hemorrhage (DIC, Waterhouse-Friderichsen syndrome), infection (TB, fungal, CMV), metabolic disease, and metastasis. The major defect is lack of glucocorticoids and mineralocorticoids.

Essentials of diagnosis

1. <u>Addisonism</u>: Weakness, paresthesia, cramping, nausea, vomiting, weight loss, **hypotension, hyperpigmentation (key difference from the secondary type)**, stress and cold intolerance, personality changes (irritable, restless, etc), and **hypothyroidism. Lab tests: Low Na and glucose, high K and ACTH**; WBC: moderate neutropenia, lymphocytosis, and eosinophilia.

Adrenal Insufficiency

Normal: cosyntropin triggers a rapid ↑ in serum cortisol

PAI: no significant rise — *exogenous ACTH*

Central adrenal insuff: blunted (minimal or suboptimal) response due to adrenal atrophy from chronically low ACTH

2. **"Cosyntropin"** (ACTH1-24) stimulation test: Best to distinguish primary and secondary insufficiency: if cortisol is high after ACTH (test positive)—it's secondary adrenal insufficiency; if cortisol remains low—it's Addison disease.

3. In mild adrenal insufficiency, cortisol and aldosterone level may be normal.

Treatment

IV hydrocortisone for adrenal crisis (abd pn, fever, hemodynamic instability)

1. **Acute insufficiency**: IV cortisol and fluid is required for acute stress periods (major surgery, infection and trauma) or **Adrenal Crisis**. Mineralocorticoid is generally not necessary.

2. **Chronic insufficiency**: Most patients will need hydrocortisone plus mineralocorticoid replacement (fludrocortisone). DHEA therapy is only for women with impaired mood despite optimal glucocorticoid and mineralocorticoid replacement.

Pheochromocytoma

It's a **rare but the most common primary benign neoplasm of the adrenal medulla in adults**. It originates from the sympathetic nerve chromaffin cells and secretes EP and NE. The clinical features are **"rules of 10%"**: 10% malignant, 10% extra-adrenal, 10% in children, 10% multiple, 10% calcified, and 10% familial (Autosomal dominant inherent, MEN 2). It may be associated with neurofibromatosis or retinal hemangioblastoma. NE is secreted by all extra-adrenal pheochromocytomas (mostly in the abdomen).

Essentials of diagnosis

1. Intermittent tachycardia, palpitation, chest and head pain, sweating, flushing, anxiety, and hypertension.

2. **Lab tests**: Elevated 24-hour urinary **VMA and HVA** (catecholamine metabolites) is the best diagnostic test. EP metabolite increase is mostly from an adrenal tumor.

3. MRI or CT best locates the adrenal tumor: if it's negative, perform a whole-body MIBG (radio-labeled I-metaiodobenzylguanidine) scan for extra-adrenal tumors.

Differential diagnosis

Essential hypertension, neuroblastoma, anxiety attacks, factitious disorder, and intracranial lesions.

Treatment

1. Alpha-R blockers: Use long-term-acting **phenoxybenzamine. Beta-R blockers alone are contraindicated** (to avoid lethal hypertension) and may only be used following alpha-R blockers to reduce hypertension.

2. Definite treatment: Surgical removal of the tumor; bilateral adrenalectomy if it's familial or malignant.

Neuroblastoma

Neuroblastoma refers to a rare spectrum of neuroblastic tumors (**including neuroblastomas, ganglioneuroblastomas, and ganglioneuromas**) that arise **from neural crest ganglia** and have the capacity to synthesize and **secrete catecholamines** (like pheochromocytomas). It is associated with mutations in the **ALK gene**, central hypoventilation, Hirschsprung disease, and neurofibromatosis type 1 (neurocristopathy syndrome). Neuroblastoma mostly develops in the **adrenal glands (#1)**, but can also begin in or spread to other areas including the chest, the spine or spinal cord regions and the abdomen. It occurs **mostly in children < age 2.**

Clinical features include **hypertension, abdominal mass and pain,** proptosis, periorbital ecchymoses ("**raccoon eyes**"), Horner syndrome, localized back pain, scoliosis, bladder dysfunction, palpable nontender subcutaneous nodules, opsoclonus myoclonus syndrome, secretory diarrhea, and systemic symptoms (fever, weakness, weight loss, anemia, etc.).

Diagnosis: CT scan, fine needle aspirate, 24-hour urinary VMA and HVA, bone scan, bone marrow biopsy, CBC, LFTs, coagulation panel, and BUN/Cr.

Treatment: Surgical excision +/- chemotherapy +/- radiation.

HYPOGONADISM

It's defined as **decreased function of the testes or ovaries**, resulting in the impairment or absence of secondary sexual characteristics and infertility.

Etiology and clinical features

1. **Primary hypogonadism—hypergonadotropic hypogonadism with elevated LH and FSH:**
It can result from **Klinefelter syndrome**, anorchia, chemo-radiotherapy, infections (mumps, TB, leprosy), or surgical or accidental castration.

2. **Secondary hypogonadism—hypogonadal hypogonadism with low/normal LH and FSH:**
This can result from aging, alcohol, chronic illness, malnourishment, constitutional delay, obesity, **hypopituitarism** (idiopathic or tumors), hypothalamic lesions, **Kallmann syndrome**, Cushing syndrome, hypothyroidism, hemochromatosis, 17-ketosteroid reductase deficiency, or **drugs** (estrogen, androgen, GnRH agonist, ketoconazole, spironolactone, marijuana)

3. **If it's prepubertal hypogonadism caused by pituitary deficiency**, patient will show underdeveloped external genitalia, high-pitched voice, and lack of beard, libido and potency.

Treatment

Treat underlying cause. Replace sex steroids to develop secondary sex characteristics, and to build and sustain normal bone and muscle mass. Pulsatile GnRH and exogenous gonadotropin therapy are used for ovulation induction in women and for induction of spermatogenesis in men.

Klinefelter Syndrome

It's the **most common primary hypogonadism**. Most patients have **47 XXY** karyotype, presenting with **lack of libido, tall figure, small testes, eunuchoid, gynecomastia**, and sterility. Intellectual disability may or may not exist. Urinary 17-KS and serum testosterone are low to normal; **LH, FSH, and estradiol are high**.

Standard diagnosis is made by analysis of the chromosome karyotypes on LC.

Treatment should focus on 3 major facets of the syndrome: hypogonadism, gynecomastia, and psychosocial problems. Testosterone replacement therapy helps with development of normal male secondary sex characteristics, and improvement of social behavior. However, testosterone therapy does not treat infertility or gynecomastia.

Kallmann Syndrome

It is a genetic **deficiency of GnRH** release by hypothalamic neurons leading to the **failure of start or completion of puberty**. It occurs in both males and females and has the additional symptoms of **hypogonadism, infertility, altered sense of smell** (anosmia or hyposmia). It is often difficult to **distinguish Kallmann syndrome or hypogonadal hypogonadism from a constitutional delay of puberty**. However, if puberty has not commenced by either 14 (girls) or 15 (boys) and one of these non-reproductive features are present, then a referral to the expert is recommended.

Diagnosis is usually made by exclusion of other causes of GnRH deficiency and delayed puberty.

Treatment includes replacing sex steroids to develop secondary sex characteristics and to build and sustain normal bone and muscle mass, and exogenous gonadotropin or pulsatile GnRH therapy to induce ovulation in women and spermatogenesis in men.

Turner Syndrome

Also known as "**Gonadal dysgenesis**", it is a female chromosomal abnormality in which all or part of one of the sex chromosomes is absent (**missing the Barr body, mostly 45 X** karyotype). In some cases, the chromosome is missing in some cells but not others, a condition referred to as mosaicism. Characteristic abnormalities include gonadal dysfunction (causing **amenorrhea and sterility**), **short stature, swelling, short 4th metacarpals, broad chest, low hairline, low-set ears, and webbed necks**. Patients also have higher risk of congenital heart disease, hypothyroidism, diabetes, vision or hearing deficits, autoimmune diseases, and a specific pattern of cognitive deficits.

Diagnosis: prenatal—mniocentesis or chorionic villus sampling; postnatal—typical symptoms plus analysis of the chromosome karyotypes.

Therapeutic guidelines for hypogonadism

1. Treat underlying cause.

2. **Hormone replacement therapy**: Use testosterone for male and estrogen-progesterone for female.

Chapter 5: High-yield Questions (HYQ)

Q1-4. 1. A 36 y/o woman at 8-week's gestation comes for her first examination. She is generally in good health except for that she is mildly overweight for her gestational age. What's the most appropriate next step?

A. Urine dipstick   B. Fasting blood glucose test   C. Random blood glucose test

D. 1-hour 50g GTT   E. 3-hour 100g GTT

2. From the above patient, 1-hour 50g GTT comes back with serum glucose = 140 mg/dL. Then a 3-hour 100g GTT is done with serum glucose = 180 mg/dL at 1 hour, 155 mg/dL at 2 hours, and 140 at 3 hours. Now what's the best next step?

A. Metformin   B. Glipizide

C. Diet control and exercise   D. Repeat 3-hour 100g GTT in a month

E. Regular insulin use and blood glucose follow-up

3. The above patient is given "Lente (70 NPH/30 regular) insulin" twice daily, 1/3 the total amount in the morning and 2/3 in the evening. At "midnight" she feels uncomfortable and wakes up. Her blood glucose is tested as 60 mg/dL. She then eats some food and sleeps better through the night. The next dawn she wakes up with discomfort again. This is most likely due to

A. the "Honeymoon" period   B. the Somogyi effect   C. the Dawn phenomenon

D. the insulin dose waning   E. unbalanced diet

4. The above patient is now at 32 week's gestation and presents with weakness, polyuria, polydipsia, lethargy, and confusion. Her vital signs are stable. Blood tests reveal glucose = 700 mg/dL, BUN and osmolality both increased, HCO_3^- = 21 mEq/L, pH = 7.30. Fetal monitoring shows "mild distress." What's the best next step now?

A. Large-volume N.S. + high-dose insulin   B. Moderate-volume N.S. + high-dose insulin

C. Large-volume N.S. + moderate-dose insulin   D. IV steroids

E. Induction of delivery

5. A 30 y/o man is found with a solitary thyroid nodule during a yearly P/E. He complains of occasional fatigue, sweating, and cough. He has a 10-year history of smoking and alcohol use, but no recent fever or radiation exposure. P/E finds warm skin and tachycardia. X-ray of the neck and chest is normal, so are other results. The most appropriate next step is

A. ultrasonography (U/S)   B. TFTs   C. fine needle aspiration (FNA)

D. I^{131} scan   E. follow-up in 3 months

6. From the above patient, TFTs reveal mildly increased T4 and decreased TSH. Now the best next step is

A. ultrasonography   B. anti-thyroid drugs   C. FNA

D. I131 scan   E. follow-up in 3 months

7. From the above patient, the I^{131} scan shows a 1.5 cm nodule with lower I^{131}-uptake within the nodule and higher I^{131}-uptake in other parts of the thyroid. FNA is performed for biopsy and reveals papillary carcinoma. Now the best next step is

A. surgery   B. anti-thyroid drugs   C. TSH suppression therapy

D. surgery + I^{131} E. follow-up in 3 months

8. A 45 y/o female presents with fever and a painful mass in the front of her neck for the past week, accompanied with anxiety, sweating, tremor, and a "pounding heart." Now she complains of lethargy, fatigue, and "always feeling cold." P/E finds normal results except for mild bradycardia and an enlarged thyroid with tenderness. Lab tests show mild TSH increase and T$_4$ decrease. The best initial treatment is

A. aspirin   B. corticosteroids   C. T$_4$ supplement

D. propranolol   E. observation

9-13: Match the following clinical scenarios with the most likely diagnosis.

A. High oral intake   B. Primary Hyper-PTD   C. Secondary Hyper-PTD

D. Tertiary Hyper-PTD   E. Vitamin (Vit) D toxicity   F. Sarcoidosis

G. Paget disease   H. Malignancy   I. Vit-D deficiency

J. Hypo-PTD   K. Pseudo-hypo-PTD

9. A 15 y/o boy has intermittent polyuria, polydipsia, polyphagia, proteinuria, bone pain, and weight loss for the past year, for which he takes insulin IM. P/E and X-ray reveal mild osteodystrophy. Blood tests reveal high levels of glucose, K, PO$_4$, creatinine, and PTH; total Ca = 6.9 mg/dL.

10. The above boy comes back for re-examination 1 year later because of progressive symptoms. P/E and X-ray demonstrate severe muscle and osteodystrophy. Urinary protein is (+++). Blood tests reveal high levels of glucose, K, PO$_4$, creatinine, PTH, and Ca (Ca = 12 mg/dL).

11. A 45 y/o female complains of 6 months of intermittent fatigue and muscle-bone pain. She follows a particular diet with a fixed range of foods. She had a history of small renal stones that were expelled spontaneously. She denies chronic diseases. Blood tests: Ca = 11.5 mg/dL, PTH is decreased; levels of glucose, creatinine, K, and PO$_4$ are all normal.

12. A 50 y/o man complains of 3 months of intermittent fever, cough, fatigue, and general muscle and bone pain. He has a 5-year history of smoking. P/E: T = 38°C; multiple reddish skin nodules on the sun-exposed areas. Blood tests: Ca = 13mg/dL; PO$_4$ is high; PTH is low; albumin, creatinine, and K levels are normal. X-ray shows bilateral pulmonary adenopathy.

13. A 50 y/o female complains of intermittent muscle cramping and convulsion, irritability and amnesia. She denies history of chronic diseases. P/E finds BP = 90/50 mmHg. Chvostek's and Trousseau's signs are both (+). ECG shows prolonged QT. Blood test results: Ca = 7.5 mg/dL; PO$_4$ is high; K, PTH, AKP, and albumin are all normal.

14. A 40 y/o female complains of 3 months of gradual fatigue, headache, upper abdominal pain, general muscle-bone pain, decreased vision, galactorrhea, amenorrhea, swelling, intermittent anxiety, dizziness, and sweating. Blood test results: Ca = 12.5 mg/dL, increased prolactin, PTH, gastrin and insulin levels; decreased PO$_4$, glucose, LH, and FSH; levels of T$_4$, TSH, calcitonin, creatinine, and K are all normal. What's the most likely Dx?

A. Pituitary adenoma   B. MEN 1   C. MEN 2A

D. MEN 2B   E. Parathyroid adenoma   F. Insulinoma

15. A 55 y/o man complains of 3 months of cough, fatigue, muscle weakness, decreased urine output, and mood lability. He has a 10-year history of "moderate" alcohol use and smoking. P/E finds hypertension, cutaneous striae, and truncal obesity. CXR shows evidence of chronic bronchitis. Blood tests reveal increased glucose, ACTH, and cortisol levels, and decreased Na and K levels. Urinary WBC, RBC, and protein are (-). The best next step is

A. 24-hour free urinary cortisol collection   B. high-dose dexamethasone suppression test

C. chest CT scan   D. aldosterone level test

E. adrenal CT scan

16. The patient in Q15 has a 24-hour free urinary cortisol level that is much higher than normal range. A high-dose dexamethasone suppression test is done the following morning and shows persistently high levels of ACTH and cortisol. Now the best next step is

A. sphenoid MRI   B. high-dose dexamethasone suppression re-tests

C. chest CT   D. aldosterone level test

E. adrenal CT

17-21: Match the following clinical scenarios with the most likely diagnosis.

A. Secondary adrenal insufficiency   B. Addison disease

C. 3-beta-hydroxylase deficiency   D. 11-hydroxylase deficiency

E. 17-hydroxylase deficiency   F. 21-hydroxylase deficiency

G. Klinefelter syndrome   H. Kallmann syndrome

I. Pituitary hypogonadism

17. A female infant is found with ambiguous genitalia, dehydration, and hypotension; decreased serum Na, cortisol, and aldosterone; increased serum K, 17-OH progesterone, DHEA, DHEAS, and ACTH.

18. A female infant is found with ambiguous genitalia, hypertension, low serum K, and high Na, DHEA, and DHEAS.

19. A male infant is found with undeveloped genitalia, hypertension, low serum K, DHEA-DHEAS and estrogen, and high aldosterone and Na.

20. A 50 y/o man presents with intermittent weakness, paresthesia, cramping, dizziness, weight loss, cold intolerance, and emotional lability. P/E finds HR = 55/min (bpm), BP = 90/50 mmHg and normal results with skin and muscles. Lab test results: serum Na = 130 mEq/L, K = 5.8 mEq/L, glucose = 70 mg/dL; ACTH is moderately decreased.

21. A 17 y/o boy comes for the P/E and is found with a tall figure, small testes, and gynecomastia. He also has poor school scores. Lab tests find urinary 17-KS and serum testosterone are mildly low; LH, FSH, and estradiol are moderately high.

22. A 50 y/o man presents with intermittent tachycardia, palpitations, headache, sweating, and anxiety for the past mo. P/E finds that the temperature is normal, HR = 120/min, BP = 160/120 mmHg. Lab tests reveal increased 24-hour urinary VMA and HVA. CT confirms an adrenal mass. What's the best treatment now?

A. Phentolamine   B. Phenoxybenzamine   C. Propranolol

D. Surgical removal   E. Phenoxybenzamine and propranolol

F. Phentolamine and propranolol

23. A 55 y/o man with lung cancer is brought to the ER after a few hours of oliguria, muscle weakness, and occasional convulsions. His vital signs are stable. Lab testing reveals that serum Na^+ = 125 and urine Na^+ = 25 (mEq/L), urine osmolality = 50 mOsm/kg. The best next treatment is

A. 3% saline followed by furosemide IV   B. diazepam in 100 ml of normal saline IV

C. demeclocycline   D. lithium

E. water and fluid restriction

24. A 55 y/o man presents with lethargy, weakness, headache, irritability, polydipsia, and polyuria with about 5 L of dilute urine per day for the past 2 days. He has a history of a mood disorder, which is recently unstable. Because of this, the patient is on a newly prescribed medicine. P/E is mostly normal. Serum Na, K, and Cl levels are all elevated, plasma osmolality is 400 mOsm/kg, and urine osmolality is 290 mOsm/kg. After water deprivation for 5 hours with ADH challenge, his urine osmolality is 300 mOsm/kg with similar volume. What's the best next step?

A. Head MRI   B. Desmopressin   C. Hydrochlorothiazide

D. Water intake increase   E. Water deprivation again

25. A 40 y/o obese woman presents with intermittent abdominal pain with rashes and loose stools for the past 5 days. Before these symptoms, she had a history of painful rash on the lips a week ago, which is now healed. P/E finds normal vital signs and body temperature. There is erythema with different-stage debris around the middle abdomen and mild tenderness in the RUQ. CBC is normal and random plasma glucose level is 160 mg/dL. Abdominal CT scan is scheduled. The most likely diagnosis is

A. somatostatinoma   B. glucagonoma   C. diabetes

D. VIPoma   E. transient hyperglycemia

Answers and Explanations

1. (D). She has 2 risk factors (>35 y/a and obesity) and thus the 1-hr 50g GTT is the best initial test to rule out DM, because she still needs this test even if 'A' (for most patients) is (+) or if 'B and C' raise suspicion. A one-step screening of 75g 2-hour GTT can also be used for suspected gestational DM.

2. (E). Patient has been confirmed by the accurate 3-hour 100g GTT for gestational diabetes (mostly Type 2 DM): ≥ 180mg/dL at 1 hour, 155 mg/dL at 2 hours, and 140 mg/dL at 3 hours, and should start regular insulin ('E') immediately to avoid future complications. Metformin is good for most diabetic patients but patients with pregnancy require regular insulin. Glipizide is contraindicated in gestational DM.

3. (B). Blood glucose decrease (Decr) at 3 a.m. and increase (Incr) at 7 am; correct treatment (Tx) is to decrease the pm insulin dose. 'A' is in IDDM, an initial episode of ketoacidosis followed by an asymptomatic interval. 'C' is a dawn hyperglycemia with insulin level normal (Nl) at 3 am but low at Dawn. 'D' has low insulin levels and high blood glucose at both 3 and 7 a.m.

4. (C). This is a state of NIDDM-HONK (Hyperosmolar nonketotic coma), with moderate hypo-insulin and non-AG acidosis requiring 'C'. 'B' is best for IDDM-DKA (with severe hypo-insulin and AG acidosis). "D and E" should follow 'C' to speed up fetal lung maturity and delivery.

5. (B). Please review "Important differential diagnostic (Dx) steps for a solitary thyroid nodule".

6. (D). When the thyroid has a nodule and displays hyperthyroidism, I^{131} scan is applied to determine if it's a "cold or hot nodule". If the nodule is 'hot', then the best Tx is 'B'. If it's "cold", FNA must be done. Ultrasound only helps determine if the nodule is cystic or solid.

7. (D) It's now the time for Tx. 'D' treats both the cancer and the hyperthyroidism, but post-radiation hypothyroidism is possible and thus TFT follow-up is necessary.

8. (A). This is typical subacute thyroiditis-- URI and brief hyperthyroidism followed by hypothyroidism. Tx is Anti-inflammation or symptomatic, with aspirin as the best option for this patient. The disease eventually returns to normal state over months. 'B' is best for Riedel thyroiditis--hypothyroidism caused by idiopathic fibrosis of the thyroid (painless, non-toxic goiter). T_4 is best for Hashimoto thyroiditis-- an autoimmune inflammatory disease of the thyroid causing a painless goiter with hypothyroidism mostly in children. 'D' is best for lymphocytic thyroiditis —a self-limited episode of thyrotoxicosis (painless goiter).

9. (C). It's secondary to Type-1 diabetic nephropathy. Correct Tx is Ca supplementation.

10. (D). It's secondary to long-term renal failure. Treat diabetes aggressively and treat renal failure with possible dialysis.

11. (A). Most likely due to excessive intake of oral Ca.

12. (F). Treat with steroids. Malignancy (lung cancer, multiple myeloma) related hyper-Ca usually is associated with progressive symptoms and Ca > 14 mg/dL.

13. (K). PTH is normal or mildly increased but with functional deficiency (probably due to G-protein defect). Tx is Vit-D and Ca supplement. Hypo-Ca can be associated with low or high PTH. Low PTH levels are seen in hereditary and acquired hypo-PTD; high PTH levels are seen in CRF and vitamin D deficiency.

14. (B). Remember it well. MEN 1 (Wermer syndrome): Pituitary, parathyroid, pancreatic tumors, and facial angiofibromas and collagenomas — "PPP". MEN 2A (Sipple syndrome): Adrenal pheochromocytoma, thyroid medullary carcinoma, and parathyroid adenoma— "ATP". MEN-IIB: Adrenal pheochromocytoma, thyroid medullary carcinoma, and mucosal neuromas — "ATM".

15. (A). Because this patient is having Cushing's syndrome and suspected with ectopic malignancy due to increased cortisol and glucose, the 24-hour urine-cortisol can be used as a screening test to replace the low-dose dexamethasone suppression test, which will only inhibit benign hypercortisolism, not the malignant.

16. (C). This patient is highly suspected with small cell lung cancer with ectopic secretion of ADH and ACTH, which was not suppressed by the high-dose dexamethasone test (This test only inhibit pituitary Cushing's). Therefore, the chest CT is the best choice here. Negative CXR cannot exclude lung cancer. Pituitary adenoma (for 'A') is usually associated with increased prolactin or GH. Adrenal Cushing's will cause decreased ACTH.

17. (F). This is the most common congenital adrenal deficiency, with masculine presentations.

18. (D). 11-hydroxylase deficiency causes increased 11-deoxycorticosterone (a potent mineralocorticoid) and DHEA (masculine signs).

19. (E). 17-hydroxylase deficiency causes both androgen and estrogen decrease and aldosterone increase, resulting in hypertension, hypogonadism and feminism. 3-beta-hydroxylase deficiency causes decrease in all three adrenal cortical steroids (mineralocorticoids, glucocorticoids, and sex steroids), resulting in low BP, low glucose, and delayed sexual development (this resembles 17-hydroxylase deficiency). It's very rare.

20. (A). "Addisonism + hypothyroidism + hypo-ACTH without hyperpigmentation" distinguish secondary adrenal deficiency from Addison's disease. ACTH stimulation is the best differential test.

21. (G). It's the #1 cause of primary hypogonadism, typically with 47 XXY karyotype. Secondary hypogonadism can result from pituitary hypogonadism (idiopathic, tumors), hypothalamic lesions and Kallmann syndrome, typically with lower LH and FSH.

22. (E). This patient has pheochromocytoma requiring immediate control of his hypertension, best with a long-acting alpha-blocker plus a beta-R blocker ('E'). When he is stable, surgery can be curative. 'A' is a short-term alpha-R blocker. A beta-R blocker alone is contraindicated here.

23. (A). This is a severe case of SIADH, with symptoms resulting from high ADH and Hypo-Na. When patient has serum $Na^+ < 120$ mEq/L or has a seizure, 'A' is required as an emergent and effective Tx (better than 'B'). "C or D" is good for chronic SIADH (slow and long-acting). 'E' is for mild cases.

24. (C). It's a case of nephrogenic DI caused by lithium intake. It can be treated effectively by stopping lithium, restricting salt, increasing water intake, and adding a thiazide. 'A' is for central DI, to search a potential pituitary or hypothalamic tumor. It would be treated with 'B' +/- surgery. In central DI: Water deprivation with ADH challenge test will decrease urine output and increase urine osmolality. 'E' is for psychogenic polydipsia, in which urine osmolality before and after an ADH analogue should be the same high level (about 700 mOsm/kg), and serum NaCl is low.

25. (B). A typical case of glucagonoma—necrotizing migratory erythema, stomatitis, glossitis, mild diabetes, and hyperglycemia; Tx is surgical resection. Somatostatinoma is a rare malignancy in the pancreas; classical triad is diabetes, gallstones, and steatorrhea. Diabetes usually shows more typical manifestations. VIPoma is a rare syndrome of watery diarrhea, hypokalemia, achlorhydria, hyperglycemia, and hyper-Ca; Tx is surgical resection.

Chapter 6

DISEASES OF THE BLOOD, LYMPHORETICULAR, AND IMMUNE SYSTEMS

Basics in Hematology

Blood Cell Differentiation (Figure 6-1 below)

—All start from hematopoietic stem cells (HSC):

Figure 6-1: Blood Cell Differentiation (Courtesy of www.wikimedia.org)

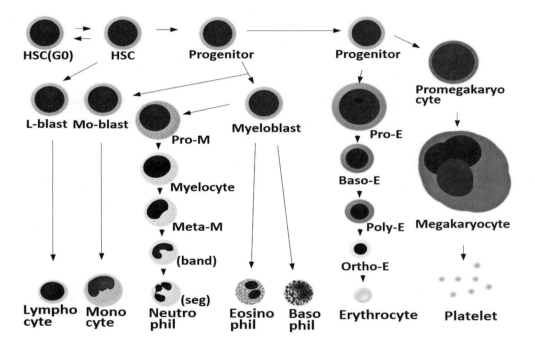

ANEMIAS

Definition: A hematocrit **(HCT) < 40%** in males or < 37% in females, or hemoglobin (Hb) <13 g/dL in males or <12 g/dL in females.

Classification by morphology

1. **Microcytic anemia**: A low mean MCV < 80. **No.1 cause is iron deficiency; others include lead poisoning, thalassemia, and sideroblastosis**. Anemia of chronic diseases can be either microcytic or normocytic.

2. **Macrocytic anemia**: Characterized by an elevated MCV > 96. This is most commonly from **vitamin B12 or folic acid deficiency** (Def). It can also result from the toxic effects of **alcohol or drugs (such as phenytoin, methotrexate, and AZT)**, liver disease, or myelodysplastic syndrome (MDS).

3. **Normocytic anemia**: Characterized by a normal MCV. It can be seen in chronic diseases, hemolysis, and early forms of above anemia.

General diagnostic points of anemia

1. History of early symptoms (when HCT is close to 30%): Fatigue, exercise intolerance, poor memory, with or without recurrent infections. It's varied individually.

2. Diagnosis is based on a low HCT or Hb. Etiologic tests include MCV, iron assay, reticulocyte count, peripheral smear, RDW, Coombs test, vitamin B12, folate levels, etc.

PEARLS—Table 6-1: Differential Diagnosis of Anemias by Lab Tests

Disease	Iron	Ferritin	TIBC	MCV	MCH	MCHC	Others
Iron deficiency anemia	<50	Low	>400	<80	<20	Normal (Nl) (20-50)	
Folate deficiency anemia	Nl	Nl (100)	Nl	>100	>35	Nl	
B₁₂ deficiency anemia	Nl	Nl (100)	Nl	>100	>35	Nl	**Neurologic symptoms**
Chronic disease anemia	<50	Nl	<250	**Nl/low**	Nl/low	<20	
Sideroblastic anemia	>150	Nl	<200	<80	Nl	Nl	**Target-C (+/-)**
Thalassemia	Nl/high	Nl/high	Nl/low	**<80**	<20	Nl	
Hemochromatosis	>150	>1000	<200	Nl	Nl	Nl	**High LFTs**
Hereditary spherocytosis	Nl	Nl	Nl	Nl	Nl	>50	

Iron (nmol/mL): Fe concentration in the serum.

TIBC: Total iron-binding capacity.

Ferritin (ng/uL): Fe-transport protein; it may increase with inflammation or malignancy.

MCV (fL/cell): Mean corpuscular volume.

MCH (pg/cell): Mean corpuscular Hb.

MCHC (g/dL): Mean corpuscular Hb concentration.

RDW (fL): Red cell distribution width, measuring variability of RBC volume/size.

Iron Deficiency Anemia

It's defined as reduced RBC and Hb with hypochromic cells, MCV < 80, and low levels of stored iron in the body. It's usually caused by an increased blood loss **(No.1 cause by GI bleeding in male and by menstrual loss in female)**. It is difficult for the body to increase the iron absorption quickly at blood loss because it's strictly regulated. Other causes include poor oral intake, malabsorption, hemolysis, etc.

Essentials of diagnosis

1. History of the above anemic symptoms, +/- brittle nails, "spoon" nails, glossitis, and pica.

2. **Lab tests**: A low serum **ferritin < 10** ng/mL is very specific and sensitive for Fe-deficient anemia as the most common diagnostic test. Serum iron, MCV and reticulocyte count are low; TIBC is high. The RDW is elevated. Blood smear shows microcytic, hypochromic RBC ("doughnut cells", **Image 136**). The **most specific** test is bone marrow (**BM**) biopsy for **Prussian blue iron staining**, but rarely used.

Treatment

1. Oral ferrous sulfate tablets are the most common treatment. Parenteral iron is used in patients with malabsorption, intolerance to oral therapy, or very high requirements.

2. Blood transfusion is the most effective treatment for severe or urgent anemia caused by blood loss.

Anemia of Chronic Disease (ACD)

It's a defect in the ability to make use of iron sequestered and stored within the reticulo-endothelial system. It can be either microcytic or normocytic. The anemia can be caused by any chronic illness-- inflammation, infection, or neoplasm. New studies suggest its association with the production of hepcidin, a master regulator of iron metabolism. ACD is the most common anemia found in hospitalized patients.

Essentials of diagnosis

1. History of chronic disease(s) and the above general anemic symptoms. Iron deficiency may coexist and worsen the symptoms.

2. Lab tests: Serum ferritin is normal or high, and serum iron, TIBC and reticulocyte count are usually low. With iron deficiency, ferritin should be low.

Treatment

Correction of underlying cause. Supplement of iron or erythropoietin (EPO) is only helpful when iron deficiency coexists (which is common) or EPO levels are very low.

Megaloblastic Anemia

It's commonly classified as the following two types by etiology—Vit-B12 and folic acid deficiencies.

I. Vitamin B12 Deficiency

Megaloblastic Anemia

It's a chronic decrease in absorption or intake of Vit-B12 that results in megaloblastic anemia and neurologic abnormalities.

Etiology

1. **The most common cause** is a **hereditary deficiency in intrinsic factor** production on an autoimmune basis, resulting in **pernicious anemia** (risk increases with age). Gastrectomy and atrophic gastritis are also common reasons for intrinsic factor reduction.

2. **Malabsorption disease:** Pancreatic insufficiency, sprue disease, Crohn disease, blind loop syndrome, and tapeworm infection (diphyllobothrium L.) can also cause Vit-B12 deficiency.

3. Diet deficit is rare and only in strict vegetarians for > 1 year (to cause the disease).

Essentials of diagnosis

1. History of anemic symptoms +/- neuropsychological symptoms: fatigue, peripheral, autonomic neuropathy (position sense abnormality, vibratory, motor, bowel, bladder, and sexual dysfunction), and psychiatric-behavioral symptoms.

2. **Lab tests**: (1) Blood smear shows macrocytosis—increased MCV, **macro-oval RBC** (differential diagnosis: round macrocytes in hemolysis, liver disease, and myelodisplasia), with many **hypersegmented neutrophils (Image 137)**. The reticulocyte count is reduced while the bone marrow is hypercellular. Pancytopenia may occur.

(2) **The most commonly used specific test is B12 level (low).** The Schilling test (most specific) for the elevated methylmalonic acid level is only done when the B12 level is uncertain. Anti-intrinsic factor (+) and anti-parietal cell Ab (+) confirm further etiology.

Treatment

Correction of underlying cause and long-term IM Vit-B12 are the best treatment. Folic acid replacement can correct the hematologic but not the neurologic symptoms.

II. Folic Acid Deficiency

Deficiency in folic acid in the body that results in megaloblastic anemia without neurologic abnormalities.

Etiology: Mostly due to **decreased dietary intake** (lack of green vegetables). Sometimes it's also due to increased requirements from pregnancy, eczema, dialysis, etc.

Essentials of diagnosis

Same hematologic manifestations as with B12 deficiency **(Image 137)** but there are **no neurologic symptoms**. The diagnosis is based on low RBC and folic acid levels, and macrocytic anemia.

Treatment: Diet correction and oral folic acid supplements.

Sideroblastic Anemia (SA)

It's a microcytic anemia caused by a defect in the Hb synthesis and characterized by trapped iron in the mitochondria of nucleated RBC. It can be congenital or acquired as a clonal bone marrow disorder. Inherited SAs (mostly X-linked) include syndromic and nonsyndromic disorders. Although it is an X-linked disorder, up to one-third of cases occur in females.

Etiology

1. **Hereditary**: From a defect in Vit-B_6 metabolism or aminolevulinic acid synthase.

2. **Acquired**: From chemicals or medications such as alcohol, isoniazid, chloramphenicol, copper deficiency, or lead poisoning. It's also associated with myelodysplastic syndrome, myeloproliferative neoplasms and refractory anemia, and occasionally may progress to AML.

Essentials of diagnosis

1. History of anemic manifestations.

2. **Lab tests**: The serum iron and transferrin saturation are high and thus TIBC is low. The serum ferritin level is normal. The most specific test is a **Prussian blue iron stain** of RBC from the BMB, revealing the ringed sideroblasts. Molecular/genetic testing may be appropriate when the bone marrow shows ring sideroblasts and a congenital sideroblastic anemia or MDS/MPN variant is suspected.

Treatment

1. Congenital SA: Remove excessive iron by phlebotomy in those with minimal anemia or use iron chelating agents in those with anemia requiring periodic blood transfusion.

2. Acquired SA: Remove the causative chemicals or drugs, use iron chelating agents with blood transfusion, treat the lead poisoning or copper deficiency, and supply Vit-B_6.

Sickle Cell Disease (SCD)

[handwritten: pt: ↓Hgb chronic pain, dx: CBC - sickle cells, Hgb electrophoresis, ↑RC, ↑bili]

[handwritten: PPx: hydroxyurea, vasoocclusive. SCD. TX: vasoocclusive crisis: IVF, O2, pain ctrl, crisis.. CBC w/ diff, bilirubin +/- infxn, f/u psychosocial stressors]

It's an **autosomal recessive** hereditary disease, characterized by irreversibly sickled cells, chronic hemolysis, and recurrent painful crises. It can be asymptomatic or presents with severe crisis, more often in the Black population. *[handwritten: baseline reticulocyte, establish baseline bili, baseline Hgb, bc they're ↑ in SCD.]*

Essentials of diagnosis

[handwritten: HbSC, carrier]

1. **"Sickle cell trait"**: >50% HbA, 35-45% HbS, and <2% HbF. It's a heterozygous form of SCD. There are no symptoms. Results of CBC and blood smear are normal. Only the ability to concentrate the urine is abnormal. Hematuria may occur occasionally. No treatment is needed for sickle cell trait.

2. **SCD (SC anemia)**: Such as **HbSS**, there is no HbA, <2% HbF, normal amounts of HbA_2, and the remainder HbS. Homozygous form (disease) is symptomatic—chronic moderate anemic symptoms, recurrent infections from Pneumococci or Hib, skin ulcers, bilirubin gallstones, osteomyelitis, retinopathy, femoral head necrosis, growth retardation, priapism, and splenomegaly followed by autosplenectomy.

[handwritten right margin: folate, from 2 deferoxamine, Iron overload from transfusion]

[handwritten: sickling → hemolysis → ↑ unconj bili → Jaundice, pigmented gallstone, cholecystectomy]

Sickle cell Disease

osteomyelitis
- sickled cells impair
blood flow thru
narrow meta physeal
vessels >7
-microinfactions
- severe as nidus
infxn.
-splenic infarcts=>
Pt susceptible
to encapsulated
orgs
- salmonella

Avascular
necrosis
bone
- conservative
mgmt, 4-6 months
- surgery

Priaprism:
- drain before
Exchange
transfusion

stroke: FND.
stroke & ACS = exchange transfusion

3. **Hemoglobin SC disease:** By Hb electrophoresis, HbS and HbC are both present.

4. **SCD painful crisis:** May occur alone and be precipitated by hypoxia, fever, infection, dehydration, and acidosis. **The acute chest syndrome** is common—severe chest pain, fever, leukocytosis, hypoxia, and pulmonary infiltrates (by CXR) and is hardly distinguishable from pneumonia. Life-threatening sickling and stroke may occur. With hemolysis in a child, concomitant G6PD or splenic sequestration should be considered. Sudden drops in hematocrit (caused by acute aplasia, not hemolysis) may be associated with Parvovirus B_{19} (PVB_{19}) infection or folate deficiency.

5. **Lab tests**: The **Hb electrophoresis** is the **most specific** test; the peripheral **smear shows sickled RBCs (Image 138)**. HPLC can also be a good option. LDH, bilirubin, and HCT are all elevated. Higher or lower HCT may be associated with folate deficiency or PVB_{19} infection. MCV is normal. Urine RBC is usually (+) and blood WBC may increase (with or without infection).

Treatment

- due to splenic autoinfarction

1. All individuals with SCD should begin **antibiotic prophylaxis (penicillin or erythromycin) in the first three months of life until age five.**

2. **Acute SCD painful crisis**: Treat with fluids, analgesics, and oxygen. Ceftriaxone and cefotaxime are used to treat or prevent Pneumococcal and Hib infections. Hydration and RBC transfusion are usually needed for severe or life-threatening conditions like acute chest syndrome, priapism, or cardiac and CNS dysfunctions.

3. **Chronic SCD**: Folic acid replacement and vaccinations against Pneumococcus and Hib. **Hydroxyurea** can decrease the frequency of the vessel-occlusive pain crisis. **Hematopoietic cell transplantation (HCT) is the only available curative option for SCD**. G-CSF is presently NOT recommended for SCD due to the risk of multiorgan failure and death.

Thalassemia

It's the hereditary, constructive **deficiency of either the α or β globin chains of the Hb molecule**, resulting in a **hypochromic, microcytic anemia**. α-thalassemia is caused by **gene deletions of 1, 2, 3 or all 4 genes (alleles) coding for the α-chain of Hb**, and is more common in Asians. β-thalassemia is mostly caused by **point mutation/substitution(s) in 1 or 2 genes coding for the Hb β-chain**, more common among Mediterranean people. **Normal Hb = 2 α-globins + 2 β-globins.**

Clinical features and diagnosis

1. Clinical manifestations are determined by the number of abnormal genes and the severity. Different types of minor thalassemias cannot be distinguished from other types of mild anemia clinically.

2. **α-thalassemia**

(1) **Silent carrier** (with 1-gene deletion): asymptomatic; the HCT, Hb level and MCV are all normal.

(2) **α-thalassemia trait** (with 2-gene deletions): mild microcytic anemia, HCT = 30-40% and a low MCV.

Thalassemia

(3) **Hemoglobin H disease** (with 3-gene deletions): more severe anemia with significantly low HCT (< 20%) and MCV; **Hb H** (tetrads of beta-chains) is positive.

(4) **Hydrops fetalis and Hb Barts** (with 4-gene deletions): fetus dies in utero secondary to gamma-chain tetrads (Hb Barts).

3. β-thalassemia

(1) **Beta-thalassemia minor: mutation in one allele causing a reduced (β^+) or absent (β^0) β-chain** (β^+/β or β^0/β); asymptomatic or showing mild anemia with a low MCV (<80 fL), low fraction of Hb A (<97.5%), and high fraction of Hb A_2 (>3.5%).

(2) **β-thalassemia intermedia** (β^+/β^+ or β^0/β^+): Patient usually shows moderate anemic symptoms and may need occasional transfusions, e.g., at times of illness or pregnancy, depending on the severity of the anemia.

(3) **β-thalassemia major: mutations in both alleles causing two absent β–chains**, resulting in increased fractions of **Hb-F and A_2** ($\alpha 2\delta 2$)—also known as **Cooley anemia.** Manifestations (if untreated) include severe microcytic anemia, growth retardation, hepatosplenomegaly, jaundice, and bony deformities early. Later symptoms include hemochromatosis, cirrhosis, and CHF from chronic anemia and transfusion complications. It progresses to death before age 20.

4. **Diagnosis**: Microcytic anemia and normal iron test results are typical. The specific **confirmation test is Hb electrophoresis.** All forms of thalassemia have low MCV, normal RDW (same sizes), and **Target cells**.

Treatment

1. **Mild thalassemia (α-thalassemia trait or β-thalassemia minor): No** specific treatment is required and should be identified to avoid repeated evaluations and treatment for iron deficiency.

2. **Hb H disease**: Folic acid supplementation; avoidance of medicinal iron and oxidative drugs (sulfonamides, etc.).

3. **β-thalassemia intermedia and major**: It usually requires **regular blood transfusions** (1-2 times/month for the "major" type). Chronic transfusions may lead to iron overload (treated with chelator **deferoxamine**). Splenectomy removes a major site of hemolysis and thus reduces needed transfusions. Appropriately selected subjects (E.g., younger age, availability of HLA-matched donor, quality of iron chelation therapy) should be considered for potentially curative hematopoietic cell transplantation (HCT).

Aplastic Anemia

Definition: Failure of all three cell lines produced in the bone marrow results in **pancytopenia**—anemia, leukopenia, and thrombocytopenia. The bone marrow is empty and without precursor cells.

Etiology

It's unknown and mostly idiopathic. Many factors can cause bone marrow failure: (1) Radiation; (2) toxins—benzene and alcohol; (3) medications—chloramphenicol and alkylating agents; (4) infections—hepatitis, HIV, CMV, EBV, or TB; (5) cancer infiltration—lymphoma, etc.

Essentials of diagnosis

1. History of exposure to any of the above toxins, drugs or infections, along with chronic fatigue, infection or bleeding with **pancytopenia on an initial CBC.**

2. A bone marrow biopsy is performed in uncertain cases to confirm the diagnosis, showing hypoplasia and fatty cell deposit without abnormal cells seen.

Differential diagnosis

<u>Fanconi anemia</u> **(FA):** FA is a rare inherited **bone marrow failure syndrome resulting from DNA damage** (interstrand crosslinks), **characterized by pancytopenia, predisposition to certain malignancies, and physical abnormalities** including short stature, microcephaly, developmental delay, café-au-lait skin lesions, etc. **Diagnosis is mostly made in childhood by assessment of chromosomal breakage. FA is sensitive to cytotoxic therapies**.

Treatment

1. Treat cytopenia with blood transfusions, antibiotics, and (rarely) growth factors. Watch for transfusional iron overload.

2. **Allogeneic hematopoietic cell transplantation (HCT)** should be performed whenever possible for the young and healthy patients. HCT can cure > 80% cases under 50 y/a. Major concerns include the possibility of developing a clonal disorder such as a myelodysplastic syndrome, acute myeloid leukemia, or paroxysmal nocturnal hemoglobinuria.

3. If HCT is not possible, **immunosuppressive** therapy **(IST)** can be tried. **Eltrombopag for six months plus IST** (usually anti-thymocyte globulin, cyclosporine, and prednisone) are recommended, with remission of about 60% of cases.

Hemolytic Anemias

It's an anemic state caused by decreased RBC survival from increased destruction of the cells by various causes. The destruction can be intravascular or extravascular (which is mostly inside the spleen).

Etiology

1. Chronic: SCD, paroxysmal nocturnal hemoglobinuria (PNH), and hereditary spherocytosis.

2. Acute: Drug-induced immune hemolysis, autoimmune hemolysis, and G6PD deficiency.

Essentials of diagnosis

1. Varied anemic symptoms (depending on the severity), along with fever, chills, chest pain, tachycardia, dyspnea, jaundice, and dark urine.

2. **Lab tests**: Increased LDH, indirect bilirubin, and reticulocyte count; normal or slightly elevated MCV. **Blood smear shows fragmented cells or schistocytes** (<u>Image 139</u>), and the haptoglobin may be low with intravascular hemolysis. Urine Hb and hemosiderin may be positive but not bilirubin.

Treatment

1. Mild cases do not need specific treatment except for avoidance of the offending agent. Hydration is useful to prevent renal toxicity by free Hb. Other therapies are based on causes.

2. Blood transfusion is needed for severe cases with very low HCT.

Specific Hemolytic Anemias

I. Drug-induced Immune Hemolytic Anemia

It is a blood disorder that occurs when a medicine triggers the body's immune system to attack its own red blood cells. Drugs that can cause this type of hemolytic anemia include **cephalosporins (most common), penicillins, rifampin, sulfa-drugs, quinidine, methyldopa and levodopa, levofloxacin, procainamide, phenazopyridine (pyridium), NSAIDs, thiazides, and dapsone**.

Clinical features are similar to those in the above hemolytic anemia.

II. Autoimmune Hemolytic Anemia (AIHA)

Also known as "**Warm or IgG hemolysis**", it occurs when IgG antibodies and activated C3 are developed against the patient's own RBCs causing autoimmune destruction and hemolysis. Usually it's idiopathic and **associated with an autoimmune disease (SLE, etc.), leukemia (CLL), lymphoma, viral infections, or ulcerative colitis**.

Clinical features and diagnosis: Extravascular hemolysis and splenomegaly; osmotic fragility and direct Coombs tests are positive. The **micro-Coombs test (positive)** is the most specific diagnostic test. Other results are similar to general hemolysis.

Treatment: Only severe autoimmune hemolysis requires treatment with initial steroids. Splenectomy is saved for patients unresponsive to steroids or immunosuppressants (rituximab over cytotoxic agents). In addition to steroids, IVIG, and splenectomy, immunosuppressants have been reported effective in some patients with <u>Evans syndrome</u> **(the combination of AIHA and ITP).**

III. Cold Agglutinin Hemolytic Anemia

It is a rare form of **autoimmune hemolytic anemia** due to **cold-reacting autoantibodies (IgM** mostly, and IgG) against polysaccharide antigens on the RBC surface. The autoimmune antibody production can be primary (idiopathic) or secondary (from infection, lymphoproliferative disease or cancer). Cold agglutinin destruction mainly occurs in the liver, which is not affected by steroids or splenectomy.

Clinical features and diagnosis: Symptoms of hemolytic anemia are typically triggered by coldness. Younger patients have milder symptoms. **Lab test**: Significant titers of a **cold agglutinin (IgM)** along with positive **Coombs' test** are the most specific diagnostic tests. Other results are similar to those for general hemolysis.

Differentiation—Cryoglobulinemia: The blood contains large amounts of cryoglobulins (mostly IG) that precipitate at T < 37°C and dissolve again if the blood is heated. It is not responsive to steroids, and is associated with hepatitis C, glomerulonephritis, multiple myeloma, and arthralgia.

Treatment: **Avoid coldness**. With symptoms, **rituximab** is administered +/- interferon, prednisone or fludarabine. Cytotoxic agents (chlorambucil or cyclophosphamide) can be used in severe cases.

IV. Hereditary Spherocytosis

It's an **autosomal dominant** disease characterized by **chronic, mild extra-vascular hemolytic anemia with spherocytes**, jaundice, and splenomegaly from a defect in the RBC membrane.

Etiology: The loss of spectrin and flexibility in the RBC membrane results in the sphere-RBC formation, which leads to hemolysis when the spheres pass the narrow passages in the spleen.

Essentials of diagnosis

1. **Significant family history, with moderate symptoms of anemia, splenomegaly, and jaundice**. Bilirubin stones and cholecystitis may occur. Severe anemia may be associated with folate deficiency or PVB19 infection.

2. **Lab tests**: Low HCT; elevated MCHC, LDH, indirect bilirubin, and reticulocyte count (similar to other hemolysis). Normal MCV and positive fragility test. **Negative Coombs test** is crucial to distinguish hereditary spherocytosis from autoimmune hemolysis (which is positive).

Treatment

1. Most patients require **no treatment but chronic folate replacement**, especially with erythropoietin (**EPO**) deficiency, which may lead to aplastic crisis. RBC cell transfusions should be given to those with symptomatic anemia.

2. **With severe anemia, splenectomy** will eliminate the site of the hemolysis, most symptoms, and the need for future cholecystectomy due to bilirubin gallstones. After splenectomy, spherocytes will remain, and patients will need vaccinations for Pneumococcus and Hib, and possible antibiotic prophylaxis.

V. Paroxysmal Nocturnal Hemoglobinuria (PNH)

PNH is a rare **X-linked** disease with **RBC membrane defect resulting in chronic, complement-induced intravascular hemolysis**, intermittent dark urine, and venous thrombosis. The defect in phosphatidyl inositol glycan A (**PIG-A gene**) allows increased binding of complement to RBCs and hemolysis, more susceptible in an acid environment and at night (hypoventilation). It affects more females than males. PNH is a clonal stem cell disease and thus has the potentials of developing into aplastic anemia and leukemia.

Essentials of diagnosis

1. Anemic symptoms, jaundice, morning dark urine (Hb urine) after sleep, **venous thrombosis** (especially in the hepatic vein: Budd-Chiari syndrome), and pain. **Suspect cases with confusing anemia**.

2. **Lab tests**: Above general hemolysis findings, along with brisk intra-vascular hemolysis and a low haptoglobin. Hemosiderinuria can be (+) if severe. **Flow cytometry (CD_{55}/CD_{59}) is the most specific diagnostic** test. Other specific tests include: Ham test (acidified-hemolysis) or sugar-water test (for RBC susceptibility to lysis by complement).

Treatment

1. **Eculizumab (a complement inhibitor) is the mainstay of therapy.**

2. In addition, all patients with ongoing hemolysis are recommended for RBC transfusions for severe anemia, supplemental iron for iron deficiency, and supplemental folic acid. If the urinary blood loss is severe, iron and corticosteroids are used. Chronic venous thrombosis is the main cause of death, which should be treated with anticoagulation as well as eculizumab for secondary prevention.

VI. Glucose-6-phosphate Dehydrogenase Deficiency (G6PD Deficiency)

It's the **X-linked** hereditary deficiency of the enzyme G6PD responsible for the reducing (antioxidant) capacity necessary for neutralizing oxidant stress to the RBC, which leads to impaired RBC integrity and acute nonimmune hemolysis.

Etiology: Various oxidant stresses result in sudden hemolysis. The most common cause is **infections**. The second cause is medicines (sulfa agents, primiquine, dapsone, quinidine, and nitrofurantoin).

Essentials of diagnosis

1. A normal person with a history of recent infection or drug ingestion, abruptly presents with severe hemolysis (jaundice, dark urine, weakness, tachycardia, and fever).

2. **Lab tests**: Evidence of **intra-vascular hemolysis** (high LDH, bilirubin and reticulocyte count with a normal MCV, low haptoglobin, and hemoglobinuria); **Heinz bodies** (precipitated Hb inclusions in RBC); **bite cells** seen on smear (Heinz body remover). The most **specific test is the G6PD level**, which is usually **low** after an episode of hemolysis.

Treatment

Episodes of hemolysis in patients with G6PD deficiency are mostly **self-limited**. Packed RBC transfusion may be necessary in cases of severe hemolysis and symptomatic anemia. The main treatment is to **avoid oxidant stress in the future.** IV hydration and blood transfusion are needed if the hemolysis is severe.

NEUTROPENIA (LEUKOPENIA)

It's defined as an absolute neutrophil count (ANC) **< 1800/uL in adults (<1500/uL in children).** ANC < 500/uL is severe neutropenia. ANC = 10 x WBC count in 1000s x (% PMNs + % Bands). Neutropenia can be caused by a combined etiology of decreased production, increased destruction or utilization, or sequestration to tissues. It can be **acute (< 3 months) or chronic (> 3 months); acquired or hereditary neutropenia.**

Etiology

1. **Acquired:**

(1) **Decreased production—aplastic anemia, malignancy, arsenic poisoning, radiation, bone marrow inhibits (ethanol, antibiotics), nutritional deficiencies (Vit B$_{12}$, folate, B$_1$ or copper deficiency);**

(2) **Increased destruction—autoimmune diseases (RA, SLE), chemotherapy;**

(3) **Medications—flecainide, phenytoin, indomethacin, propylthiouracil, carbimazole, chlorpromazine, trimethoprim-sulfamethoxazole, clozapine, ticlodipine;**

(4) **Others—infections, bone marrow-infiltrating diseases, metabolic diseases (hyperglycinuria, ketoacidosis, hypothyroidism, Gaucher disease, etc.), or idiopathic.**

2. **Intrinsic:** Hereditary disorders (benign congenital or familial neutropenia/leukopenia, cyclic neutropenia), Chediak-Higashi syndrome, dyskeratosis congenita, Fanconi anemia, etc.

Clinical features and diagnosis

1. **Acute neutropenia:** Increased infections and sepsis by Staph-aureus, Pseudomonas, E. coli, Klebsiella, or Proteus.

2. **Chronic and autoimmune neutropenia:** Recurrent sinusitis, gingivitis, stomatitis, and perianal infections (rather than sepsis).

3. **Diagnosis: History, P/E and CBC** are the most important basis of diagnosis. Bone marrow biopsy is needed if anemia and thrombocytopenia are co-existent. Tests of serum IG and ANA levels may be helpful with further diagnosis.

Treatment

Any fever should be treated with **broad-spectrum antibiotics** after samples are taken for culture and sensitivity tests. Suspected fungal infection should be treated with anti-fungal agents. **IVIG helps with acute disease.** Recombinant Granulocyte-colony stimulating factor 3 (G-CSF 3) can be effective in chemotherapy patients and in patients with congenital neutropenia, and help shorten the duration of neutropenia. Bone marrow transplantation is the hopeful therapy for recalcitrant cases.

COAGULOPATHY

[handwritten: Inhibitor development: immune system recognizes infused factor VIII (tx of hemophilia A) as foreign, forming antibodies that interfere w/ factor fxn.
~ ↑ bleed freq or hemorrage refractory to tx in hemophilia A pt rec. factor replacement. 25%]

Hemophilia A and B

It's an **X-linked** recessive disease with the deficiency of coagulation **factor 8 in hemophilia A and factor 9 in hemophilia B** resulting in an increased risk of deep tissue bleeding. Hemophilia A is far more common than Hemophilia B. They are only expressed in male patients. Females are carriers of the disease but do not express the disease because the diseased female would be a homozygote resulting in intrauterine fetal death.

Essentials of diagnosis

1. Mild deficiency may cause bleeding symptoms only with trauma or during surgery. More severe deficiency can result in spontaneous deep tissue bleeding, such as deep bruising, hemarthrosis, and GI, UT or CNS bleeding. *[handwritten: recurrent]*

2. **Lab tests**: Typically showing a **prolonged aPTT** (activated partial thromboplastin time) **but normal PT** (prothrombin time) **and BT** (bleeding time, indication of platelet function). "Mixing study" can determine if a factor deficiency is present. Testing of factor 8 or 9 levels determines the specific type of diseases. *[handwritten: factor VIII def]*

Treatment

1. **Mild bleeding**: Use desmopressin during bleeding and prior to surgery. **Desmopressin (DDAVP)** promotes subendothelial releasing of factor 8 and is only effective for mild **hemophilia A deficiency**.

2. **Severe bleeding**: Replace the specific factor 8 or 9.

Vitamin K Deficiency

[handwritten: celiac IBD, leafy veggies]
[handwritten left margin: biliary atresia]

Vitamin K (Vit-K) deficiency is usually due to the dietary deficiency, malabsorption (including bile duct obstruction), prolonged use of antibiotics (over-killing of colon bacteria that produce Vit-K), or intake of a vitamin K1-antagonist (coumadin), resulting in **decreased clotting factors 2, 7, 9, and 10,** and in bleeding. *[handwritten: & Protein C & S]*

[handwritten right margin: ↓ADEK, exocrine pancr insuff, cystic fibrosis → rep. pancr enzyme supp, also vit K supp, ↓ resp tract infxns = ↑ abx ⇒ more vit K def]

Essentials of diagnosis

1. Presentations include hemophilia-like bleeding—ecchymosis, petechiae, hematomas, oozing of blood at surgical or puncture sites; risk of massive uncontrolled bleeding; stomach pains; malformation of developing bones (particularly in infants). *[handwritten: typically normal, prolonged in severe Vit. K def]*

2. **Lab tests**: Both the **PT and aPTT are prolonged**, with the PT prolonged first and more severely. BT is normal. Diagnosis is confirmed by correction of the PT and PTT in **response to given Vit-K**.

Treatment

1. Mild bleeding: Treat with Vit-K and correct underlying causes.

2. Severe bleeding: Give IV infusions of fresh frozen plasma FFP along with Vit-K.

fibrinogen disorder?

Hemorrhage Caused by Liver Diseases

Any liver disease or damage that causes acute or chronic hepatic failure can lead to hemorrhage **similar to that from Vit-K deficiency**. This is due to a **decrease in most of the clotting factors made in the liver (except for factor 8 and von Willebrand factor) resulting mainly in GI tract bleeding**.

Lab tests: Similar to that of Vit-K deficiency—prolonged PT and aPTT.

Differential diagnosis

Hemorrhage from Vit-K deficiency will be improved with Vit-K supplements but **hemorrhage caused by liver diseases** will not.

Treatment

1. Treat the original disease.

2. IV administration of fresh frozen plasma (FFP) for severe bleeding (melena, etc). **FFP** is helpful because **it contains all clotting factors except platelets**.

von Willebrand Disease (vWD)

It's a genetic disease with **decreased v-W factors (vWF)** that cause a **defective ability of platelets to adhere** to the endothelial lining of vessels and an increased predisposition to **platelet-type bleeding**. The platelet aggregation is normal because it's mediated by fibrinogen.

Essentials of diagnosis

1. **Superficial** mucosal and skin bleeding such as epistaxis, petechiae, bruising, and menstrual abnormalities; worse after the use of aspirin.

2. **Lab tests**: BT is prolonged. The vWF (known as **factor 8 antigen**) is low. The platelet counts and shape are normal. PTT may be prolonged if factor 8 decreases concomitantly. The **ristocetin-induced platelet aggregation test** is the most specific diagnostic test, which demonstrates abnormal platelet binding ability.

Treatment

1. For minor bleeding or surgery, **desmopressin (DDAVP) is the best initial therapy**, which releases subendothelial stores of vWF. Additional treatment for vWD includes antifibrinolytic agents, topical hemostatic agents, estrogen, and recombinant factor VIIa.

2. **For major bleeding or surgery, factor VIII or vWF replacement is needed. Aspirin should be avoided,** and FFP is ineffective.

Disseminated Intravascular Coagulation (DIC)

P AS| 798 — *fibrinogen disorder?*

P tissue factor secretion from tumor malignancy

It's a consumptive coagulopathy with a pathological activation of coagulation from a major disease, resulting in thrombosis, hemorrhage of both platelet and clotting-factor type, microangiopathic hemolysis, marked production of fibrin degradation products (FDPs, such as d-dimers), and systemic malfunctioning. It may develop multiple organ failure and death.

P risk of arterial r venous thrombosis

DIC

Etiology

An idiopathic disorder induced by a major underlying disease. **The most common cause is sepsis.** Others include trauma, burns, pancreatitis, rhabdomyolysis, hemolysis from transfusion reactions, promyelocytic leukemia (M3 AML), adenocarcinoma, placental abruption, amniotic fluid embolism, etc. The disease can cause cellular destruction and initiate the cascade of consumption of platelets as well as clotting factors.

Essentials of diagnosis

1. Acute DIC: History of a serious disease (sepsis, AML, ABO-incompatibility, burn, or trauma), followed by bleeding, hemolysis, fever, shock, or/and renal dysfunctions. Small hemorrhage or **purpura fulminans** on the skin may be present (**Image 34**).

↑ tissue factor secretion activates coag cascade

2. Chronic DIC: History of a malignancy (especially pancreatic, gastric, ovarian, or brain cancer), followed by hemorrhagic purpura, venous or arterial thromboembolism, anemia, renal dysfunctions, etc.

3. **Lab tests:** (1) **Increased BT, PT, aPTT, D-dimers, and FDPs**; decreased platelet count and fibrinogen level. (2) **Peripheral blood smear** often shows the **schistocytes as fragmented cells (Image 139)** consistent with intra-vascular hemolysis. Chronic DIC may show milder changes in the above lab tests than acute DIC.

4. DIC is a clinical and laboratory diagnosis, based on findings of coagulopathy and/or fibrinolysis in the appropriate setting.

Differential diagnosis

Similar conditions include severe liver disease or heparin-induced thrombocytopenia, other causes of microangiopathic hemolytic anemia, TTP, etc.

Treatment

1. A major principle in the treatment of DIC is to correct the underlying cause in order to eliminate the stimulus for ongoing coagulation and thrombosis.

2. IV **FFP and platelet** transfusions are necessary for most patients with serious bleeding (platelet count < 10,000/mL). Heparin is rarely used except for patients presenting mainly with thrombosis. Patients with purpura fulminans appear to benefit from the use of protein C concentrate. Administration of antifibrinolytic agents (tranexamic acid, epsilon-aminocaproic acid, or aprotinin) is generally contraindicated.

PLATELET DISORDERS

Pathoma 32, P IAS) 397

Immune Thrombocytopenic Purpura (ITP)

It has been called "**Idiopathic thrombocytopenic purpura, immune thrombocytopenic purpura, or autoimmune thrombocytopenic purpura (AITP)**". Etiology is unclear. It's likely that idiopathic antibodies attack the platelets, resulting in platelet removal by macrophages through the spleen. ITP is

- acquired formation of autoantibodies vs. platelet surface glycoproteins => ↑ splenic clearance => inhibition of megakaryocytosis. => platelet counts < 100K, prolonged skin/mucosal bleeding, ecchymosis, & petechiae

Immune Thrombocytopenic Purpura

frequently associated with lymphoma, CLL, HIV, and autoimmune diseases. **Female** has higher prevalence than male.

Evans syndrome: It's a disorder of ITP combined with autoimmune hemolytic anemia.

1° ITP: no cause

Essentials of diagnosis   2°: HIV, HCV, SLE

1. Usually a young, healthy female presents with superficial bleeding such as epistaxis, bruising, hematuria, or dysfunctional uterine bleeding. P/E commonly finds petechiae, purpura, or ecchymoses; usually there is no splenomegaly or fever.

2. **Lab tests**: Decreased platelet counts (thrombocytopenia) and prolonged bleeding time (BT) are the major findings. Note that normal BT may not exclude ITP. Antiplatelet antibody test is highly sensitive but lowly specific. Bone marrow biopsy usually reveals abundant megakaryocytes, indicating a mechanism of peripheral platelet destruction rather than platelet production.

Differential diagnosis

Henoch–Schönlein purpura (HSP):

HSP, also known as **anaphylactoid purpura**, purpura rheumatica, is a systemic vasculitis more common in children. It is characterized by deposition of IgA immune complexes following an URI, presenting with palpable purpura (small hemorrhages, **Image 58**) and joint and abdominal pain, with or without renal involvement (hematuria or proteinuria). It usually resolves within several weeks.

Other differentiations: Excluding cancer metastasis, infection, medications, etc.

Treatment

1. **Prednisone is the initial treatment** for most patients.

2. **Rituximab or splenectomy** is for patients with continuous platelets < 20 x 10³/μL despite repeated steroid use.

3. **Thrombopoietin receptor agonists (romiplostim, eltrombopag)** are used when the above therapies are failed. IVIG or Rhogam is used with rapid effects when patient has profoundly low platelets (< 10 x10³/μL) and life-threatening bleeding. Platelet transfusions are only rarely used in life-threatening bleeding when the above treatment all fails.

Thrombotic Thrombocytopenic Purpura (TTP)

It's a syndrome of **F**ever, microangiopathic hemolytic **A**nemia, **T**hrombocytopenic, **R**enal dysfunctioning, and **N**eurologic symptoms ("**FAT RN**") without known etiology. Risk factors include OCP use, pregnancy, SLE, and infections. No anti-platelet antibody is present with TTP.

Essentials of diagnosis

1. "**FAT RN**": Fever, anemia (hemolytic), thrombocytopenic purpura or petechiae, renal dysfunction, neurological symptoms (headache, mental status change, aphasia, seizures, or hemiparesis), and splenomegaly.

TTP

2. **Lab tests**: Low levels of RBC, Hb, and platelets; high levels of indirect bilirubin, LDH, and creatinine; schistocytes; prolonged BT. Coagulation and Coombs' tests are (-).

Treatment

1. **Urgent plasma exchange**—large volume **plasmapheresis** with FFP to supply factors 2, 5, 7, 8, 10, and platelets, and remove autoimmune antibodies, extra vWF and defective enzymes. Administration of platelets alone may worsen the thrombosis.

2. **Corticosteroids**, aspirin (to inhibit platelets), and dextran are helpful. **Rituximab** may be used with severe TTP.

3. **Splenectomy** is performed if it's refractory to the above treatment.

HEMATOPOIETIC NEOPLASMS

PEARLS: According to WHO, 2016, **hematopoietic neoplasms** include lymphomas, leukemias, myelo-proliferative neoplasms, plasma cell dyscrasias, histiocytic tumors, and dendritic cell neoplasms. **Lymphoid neoplasms** include precursor B lymphoblastic leukemia/lymphomas and mature B or T cell lymphomas. **Myeloid neoplasms** include **acute myeloid leukemias** (AMLs), **myeloproliferative neoplasms** (MPNs), and **myelodysplastic syndromes** (MDS).

Leukemia (LK) is malignant proliferation of hematopoietic cells (mainly generating immature WBCs called "blasts"), and can be acute or chronic, lymphocytic or myelogenous. Leukemia is the most common form of cancer in childhood.

Several entities previously considered distinct are now grouped together under single diagnostic categories: chronic lymphocytic leukemia and small lymphocytic lymphoma; precursor B cell lymphoblastic leukemia and pre-B cell lymphoblastic lymphoma; pre-T cell lymphoblastic leukemia and pre-T cell lymphoblastic lymphoma.

Tumor lysis syndrome (TLS):

TLS is an oncologic emergency that is caused by massive tumor cell lysis and the release of large amounts of potassium, phosphate, and uric acid into the systemic circulation. Deposition of uric acid and/or calcium phosphate crystals in the renal tubules can result in acute kidney injury, which results in oliguria or anuria. TLS occurs frequently in patients with aggressive lymphomas and ALL following the initiation of cytotoxic therapy, hyperkalemia, hyperphosphatemia, and hyperuricemia. **Treatment:** Hydration (IV fluids), diuretics, urinary alkalinisation, allopurinol, and reduced phosphate intake. The best treatment is prevention based upon a disease-specific estimated risk.

LYMPHOID NEOPLASMS

Lymphoid neoplasms include **precursor B lymphoblastic leukemia/lymphomas, mature B cell neoplasms (including chronic lymphocytic leukemia or small lymphocytic lymphoma, lympho-plasmacytic lymphoma, B cell prolymphocytic leukemia, diffuse large B cell lymphoma, follicular lymphoma, mantle cell lymphoma, and hairy cell leukemia), Hodgkin lymphoma, and mature T cell or NK cell lineage lymphomas.**

Hodgkin Lymphoma (HL)

Also called Hodgkin disease, HL is a malignant transformation and proliferation of lymphocytes (mainly B cells and in lymph nodes—LN), characterized by the presence of **multinucleated Reed-Sternberg cells (Image 140)** on histology.

Etiology

Unknown; may be associated with EBV and some genetic factors. There are **two peak ages**—30's (mainly nodular sclerosing type) and 60's (mainly lymphocyte-depleted type). **Male** has higher prevalence than female.

Staging

The same for both Hodgkin and non-Hodgkin lymphoma (NHL).

Stage 1: One lymphatic group.

Stage 2: Two lymphatic groups on the same side of the diaphragm.

Stage 3: Lymphatic groups on both sides of the diaphragm, or any extra-lymphatic organ contiguous to the primary nodal site.

Stage 4: Widespread metastases involving extra-lymphatic sites (bone marrow, liver, etc.).

Essentials of diagnosis

1. **Most patients are found at stage 1-2 (local) disease. Regional adenopathy**—Pathologic mark: enlarged, rubbery, non-erythematous, **nontender LN** (mostly cervical, supraclavicular, and axillary), along with **systemic "B" symptoms**—night sweats, pruritus, weight loss, and hepatosplenomegaly. **Pel-Ebstein fever** (1-2 week alternating high fever and no fever) and **alcohol-induced LN pain** are rare but specific signs for HL.

2. **Lab tests**: Excisional LN biopsy is the first diagnostic step, mostly showing typical multinucleated **R-S cells ("Owl Eye Cells", Image 140)** and many inflammatory cells. Other lab findings include anemia, increased WBC, eosinophil, and platelet count. High LDH level indicates an adverse prognosis.

3. A CXR film, or chest/abdomen CT or MRI scan is used to determine if the disease is localized or metastasized. Staging is done to guide treatment, which is radiation or chemotherapy.

Treatment—based on stages

1. Localized disease (like Stage 1A and 2A) is treated with radiation directly toward the LN plus the next contiguous region. It's more effective with combined chemotherapy.

2. All patients with evidence of "B" symptoms and > stage 3 disease are treated with chemotherapy. The most effective combination and standard chemotherapy is **ABVD** (adriamycin/doxorubicin, bleomycin, vinblastine, and dacarbazine), which is superior to MOPP (meclorethamine, oncovin or vincristine, prednisone, and procarbazine) because of fewer adverse effects (such as secondary leukemia, aplastic anemia, permanent sterility, and peripheral neuropathy).

Classification and prognosis

1. According to WHO, Hodgkin lymphoma is currently classified into nodular lymphocyte-predominant (**NLPHL**) and classical Hodgkin lymphoma (**CHL**). The classical Hodgkin lymphoma is further divided into four subtypes: nodular sclerosing HL (the most common type), lymphocyte-rich CHL, mixed-cellularity HL, and lymphocyte-depleted HL.

2. **The lymphocyte-rich classical HL has the most favorable prognosis; the lymphocyte-depleted type has the worst**. 5-year survival rates are mostly good: 90% for stage 1-2 HL; 84% for stage 3; 65% for stage 4 HL.

Non-Hodgkin Lymphoma (NHL)

It's malignant transformations and clonal expansion of lymphocytes variously derived from B cell progenitors, T cell progenitors, mature B cells, mature T cells, or (rarely) natural killer cells, causing the accumulation of neoplastic cells in both lymph nodes (LNs) and extra-LN organs (the spleen and blood). NHL is the **most common hematopoietic**, **high-grade** neoplasm, and **much more common than HL**. Common aggressive types include **diffuse large B cell lymphoma** (#1), Burkitt lymphoma, adult T cell leukemia-lymphoma, and precursor B and T lymphoblastic leukemia/lymphoma.

Etiology

Unknown. Chromosomal translocations at t(14, 18) may be involved. It may be associated with the inactivation of tumor suppressor genes, or oncogenic viruses—EBV (Burkitt lymphoma), HTLV-1, HCV, and HIV, or H. pylori, or autoimmune disease.

Essentials of diagnosis

1. **Most patients are found at stage 3-4 disease. Diffusively enlarged, painless LNs** mostly involve extra-lymphatic sites (such as spleen, skin, stomach, lung, CNS) as well as the blood, similar to CLL. HIV (+) patients commonly have CNS lesions. **Systemic "B" symptoms** include fever, weight loss, hepatosplenomegaly, etc.

2. **Lab tests: Excisional lymph node biopsy** confirms the diagnosis, which shows monomorphic neoplastic lymphocytes. Then staging is performed (same as for the HL) for early treatment because it's easily widespread at initial diagnosis. The bone marrow (BM) biopsy is often needed for the staging. Other findings include anemia, leukocytosis, eosinophilia, and high LDH.

Treatment

1. As with HL, local disease such as **Stage 1A and Stage 2A are treated with radiation**. Most patients with advanced disease (stage 3-4) should receive combined chemotherapy with three cycles of "R-CHOP" (cyclophosphamide, doxorubicin, vincristine, and prednisone plus rituximab) followed by locoregional radiation therapy.

2. As a general strategy, low-grade symptomatic NHL is treated with a palliative approach, and high-grade disease is treated aggressively with a curative strategy. CNS lymphoma is often treated with radiation in addition to CHOP. Relapses of NHL can be controlled with bone marrow transplantation.

Acute Lymphoblastic Leukemia (ALL)

ALL (Image 141) is the most common malignancy in children [*Lymphoblasts*] with overproduction of immature lymphocytes in the bone marrow. It's more common in < 10-year children, five times more common than acute myeloid leukemia (AML). Children with certain genetic and immunodeficiency syndromes are at increased risk **These risk factors include Down syndrome, neurofibromatosis type 1, Fanconi anemia, SCID, Bloom syndrome, and ataxia telangiectasia. Prior radiation** exposure increases risk of all leukemias.

Bloom syndrome: It is a rare, autosomal recessive chromosomal instability disorder that is caused by mutations in the BLM gene. It is more often seen in E. European Jewish descendants. It is characterized by short stature, a skin rash following sun exposure, and a greatly increased risk of cancer.

Essentials of diagnosis

1. The most common symptoms are nonspecific but persistent fever, infection, bleeding, bone pain, or lymphadenopathy in children.

2. It's more often associated with infiltration of other organs. **Peripheral blood smear** shows large, uniform **lymphoblasts (>20%).** Periodic acid-Schiff stain **(PAS) is positive. Neutrophils are low while total WBCs may be high or low.** Common ALL-antigen **(CALLA)** and terminal deoxynucleotidyl transferase **(TdT)** are usually present. High WBCs may be associated with worse prognosis.

3. Clinically it's similar to AML and thus histologic diagnosis is important. By the French-American-British (FAB) classification system, ALL is further classified into **L1, L2, and L3 ALL.**

Treatment

Standard chemotherapy is daunorubicin, vincristine, prednisone, and asparaginase. **Add intrathecal methotrexate** to prevent the CNS relapse. Most children with ALL are treated on "research protocols" with improve survival rates (5-year may be >80%). Regular follow-up after the chemotherapy is needed.

Chronic Lymphocytic Leukemia (CLL)

It's a **lymphoid malignancy** with overproduction of functionally incompetent, leukemic, **well-differentiated B cells** that accumulate in the bone marrow, blood, lymph nodes, spleen, and liver. It is the **most common type of leukemia in adults and with an extremely heterogeneous course.**

Etiology

Unknown. It's more common in older men (> 60 y/a) and with some genetic trends.

Essentials of diagnosis

[*Lymphocytosis & smudge cells*]

1. Most patients present as an **asymptomatic elevation of WBC** found on routine evaluation and relatively in early stage. Many patients also have fatigue, lethargy, **infection, and enlarged lymph nodes** (80%) and spleen or liver (50%). Bone pain can be present in a later stage.

2. **Lab tests**: (1) Specific tests are **flow cytometry** demonstrating the presence of B cell antigens **CD19, CD20, and CD5** (this is usually only on T cells).

CLL

Chronic Lymphocytic Leukemia

(2) WBC (mainly B cells) mostly > 50 x $10^3/\mu L$. **Blood smear** usually reveals numerous, small, normal-appearing (mature) lymphocytes and **typical ruptured "smudge cells" (Image 143)**. Leukemic cell infiltration can cause hypo-IG, anemia, granulocytopenia, and thrombocytopenia.

3. Staging and prognosis for CLL:

Stage 0—lymphocytosis alone; stage 1—lymphadenopathy; stage 2—splenomegaly; stage 3—anemia; stage 4—thrombocytopenia.

Treatment

1. There is no significant survival benefit of treating early stage, asymptomatic CLL. Thus observation rather than immediate treatment is recommended.

2. Therapy is indicated for patients with "active disease" as manifested by advanced stage, high tumor burden, severe disease-related "B" symptoms, or repeated infections.

(1) Localized (stage 1 and 2): Involved-field radiation therapy alone is preferred.

(2) > Stage 2 CLL with symptoms should be treated with palliative chemotherapy. 1) Younger patients: fludarabine +/- rituximab +/- cyclophosphamide. 2) Older patients: chlorambucil plus a novel anti-CD20 antibody (obinutuzumab or ofatumumab); if no response, fludarabine-based regimens.

Prognosis

Although CLL is incurable, long-term survival can still be expected, which mainly depends on staging. The survival time of untreated stage 0 and stage 1 CLL is 10-12 years. The survival length of stage 3 and stage 4 diseases is 1-2 years.

Hairy Cell Leukemia (HCL)

HCL is an **uncommon chronic B cell lymphoid malignancy**. It is characterized by progressive accumulation of clonal small mature B cells **with "hairy" projections on the cell** surface in the blood, bone marrow, and spleen. It occurs mostly in the elderly and the etiology is unknown.

Essentials of diagnosis

1. Common presentations include weakness, weight loss, bruising/petechiae, abdominal pain, infection (more common with atypical mycobacteria like MAI), possible splenomegaly, but rarely with LN enlargement.

2. **Lab tests**: (1) CBC reveals **pancytopenia. Blood smear** typically shows **leukopenia with hairy cells** (mononuclear cells with abundant pale and projected cytoplasm, **Image 145**), which can be confirmed by the specific tartrate-resistant acid phosphatase (**TRAP**) staining.

(2) **Bone marrow biopsy** confirms well-differentiated B-cell infiltration with hairy cells.

Treatment

Many patients with HCL are asymptomatic and can be observed for months and occasionally years after diagnosis.

Hairy Cell Leukemia

1. Indications for treatment:

(1) Significant pancytopenias: neutrophil count <1000/mL with repeated infections, symptomatic anemia with Hb <11.0 g/dL, or bleeding due to a platelet count <100,000/mL; (2) Splenomegaly or adenopathy; (3) Systemic symptoms (E.g., fever, night sweats, fatigue, and weight loss).

2. Initial therapy is a nucleoside analogue—**cladribine**, which can effectively induce remission in symptomatic patients. Splenectomy and interferon may also help. About 10% of cases remain benign even without treatment.

MYELOID NEOPLASMS

Acute Myeloid (Myelocytic) Leukemia (AML) *neutrophil - predominant*

AML is the rapid malignant proliferation of myeloid lineages (mainly abnormal WBCs) and bone marrow failure from the derangement of the pluripotent stem cell, resulting in destruction of the normal production of the entire bone marrow. AML is the most common acute leukemia affecting adults, and its incidence increases with age.

Etiology

Unknown for most cases. Well-known **risk factors** are **radiation exposure, benzene, chemo-drugs (melphalan, etoposide, etc), and retroviruses**. Genetic susceptibility includes Down syndrome and Klinefelter syndrome. Myelodysplasia and sideroblastic anemia can also develop into acute leukemia.

Essentials of diagnosis

1. Most presentations result from marked **pancytopenia**—Anemia (fatigue, dyspnea on exertion, pallor), excess bleeding (gum, nose) or bruising, and infection (due to WBC deficiency) are most common; enlarged liver, spleen and LN, and bone pain (tumor cell infiltration) are also common.

↑↑↑ myeloblasts on peripheral smear.

2. **Lab tests**: (1) CBC usually shows that **all three cell lines are suppressed**; WBC count can be low (mostly), normal or high; platelets and Hb are mostly low. (2) A **bone marrow biopsy with > 20% blasts confirms the diagnosis** of AML. (3) **Accurate diagnosis is by use of monoclonal antibody**—to determine specific types of AML. (3) **AML (Image 142)** in histology is characterized by **large myeloblasts with notched nuclei and Auer rods (bar, body)** in peripheral blood smear, with **positive TdT, myeloperoxidase (MPO),** and esterase. Increased LDH and uric acid are nonspecific changes.

3. By the **FAB system, AML is further classified into M0-M7 subtypes:**

(1) **FAB M0**—AML with minimal differentiation.

(2) **FAB M1—AML** without maturation.

(3) **FAB M2—Acute myeloblastic leukemia** with maturation: Predominant peripheral myeloblasts.

(4) **FAB M3—Acute promyelocytic leukemia:** Associated with Auer bars, granulocytosis, and DIC.

AML

(5) **FAB M4—Acute myelomonocytic leukemia:** Marked WBC increase, with 80% blasts, alpha-naphthyl esterase (+) and possible CNS involvement.

(6) **FAB M5**—Acute monoblastic and monocytic leukemia.

(7) **FAB M6—Acute erythroid/erythroblast leukemia:** Predominant erythroblasts, with irregular outline and increased nucleus:plasma ratio.

(8) **FAB M7**—Acute megakaryoblastic **leukemia**.

4. **By WHO, AML is divided into four main groups:**

(1) AML with recurrent genetic abnormalities.

(2) AML with myelodysplasia-related features.

(3) Therapy-related AML and MDS.

(4) AML, not otherwise specified.

Treatment

1. **Combined chemotherapy (daunorubicin/idarubicin plus cytarabine)** is the main initial treatment for all acute leukemias (especially when cytogenics is good) to induce a remission for further consolidation.

(1) For younger patients: Remission induction treatment is done with daunorubicin or idarubicin for 3 days and standard dose of cytarabine (Ara C) for 7-10 days. If a patient relapses after initial chemotherapy or if cytogenics is poor, consider bone marrow transplantation. Prior to the therapy, adequate hydration plus **allopurinol** should be started to prevent hyperuricemia and renal failure caused by blast lysis (**tumor lysis syndrome**). **(2) For older patients** with severe comorbidity and unfavorable risk disease, supportive care (blood transfusion, antibiotics) alone or less intensive chemotherapy rather than induction chemotherapy is suggested to reduce mortality.

2. For **M3 AML: Add** Vit-A derivative all-trans-retinoic acid (**ATRA**).

3. **Leukostasis syndrome**: It's the crisis from extremely high WBC level, and treated with **hydroxyurea along with leukapheresis** to reduce WBC rapidly.

MYELOPROLIFERATIVE NEOPLASMS (MPNs)

MPNs, previously termed the **myeloproliferative disorders**, are characterized by the **clonal proliferation of one or more hematopoietic cell lineages**, predominantly in the bone marrow, but sometimes in the liver and spleen. **In contrast to myelodysplastic syndromes** (MDS), MPNs demonstrate terminal myeloid cell expansion into the peripheral blood. **The MPNs include polycythemia vera (PV), essential thrombocythemia (ET), chronic myeloid leukemia (CML), primary myelofibrosis (PMF), chronic neutrophilic leukemia (CNL), chronic eosinophilic leukemia (CEL) or hypereosinophilic syndrome (HES),** and **mast cell disease** (systemic mastocytosis and mast cell leukemia).

Polycythemia Vera (PV)

Polycythemia is defined as abnormal elevation of hematocrit that causes erythrocytosis, also with increased WBCs and platelets. It can be caused by primary increase in RBC production or be secondary to decrease in plasma volume (hemoconcentration). **PV is a myeloproliferative neoplasm caused by clonal proliferation of pluripotent bone marrow stem cells.** It is associated **with a low serum level of erythropoietin (EPO).** PV cells have a mutation in the tyrosine kinase (JAK2), which make the cells hypersensitive to EPO.

Etiology

1. **Primary erythrocytosis**: Usually caused by hypoxia (from smoking, lung disease, or high attitude), or EPO-producing tumors or polycythemia vera.

2. **Secondary erythrocytosis**: Excessive diuresis, severe diarrhea, and burns.

Essentials of diagnosis

1. Patient usually presents with "**hyperviscosity syndrome**": Pruritus (after bath), fatigue, plethora, easy bruising/bleeding, blurred vision, neurologic signs, hepatosplenomegaly, and even CHF.

2. **Diagnosis** is based on above clinical presentations and CBC results: Elevated RBC, HCT, WBC, and platelets. **The most accurate and confirmative test is TAK2 mutation assay (accurate in 95% of patients).** EPO levels can help distinguish PCV (with **low EPO**) from other causes (with high EPO). Vit-B$_{12}$ levels are usually high (unclearly).

Treatment

1. First treat underlying cause. Supportive care includes control of severe pruritus, hyperuricemia and gout, erythromelalgia, and bleeding.
2. **Phlebotomy** is the most effective treatment to relieve most symptoms of primary erythrocytosis. Myelosuppressive agent hydroxyurea is recommended for patients with high risk of thrombosis (and leukocytosis), along with aspirin or anti-thrombotic ASA (acetylsalicylic acid).

Essential Thrombocythemia (ET)

It's an uncommon **myeloproliferative neoplasm** characterized by marked increase in megakaryocytes in the bone marrow and platelets in the blood. Similar to PV, it's associated with JAK2 gene mutations.

Essentials of diagnosis

1. Most patients are about 50-60 y/a, found with high levels of platelets without symptoms and other causes. Patients may occasionally present with signs of thrombosis or bleeding. It can be difficult to be distinguished from reactive high platelets from iron deficiency, infection, or cancer.

2. **Lab tests**: Elevated platelet count (can be $> 2 \times 10^6/\mu L$); normal REC mass. Bone marrow smear shows increased megakaryocytes without other morphologic abnormalities.

Treatment

Oral **hydroxyurea** is the drug of choice to effectively reduce the platelets and risk of thrombosis. If RBC is suppressed, anagrelide can be added. With erythromelalgia (burning in hands/feet + erythema/pallor/cyanosis + palpable pulses), aspirin is added with better effects.

Primary Myelofibrosis (PMF)

It's an uncommon **myeloproliferative neoplasm** characterized by ineffective erythropoiesis and the deposition of fibrous connective tissue (fibrosis) of the bone marrow, leukoerythroblastic and teardrop poikilocytosis in peripheral blood smear, and marked splenomegaly. It's also associated with JAK_2 gene mutations.

The related MPNs essential thrombocythemia (ET) and polycythemia vera (PV) can both undergo delayed disease transformation into a fibrotic state with similar manifestations called **post-ET myelofibrosis or post-PV myelofibrosis**, respectively.

Essentials of diagnosis

1. **Anemic presentations** (pallor, weakness); **marked splenomegaly**; early satiety; **hypercatabolic** symptoms (severe fatigue, low-grade fever, night sweats, and weight loss).

2. **Lab tests**: Leukoerythroblastic and **teardrop poikilocytosis** in peripheral blood smear; giant, **abnormal platelets**; variable WBC counts; **nucleated RBC**; hypercellular bone marrow with reticulin or collagen **fibrosis**; bone marrow usually cannot be aspirated ("**dry tap**").

Treatment

1. Mild cases may only need symptomatic treatment and occasional transfusion support.

2. Low-risk disease: Hydroxyurea; high-risk disease: JAK2 inhibitor ruxolitinib. Lenalidomide or thalidomide as mainly for multiple myeloma may improve symptoms with acceptable toxicity. Erythropoietin may help with anemia.

3. Allogeneic hematopoietic cell transplantation (HCT) is the only therapy with a curative potential in PMF. However, most patients will not be candidates for HCT and will only get palliative care.

Chronic Myeloid Leukemia (CML)

It's a chronic **myeloproliferative neoplasm** characterized by the **massive overproduction of myeloid cells**. These cells retain most of their function until later in the course of the disease.

Etiology

Unknown. Philadelphia chromosome translocation **t(9, 22)** is a known feature, resulting in a gene producing an enzyme with **tyrosine kinase** activity. It is a clonal disease of myelocytes.

Essentials of diagnosis

CML

1. Mostly a middle-aged patient presents with fatigue, **night sweats, pruritus** after bath, and low-grade fever. Later, abdominal pain (from **splenomegaly**) and bone pain (from WBC infiltration) often occur. Infection, bleeding or enlarged lymph nodes (LN) are uncommon. A rare leukostasis reaction may occur with extremely high WBC (20-50 x 10^3/μL), resulting in vascular clots, dyspnea, blurry vision, priapism, thrombosis, and stroke.

2. **Lab tests**: Demonstration of the **Ph-chromosome is the most specific** test (> 90%), which is **BCR-ABL** assay for Ph t(9, 22) translocation. Other results include **marked elevation of WBC,** mostly neutrophils with a left shift and with rare blasts. Basophils, platelets, LDH, uric acid and B12 are high and the **WBC-AKP is low. Bone marrow biopsy usually shows small megakaryocytes with hypolobulated nuclei ("dwarf megakaryocytes"; <u>Image 144</u>).**

Differential diagnosis

<u>Leukemoid reactions:</u> A benign WBC disorder; may be a pre-leukemia state, or secondary to an infection or leukemia; **no Ph t(9, 22).** Patient presents with fever, infection, **marked increase in AKP, leukocytosis** with granules of precursors and "left shift", promyelocytes, and myelocytes. **Treatment is leukapheresis** to remove excessive WBC immediately.

Treatment

1. **Chronic:** A BCR-ABL **tyrosine kinase inhibitor (TKI)** —imatinib, dasatinib, or nilotinib—**is the best initial therapy** to improve CML outcome. The **second-generation TKIs nilotinib and dasatinib** have shown better effects in early treatment of CML. Hydroxyurea may be added for recalcitrant cases.

2. If the patient does not respond well or patient is < 60 y/a and with a matched sibling donor, BM-transplantation is attempted early for a cure (60%) and to prevent it from converting to acute leukemia.

3. Acute blast: Treat as for acute leukemia, plus dasatinib.

4. Other therapies: alpha-interferon helps eliminate the Ph-chromosome. If no response, hydroxyurea is used to reduce WBC and treat leukostasis syndrome.

Chronic Neutrophilic Leukemia (CNL)

CNL is a rare **myeloproliferative neoplasm** characterized by **mature granulocytic proliferation** in the blood and marrow, and infiltration into the organs resulting in hepatosplenomegaly. There is usually toxic granulation in the neutrophils, nuclear hypersegmentation and an increased leukocyte alkaline phosphatase (**LAP**) score. The pathology is associated with point mutations in the CSF3R gene. The Ph chromosome and its products are mostly not detected in patients with CNL. Although these patients do not usually progress to AML, their **survival is short and usually less than two years.**

Essentials of diagnosis

1. The most common clinical finding is **hepatosplenomegaly**. Pruritus, gout, and mucocutaneous bleeding are occasionally seen.

2. Lab tests: Peripheral blood neutrophilia (absolute neutrophil counts ANC >7700/μL with a total WBC <11,000/μL) with myeloid precursors (promyelocytes, myelocytes) comprising < 5% of leukocytes. Bone marrow biopsy will show a hypercellular marrow with an increased myeloid:erythroid ratio of 20:1 or greater. Myelocytes and neutrophils are increased, and blasts and promyelocytes are not increased.

Differentiation

Neutrophilic leukocytosis is commonly seen in infection, stress, smoking, pregnancy, and following exercise. It can also occur in the polycythemia vera and chronic myeloid leukemia.

Treatment

Similar to CML. Effective treatment is uncertain. Some patients may respond to interferon and the JAK1/2 inhibitor ruxolitinib.

Chronic Eosinophilic Leukemia (CEL) or Hypereosinophilic Syndrome (HES)

CEL or HES is a rare **myeloproliferative neoplasm** characterized by **primary hypereosinophilia, anemia, thrombocytopenia,** hepatomegaly, and splenomegaly due to eosinophilic infiltration and mediator release causing damage to multiple organs. It is often associated with mutations that activate the tyrosine kinase activity of either the PDGFR-alpha or PDGFR-beta receptor. Eosinophilic myocarditis is a major cause of morbidity and mortality among patients with HES.

Essentials of diagnosis

Various history and P/E findings along with CBC and differentiation (including CSF analysis).

1. Clinical presentations vary and may include fever, fatigue, cough, myalgias, pruritis, diarrhea, hepatomegaly, splenomegaly, **hypereosinophilia, anemia, and thrombocytopenia.**

Hypereosinophilia is defined as the eosinophil count in the peripheral blood exceeding 1.5×10^9/L (1500/μL, or evidence of extensive tissue infiltration by eosinophils and/or marked deposition of eosinophil granule proteins.

2. Some patients have no symptoms and are found out accidentally during a routine blood test.

Classification and differentiation

1. **Acute eosinophilic leukemia (AEL):** marked increase in the immature eosinophil counts in the blood and/or bone marrow with its infiltration of tissues; > 10% blast forms in the bone marrow; a clinical course similar to other acute leukemias, with pronounced anemia, thrombocytopenia, and susceptibility to infection. Cardiac and neurologic complications may develop.

2. **Secondary eosinophilia:** an IL-5 reactive phenomenon caused by allergic disorders (more common in developed countries, with coexistent IgE elevation, including drug reactions, asthma, hay fever, urticaria, aspergillosis, pemphigus, and dermatitis herpetiformis), parasitic/fungal infections (more common in developing countries), vasculitis and collagen diseases (angioedema with eosinophilia, Loeffler syndrome, Churg-Strauss syndrome, and eosinophilic granuloma), and lymphoid neoplasms, etc.

3. **Hereditary (familial) eosinophilia**: an autosomal dominant disorder with stable eosinophilia and benign clinical course.

4. **Eosinophilia-myalgia syndrome**: an incurable syndrome with flu-like myalgias, neurological symptoms and eosinophilia after ingestion of poorly produced L-tryptophan supplements.

Treatment

1. **Imatinib** is the initial therapy for most CEL and AEL patients with myeloproliferative features. Otherwise, for cases without myeloproliferative features, **corticosteroids** are used. Recurrent cases are treated with **hydroxyurea** +/- interferon-alpha, etc.

2. For secondary diseases: Treat underlying cause—such as a parasitic/fungal infection, allergic disorder, or neoplastic disease.

MYELODYSPLASTIC SYNDROMES (MDS)

These are a group of acquired, **heterogeneous, malignant**, clonal disorders of the hematopoietic stem cells. MDS are usually idiopathic and characterized by **peripheral cytopenias, a hypercellular marrow, and some morphologic and cytogenic abnormalities in two or more hematopoietic cell lines**. MDS can also be late results of cytotoxic chemotherapy and may evolve into AML, and thus were called "preleukemia". **They include "refractory anemia, refractory anemia with excess blasts, chromosome 5q (deletion) syndrome, and chronic myelomonocytic leukemia."**

Essentials of Diagnosis

1. Patients are usually over 60 y/a and diagnosed by **abnormal lab tests without symptoms**. Some may have anemic symptoms (pallor, weakness), fever, infection, or bleeding.

2. MDS must be distinguished from other entities that may also present with cytopenias and/or dysplasia. Common conditions that present with features similar to MDS include HIV infection, deficiencies of vitamin B_{12}, folate, or copper, and zinc excess.

3. **Lab tests**: Peripheral blood—markedly low RBC; normal or increased MCV; neutropenia. BM smear—hypercellular, erythroid hyperplasia with megaloblastic, multinucleated features; ringed sideroblasts; abnormal granules.

Treatment

1. Patient needs immediate supportive care. **Erythropoietin** is helpful with refractory anemia; **lenalidomide** is helpful with transfusion-dependent anemia. **Azacitidine or decitabine** is the drug of choice to alleviate myelodysplasia and improve survival for patients with a low IPSS-R score (<3).

2. **Prognosis**: Unless bone marrow transfusion is attempted for a cure, myelodysplasia is eventually **fatal**.

Special Neoplasm-Associated Disorders

Some disorders have special connections with certain neoplasms, summarized below.

PEARLS——Table 6-2: Special Neoplasm-associated Disorders

Disorder	Neoplasm
Actinic keratosis (**Image 59**)	SCC of the skin
Acanthosis nigricans (**Image 63**) (Hyperpigment and thickening of skin)	Elder: Visceral cancers (stomach, lung, breast, uterus); Young: diabetes
Autoimmune disease (Hashimoto thyroiditis, Myasthenia gravis)	Thymomas (benign and malignant)
AIDS	Aggressive lymphomas (Non-Hodgkin), Kaposi sarcoma
Barrett's esophagus (Chronic GI reflux)	Esophageal adenocarcinoma (AdC)
Chronic atrophic gastritis/pernicious anemia	Gastric AdC
Cirrhosis (alcoholic, hepatitis B or C)	Hepatic carcinoma
Down syndrome	ALL ("ALL—DOWN")
Dysplastic nevus (**Image 61**)	Malignant melanoma
Immunodeficiencies	Malignant lymphomas, ALL
Paget disease of the bone	Secondary osteosarcoma and fibrosarcoma
Plummer-Vinson syndrome	SCC of the esophagus
Ulcerative colitis	Colonic AdC
Tuberous sclerosis	Astrocytoma, cardiac rhabdomyomas, renal cell carcinoma (RCC)
Xeroderma pigmentosum (**Image 55**)	SCC and BCC of the skin

PLASMA CELL DISORDERS

Multiple Myeloma (MM)

It's a rare clonal, malignant proliferation of plasma cells at varying stages to replace the bone marrow, resulting in excessive production of large quantities of **functionless monoclonal IG**. It mostly affects the elderly, with various systemic involvements such as bone, kidney, and infection. The etiology is unknown. **Risk factors** include radiation, monoclonal gammopathy of undetermined significance (MGUS), and certain chemicals (pesticides, petroleum, etc.).

Essentials of diagnosis

1. Most patients are > 60 y/a, with **bone pain** as the commonest symptom (back and ribs, secondary to pathologic fracture). Other symptoms include **infection** (especially **Pneumococcus and Hib), anemia** (weakness and pallor), **renal failure**, and **hyper-Ca** (polyuria, polydipsia, and altered mental status).

2. **Lab tests**: (1) Blood protein electrophoresis shows markedly elevated monoclonal **M proteins** (**IgG** most, then IgA, IgD).

(2) Typical **hyper-Ca** (> 13 mg/dL), **Bence-Jones protein** (urine), and **increased BUN, creatinine, and urine acid**.

(3) **Bone marrow biopsy with > 10% plasma cells confirms the diagnosis**.

(4) Others: **Lytic bone lesions** (X-rays); normocytic anemia.

Differential diagnosis

MM should be distinguished from patients with monoclonal gammopathy of undetermined significance (MGUS) and smoldering multiple myeloma (SMM) who do not need therapy.

Other diseases with increased M-proteins: MGUS, Waldenstrom macroglobulinemia, amyloidosis, CLL, and lymphoma.

Treatment

1. Most patients are treated initially with combined chemotherapy of **VRd: bortezomib, lenalidomide, and low-dose dexamethasone**. Melphalan is for the elderly who cannot tolerate adverse effects.

2. Because myeloma cells tend to be resistant to the chemicals by an MDR gene, autologous **HCT** should be prepared for early curative attempt, especially for younger patients.

Monoclonal Gammopathy of Undetermined Significance (MGUS)

It's a condition with the excessive production of particular IGs **(IgG, IgM) by plasma cells without the systemic manifestations of myeloma**, such as bone lesions, renal failure, anemia, and hypercalcemia. It's the #1 monoclonal gammopathy (60%), with 1-3% prevalence in the elderly. Etiology is unknown.

Essentials of diagnosis

1. Most patients are asymptomatic and found out on random blood testing: elevated serum total proteins and IG levels (lower than those in myeloma); M-spike in protein electrophoresis.

2. No abnormal Ca, BUN, Hb, or lytic bone lesions. Bone marrow biopsy shows < 5% plasma cells.

Treatment

Treatment is neither necessary nor effective. About 1% of cases transform into myeloma. More M-spike IG indicates more risk.

Waldenstrom Macroglobulinemia

It's a malignant B-lymphocyte (pre-plasma) and plasma cell disorder that results in monoclonal IgM gammopathy, characterized by increased IgM, hyperviscosity syndrome, abnormal coagulation, cryoglobulinemia, amyloidosis, and cold agglutinin disease (with hemolytic anemia). The disease is also referred to as lymphoplasmacytic lymphoma with IgM gammopathy. It's a chronic, indolent disease of the elderly with potential turnover from MGUS.

Essentials of diagnosis

1. Fatigue and weight loss followed by **Raynaud** phenomenon (from cryoglobulinemia), engorged blood vessels in the eye, **mucosal bleeding**, and even **hyperviscosity syndrome** (thrombosis, pulmonary edema, blurred vision, sensational and mental changes, stupor, and coma). Multi-organ enlargement and dysfunction can also be present.

2. **Lab tests**: (1) Serum or urine protein electrophoresis typically shows **elevated IgM**.

(2) Bone marrow biopsy and aspiration confirm the diagnosis, revealing small numbers of abnormal plasma cells with Dutcher bodies (PAS-positive IgM around the nucleus).

(3) Others: Increased LDH, uric acid, AKP, and ESR. Lytic bone lesion is absent in X-ray.

Treatment

1. Many patients are asymptomatic for months or years without the need of treatment.

2. Symptomatic patients are usually treated initially with **rituximab** (Anti-CD$_{20}$). Dexamethasone and cyclophosphamide may be added for advanced disease and underlying malignancy—lymphoma. Emergent **plasmapheresis** is used to remove excessive IG in case of hyperviscosity syndrome.

Cryoglobulinemia

It's a condition that the blood contains large amounts of cryoglobulins—mostly IG proteins that become insoluble at reduced temperatures. Cryoglobulins typically precipitate at temperatures below normal body temperature (37°C) and will dissolve again if the blood is heated. It is often associated with disorders with blood cell dyscrasia such as chronic hepatitis C (most commonly), endocarditis, some autoimmune disorders (SLE, RA, Sjogren syndrome), multiple myeloma, etc. It's grouped into three subtypes.

Essentials of diagnosis

1. Clinical manifestations include joint pain, glomerulonephritis (edema, hypertension, proteinuria), purpuric skin lesions, and neurologic signs.

2. Lab tests: RF (+) and cold precipitable immune complex (+).

Differentiation

Cold agglutinin disease:

It's associated with EBV, Mycoplasma infections, lymphoma, etc; mainly cause **agglutination of RBCs and hemolytic anemia**. **Treat with warmness, rituximab**, and cyclophosphamide or cyclosporine.

Treatment

Treat underlying cause, especially **hepatitis C** (with interferon and ribavirin) and occasionally hepatitis B. Immunosuppressive therapy usually combines a short course of **glucocorticoids with rituximab** or cyclophosphamide and, in some patients, plasmapheresis.

Amyloidosis

Amyloidosis is an uncommon disorder where a protein abnormally deposits in tissue resulting in organ dysfunction and ultimate organ failure. There are 2-4 categories of amyloidosis:

1. **Systemic (Primary)**—IG light chain (AL) amyloidosis, most common in developing countries.

2. **Secondary**—serum protein A amyloidosis, produced in inflammatory conditions (AA), most common in developed countries.

3. **Hereditary**—transthyretin (TTR) type; senile amyloid (atrial natriuretic peptide).

4. **Renal failure type**—beta2-microglobulin, not filtered out by dialysis membranes (A-beta2-M).

Essentials of diagnosis

— Cerebral Amyloid Angiopathy

1. Localized amyloidosis: Local organ dysfunctions—hoarseness, proptosis, visual disturbances, etc.

2. Systemic amyloidosis: Usually unexplained heart failure (infiltrative or restrictive cardiomyopathy), nephrotic syndrome, hepatic dysfunction, malabsorption, weight loss, autonomic insufficiency, carpal tunnel syndrome (bilateral), and peripheral neuropathy. Other presentations include enlarged tongue, waxy or rough plaques on skin, dyspnea, etc.

3. **Lab tests**: Tissue biopsy confirms diagnosis by demonstrating pink deposition (H&E stain, Congo red amyloid protein). In primary amyloidosis, the amyloid protein is kappa or lambda IG light chain. Light chain paraprotein can be found in serum or urine testing. Abnormal results from cardiac, renal and hepatic tests are helpful.

Differential diagnosis

Multiple myeloma and MGUS: They have some overlapping manifestations with primary amyloidosis and must be distinguished. About 12% of MGUS will convert to primary amyloidosis.

Treatment

Similar therapies as for multiple myeloma may be needed. Patients eligible for HCT should be treated with high-dose **melphalan followed by hematopoietic stem cell** rescue rather than chemotherapy. It should aim at the underlying infection in AA amyloidosis, at the underlying plasma cell dyscrasia in AL amyloidosis, at renal transplantation in dialysis-related amyloidosis, and at liver transplantation in certain hereditary amyloidosis.

Prognosis: There is **no cure** for primary amyloidosis presently. Treatment can only slow progress.

IMMUNOLOGIC DISEASES

ALLERGIC DISEASES

Hypersensitivity Reactions

It's defined as an inappropriate and excessive immune reaction to an allergen (as pollen, dust, animal hair, certain foods, chemicals, and proteins). The severity ranges from mild allergy to severe systemic reactions leading to anaphylactic shock. There are four types of them summarized below.

Table 6-3: Summary of Hypersensitivity Reactions

Type I   IgE-mediated (immediate) hypersensitivity
With inherited tendency; antigen (Ag) reacts with IgE on mast cells and basophils, causing the release of vasoactive and muscle-active substances (histamine, etc.). The reaction develops rapidly after antigen exposure due to preformed antibodies (Ab) and results in itchy rashes, throat swelling, and low BP. Two clinical subgroups: (1) Atopy: **"Atopic triad" —asthma, eczema, and hay fever**; others including allergic rhinitis, atopic dermatitis, and allergic gastroenteropathy. (2) **Anaphylaxis**: induced by certain drugs, foods, latex, or insect bites; causing potentially fatal (a) hypotension/shock, (b) bronchospasm, (c) GI-uterine muscle contraction, (d) urticaria or angioedema.
Type II   Cytotoxic (Antibody-mediated) hypersensitivity
Antibodies (IgG, IgM) bind to antigens that are intrinsic components of cell or basement membranes, resulting in direct damage, or formation of membrane attack complex (MAC) with complement causing cell lysis or phagocytosis. Patients usually present as hemolytic anemia, thrombocytopenia, or neutropenia. E.g., **autoimmune or drug-induced hemolytic anemia, Rh disease (hemolysis), Goodpasture syndrome, rheumatic fever**, etc.
Type III   Immune complex-mediated hypersensitivity
Insoluble complement-bound aggregates of Ag + Ab complexes are deposited in vascular walls or on serosal surfaces, attracting neutrophils to release lysosomal enzymes, PGs, and kinins. Clinical features include purpura and/or petechiae, LN swelling, low complement levels and increased ESR. Examples: (1) **Serum sickness:** More often involves the heart, joint, and kidney. (2) **The Arthus reaction:** A localized subacute immune complex reaction, presenting with edema, necrosis, etc.; e.g., hypersensitivity pneumonia; thermophilic actinomycetes. (3) **Vasculitis** and others: drug-induced, immune complex **glomerulonephritis, SLE, RA, polyarteritis nodosa**, etc.
Type IV   Delayed or (T) Cell-mediated hypersensitivity
Sensitized $CD4^+$ T-cells meet Ag and release lymphokines that activate macrophages or $CD8^+$ T-cells. Activated $CD8^+$ T cells destroy target cells on contact, whereas activated macrophages produce hydrolytic enzymes and transform into multinucleated giant cells. The reaction takes 2-3 days to develop. E.g., **contact dermatitis** (poison ivy), **TB skin testing, transplant rejection, drug fever, drug-induced hypersensitivity syndrome, Stevens-Johnson syndrome and toxic epidermal necrolysis**, maculopapular (including morbilliform) eruptions, and acute generalized exanthematous pustulosis
PERALS: Drugs can induce any type of the above hypersensitivity reactions.

PRIMARY IMMUNODEFICIENCY DISORDERS

In immunodeficiency, infections are characterized by increased frequency and severity, a prolonged course, and often by unusual microorganisms.

Table 6-4: Important Immunodeficiencies

I. B Cell Deficiency (Def)
IgA Deficiency
Features: #1 common isolate IG deficiency (both IgG and IgM); usually with mild, **recurrent mucous infections, atopic diseases, and transfusion reactions** (due to anti-IgA Ab); increased risk of lymphoma and autoimmune diseases. **Dx:** Test IgA levels (may be low or normal). **Tx:** Antibiotic treatment for recurrent infections. If it fails, subcutaneous (SC) IG or IVIG may be used but it may provoke anaphylaxis.
X-linked Agammaglobulinemia (Bruton Agammaglobulinemia)
Features: 1. **Boys only**; deficiency in the X chromosome (q22) of **B cells causing most IG deficiencies**. If it's a female, autosomal-recessive pattern of inheritance should be suspected. 2. **Risk of life-threatening bacterial infections**: encapsulated Pseudomonas, Pneumococcus, Hib, etc. **Dx:** 1. Test IG levels; if low, confirm diagnosis with subsets of B cells and T-cells (B cells absent, T cells high). 2. **Tonsil, adenoids, lymph nodes (LN), and spleen may be absent.** **Tx:** Regular prophylactic antibiotics and SCIG or IVIG replacement.
Common Variable Immunodeficiency
Features: 1. **Combined B-cell and T-cell deficiencies; B cells are about normal in number but deficient in production of IG**; IgG, IgM and IgA levels drop in the 20-30s. 2. Increased or recurrent pyogenic upper and lower respiratory infections—sinusitis, otitis media, bronchitis, and pneumonia; increased risk of lymphoma and autoimmune diseases; Giardiasis, malabsorption, etc. **Dx:** Test IG levels and confirm with B-cell and T-cell subsets. **Tx:** Therapeutic antibiotics for infections and regular SCIG or IVIG for chronic maintenance.
IgG Subclass Deficiency
Features: 1. A **low IgG subclass (G1—G4)** and a deficient antibody response to that subclass, while the total blood IG levels may be normal or high. Most patients with IgG2 deficiency also have IgA deficiency, which can be a marker for general immune dysfunction. 2. Presents with frequent **sinopulmonary infections**, but the child has a normal growth pattern. **Diagnostic tests**: Quantitation of IgG subclasses. There is age-dependent variation, and thus standards should be age-appropriate. **Tx:** Antibiotics and SCIG or IVIG are used for severe infections.
II. T Cell Deficiency
Thymic Aplasia (DiGeoge syndrome)
Features: "**Poor George has no thymus**." **Mainly T-cell deficiency**. First-day **newborn tetany** due to hypo-Ca. Increased infections by viruses, fungi, and PCP. **Dx:** Absolute LC count; mitogen stimulation response; delayed hypersensitivity skin test. **Tx:** 1. IVIG and **hematopoietic cell transplantation (HCT)** to alleviate antibody deficiencies. 2. PCP prophylaxis. 3. Thymus transplantation.

III. Combined Lymphocyte Deficiency

Severe Combined Immunodeficiency (SCID)
Features: Severe deficiencies in both B cells and T cells. B-cell deficiencies cause recurrent, severe **sinopulmonary infections** (as early as 6-mo of age); T-cell deficiencies cause frequent, chronic viral, fungal or/and opportunistic infections (**varicella, candida, PCP**). **Tx:** 1. Early IVIG and **hematopoietic cell transplantation (HCT)** are widely tried as the cure. If the transplantation is not available, gene therapy may be the cure. Adenosine deaminase (ADA) deficiency may be treated with enzyme replacement therapy. 2. Fungus and PCP prophylaxis.

Ataxia-Telangiectasia
Features: 1. Autosomal recessive heredity; a syndrome of oculocutaneous telangiectasias and progressive cerebellar ataxia mostly **with IgA deficiency**. 2. Cause: Chromosome 11 DNA repair deficiency. 3. Increased risks of leukemia, non-Hodgkin lymphoma, and gastric carcinoma. **Tx:** Only alleviative; give IG if IG deficiency is severe.

Wiskott-Aldrich Syndrome
Features: 1. **X-linked, less severe B-cell and T-cell deficiencies**. 2. Low IgM and IgA, high IgE:IgA, **thrombocytopenia, bleeding, eczema,** and recurrent otitis media. 3. Increased risk of **atopic diseases**, aggressive bacterial infections (Pneumococcus, Staph-aureus, Hib), leukemia, and lymphoma. **Tx:** 1. IVIG + antibiotics for severe infections. 2. **HCT** is the only cure. Most patients die during childhood.

IV. Phagocytic Deficiency

Chronic Granulomatous Disease (CGD)
Features: 1. **2/3 cases are X-linked**; 1/3 are autosomal recessive heredity; superoxide deficiency in PMNs and macrophages. 2. Anemia, lymphadenopathy, and hyper-IG. 3. Chronic respiratory, GI, and UT infections; skin infections, granulomas, and ulcerations; Aspergillus, hepatitis, and osteomyelitis. 4. **Lab tests**: Pathogens are catalase (+); neutrophil count and assays; **NTT** (nitroblue tetrazolium test) confirms **Dx of CGD. Tx:** 1. Daily TMP-SMX for prevention. Other antibiotics for specific infections. γ–IFN decreases severe infections. 2. **HCT** and gene therapy are potential cures.

Leukocyte Adhesion Deficiency (LAD)
Features: 1. **Deficiencies in the leukocyte chemotaxis**; minimal inflammation and no pus in wounds. 2. Recurrent skin, mucosal and respiratory infections; may be with delayed umbilical cord separation and omphalitis in a newborn. 3. **Lab tests**: High WBCs in blood. **Tx: HCT** is the cure.

Chediak-Higashi Syndrome
Features: 1. Autosomal recessive; **Deficiencies in neutrophil chemotaxis; a syndrome with neutropenia, albinism, and neuropathy**. 2. Increased risk of overwhelming infections with Strep-pyogenes, Staph-aureus, and Pseudomonas-spp. **Tx: HCT** is the best Tx.

V. Complement Deficiency

C1 Esterase Deficiency (Hereditary Angioedema)

Features: 1. Autosomal dominant. 2. Recurrent angioedema provoked by stress/trauma, lasting 3 hours—3 days and can cause life-threatening airway edema. 3. **Lab tests**: Total hemolytic complement (CH50): quantity and function test. **Tx:** Purified C1 esterase and FFP are helpful before surgery.

Terminal Complement Deficiency (C5-9)

Features: 1. Deficiency in forming membrane attack complex (MAC). 2. Causing **recurrent meningococcal or gonococcal infections**. Rarely, it may cause lupus or glomerulonephritis. **Tx:** Prevention with meningococcal vaccine and specific antibiotics.

TRANSPLANTATION MEDICINE

Stem cell transplantation (**hematopoietic cell transplantation, HCT**) is a highly valuable treatment, even the only curative option, for many hematologic malignancies and non-malignant diseases. Its basis is the ability of the hematopoietic stem cell to restore the bone marrow (BM) function and formation of all blood components completely, including re-formation of the immune system. Direct BM transplantation is now more commonly replaced by using peripheral blood treated by G-CSF (filgrastim) (to get stem cells from the BM). The dose-limiting toxicity of all chemotherapy is myelosuppressive and it can be restored by transplanted stem cells. This allows both chemotherapy and new BM to work better against the disease.

There is also an increasing need of using tissue or organ transplantation in many recalcitrant or end-stage diseases, and thus it's important to understand some basic concepts in transplantation medicine. Organs that can be transplanted include the heart, kidneys, liver, lungs, pancreas, intestine, and thymus. Tissues include bones, tendons (both referred to as musculoskeletal grafts), cornea, skin, heart valves, nerves, and veins. The kidneys are the most commonly transplanted organs, followed by the liver and then the heart. The cornea and musculoskeletal grafts are the most commonly transplanted tissues, which far outnumber organ transplantation. Transplantation medicine is one of the most challenging and complex areas of modern medicine, with transplant rejection as the key problem that can be reduced through serotyping to determine the most appropriate donor-recipient match and through the use of immunosuppressant drugs.

Types of transplantation and rejection reactions

1. Autologous (Autograft)

It's the transplantation of an organ or tissue to the same person. No rejection reaction occurs under this condition. Examples include skin grafts, vein extraction for CABG, stem cell autograft, and storing blood in advance of surgery.

2. Syngeneic (Isograft)

It's the transplantation from a donor to a genetically identical recipient, or between identical twins. **Rejection reaction** is very rare and only due to prior host sensitization (preformed antibodies).

3. Allogeneic

It's the transplantation of an organ or tissue between two genetically non-identical members of the same species. Prerequisite conditions are ABO and HLA matching the donor and recipient. Three types of rejection reactions can occur even with antigenic matching and immunosuppressants: hyperacute (within minutes, with preformed antibodies), acute (days—months), and chronic (months—years).

4. Graft-versus-host disease (GVHD)

It's a condition specific to allogeneic bone marrow transplantation, in which donated T-cells attack host tissues. It may be caused by minor histocompatibility antigens. It can occur as acute (within 3 months) or chronic (> 3 months). Common presentations are skin changes, GI symptoms, cholestatic liver dysfunction, and obstructive lung disease. It's usually treated with high-dose steroids.

Graft-versus-leukemia effect: It's a variant of GVHD. It is found that leukemia patients treated with allogeneic bone marrow transplantation have much lower relapse rates than those treated with autologous transplantation. This may be explained by a reaction of donated T-cells against leukemic cells.

5. Xenograft and xenotransplantation

It's the transplantation of organs or tissues from one species to another. An example is porcine heart valve transplant, which is quite common and successful now. However, xenotransplantation is generally considered dangerous because of the increased risk of non-compatibility, rejection, and disease carried in the tissue.

Chapter 6: High-yield Questions (HYQ)

1. A 30 y/o Asian woman has a 6-month history of fatigue, skin ulcers, bilirubin gallstones, and recurrent pneumonia. She's been a strict vegetarian for the past 3 months. Last week, she had fever, cough with sputum, and chest pain again and was started on antibiotics. Physical examination (P/E) finds a pale face, moderate fever, tachypnea, tachycardia, and normal (Nl) BP. Lab test results: sickled RBC, normal MCV, reticulocytes, and WBC counts; elevated LDH and bilirubin; hematocrit (HCT) = 30% (HCT was 45% a week ago). What's the most likely cause of the low HCT?

A. Acute hemolysis

B. Acute aplasia

C. G6PD deficiency

D. Vitamin B$_{12}$ deficiency

E. Infection

2. A 60 y/o man complains of lower limb pain and easy bruising for the past 3 days. The pain is not relieved by rest. He has 4-5 years of history of smoking, hyperlipidemia, and vasculitis and was on heparin for DVT prophylaxis 2 weeks ago. P/E finds stable vital signs and multiple bruises on the lower limbs. Lab tests reveal normal RBC and WBC; platelets = 50 x 10^3/uL, aPTT (activated partial thromboplastin time) = 30 sec, PT (prothrombin time) = 20 sec, BT (bleeding time) = 8 min, and LDL = 200 mg/dL. The best next step is to

A. start warfarin

B. start lovastatin

C. start lepirudin

D. stop heparin

E. infuse platelets

3. A 30 y/o female comes to you for a bruise on the right ankle. She had mild trauma to the ankle yesterday. She has had three spontaneous abortions in the past year. P/E shows normal vital signs and a swollen bruise with tenderness on the right ankle. Blood tests reveal normal BT, PT, and aPTT. What's the most likely clotting deficiency?

A. Factor 7

B. Factor 8

C. Factor 13

D. Platelet

E. Lupus anti-coagulant

4. A 60 y/o female is brought to you for fever, weakness, and right foot pain following an ankle injury a week ago. She denies history of chronic disease. P/E results are: T = 39.5°C, HR = 100/min, normal BP; swollen right ankle with tenderness at extending to nearby bone. Lab test results: ESR = 120, WBC = 25 x 10^3/uL, with granules and "left shift"; multiple promyelocytes on the blood smear, and markedly increased AKP. Ph-chromosome report is (-). What's the most appropriate next step for early diagnosis (Dx) and treatment (Tx)?

A. Tech^{99} scan

B. Bone marrow biopsy

C. Blood samples for culture and sensitivity

D. Diagnostic antibiotics

E. Diagnostic hydroxyurea and leukapheresis

5-12: Match the following clinical scenarios with the most likely cause or diagnosis.

A. Iron deficiency

B. Intrinsic factor deficiency

C. Autoimmune IgM antibody (Ab)

D. Chronic disease

E. Hb synthesis deficiency

F. 2 α-gene deletions

G. 1 β-gene deletion

H. 1 α-gene deletion

I. G6PD deficiency

J. RBC sickling

K. Aplastic anemia

L. Autoimmune IgG antibody

M. X-linked deficiency with RBC membrane

N. Autosomal dominant deficiency with RBC membrane

5. A 60 y/o man presents with recurrent URIs, weight loss, multiple lymph node (LN) enlargements without tenderness, and hepatosplenomegaly. Blood tests reveal WBC = 70 x 10^3/uL with predominant LC and multiple "smudge cells". LDH, bilirubin, and reticulocytes are increased. HCT is low; MCHC% is high. Coombs' test is (+).

6. A 50 y/o female presents with progressive fatigue, stomach discomfort, irritability; decreased appetite, position sense, urination sense, vision, and memory for the past year. Her diet is regular. Lab tests: MCV = 110%, HCHb = 40g/dL, platelets = 10 x 10^3/uL, with predominant macro-oval RBCs and many hypersegmented WBCs. The reticulocyte count is reduced.

7. A 40 y/o female presents with fatigue and decreased appetite for the past 3 months. P/E results are unremarkable except for pale skin and mucosa. Lab tests reveal normal (Nl) WBC and platelets; Hb = 10 g/dL, MCV = 75 fL/cell, HCH = 19 pg/cell, TIBC = 400, and decreased reticulocyte count.

8. A 60 y/o man presents with 3-month of fatigue, weight loss, and lymph node enlargements diagnosed as "lymphoma". He has skin yellowing for the past 3 days and his symptoms change with the weather. Lab tests: MCV = 90 fL/cell, HCH = 20 pg/cell; LDH, bilirubin, and reticulocytes are all increased; HCT is low; Coombs' test is (+).

9. A 20 y/o man presents with 3-month of progressive fatigue and weakness. P/E finds a pale, weak man. Blood tests: normal WBC and platelet counts; normal levels of ferritin and HCHb; decreased HCT, MCV, and TIBC; multiple target cells. Hb-electrophoresis is normal.

10. A 30 y/o man has a 3-month history of periodic jaundice, fatigue, and RUQ pain. His uncle has a similar history. Ultrasound shows gallstones. Lab tests: normal WBC counts, MCV, LDH, and haptoglobin; decreased Hb and HCT; elevated MCHC, indirect bilirubin, and reticulocyte count; fragility test is (+) and Coombs test is (-).

11. A 30 y/o man takes a long nap after a 2-hour swimming. When he wakes up, he has weakness, yellowing skin, dark urine, and persistent left foot pain. P/E finds a cold, pale left foot with tenderness. Lab tests: normal WBC and MCV; decreased HCT, Hb, haptoglobin, and CD_{59}; elevated indirect bilirubin and reticulocyte count; fragility test is (+) and Coombs test is (-).

12. A 30 y/o Asian female presents with fatigability after exertion. She is otherwise feeling well. Blood tests reveal Hb = 10.5 g/dL, HCT = 35%, and MCV = 75%. Hb-electrophoresis shows $\alpha 2\beta 2$ globins.

13-17: Match the following clinical scenarios with the best initial treatment.

A. Vitamin K	B. Desmopressin	C. Clotting factor 8 and 9
D. IV platelets	E. Fresh frozen plasma (FFP)	F. FFP + platelets
G. vWF	H. Prednisone	I. Splenectomy
J. IVIG	K. Aspirin	L. Plasmapheresis
M. Heparin	N. Blood transfusion	

13. A 25 y/o female presents with epistaxis, easy bruising, and dysfunctional uterine bleeding for the past month. P/E finds multiple superficial petechiae and purpura; other results are normal. Lab tests reveal Hb = 10 g/dL, platelets = 50 x 10^3/uL; BT = 8.5 min; PT and aPTT are normal; antiplatelet antibody is (+) and Coombs' test is (-).

14. A 40 y/o female presents with fever, headache, and dry cough followed by weakness, confusion, and yellowing skin with purpura for the past 3 days. P/E finds moderate fever, tachycardia, jaundice, multiple superficial

petechiae, and splenomegaly. Lab test results: Hb = 9 g/dL, platelets = 40 x 10^3/uL; increased indirect bilirubin, creatinine, and BT; PT and aPTT are normal. Antiplatelet antibody and Coombs' tests are both (-).

15. A 10 y/o boy presents with easy bruising and joint swelling after a mild injury for the past month. His uncle and he himself both have history of periodic diarrhea and fatigue. Lab results: CBC is normal; PT and aPTT are prolonged; BT is normal.

16. An 18 y/o girl presents with easy epistaxis, petechiae, and prolonged menstruation for the past 3 months. She is otherwise fine. She says that her aunt has a similar history in the past. Lab results: CBC, platelet count, PT, and aPTT are normal; BT is 8 min.

17. A 30 y/o man presents with progressive fatigue, bone pain, confusion, and easy bleeding from his gums and nose for the past 2 weeks. P/E finds moderate fever, tachycardia, hypotension, petechiae, and an enlarged liver, spleen, and lymph nodes. Blood tests reveal pancytopenia, with predominant promyelocytes with granules and special bars. His BT, PT, aPTT, and d-dimers are all elevated.

18-25: Match the following clinical scenarios with the most likely diagnosis.

A. Hodgkin lymphoma (HL) stage 2	B. HL stage 3	C. Non-Hodgkin lymphoma (NHL)
D. CML	E. CLL	F. AML M3
G. AML M4-5	H. AML M6	I. Hairy cell leukemia
J. ALL	K. Leukemoid reaction	L. Multiple myeloma (MM)
M. Polycythemia	N. Waldenstrom macroglobulinemia (WM)	
O. Monoclonal gammopathy of undetermined significance (MGUS)		P. Aplastic anemia

18. A 30 y/o man presents with fatigue, night sweats, abdominal distension, and several painless masses around the neck for the past 2 months. P/E finds fever, weight loss, hepatosplenomegaly, and multiple enlarged lymph nodes on both sides of the neck without tenderness. Blood tests show anemia, high LDH, and WBC of 30 x 10^3/uL with predominant small lymphocytes (LC). CT reveals additional enlarged lymph nodes in the abdomen.

19. A 30 y/o man presents with fatigue, night sweats, pruritus, abdominal distension, and several painless masses around the neck for the past 2 months. P/E finds mild weight loss and multiple enlarged lymph nodes on both sides of the neck without tenderness. Blood tests reveal anemia, high LDH, and WBC of 30 x 10^3/uL with predominant small lymphocytes. CT result is consistent with that of P/E. Lymph node biopsy confirms the Dx.

20. An 8 y/o boy presents with fever, weakness, and frequent spontaneous nose bleeds over several days. P/E finds multiple enlarged lymph nodes around the neck and hepatosplenomegaly. Blood tests reveal pancytopenia, numerous lymphoblasts, and positive PAS and TdT. Bone marrow (BM) biopsy confirms the Dx.

21. A 15 y/o boy presents with weakness, fever, night sweats, reddish skin, and frequent spontaneous nose bleeds for the past week. P/E finds multiple painless, enlarged lymph nodes around the neck, and hepatosplenomegaly. Blood tests reveal elevated RBC and WBC counts, and both RBCs and WBCs show predominantly irregular outlines and increased nucleus/plasma ratio.

22. A 35 y/o man presents with progressive fatigue, night sweats, low-grade fever, bone pain, priapism, and hepatosplenomegaly for the past month. Lab results: WBC = 250 x 10^3/uL, with predominant normally-shaped

neutrophils with left shift and low AKP; basophils, platelets, LDH, uric acid and B_{12} levels are all elevated. CD_5 on T-cells is (+) but on B-cells is (-).

23. A 60 y/o man presents with progressive fatigue, pallor, petechiae, fever, bone pain, and hepatosplenomegaly for the past month. Lab results: CBC reveals pancytopenia; blood smear shows well-differentiated B cells and mononuclear cells with abundant pale and projected cytoplasm; TRAP staining is (+). BM biopsy confirms the Dx.

24. A 60 y/o man complains of periodic fatigue and muscle soreness for the past month. X-Rays show normal lungs and bone density. Lab results: Mild elevation of IG levels, total protein = 8.5 g/dL, Ca = 11 mg/dL, BUN = 18 mg/dL; M-spike is shown in protein electrophoresis. BM biopsy shows 4% plasma cells.

25. A 60 y/o man presents with progressive fatigue, cold limbs with bone pain, periodic priapism, sensational changes, and hepatosplenomegaly for the past month. X-ray shows normal lungs and bone density. Lab tests: Elevated serum protein, IG and BUN levels; M-spike in protein electrophoresis. BM biopsy: 7% abnormal plasma cells; PAS is positive.

26. A 11 y/o boy with acute lymphoblast leukemia (ALL) is treated with combined chemotherapy with daunorubicin, vincristine, prednisone, asparaginase, and methotrexate. On the third day, his serum Ca, BUN, and creatinine levels are elevated. His vital signs are stable. The most likely cause of the acute kidney injury is

A. daunorubicin   B. vincristine   C. Hyper-Ca

D. hyperuricemia   E. prednisone   F. asparaginase

G. methotrexate

27-32: Match the following clinical scenarios with the most likely diagnosis.

A. Thymic aplasia   B. IgA deficiency (Def)
C. IgG subclass deficiency   D. Ataxia-Telangiectasia
E. X-linked agammaglobulinemia (Bruton's)   F. Wiskott-Aldrich syndrome
G. Common variable immunodeficiency   H. Severe combined immunodeficiency (SCID)
I. Leukocyte adhesion deficiency (LAD)   J. Chediak-Higashi syndrome
K. Chronic granulomatous disease (CGD)   L. C_1 esterase deficiency
M. Terminal complement deficiency

27. A 3 y/o boy is brought to the physician for ear and knee pain. This is the third time this year that he has had these pains. P/E finds T = 39°C, HR = 100/min, swelling and tenderness of the left middle ear and the right knee, with erythematous rashes. Lab tests reveal (+) ANA and HLA-B_{27}, and increased WBCs.

28. A 4 y/o boy is brought to the physician for a sore throat, the third time this year that he's had this problem. P/E finds T = 39°C, HR = 100/min, swollen tonsils with pus, and a painful right knee with erythematous rashes. He also had two "common colds" in the past month. Lab tests reveal ANA (+) and low levels of lymphocytes and IG.

29. A 7 y/o boy is brought to the physician for ear pain and nose bleeding for the third time this year. P/E finds T = 39°C, HR = 100/min, swelling and tenderness of the left middle ear, and erythematous rashes on the limbs. Lab tests reveal low lymphocytes, platelets, and IgM; high IgE and IgA; and ANA (+). His uncle has a similar history.

30. A 7 y/o boy is brought to the physician for recurrent "painful red skin nodules". P/E finds pale conjunctiva and lips, several swollen lymph nodes, and multiple erythematous nodules with tenderness on the limbs. Lab tests reveal low Hb, high IG levels, and normal WBC count. Catalase and NNT are (+). His uncle has a similar history.

31. A 2 y/o boy is brought to the physician for recurrent sore throat and fever. P/E finds T = 39°C, HR = 100/min, and swollen throat with purulent exudate without tonsils seen. He was hospitalized twice for pneumonia in the past 3 months. Lab tests reveal very low levels of B cells and high levels of WBCs and T-cell subsets.

32. A 5 y/o boy is brought to the physician for recurrent sore throat and a persistent, swollen, painful lesion on the left hand, for which he had a paper cut 3 weeks ago. He had a similar sore throat and unhealed cut for the past 5 weeks. P/E finds T = 38.5°C, swollen tonsils without pus, and a swollen, tender cut without pus on the hand. WBCs including B- and T-cell subsets are increased.

Answers and Explanations

1. (B). Most likely it's SCD with acute aplasia triggered by a new respiratory infection. Both "A and C" are possible if LDH, bilirubin and reticulocytes are all elevated. It takes about 1 year for a vegetarian to develop B_{12} deficiency (Def) ('D'). 'E' may be a trigger for the symptoms but must work through "A, B, or C" to cause HCT decrease.

2. (D). This is an uncommon case of heparin-induced thrombocytopenia due to anti-platelet factor 4 complex causing decreased platelets and increased BT. The first step is to stop heparin and wait for the platelets to recover to > 100 x 10^3/uL before adding warfarin. Warfarin alone without heparin may induce limb gangrene in a patient with DVT. "C and B" should be the next step after heparin is stopped. 'E' is reserved for more severe bleeding.

3. (C). Delayed hemorrhage (bruising, recurrent spontaneous abortions) is usually caused by instability of clot due to factor 13 deficiency— deficiency of fibrin cross-linking. 'E' can cause a false aPTT increase and is one condition in the anti-phospholipid syndrome, which includes anti-phospholipid Ab (causing false positive VDRL), anti-cardiolipin Ab (causing platelet decrease), and recurrent A-V thromboses and abortions. Normal (Nl) BT, PT and aPTT exclude all other choices.

4. (A). This is most likely acute osteomyelitis with a leukemoid reaction, a benign WBC disorder similar to CML but without the Ph-chromosome and leukemic cells. Tech[99] scan is the most used tool for a fast diagnosis (Dx) of osteomyelitis, although BM biopsy is the definite diagnostic means (not always done). Antibiotics should be started after 'C'. 'E' is for treating leucostasis syndrome from leukemia.

5. (L). Most likely ALL-induced autoimmune hemolytic anemia; osmotic fragility and direct Coombs' tests (+).

6. (B). Megaloblastic anemia caused by intrinsic factor and B_{12} deficits, often from atrophic gastritis or gastrectomy.

7. (A). It is a common case of iron deficiency anemia—microcytic, hypochromic anemia. Decreased ferritin is the No.1 test used for Dx when a patient has low HCT and MCV.

8. (C). It is a form of autoimmune hemolytic anemia due to cold-reacting autoimmune Ab (IgM, IgG) against polysaccharide antigens on the RBC surface. The autoimmune Ab production can be primary or secondary.

9. (E). Sideroblastic, microcytic anemia is caused by Hb synthesis deficiency. It can be hereditary (Vit-B$_6$ Def) or acquired (alcohol, INH, lead poisoning, etc.). Fe-stain of BM RBC is the most specific test. Treat with B$_6$.

10. (N). It's hereditary spherocytosis with mild extra-vascular hemolytic anemia. Treat it with folate, EPO, or/and splenectomy.

11. (M). This is PNH with thrombosis. It differs from spherocytosis due to deficiencies in the X-linked PIG-A gene and CD$_{59}$ (No.1 specific test). Give iron and corticosteroids if severe and treat thrombosis.

12. (F). Alpha-thalassemia trait: mild microcytic anemia, HCT = 30-40%. 1 alpha–gene deletion = silent carrier; 3-gene deletions = Hb disease; 4-gene deletions—intrauterine death. Beta-thalassemia minor = 1 beta–gene deletion; beta–thalassemia major = 2 beta–gene deletions (Hb-F and Hb-A$_2$).

13. (H). ITP is an idiopathic autoimmune thrombocytopenia caused by antiplatelet Ab. Prednisone is the best initial Tx. Splenectomy is indicated when platelets are $< 20 \times 10^3$/uL despite repeated steroids. IV IG, RhoGam, or platelet transfusion is used when platelets are $< 10 \times 10^3$/uL and with life-threatening bleeding.

14. (L). TTP is best treated with plasmapheresis—plasma exchange with FFP with all clotting factors added and autoimmune antibodies (Ab), extra vWF, and defective enzymes removed. Steroids and aspirin also help, but platelets may worsen it.

15. (A). Most likely a Vit-K deficiency caused by chronic diarrhea (colitis, sprue, etc). Treat underlying disease and give Vit-K (to correct PT, aPTT). Hemophilia has similar symptoms, but would have normal PT and low aPTT.

16. (B). Most likely vWD; an abnormal ristocetin platelet aggregation test is the #1 specific diagnostic test. For minor bleeding, desmopressin is the best initial Tx to release subendothelial vWF. For serious bleeding or surgery, vWF supply is needed.

17. (F). It's a case of M3--promyelocytic leukemia complicated with DIC. The best immediate Tx is large volume of IV fluid with FFP + platelets for DIC and shock, followed by antibiotics and chemotherapy.

18. (C). NHL is a high-grade malignant expansion of B cells mainly and involves both the lymph node (LN) and extra-LN organs. LN biopsy confirms the Dx. This case is > stage 3 and treated with radiation + chemotherapy.

19. (A). HL is a malignant expansion typically of B cells and primarily involving LNs. Excisional LN biopsy confirms the Dx, which will show characteristic R-S cells, etc. This case is at an early stage and can be treated with local radiation. Higher-stage disease is usually treated with ABVD.

20. (J). An ALL with uncommonly low WBC, but with characteristic peripheral lymphoblasts, CALLA, and TdT. Clinically it's hardly distinguishable from other acute leukemias and aplastic anemia. Chemotherapy is the main treatment (Tx).

21. (H). AML M6—erythroblast leukemia, with predominant erythroblasts, showing irregular outlines and increased nuclear:plasma ratio. AML M3--promyelocytic leukemia: associated with Auer rods, granulocytes, and DIC. M$_4$ and M5—monocytic leukemia: with marked WBC increase, 80% blasts and α-naphthyl esterase (+).

22. (D). CML is usually diagnosed by the most specific test--Ph-chromosome (+). Other lab results also support the Dx. Imatinib is the best Tx. CD$_5$ (+) on B-cells (not T-cells) is a specific marker for CLL, as with CD$_{19-20}$.

23. (I). HCL is a rare malignant disease of well-differentiated B cells in the elderly, characterized by pancytopenia and mononuclear "hairy cells".

24. (O). Monoclonal gammopathy of undetermined significance (MGUS) —the over-production of IgG and IgM by plasma cells without the systemic symptoms of MM. Most patients are asymptomatic and discovered by routine or random blood testing. No Tx is needed. MM will have much higher levels of total protein, IG, Ca, and BUN, along with lytic bone lesions and serious systemic symptoms.

25. (N). WM is a malignant B cell and plasma cell disorder causing increased monoclonal IgM. Patients may have fatigue, Raynaud phenomenon, thrombosis, and neurologic symptoms. Tx is plasmapheresis along with chemotherapy.

26. (D). Acute renal insufficiency in a patient with hematologic cancer is most likely caused by hyperuricemia from tumor lysis syndrome. Daunorubicin (#1 toxicity is cardiac), vincristine, Hyper-Ca, prednisone, asparaginase, and methotrexate are all potentially nephrotoxic but may take > 5 days (and high doses) to result in renal failure.

27. (B). IgA deficiency is the #1 common immunodeficiency, associated with increased autoimmune disease and certain cancers. Most cases require antibiotic Tx. Note that most patients with IgG_2 deficiency or Ataxia-Telangiectasia also have IgA deficiency.

28. (G). Common variable immunodeficiency is characterized by combined B-cell and T-cell deficiencies, low IG levels, increased pyogenic and viral respiratory infections, and increased risk of lymphoma and autoimmune disease. Tx is IVIG along with preventive antibiotics.

29. (F). Wiskott-Aldrich syndrome is X-linked, less severe B-cell and T-cell deficiencies, with increased risk of atopic disease, aggressive bacterial infections (Pneumococcus, S. aureus, Hib), leukemia, and lymphoma. Tx is IVIG, antibiotics, and bone marrow transplants.

30. (K). Chronic granulomatous disease (CGD). 2/3 of cases are X-linked; superoxide deficiency in PMNs and macrophages; anemia, lymphadenopathy, and hyper-IG; chronic infections; (+) catalase and NTT (nitroblue tetrazolium test) confirm diagnosis. Give daily TMP-SMX for prevention.

31. (E). X-linked agammaglobulinemia (Bruton's) occurs in boys only; with B-cell and most IG deficient and life-threatening bacterial infections. T-cells may be high. Tonsil, adenoids, lymph nodes, and spleen may be absent.

32. (I). Leukocyte adhesion deficiency is characterized by deficiency in the leukocyte chemotaxis, recurrent skin, mucosal, and respiratory infections, and minimal, nonpurulent inflammation in wounds. WBC counts are normal.

Chapter 7

RENAL, UROGENITAL,

ACID-BASE AND ELECTROLYTE DISORDERS

ACID-BASE DISORDER

Common acid-base disorders are summarized in Table 7-1.

PEARLS—Table 7-1: Summary of Acid-base Disorders

Category	pH	PCO$_2$ (mmHg)	[HCO$_3$] (mEq/L)	Compensation
Metabolic Acidosis	<7.35	<35	<24	Hyperventilation; pH may be normal with coexisting respiratory alkalosis
Respiratory Acidosis	<7.35	>45	>28	Renal HCO$_3$ reabsorption
Respiratory Alkalosis	>7.45	<35	<24	Renal HCO$_3$ secretion
Metabolic Alkalosis	>7.45	>45	>28	Hypoventilation

Note: pH and PCO$_2$ (mmHg) are the two most important values to judge the acid-base disorder.

Henderson-Hasselbalch equation: pH = pKa + log {[HCO$_3$]/0.03 PCO$_2$}

P$_{CO2}$ = 1.5 [HCO$_3$] + 8 (mmHg);

P$_{CO2}$ increases (Incr) by 10, HCO$_3$ increases by 1 mEq/L (acute) or by 4 mEq/L (chronic).

P$_{CO2}$ decreases (Decr) by 10, HCO$_3$ decreases by 2 mEq/L (acute) or by 5 mEq/L (chronic).

New Reference Anion gap (AG) = [Na$^+$] - {[Cl$^-$] + [HCO$_3$]} = **3-10** mEq/L. If K$^+$ is a considered factor, it should be added with Na$^+$. **Note that hypoalbuminemia, hyperkalemia, hypercalcemia and/or hypermagnesemia may reduce the AG.**

Classification

1. Metabolic Acidosis

(1) AG acidosis (AG >10): Causes include salicylates, Fe, INH, lactic acidosis, diabetic ketosis, methanol, ethanol, paraldehyde, ethylene glycol (causing urine Ca-oxalate crystal), and uremia.

(2) Non-AG acidosis (AG is normal): Diarrhea, hyper-Cl metabolic acidosis, RTA, TPN (total parenteral nutrition), acetazolamide or spironolactone intoxication, and Addison disease. **First test is urinary AG (UAG).**

UAG = Urine [Na$^+$ + K$^+$] – Urine [Cl$^-$]; normal range: 0 to –50. A positive UAG indicates low or normal NH4 secretion. A negative UAG means increased NH4 secretion.

Treatment

(1) Increase blood volume by IV infusion of normal saline (N.S.).

(2) Treat underlying causes as listed above.

(3) Supply NaHCO3 only when pH < 7.2.

2. Respiratory Acidosis

Hypoventilation due to CVA, COPD, restrictive pulmonary disease, foreign body obstruction, narcotics/sedatives, pneumothorax, pleural effusion, flail chest, and head trauma.

Treatment

(1) Supply O2 and IV fluid and correct underlying causes.

(2) Chronic: Mechanical ventilation along with O2 supplement.

3. Metabolic Alkalosis

The most common type of acid-base disorders for in-patients.

(1) **Responsive to NaCl:** Due to vomiting, contraction alkalosis, diuretics, low blood volume, or villous adenoma. Treat with N.S. along with KCl.

(2) **Unresponsive to NaCl:** Due to primary hyperaldosteronism, Cushing syndrome, or Barter syndrome (Cl$^-$ absorption decreases, renin increases, etc.).

Treatment

(1) **Treat underlying etiology**: Cause of vomiting or gastric loss; stopping loop/thiazide diuretics or exogenous sources of alkali; correcting hypokalemia.

(2) **The most effective therapy is volume expansion with normal saline (primary Tx) plus KCl and spironolactone or acetazolamide (if severe).** IV infusion of HCl is used rarely and only with persistent metabolic alkalosis.

4. Respiratory Alkalosis

Hyperventilation due to anxiety, pain, head trauma, CVA, asthma, CHF, PE, ASA intoxication, pneumonia, thyrotoxicosis, mechanical ventilation, pregnancy (high progesterone), or hepatic failure (high progesterone).

Treatment

Treat and correct underlying causes.

TUBULOINTERSTITIAL DISEASES

Renal Tubular Acidosis (RTA)

Definition: RTA is a net decrease in either tubular H^+ secretion or HCO_3^- reabsorption, which results in non-AG metabolic acidosis. There are three main types as summarized below.

PEARLS—**Table 7-2: Summary of Renal Tubular Acidosis**

Type 1 (distal)	**Deficiency (Def): NH4Cl and H$^+$ secretion.** Urine pH > 5.3, serum K^+ is low; urine K^+ is high; serum HCO_3^- = 16-20. **Etiology:** Hereditary, SLE, Sjogren syndrome, amphotericin B, cirrhosis, nephro-calcification. **Treatment (Tx): Supplement of KHCO3.**
Type 2 (proximal)	**Deficiency: KHCO3 reabsorption decrease.** Urine pH < 5.3, serum K^+ is low; urine K^+ is high; serum HCO_3^- < 15. It's the only RTA type with **AG acidosis.** **Etiology:** Hereditary, sulfonamides, Vit-D deficiency, carbonic anhydrase inhibitor, amyloidosis, chronic hypo-Ca, chronic hepatitis, Wilson disease, Fanconi syndrome, myeloma, heavy metals. **Treatment: Supplement of KHCO3;** thiazide diuretics.
Type 4 (distal)	**Deficiency: Aldosterone insufficiency, No.1 common in chronic renal failure (CRF).** Urine pH < 5.3, serum KCl is high, urine K^+ is low, and serum Na^+ is low. **Etiology:** Hypo-renin hypoaldosteronism, Addison disease, diabetes, hypertension, Sickle cell disease, chronic interstitial nephritis, aldosterone resistance. **Treatment: Fludrocortisone, NaHCO3; K restriction.**

Acute Tubular Necrosis (ATN) and Acute Interstitial Nephritis (AIN)

Etiology

It is complex, including ischemia, drugs, toxins, and autoimmune damages, etc. These causes can also lead to tubulointerstitial nephritis.

1. **Ischemia**: Severe fluid or blood loss.

2. **Toxins and drugs:**

(1) **Pigment—hemoglobinuria (from hemolysis); myoglobinuria (from rhabdomyolysis** by surgery, trauma, seizure, etc). **Diagnostic tips for rhabdomyolysis**: urine dipstick test will only be (+) for significant hematuria, but no RBC will be seen under microscope. Serum CPK (markedly), potassium and uric acid levels are increased, and calcium is decreased (due to the Ca binding to damaged muscle). **Treatment**: (a) saline hydration; (b) mannitol for osmotic diuresis; (c) NaHCO3 for reducing Hyper-K and renal precipitation of myoglobin.

Note: Urine dipstick analysis cannot distinguish among hemoglobin, myoglobin, and RBC.

(2) **Contrasts: can cause immediate renal toxicity,** especially with old age, dehydration, diabetes, renal disease, and myeloma; **preventable with saline hydration.**

(3) **Metals**: Lithium, lead, mercury, or gold can **cause nephrogenic DI.**

(4) **Protein:** Myeloma—Bence-Jones protein is directly toxic to renal tubes.

(5) **Analgesics**: Female:male = 5:1. Phenacetin (and its metabolite acetaminophen) and aspirin (with synergism) are common. NSAIDs cause a combination of interstitial nephritis, direct toxic effect, papillary necrosis, and inhibition of vasodilators (by PG inhibitors). Analgesics can cause ATN or/and papillary necrosis more easily with renal underperfusion or ischemia.

Diagnosis of analgesic nephropathies: (a) History of ingestion 1g/d for 1-3y; (b) sterile pyuria, hematuria, flank pain, and mild proteinuria. Treatment is supportive.

(6) **Antibiotics – usually non-oliguric: aminoglycoside** (10-30% cases, usually with 1-week delayed reactions), **cephalosporins, tetracycline, methicillin, and amphotericin B. Hypo-K or hypo-Mg may increase risk of the drug toxicity, which is mostly dose-dependent.**

(7) **Anti-cancer drugs—non-oliguric:** cisplatin, methotrexate, cyclosporine, and mitomycin.

(8) **Hyperuricemia**: usually from acute tumor lysis syndrome. Long-standing hyperuricemia from gout can result in chronic renal failure.

3. **Autoimmune diseases:** Goodpasture syndrome, Wegener granulomatosis, polyarteritis nodosa, Henoch-Purpura, etc.

4. **Radiation**: With doses above 2,000 rads to the kidneys.

Clinical features of ATN—three phases (after renal ischemia)

1. Prodromal: The time between the damage and the onset of renal failure.

2. Oliguric (< 400 mL/d) or anuric (< 100 mL/d).

3. Post-oliguric: A recovery diuretic phase.

Clinical features of AIN

1. Mostly caused by drugs --NSAIDs, penicillins (PCN), sulfonamides (antibiotics and diuretics), anti-TB drugs (rifampin as No.1), vancomycin, ciprofloxacin, erythromycin, tetracycline, allopurinol (also associated with hepatic injury), etc. Some are due to infections or idiopathic reasons.

2. Common presentations include fever, rash, and abnormal urine.

3. Lab tests: Blood—Increased IgE and eosinophils; urine—eosinophiluria, hematuria, and proteinuria (< 2g/24h). Biopsy usually shows normal glomeruli with interstitial edema and eosinophils.

Treatment of ATN and AIN

1. Potentially offending agent should be immediately discontinued. Adequate IV fluid +/- short-term diuretics is the main prevention and therapy for ATN. Treatment of underlying cause and symptoms should be addressed. No additional therapies are required in most cases of ATN and AIN with minimal elevations in the serum creatinine due to their self-limited nature.

2. Biopsy-confirmed or moderate to severe cases of acute interstitial nephritis should be treated with short-term glucocorticoids, except for NSAID-induced AIN, which has a poor response.

Acute Kidney Injury (AKI)

AKI, previously called acute renal failure (ARF), is an abrupt loss of kidney function and increase in BUN and creatinine that develops usually in 7 days. By its various etiologies, it can be divided into **pre-, intra- and post-renal azotemia**.

The two major causes of acute kidney injury (AKI) developing in the hospital are prerenal disease and acute tubular necrosis (ATN). Decreased kidney function due to prerenal disease occurs when renal ischemia is part of a generalized decrease in tissue perfusion and when there is selective renal ischemia. ATN can occur with prolonged and/or severe ischemia. This can result in histologic changes, including necrosis.

PEARLS—Table 7-3: Summary of Acute Kidney Injury

1. Prerenal azotemia
Etiology: Any cause of **decreased renal perfusion**. (1) **Blood volume deficits**: Bleeding, poor intake, burns, diuretics, GI-GU loss (vomiting, diarrhea, diabetes), "the third spacing" of fluids (pancreatitis, peritonitis), sweating, and Addison disease. (2) **CVS**: CHF, shock, sepsis, pericardial diseases (constrictive pericarditis, tamponade), coarctation of the aorta, and renal artery stenosis (particularly with ACEI use). (3) **Drugs**: NSAIDs (direct toxicity can cause papillary necrosis in a day), gentamycin (dose-dependent). (4) Others: Low oncotic pressure (nephrotic syndrome, catabolic states), hepatorenal syndrome. **Lab tests:** Urine osmolality > 500 mOsm/kg, gravity > 1.020, urine Na^+ < 20 mEq/L, serum BUN/creatinine ratio > 20, Na-fraction-excretion (FENa%, most precise) < 1%; urine sediment: normal (hyaline +/-).
2. Intrarenal (Intrinsic) azotemia
Etiology: Very complicated; including acute tubulointerstitial necrosis (ATN), acute interstitial nephritis, nephrotic syndrome, glomerulonephritis, thromboembolism, etc. **Lab tests:** urine osmolality < 500 mOsm/kg, gravity < 1.010, urine Na^+ > 40 mEq/L, serum BUN:creatinine < 20, FENa% > 1%, urine sediment: RBC/granule cast (glomerulonephritis), protein cast (> 3.5g/24h, nephrotic syndrome).
3. Postrenal azotemia
Etiology: Any **obstruction to the outflow** of urine. This type only accounts for about 5% of cases. Prostate hypertrophy or cancer, kidney stones, pelvic tumors, ureter clot or strictures, and neurogenic bladder (functional obstruction), etc. **Dx:** (1) P/E. (2) Urinalysis (UA). (3) Ultrasound (U/S). Lab results are variable.

PEARLS—Table 7-4: Urinary Sediments and their Significance

Hyaline casts: Prerenal renal failure; normal concentrated urine, febrile disease, strenuous exercise, diuretic use
RBC (casts), +/- protein: Glomerulonephritis
WBC (casts), +/- eosinophils: Pyelonephritis; tubulointerstitial nephritis
Granular/epithelial/tubular cast (muddy): ATN or nonspecific
Fatty cast: Nephrotic syndrome
Broad waxy cast: CRF (indicative of stasis in enlarged collecting tubes)

GLOMERULAR DISEASES

There are many causes of glomerular disease and most patients present with either nephrotic or nephritic pattern, which is based upon the urine sediment and the degree of proteinuria. Hepatitis C-associated nephropathies include membranous nephropathy, mixed cryoglobulinemia syndrome, and polyarteritis nodosa.

General diagnostic points for kidney diseases

Urinalysis, the blood urea nitrogen (BUN) and creatinine (Cr) are the best initial tests to evaluate renal function.

Transient proteinuria including orthostatic proteinuria exists in < 10% of the population as a benign state. Persistent proteinuria may indicate pathology and the need of a kidney biopsy. Protein:creatinine ratio is more accurate than 24-hour collection of protein in the urine.

WBC in the urine indicates inflammation and infection (neutrophils) or allergic interstitial nephritis (eosinophils, by W&H stains).

Hematuria indicates stones in the kidney, ureter, or bladder; glomerulonephritis, infection (cystitis, pyelonephritis), cancer (kidney, ureter, or bladder); coagulopathy; medications (cyclophosphamide causing hemorrhagic cystitis); trauma (contusion of the kidney or bladder).

False positive hematuria may be caused by hemoglobin or myoglobin in the urine.

Nephritic Syndrome

GN 1.5+6

Nephritic => inflammatory

PEARLS—Classic features (triad) of nephritic syndrome:

+RBC casts

(1) Peripheral edema; (2) Hematuria; (3) Hypertension (HTN).

from salt retention

Also, proteinuria (less than nephrotic due to ↓ GFR)
— azotemia
– oliguria

P482 p 596

Table 7-5: Summary of Nephritic Syndrome

---

1. IgA nephropathy (Berger disease)

It's the most common glomerulonephritis.
Etiology: Abnormal IgA glycosylation; associated with infection and Henoch-Schönlein purpura; usually <30 y/a.

Dx: (1) Gross hematuria after 1-3 day's URI or GI infection; no protein or WBC in the urine, normal (Nl). **complements** (BP may be Nl). **(2) Lab:** Increased serum BUN, IgA, and renal deposits of IgA, IgG, and IgM (by immunostaining). **Renal biopsy** is the confirmative means of diagnosis.

Tx: BP control; steroids +/- immunosuppressants help with acute flares. **Prognosis:** 80% of cases are good; 20% may progress to end-stage CRF.

---

2. Post-streptococcal glomerulonephritis (Acute glomerulonephritis) *mesangial immune complex deposits*

Etiology: Mostly associated with **Strep-A** (beta-hemolytic) **infection** (pharyngitis or impetigo).

Dx: (1) After 1-3 weeks, with edema, hypertension, oliguria, and brown urine (hematuria and proteinuria). (2) Lab: Low serum C3, high ASO and hyaluronidase titer; lumpy-bumpy glowing immune complexes.

Tx: (1) Anti-Strep (PCN-V; cephalexin or cefadroxil). **(2)** Supportive (rest, salt-fluid restriction, anti-hypertension). **Prognosis:** Mostly self-limited, with good prognosis.

---

3. Idiopathic rapidly progressive glomerulonephritis *crescentic*

Etiology: Associated with SLE, mixed cryoglobulinemia, subacute infectious endocarditis, and shunt infections. It is an idiopathic form of severe GN characterized by **numerous crescent** formation (by renal biopsy), **acute renal failure**, and **(+) pANCA**; trapped immune complexes (with IG, C3). *in most glomeruli*

Dx: Clinical manifestations, lab tests, and renal biopsy.

Tx: (1) Symptomatic and supportive Tx. **(2)** Pulse prednisone +/- cyclophosphamide +/- plasmapheresis (to remove circulating antibody). Patient's response is limited. **Prognosis:** Poor.

Differential diagnosis

Granulomatosis with polyangiitis (Wegener granulomatosis; also see Chapter 8, Page 332):

Definition and etiology: Granulomatous inflammation of the respiratory tract with necrotizing vasculitis of small and medium-sized vessels, a form of polyarteritis nodosa.

Diagnosis: (1) URI (sinusitis, stomatitis, otitis) + **hemoptysis +/- hematuria** (renal vessel lesions). **(2) CXR: Lower respiratory infection/inflammation (bilateral pulmonary lymphadenopathies). (3) Lab: Hematuria, cANCA (+),** and cell-mediated immunoreactions.

Treatment: High-dose steroids and cytotoxics. Prognosis: May relapse after remission.

Anti-GBM antibody (Goodpasture) Disease: *— pulm hemorrhage & glomerulonephritis*

Goodpasture

Definition and etiology: An idiopathic glomerulonephropathy (GN) with pulmonary capillary hemorrhage caused by anti-GBM and anti-pulmonary capillary membrane antibodies, a type 2 hypersensitivity reaction. It's also considered an alveolar filling disease (see Chapter 3).

Diagnosis: (1) Dyspnea, hemoptysis (peripheral pulmonary capillary infiltration), **respiratory failure, and hematuria. (2) Worsened CXR (pulmonary infiltrates). (3) Lab: Hematuria, proteinuria, anti-GBM antibody (+), oliguria, renal failure (high BUN/Cr ratio).** Iron-deficiency anemia, hemosiderin-filled macrophages in sputum. **Renal biopsy:** Linear deposit of immuno-complex. *IgG*

Treatment: (1) If renal biopsy show < 30% crescents: Pulse prednisone +/- cyclophosphamide. **(2)** If biopsy shows > 70% crescents: Prednisone + cyclophosphamide + plasmapheresis. **Prognosis:** Variable.

Nephrotic Syndrome *FA slp·541*
—edema
—fatigue
—proteinuria
—abd pn from rapid fluid accumulation

Nephrotic syndrome is a result of injury to the glomerular filtration barrier, which increases its permeability and generates two characteristics—urine protein excretion and hypoalbuminemia.

PEARLS—Classic features of nephrotic syndrome:

(1) Peripheral edema; (2) Proteinuria (> 3.5 g/24h) and lipiduria; (3) Hypoalbuminemia (serum albumin < 3 g/dL) and hyperlipidemia; (4) Oval fat bodies and bland sediment in the urine.

Etiology

All vasculitides and glomerular nephropathies (GN), as well as diabetes, SLE, amyloid disease, and multiple myeloma, etc, can lead to nephrotic syndrome, and eventual renal failure. Hepatitis C-associated nephropathies include membranous nephropathy, mixed cryoglobulinemia syndrome, and polyarteritis nodosa.

Table 7-6: Summary of Nephrotic Syndrome

> **1. Minimal change disease (MCD, Nil disease)**
>
> **MCD is the most common form of idiopathic nephrotic syndrome in childhood** (90%). Patient has some clinical features of nephrotic syndrome plus **minor changes without immune deposition** on light microscopy **(LM)** and characteristic **fusion of foot processes** on electronic microscopy **(EM). Tx: Prednisone** is usually effective in >80% children and adults. *→flattening, effacement*
>
> **PEARLS: Minimal change (disease) variants** that initially show only minor changes on LM include: **(1) Idiopathic mesangial proliferative glomerulonephritis; (2) IgM nephropathy; (3) C1q nephropathy**. All these disorders are **diagnosed by biopsy. Idiopathic mesangial proliferative glomerulonephritis** is characterized by mesangial proliferation, global increase in mesangial cells and matrix, and the absence of IgG or IgA immune deposits. Clinically it shows very variable hematuria and proteinuria. **Treatment** is prednisone +/- cytotoxics. Effects and prognosis vary.

Normal findings. Also on IF.

edema + proteinuria

LM:
localized regions of mesangial sclerosis & Bm collapse

2. Focal segmental glomerulosclerosis (FSGS)

FSGS is a histologic lesion rather than a disease. It's the most common form of primary/idiopathic nephropathy in adults. Primary FSGS typically presents with the nephrotic syndrome. **Secondary FSGS** typically presents with non-nephrotic proteinuria and renal insufficiency, caused by infections (particularly with IVDA and HIV), toxins (including heroin, interferon, cyclosporine, and pamidronate), genetic abnormalities, and renal atheroembolic disease. Complex manifestations of FSGS include hematuria, increased BUN:creatinine ratio and lipids, hypercoagulability (antithrombin III loss), heavy proteinuria (> 3.5g/d), and lipiduria. Histology typically shows **focal segmental immune deposits**, with scarring and shrinking of the kidney.

Tx: (1) Salt restriction, diuretics, statins for hyperlipidemia, and heparin and coumadin for hypercoagulability. (2) Prednisone is the initial Tx, effective in about 20% patients. Cytotoxics are more helpful with refractory cases. **Prognosis**: Mostly progresses to end-stage CRF over 5-10 years.

3. Membranous nephropathy (MN)
- glomerulonephritis
- GBm thick

MN is **among the most common causes** of the nephrotic syndrome in nondiabetic adults. MN can be either **idiopathic or secondary** to drugs (**gold, penicillamine**) and diseases such as **hepatitis B & C**, syphilis, malaria, autoimmune disease (**SLE**), cancer (except Hodgkin disease). **EM**: Immune complex and granular deposits (**IgG and C3) on the GBM**, with "**spike and dome**" appearance. GFR is normal but the urinary loss of anti-thrombin III may result in **hypercoagulability**. *"subepithelial spikes"*

Tx: (1) Salt restriction, ICE-I for hypertension and persistent proteinuria, statins for hyperlipidemia, heparin and coumadin for hypercoagulability. (2) Steroids plus cytotoxics may help in severe disease. **Prognosis**: 80% can be stable and 20% may progress.

Differentiation

Membranoproliferative glomerulonephritis (MPGN)

→ uworld: nephritic > nephrotic

Also known as **mesangiocapillary glomerulonephritis**, MPGN is a heterogeneous chronic glomerulonephritis that **share mixed nephritic and nephrotic features** and microscopic findings. They mostly affect children. The main cause is immune complex deposition that is idiopathic or secondary to a systemic disorder. It is also associated with some viral infections such as hepatitis B and C. *C3 nephritic factor*
stabilizes C3 convertase
↓ C3 levels

Clinical features and diagnosis

1. It is often associated with or **secondary to SLE (lupus nephritis) or HCV** or/and other viral/bacterial infections, clinically with very variable hematuria, proteinuria, and hypertension.

2. **Lab** tests typically show **hypocomplementemia** (especially **low C3), which indicates the disease activity**. Diagnosis is made by renal biopsy, which will show **immune complex (IgG and C3) deposits** in the glomerulus and thickening of the glomerular basement membrane under light microscopy.
"tram track" appearance from GBM splitting from "mesangial hypercellularity"

Treatment

Symptomatic treatment along with prednisone or/and cytotoxics. **Prognosis** varies and usually progresses to end-stage chronic kidney disease.

Chronic Kidney Disease; Chronic Renal Failure (CKD; CRF)

Chronic kidney disease (CKD), also known as chronic renal failure (CRF), is a progressive loss in renal function over a period of months or years due to varieties of causes.

Etiology

1. Diabetes—No.1 cause of CRF with over 7 years of proteinuria.

2. Hypertension—Most common in cases without diabetes but with renal artery sclerosis.

3. Glomerulonephritis and glomerulonephropathy.

Essentials of diagnosis

1. History of chronic renal diseases, diabetes, or CVD; commonly presenting with edema, hypertension, anemia, GI symptoms, neuropsychologic changes, etc.

2. **Lab tests**: Increased BUN:creatinine ratio, phosphate (P_2), and K^+; decreased Ca^{2+}, HCO_3^-, and Hb. Urine analysis: proteinuria, tubular cast; urine gravity = 1.010 (same as in the serum).

Treatment

1. Cessation of offending agents. Restriction of protein intake and **early use of ACE-I** are important treatment to reduce mortality. However, if creatinine > 3 and urine protein > 3^+ with hypertension, ACE-I may worsen renal function, thus only protein restriction is indicated.

2. Symptomatic treatment: Supply Ca, $NaCO_3^-$, glucose, and insulin. **Add Ca** in food if PTH and phosphate (P_2) are high and Ca^{2+} is low in the blood.

3. **Erythropoietin** helps with anemia. Adverse effects: (1) Hypertension; (2) headache; (3) Flu-like symptoms.

4. **Dialysis**: Indications—"**AUOK**": **A**cidosis, **U**remic syndrome, **O**verloaded (fluid), $K^+ > 6.5$ **mEq/L.** Hemodialysis is better than peritoneal dialysis.

5. Kidney **transplantation** should be prepared early because of its great potential for cure.

Complications—End-stage renal failure

1. **MI: Now it's the No.1 cause of death in renal failure; infection is the No.2**. Platelet dysfunction is the No.1 cause of bleeding in uremic syndrome.

2. **Uremic syndrome:**

(1) CVS dysfunction: pericarditis, hypertension, CHF, and atherosclerosis.

(2) Hematologic: anemia, low lymphocytes (increased infection), and increased bleeding time (BT).

(3) GI dysfunction: nausea and vomiting.

(4) Neurologic: polyneuritis, encephalitis, and seizure.

(5) Osteodystrophy: secondary PTH increase, metastatic calcification, bone pain, osteomalacia and osteitis fibrosa. **Treat** it with Vit-D, Ca, and P_2-binders (Amphojel).

(6) Hyperuricemia (itchy).

Treatment of uremia: (1) Diet: Protein, K, Na and fluid restriction. (2) Dialysis. (3) Renal transplantation.

3. **Electrolyte disorder—"3 highs 3 lows":** High K^+, phosphate (P_2), and Mg^{2+}; low Na^+, Cl^-, and Ca^{2+} in the serum.

(1) **Hypo-Ca and hyper-P_2**: Due to decreased 1, 25 $(OH)_2$ D_2 in the kidney and peripheral resistance to PTH, resulting in increased fecal loss of Ca, decreased urinary P_2-secretion, and the deposition of Ca-P_2 in soft tissue. The secondary hyper-PTH eventually leads to Ca leaching from bones.

(2) **Hyper-Mg**: Secondary to reduced urinary secretion. Treatment is avoiding Mg-containing drugs.

FLUID AND ELECTROLYTE DISORDERS

Hyponatremia

Definition: Serum Na^+ <135 mEq/L without hyperglycemia or hyperlipidemia.

Etiology

1. Hypervolemic status: Secondary to decreased intra-vascular volume (Baro-receptor reflex), ADH production, and free-water clearance; commonly seen in CHF, nephrotic syndrome, cirrhosis, and renal insufficiency.

2. Hypovolemic status: GI losses (vomiting, diarrhea, nasogastric suction), diuretics, sweating, burns, hypotonic over-fluid, and Addison disease.

3. Euvolemic status: Psychogenic polydipsia (>10 L/d intake), hypothyroidism, SIADH, CNS and pulmonary disorders (infection, embolus, tumor, trauma, shock, asthma, etc.), and drugs (oral hypoglycemics, anti-metabolics, etc.).

4. Pseudohyponatremia: Hyperlipidemia and hyperglycemia.

Essentials of diagnosis

1. Symptoms appear when Na^+ < 125 mEq/L, all neurologic: headache, lethargy, obtundation, and eventual coma and seizures. Severe manifestations occur if Na^+ < 120 mEq/L.

2. Serum Na^+ < 135 mEq/L; urine osmolality > serum osmolality; urine Na^+ > 40 mEq/L.

Treatment

Na correction should be gradual. Rapid correction can result in central pontine myelinolysis—brainstem lesion, showing paraparesis, dysarthria, or dysphagia.

1. Mild (serum Na^+ = 120-130 mEq/L): Fluid restriction to < 1L.

2. Moderate ($Na^+ = 110$-120 mEq/L): Loop diuretic and normal saline (N.S.) to remove net free-water.

3. Severe ($Na^+ < 110$ mEq/L plus symptoms): Hypertonic saline IV.

Hypernatremia

Definition: Serum $Na^+ > 155$ mEq/L.

Etiology: Mostly due to insensible losses.

1. Extra-renal loss: Increased loss through the skin (sweating, burns, fever, and exercise), respiratory or GI tract infections, or osmotic/infectious diarrhea.

2. Renal: **Idiopathic (most common)**, nephrogenic DI (including lithium use), chronic glomerulopathy, hyper-Ca, hypo-K, demeclocycline, sickle cell disease, central DI, trauma, infection, tumor, osmotic dieresis—diabetic ketoacidosis, nonketotic hyperosmolar coma, mannitol, or diuretics.

Essentials of diagnosis

1. Primarily with neurologic symptoms: Lethargy, weakness, irritability, seizures, and coma are present with any severe hyper-Na.

2. DI gives a dilute diuresis of 3-20 L/day.

Treatment

1. Acute: Isotonic fluids IV. Correction of Na should be less than 1 mEq/2hour. Complications of overly rapid correction include cerebral edema, permanent neurologic damage, or seizures.

2. **Central diabetes insipidus**: Give vasopressin (ADH) and try to correct the underlying cause.

3. **Nephrogenic diabetes insipidus:** Stop irritable agents and give thiazides or NSAIDs, which work by inhibiting prostaglandins (PGs, which impair concentrating ability) and enhancing ADH actions.

Hypokalemia

Definition: Serum $K^+ < 3.5$ mEq/L.

Etiology

1. Alkalosis—transcellular shift: H^+ out and K^+ in. Increased insulin promotes K^+ into cells with glucose.

2. GI Loss: Vomiting, diarrhea, and tube drainage; low oral intake (rare).

3. Increased urinary loss: Primary hyperaldosteronism (Conn syndrome), diuretics, diabetic ketoacidosis, Cushing disease, licorice, renal tubular acidosis, etc.

4. **Bartter syndrome**: Due to primary deficiency in Na^+-Cl^- reabsorption from Loop of Henle, it causes high levels of renin and aldosterone but normal BP.

Essentials of diagnosis

1. (1) Symptoms start when $K^+ < 3.0$ mEq/L—muscle weakness, paralysis, cardiac arrhythmias. (2) ECG shows U-wave and T-wave flattening (**Image 4**). Nephrogenic diabetes insipidus may or may not be present.

2. **Bartter syndrome**: There are high levels of renin and aldosterone, normal BP, and severe hypo-K and hypo-Cl alkalosis.

Treatment

1. Correction of underlying cause and oral supply of KCl is the best treatment.

2. IV KCl should be very slow and only for severe hypo-K, with N.S. or ½ tension N.S. Potential complication of too rapid KCl infusion is fatal arrhythmia.

Hyperkalemia

Definition: Serum K^+ is > 5.5 mEq/L.

Etiology: Increased oral or IV intake along with impaired renal excretion (renal failure).

1. Acidosis (H^+-K^+ exchange): High H^+ into cells and K^+ out; insulin deficiency.

2. Tissue breakdown: Rhabdomyolysis, tumor lysis, or post-seizures or vigorous exercise.

3. Hypo-aldosteronism: Type 4 renal RTA, ACE-I, heparin inhibition of aldosterone, Addison disease, adrenalectomy, K-sparing diuretics (triamterene, amiloride, spironolactone), or NSAIDs.

4. Periodic paralysis: Recurrent, mild, brief episodes of muscle weakness with mild increase in K^+. Family history is usually present.

Essentials of diagnosis

1. Muscular weakness (usually $K^+ > 6.5$ mEq/L) and hypoventilation.

2. **ECG: Peaked T** waves, **widened QRS**, short QT, or prolonged PR (**Image 4**). Abnormal cardiac conduction is the No.1 cause of death.

Treatment

1. $CaCl_2$ IV: In urgent case with abnormal ECG, giving immediate and short-lived effect on membrane stabilization.

2. $NaHCO_3$ IV: Alkalosis drives K^+ into cells. Avoid giving it together with Ca^{+2} (because it will form $CaCO_3$ precipitate).

3. Glucose and insulin IV: Drives K^+ intracellularly, takes > 30 min to work.

4. Others: Diuretics are commonly used to excrete K^+ and Na^+. Kayexalate (Cation exchange resins) absorbs K and releases Na effectively; given with sorbitol (to prevent constipation) and combined with the above treatment. Beta-R agonists also have anti-hyper-K effect.

5. Dialysis: Indicated when $K^+ > 6.5$ despite other treatment.

Hyperk

Contraindication

NSAIDs should never be used with K-saving diuretics or ACE-I in elderly patients or with renal failure, to avoid fatal hyperkalemia!

Hypomagnesemia (Hypo-Mg) — *induces PTH resistance & ↓PTH secretion => hypocalcemia*
- variable PTH levels

Definition: Serum Mg is < 1.8 mg/dL.

Etiology

1. GI causes: Malabsorption, steatorrheic states (most common cause); prolonged fasting; fistulas.

2. Alcoholism (No.1 common).

3. Renal losses: SIADH, diuretics, Bartter syndrome, drugs (gentamicin, amphotericin B, cisplatin), renal transplantation.

Essentials of diagnosis

1. Marked neuromuscular and CNS hyperirritability: (1) Muscle twitching, weakness, tremors; (2) hyperreflexia, seizures; (3) mental status changes.

2. Effects on Ca^{2+} and K^+ levels: Commonly coexisting with hypo-Ca^{2+} (because of decreased PTH and bone resistance to PTH with hypo-Mg); 50% coexisting with hypokalemia.

4. ECG changes: prolonged QT interval, T wave flattening, and eventual torsade de pointes.

Treatment

1. For mild hypo-Mg: oral magnesium oxide (MgO).

2. For severe hypo-Mg: IV $MgSO_4$.

Hypermagnesemia (Hyper-Mg)

Definition: Serum Mg is > 2.5 mg/dL.

Etiology

1. Renal failure (No.1 common); adrenal insufficiency.

2. Early-stage burns, massive trauma or surgical stress, rhabdomyolysis, severe ECF volume deficit, severe acidosis, excessive ingestion of Mg-containing agents.

Essentials of diagnosis

1. Nausea, weakness; facial paresthesia; progressive loss of deep tendon reflexes; later—muscular paralysis and coma. Death is usually caused by respiratory failure or cardiac arrest.

2. ECG changes resemble those with hyperkalemia—prolonged P-R interval, widened QRS complex, and elevated T waves.

Treatment

1. Stop exogenously administered Mg, along with normal saline and furosemide.

2. IV administration of Ca-gluconate for severe symptoms (cardioprotection).

3. Dialysis is indicated in renal failure cases.

NEPHROLITHIASIS

Nephrolithiasis refers to renal stone formation due to increased Ca, P_2, oxalate, uric acid, and cysteine in the body. It occurs in 1-5% of the population. Composition of stones: **Ca-oxalate 70%**, Ca-phosphate 10%, Mg/Al-phosphate (Struvite) 5-10%, uric acid 5%, and cysteine 1%.

Etiology

1. **Hypercalcemia**: (1) Increased absorption; (2) Vit-D intoxication +/- granulomatous disease; (3) familial or idiopathic renal hypercalciuria; (4) Hyper-PTH (Ca-phosphate); (5) cancer: multiple myeloma, or metastasis to bone.

2. **Hyperoxaluria**—mainly idiopathic: (1) With fat malabsorption, Ca binding with fat and increased oxalate reabsorption; (2) hypocitraturia: decreased citrate-Ca binding and increased Ca absorption (facilitated by **acidic** conditions).

3. **Uric acid stones**: Formed in **acidic** conditions (pH < 5.5) and associated with diseases such as gout, Crohn disease, and hematologic cancers. It's the only **radiolucent** stone here.

4. **Struvite stones**: UTIs with urease-producing organisms (Proteus, Staphylococcus, Pseudomonas, and Klebsiella) generates highly **alkaline** urine that produces struvite stones.

5. **Cystinuria**: Only associated with genetic disorders.

Essentials of diagnosis

1. **Constant or paroxysmal flank pain**—non-colicky, waxes and wanes, radiating to groin; gross or microscopic hematuria; often accompanied with nausea, vomiting, dysuria, and urinary urgency.

2. **More than 80% stones can be found by an initial ultrasound and plain x-ray** examination. Some patients are diagnosed asymptomatically during imaging for other purposes.

3. **Intravenous pyelogram (IVP) is the best means to confirm diagnosis (stone or tumor).** Helical CT can help diagnose other causes of flank pain (tumor, abscess, etc.). Testing of serum and urine Ca may also help determine etiology.

Treatment

1. Analgesia, hydration and bed rest are the major treatment. **Stones ≤ 5 mm can usually pass spontaneously—observation. Both tamsulosin and nifedipine have been shown to increase the likelihood of stone passage for sizes ≤ 10 mm.**

2. **For stones 5-10 mm with symptoms: Shockwave lithotripsy** is the best initial therapy. If stones and symptoms persist or/and **stones > 10mm**, percutaneous nephrolithotomy can be the effective therapy.

3. Complications: Persistent renal obstruction and even permanent renal damage may occur if left untreated.

RENAL CYSTIC DESEASES

Polycystic Kidney Disease (PKD)

AKD is inherited as an autosomal dominant or recessive trait. Autosomal dominant PKD (ADPKD) is caused by mutations of either PKD1 or PKD2 genes. PKD1 mutations are more common and cause more severe disease than PKD2 mutations. Autosomal dominant PKD as for most adults may end in renal failure by 60 y/a in about 50% cases. The autosomal recessive PKD is rare and mostly found in infants and young children that may lead to early-year death. Etiology is unclear.

Essentials of diagnosis

1. Family history, flank pain, hematuria (micro and gross), infections, and evidence of calculi. It may also be found asymptomatic on screening of family members. Extra-renal manifestations include **hypertension** (No.1), hepatic cysts (50%), colonic diverticula, intracranial aneurysm, or mitral valve prolapse. Family history is helpful but not necessary.

2. P/E may find large, palpable kidneys, combined with hypertension: suggestive of the disease.

3. Ultrasound or CT scan confirms diagnosis by showing multiple cysts in bilateral kidneys; total number depends on age.

Treatment

1. Conservative therapies of early, strict control of blood pressure (ACE-I), UTI and calculi, a low-salt and low-protein diet, and use of statins are major steps of treatment to prevent symptoms and cardiovascular complications.

2. Dialysis or renal transplantation is indicated in end-stage renal failure (a frequent complication).

Differential diagnosis

Simple renal cysts:

It is common and may have similar, milder manifestations of ADPDK but normal kidney size and BP, occasional hematuria, and less family history. If there is a smooth wall without debris in the cyst, no further therapeutic or diagnostic tests are needed. Persistent cysts with irregular walls or debris inside should be aspirated for pathologic examination to exclude malignancy.

Acquired renal cysts:

Usually in patients with dialysis with small kidney size, occasional hematuria, variable hypertension; may be associated with adenocarcinoma in cysts; always leading to renal failure.

Medullary sponge kidney:

A rare, non-inherited disease; 40-60 y/a; normal kidney size, cysts may exist in collecting ducts; associated with renal calculi and UTI; usually not associated with hypertension, hematuria, or renal failure.

Medullary cystic kidney:

Rare, autosomal dominant inheritance, adulthood onset; small kidney size with cysts; normal BP, polyuria, salt wasting, always leading to renal failure.

Urinary stone disease:

(1) Flank pain and hematuria; (2) Nausea and vomiting; (3) Diagnosed by CT scan.

UROGENITAL NEOPLASMS

Renal Cell Carcinoma (RCC)

RCC is the most common form of kidney cancer arising from the renal tubule. It occurs more common in male over 55 y/a. Etiology is unknown. The **No. 1 risk factor is smoking**. Others include family history, inherited disease (such as von Hippel-Lindau disease), etc.

Essentials of diagnosis

1. The **classic triad** is **painless hematuria, flank pain, and an abdominal mass**, but now known as the "**late triad**" beyond a curative stage. Most cases are asymptomatic and accidentally detected on imaging for other purposes.

2. Other symptoms include fever, sweats, malaise, constipation, anemia or plethora (due to decreased or increased erythropoietin), hypertension, Hyper-Ca, weight loss, visual deficiency, female hirsutism, and varicocele (mostly on the left, due to tumor blockage of the left gonadal vein and left renal vein).

3. **Diagnostic steps**:

(1) If no mass is palpable, ultrasound can be the initial diagnostic test.

(2) If P/E reveals a mass: CT can be the best initial exam.

(3) IVP with cystoscopy is the most precise method to define the tumor (and stones, cysts).

(4) Asymptomatic screening by ultrasound +/- CT can be considered in patients with 1) inherited conditions (Von Hippel-Lindau syndrome and tuberous sclerosis); 2) end-stage renal disease; 3) a strong family history of RCC; 4) prior kidney irradiation.

4. **Staging (Anatomic stage/prognostic groups)**:

I (T_1): Within the capsule, 5-year survival 75%;

II (T_2): Outside capsule but within Gerota's fascia, 5-year survival 50%;

III (T_1N, T_2N or T_3+/-N): Metastasis to lymph nodes (LN);

IV (T_4N+/-M): Metastasis to distant organs.

| PEARLS | Differential diagnosis of hematuria |

1. Urethra (injury): Initial hematuria.

2. Bladder (injury, cancer): Terminal hematuria.

3. Above the bladder (renal injury or cancer): Mixed hematuria.

Treatment

1. Surgical resection is the most effective treatment of RCC (Stage I, II, or III). RCC is resistant to most Chemo-/radio therapies.

2. For elderly patients and those with significant comorbid disease, ablative techniques (cryoablation, radiofrequency ablation) are an alternative.

3. For advanced clear cell RCC: immunotherapy with high-dose interleukin-2 (IL-2), pazopanib or sunitinib is the first-line treatment.

Wilms Tumor

Wilms tumor is the most common renal malignancy in children and is one of the most common cancers in early childhood. Almost all cases are diagnosed before age 10, and two-thirds before 5. It may occur as a part of a multiple malformation syndrome including **Beckwith-Wiedemann, WAGR, and Denys-Drash syndromes.** Wilms tumor is associated with mutations of a number of genes including WT1, p53, FWT1, and FWT2 genes.

Essentials of diagnosis

1. The most common presentation is an **asymptomatic abdominal mass or swelling, a solitary tumor** in a single kidney. Others findings (later) may include abdominal pain, hematuria, and hypertension.

2. Screening for Wilms tumor with serial abdominal **ultrasonography** is performed in high-risk patients. Contrast-enhanced **CT or MRI** is obtained to evaluate the nature and extent of the mass. The **diagnosis is made by histologic confirmation after surgery or biopsy**. Tumor histology is linked to the outcome. The classic favorable histology Wilms tumor is comprised of three cell types (blastemal, stromal, and epithelial cells). **Anaplasia is associated with poor outcome**.

Staging of Wilms tumor is based upon the anatomic extent of the tumor without consideration for genetic, histologic, or biological markers.

Treatment—based on staging

1. Surgical excision for all patients with resectable tumors.
2. Chemotherapy for all patients except those with very low risk tumors.
3. Radiation therapy as indicated by stage and/or histology.

Benign Prostate Hyperplasia (BPH)

BPH is an increasingly common benign prostate enlargement as part of the aging process usually after 50 y/a. It may lead to partial obstruction of the urethra with related symptoms. The pathologic feature is **central hyperplasia** of the epithelial component (compared to prostate cancer with peripheral dysplasia). Etiology is unknown.

Essentials of diagnosis

1. Obstructive symptoms in an elder patient: Urinary hesitancy or retention, intermittent stream, and terminal dribbling; irritative voiding symptoms +/- opening hematuria.

2. DRE (digital rectal exam): Smoothly enlarged prostate; mild hyperplasia may not be detected.

3. Urine analysis (U/A) +/- culture can rule out infection or hematuria due to cystitis or prostatitis. Creatinine test is done for suspicious obstruction and renal failure.

4. Ultrasound-guided biopsy of suspicious mass. Upper UT-imaging or PSA testing is little helpful.

Treatment

1. Watchful waiting: Observe and monitor mild symptoms, as many cases may shrink with age.

2. Medications**:**

(1) **The No.1** choice is **alpha-R blocker tamsulosin,** with high selectivity on prostate and bladder smooth muscle and least S/E.

(2) **Terazosin** can also be used with gradual dosing to reduce S/E (BP decrease, reflux ejaculation).

(3) **Finasteride** (5-alpha-reductase inhibitor) is effective in reducing blood flow and obstruction when the prostate is > 40g, with similar therapeutic effects as tamsulosin.

3. Surgery:

(1) For patient with moderate symptoms, transurethral resection is indicated.

(2) With severe obstructive symptoms, open prostectomy is recommended.

Prostate Cancer

It's the **most common cancer (in male) and second cause of cancer death in male.** It is mostly an **adenocarcinoma** originated from the peripheral zone of the prostate. It commonly **metastasizes to bone.**

Risk factors: There is no clear single risk factor; may be associated with high level of testosterone and sexual activity, smoking, senior age, diet, occupation, family history, Black race, etc.

Essentials of diagnosis

1. Patient is usually asymptomatic until obstructive symptoms on voiding similar to benign prostatic hypertrophy appear, with progressive urine retention, decreased urinary stream, weight loss, and back/bone pain (bone metastasis— "Mets").

2. DRE (digital rectal examination) may reveal an asymmetric, rock-hard, discrete peripheral nodule if beyond early stage. Biopsy is required with an abnormal DRE result found, regardless of PSA levels.

3. PSA (prostate specific antigen) is usually markedly elevated (> 4 ng/ml) with prostate cancer. A PSA level substantially above normal for a certain age may be an indication for biopsy. A change from prior values (more than 0.35 ng/mL/year for a PSA of < 4.0 or 0.75ng/mL if the PSA is > 4.0) is suspicious. Transrectal ultrasound-guided **biopsy is required to confirm the diagnosis**.

4. CT helps determine lesion extent and therapy. With bone pain (metastasis), it is best diagnosed by bone Scint[99]-scan. Gleason histology system helps determine the cancer grade.

5. Staging: Combined TNM and anatomic (I-IV) staging systems are used for therapeutic guidelines and prognosis. Nomograms are accurate predictive tools to assist in choosing the optimal therapy.

Management

1. Patients > **age 70** with a suspicious nodule or cancer, no PSA or FNB is needed and just **let it go** naturally, because most patients with prostate cancer die of other diseases and many cases with well-differentiation do not progress without treatment.

2. For **Stage I (T1a) —IIa (T1c-T2b) tumor**:

(1) > age 65: Follow up PSA and DRE per 6-12 months.

(2) < age 65: radical prostectomy plus radiation. Common complications after surgery include incontinence and erectile dysfunction. Nerve-sparing surgery can reduce adverse effects.

3. **Stage IIb (T2c) —III (T3a/b): Radiation**.

4. **Stage IV** (T4+/-N1+/-M, distant metastasis):

(1) Choose palliative radiation along with androgen ablation therapy—GnRH agonist **leuprolide** (No.1) **plus** androgen-R blocker **flutamide**, to avoid "flare phenomenon".

Flutamide S/E: Male breast enlargement, hepto-toxicity, GI-toxicity, increased warfarin-toxicity.

(2) Orchiectomy is another option. This and hormonal therapy can help control the size and progression of metastases, but cannot prevent recurrences.

5. **Gleason grading**: It's a measure of the malignant potential of prostate cancer. A high Gleason grade suggests a greater benefit of surgical resection of the prostate (early).

6. **PSA follow-up is beneficial for prognosis** in all post-treatment patients. PSA screening among healthy men has not shown clear mortality benefit; a normal PSA does not exclude the possibility of prostate cancer.

7. Non-beneficial management: "screening imaging study", lumpectomy, or chemotherapy. None of these has a clear mortality benefit.

Prevention and screening

According to USPSTF, men are generally **not recommended to be screened for prostate cancer** because there is moderate certainty that the (survival) benefits of such screening do not outweigh the harms. If a patient with risk factors has discussed with the physician and decided to be screened, PSA tests at intervals of 2-4 years are recommended. DRE is not recommended as part of the screening. Screening should be stopped after age 69 or earlier when comorbidities limit life expectancy to <10 years.

Bladder Cancer

It's the **second most common urologic cancer**. 90% of bladder cancers are transitional cell carcinomas. The most common route of spread is local extension to surrounding tissues. The prevalence pattern is male more than female and mostly older than 60 y/a.

Risk factors: smoking, industrial carcinogens (**aniline dye, azo dyes**), radiation, long-term use of cyclophosphamide, chronic bladder infections, urinary stones, biologic agents (artificial sweeteners), etc.

Essentials of diagnosis

1. The most common presentation is painless, gross hematuria at terminal urine, +/- irritative voiding symptoms (frequency, urgency, and dysuria). In early stage, most patients are asymptomatic.

2. Urine analysis is useful in showing macro- or microscopic hematuria and ruling out infection. **Cystoscopy plus biopsy** are diagnostic (detecting malignancy). IVP can be used to determine upper UT lesion, with possible bladder filling defects.

Treatment—Depending on combined TNM and anatomic (0—IV) staging

1. Stage 0a (Ta), superficial, limited to mucosa, diameter of about 1 cm: Complete transurethral resection the tumor plus intravesical chemotherapy is the best treatment. It is likely to recur after removal.

2. Stage 0is (Tis), larger, high-grade recurrent cancer and muscle invasive carcinoma-in-situ: Intravesical chemotherapy—gemcitabine plus cisplatin or the methotrexate, vinblastine, doxorubicin, cisplatin (MVAC) regimen. Post-chemotherapy cystectomy is generally preferred.

3. Beyond stage I (T_1, involving lamina propria) and invasive cancer without metastasis (Stage II—$T_{2a/b}$; Stage III—$T_{3a/b}$; T4a): Aggressive resection plus chemotherapy.

4. Stage IV (T_{4b} +/- N_1+/- M_1) —cancer with distant metastasis: Chemotherapy only.

Testicular Carcinoma

It is a rare cancer of the testis, mainly affecting young men (20-35 y/a). 95% of cases are testicular germ cell tumors (GCTs, seminoma and nonseminoma), and the rest are nongerminal (Leydig-cell, Sertoli-cell gonadoblastoma). Almost **all testicular nodules are malignant**. Testicular germ cell tumors (GCTs) are among the most curable solid neoplasms, with about 95% of five-year survival rates.

Essentials of diagnosis

1. Patient usually presents with a (right-side) painless nodule accidentally found, **confirmed by ultrasound** (no transillumination) **and orchiectomy. Do not perform fine needle biopsy (FNB)** to avoid spreading.

2. Blood testing for **tumor markers and follow-up**: PLAP, alpha-FP, beta-hCG, etc. LDH and CEA may increase non-specifically.

(1) **Germ Cell tumors (95% of cases):**

Seminoma: Placental alkaline phosphatase (PLAP) increases markedly.

Embryonic carcinoma: Alpha-FP increases markedly; beta-hCG increases in 50% of patients.

Choriocarcinoma: Beta-hCG increases markedly.

(2) **Sex cord/gonadal stromal tumors—nongerminal tumors (5%):**

Leydig-Sertoli cell tumor and gonadoblastoma cause **increased testosterone. Granulosa cell tumor causes high estrogen.**

3. **Staging**: CT scan of the chest, abdomen, and pelvis should be performed for staging. The metastasis is usually going through the lymphatic channels in the retroperitoneum up to the chest.

Treatment

1. If a testicular cancer is suspected based on physical examination or ultrasound, the testicle should be radically resected by the inguinal route (without cutting the scrotum to avoid spreading) followed by radio- or chemo-therapy (a single-agent carboplatin). For a stage I seminoma, a high cure rate can be achieved with radical orchiectomy. After the orchiectomy, biopsy should be performed for confirmation. As active surveillance, beta-hCG and AFP levels should be followed to compare with the preoperative values.

2. Patients with stage II seminoma are effectively treated with radiotherapy or cisplatin-based combination chemotherapy. Radiotherapy is used for local disease and chemotherapy is for widespread disease. Most testicular cancers (seminomas) are especially **radio- or chemo-sensitive** (platinum-based), making the treatment for this cancer promising, even with metastasis.

3. Further surgery for lymph node dissection may be needed in some cases, such as non-seminomas.

Penile Cancer

Clinical features and diagnosis

1. It is a rare malignancy of the penis and the peak incidence is in 70's men, may be associated with HSV and HPV18 infections. Circumcision has a protective effect according to statistics.

2. It presents as an exophytic mass on the penis.

Treatment

1. Surgical excision for Tis, Ta, or T1 penile cancer carries a good prognosis with a low risk of recurrence, and thus a limited excision is recommended.

2. Men with stage T2 to T4 tumors are considered to have a higher risk of recurrence with an organ-preserving therapy, and thus penile amputation with a negative surgical margin is recommended.

MISCELLANEOUS DISORDERS

Cryptorchism

It is the absence of one or both testes from the scrotum, a common birth defect in male. It can be found anywhere from retroperitoneal abdomen to the inguinal canal (90%). **Risk factors** may include premature infants, lower weight, alcohol consumption and smoking, obesity, diabetes during pregnancy, and family history.

Undescended testes are associated with increased risk of infertility, testicular germ cell tumors, testicular torsion and infarction, inguinal hernias, and psychological problems when the boy is grown. In most cases the testicle will descend into the scrotum spontaneously during the first year of life.

Treatment

Initial management is watchful waiting for its high spontaneous resolution. If this fails (> 6 months), surgical **orchiopexy** is the effective treatment to avoid the above risks. ﹛↓ risk of subfertility ﹜ testicular cancer.

[handwritten margin notes: Intra-abd testis >> 10x risk for torsion. -severe abd pn ﹜ vomiting. -If it's in the inguinal canal = inguinal swelling + pain]

Urinary Incontinence

It's defined as the inability to hold urine, producing involuntary urinary leakage. It's more common in childbearing and elder females. Urinary incontinence is classified and summarized in Table 7-7.

Essentials of diagnosis

1. Etiologic analysis of the symptoms and history. Use voiding diary and urodynamic testing.

2. Lab tests:

(1) Urine analysis and culture to exclude UTI.

(2) Cystogram to exam fistula and bladder abnormalities.

(3) Serum creatinine test to exclude renal dysfunction.

Table 7-7: Summary of Urinary Incontinence

Category / Clinical features, diagnosis, and treatment
1. Stress Incontinence #1 form of true urinary incontinence. **Etiology:** High bladder pressure due to increased intra-abdomen pressure. **Dx**: Loss of urine occurs in small spurts simultaneously with coughing or sneezing only during the day. P/E may reveal a cystocele. The Q-tip test is (+). **Tx**: 1. Conservative Tx: Kegel exercises and estrogen replacement in postmenopausal female. 2. Surgery: Elevation of the urethral sphincter (urethropexy), with > 85% success.
2. Irritative Incontinence **Etiology:** Involuntary rises in bladder pressure by irritation from infection, stone, tumor, or a foreign body. **Dx**: Above etiology, along with loss of urine occurring with urgency, frequency, and dysuria; day or night. P/E may show suprapubic tenderness or (-). **Tx**: Treat underlying cause.
3. Hypertonic (Urge) Incontinence **Etiology:** Involuntary rises in bladder pressure occur from idiopathic detrusor contractions that cannot be suppressed voluntarily. **Dx**: Urgent loss of urine occurs in large amounts usually without warning; day or night. P/E, urinary analysis and culture are all normal. Cystometric studies show normal residual volume, but involuntary detrusor contractions are present even with small volumes of urine. **Tx:** An anticholinergic or NSAID to inhibit detrusor contractions; TCA; Ca-R blocker.
4. Hypotonic (Overflow) Incontinence **Etiology:** Bladder pressure rises gradually from an overdistended, hypotonic bladder. Involuntary urine loss occurs when the bladder pressure exceeds the urethral pressure. **Dx**: Pelvic fullness, with intermittent loss of urine in small amounts both day and night. P/E, urinary analysis and culture may be normal. Cystometric studies will show markedly increased residual volume without involuntary detrusor contractions. **Tx**: Intermittent self-catheterization may be necessary. Stop offending drugs. Use cholinergics to stimulate bladder contractions and an alpha-R blocker (tamsulosin) to relax the bladder neck.

---

5. Total Incontinence

Etiology: Lost sphincter efficiency (damaged by surgery, neurologic injury, cancer); UT defects, etc.

Dx: Uncontrolled urine loss at all times and in all positions.

Tx: Surgery.

Male Infertility

Definition: The inability to achieve pregnancy in one year of normal sexual activities without contraception. It affects 15% of couples, and male factors account for 40% of infertility among couples.

Essentials of diagnosis

1. A **full history** of the couple is essential, including drug effects, surgeries, infections, injuries, poor coital skills, and psychosocial factors.

2. **P/E**: Search anatomic defects—hypospadias, epispadias, varicocele, etc.

3. **Necessary lab tests**: CBC, urine analysis, testing for STD, antisperm AB, and thyroid function.

4. **Ejaculation analysis**: It's the most important fertility testing. Normal volume is 1.5-5 mL; < 25 million/mL is abnormal. Semen should be examined within 1-2 hours after collection.

Treatment

1. Education: Proper timing for intercourse in relation to the female reproductive cycle.

2. Endocrine therapy is for patient with pituitary disease. Surgery is needed for anatomic defect.

3. Special technology: Intrauterine insemination or in vitro fertilization can be used for patients with low sperm counts.

Chapter 7: High-yield Questions (HYQ)

1. A 30 y/o female has severe diarrhea 1 week after receiving antibiotic treatment for acute asthma and pneumonia. Her vital signs are stable. Blood gases and biochemistry show $PO_2 = 90$ and $PCO_2 = 34$ (mmHg), $[HCO_3^-] = 22$ mEq/L, and pH = 7.4. What's her acid-base status?

A. Normal with compensation   B. Respiratory alkalosis   C. Metabolic acidosis

D. Mixed respiratory acidosis and metabolic alkalosis

E. Mixed respiratory alkalosis and metabolic acidosis

2. A 30 y/o man is brought to the ER for a grand mal seizure. His vital signs are stable, with mild tachypnea and tachycardia. There are no other abnormal findings. What's his most likely acid-base status?

A. Low pH, PCO_2, and HCO_3^-

B. High pH, PCO_2, and HCO_3^-

C. Low pH and HCO_3^-, high PCO_2

D. Low pH and PCO_2, high HCO_3^-

E. Low pH, high PCO_2 and HCO_3^-

3. What type of acid-base disorder will be present for triple diseases with severe pneumonia, asthma, or coughing, along with diabetic ketosis and vomiting?

A. Respiratory alkalosis with normal metabolic compensation

B. Mixed respiratory alkalosis and metabolic acidosis

C. Mixed respiratory alkalosis and metabolic alkalosis

D. Metabolic acidosis and metabolic alkalosis mixed

E. Mixed respiratory alkalosis, metabolic acidosis, and metabolic alkalosis

4. A 50 y/o man is diagnosed with chronic hepatitis B and cirrhosis, complicated by renal dysfunction. Lab tests reveal $PO_2 = 95$, $PCO_2 = 33$ (mmHg), serum K = 3.3 (mEq/L), $[HCO_3^-] = 14$ (mEq/L), AG = 14, pH = 7.2; urine pH = 5.0, urine protein is (+), and KCl is increased. What's the most likely diagnosis (Dx)?

A. Non-anion-gap (AG) metabolic acidosis

B. Type 1 RTA (renal tubular acidosis)

C. Type 2 RTA

D. Type 4 RTA

E. Respiratory and metabolic acidosis

5. A 60 y/o woman is diagnosed with chronic renal disease. Lab results: $PO_2 = 95$, $PCO_2 = 33$ (mmHg), serum Na = 135 mEq/L, K=5.7 mEq/L, $[HCO_3^-] = 14$, AG = 10, pH = 7.25; urine pH = 5.0, urine protein is (+) and KCl is decreased. What's the best next treatment (Tx)?

A. Thiazide   B. IV $NaHCO_3$ C. Large volume of IV fluid

D. Fludrocortisone   E. Blood dialysis

6. A 10 y/o boy in poor health condition presents with 5 days of fever, headache, and right ear pain followed by foot pain, rash, and cough with sputum and threads of blood. P/E shows T=38°C, nodular, erythematous rash on both feet, and stable vital signs. CXR reveals bilateral pulmonary lymph node infiltrates. Urinalysis shows RBC (+) and protein (+). Blood tests show lymphocytosis and cANCA (+). TB skin test is (+/-). The most likely diagnosis is

A. Acute pulmonary TB   B. Polyarteritis nodosa   C. Allergic interstitial nephritis

D. Goodpasture syndrome   E. Allergic pneumonia

7-12: Match the following clinical scenarios with the most likely diagnosis.

A. Minimal change disease

B. Granulomatosis with polyangiitis

C. Acute glomerulonephritis

D. Goodpasture syndrome

E. Allergic interstitial nephritis

F. Membranous nephropathy

G. Membranoproliferative glomerulonephritis

H. Mesangial proliferative glomerulonephritis

I. Focal segmental glomerulosclerosis

J. IgA nephropathy (Berger disease)

K. Idiopathic rapidly progressive glomerulonephritis

7. A 40 y/o female presents with abrupt onset fever, dyspnea, cough with sputum and threads of blood, dark urine, and oliguria. P/E shows T = 38°C and stable vital signs. CXR reveals diffuse pulmonary infiltrates. Urine analysis shows RBC casts. Blood tests reveal decreased RBC and increased BUN.

8. A 40 y/o female presents with fever, sore throat, abdominal pain, joint pain, generalized rash, and gross hematuria for 3 days. P/E results: T = 38°C, stable vital signs, multiple joint tenderness, and generalized purpura. Lab results: decreased RBC and platelets; numerous RBC but no WBC or protein in the urine; increased BUN and monoclonal IgA in the serum, and renal deposits of IgA, IgG, and IgM (by immunostaining).

9. A 60 y/o man presents with decreased appetite, variable hematuria and proteinuria, and recurrent deep foot pain that has been relieved by exercise and heparin for the past 2 months. He has had "chronic hepatitis" for the past few years. Lab tests reveal anemia, increased BUN, decreased IgG and C3, and anti-HCV (+). Renal biopsy shows "spike and dome" immune complex deposits.

10. A 10 y/o boy presents with generalized edema, hypertension (HTN), oliguria, and brown urine for the past 3 days. He had fever and a sore throat 1 month ago. Lab test results: hematuria, proteinuria, low RBC and serum C3, and high hyaluronidase titer.

11. Continued from Q10: Most of the boy's symptoms disappear after 3-months supportive Tx. However, follow-up lab tests reveal proteinuria, hypoalbuminemia, and hyperlipidemia. Renal biopsy by light microscopy is normal. His vital signs are normal.

12. A 35 y/o female with a 3-yr history of IV drug abuse presents with 3-month of abdominal discomfort, headache, dark frothy urine, and decreased energy, appetite and weight. P/E finds stable vital signs. Lab results: beta-hCG (+); Hb = 9.5 g/dL, WBC = 10,000/ul with predominant lymphocytes; increased BUN, HbsAg (+), anti-HBs (-), anti-HCV (+), LDL = 350 mg/dL, and decreased albumin, IgG, and C3; urinary casts of RBC and protein.

13. Continued with Q12: This patient is hospitalized and put on bed-rest for pregnancy. Apart from the treatment of her nephrotic syndrome, the most important next step in treatment is

A. alpha-interferon and ribavirin   B. regular heparin   C. coumadin

D. low-molecule-weight heparin   E. steroids

14. A 60 y/o woman with a 5-year history of diabetes and chronic glomerulonephritis is hospitalized for systemic edema, hypertension, fatigue, nausea, and mood changes. Lab test results: blood pH = 7.25, K = 5.8 mEq/L, Na = 130 mEq/L, total Ca = 8 mg/dL, [HCO_3^-] = 20 mEq/L, albumin = 3 g/dL, creatinine = 3.1 mg/dL, Hb = 9.5 g/dL; urine protein = +++, tubular cast (muddy), urine gravity = 1.010. What's the most appropriate next step of treatment?

A. ACE-I	B. Protein restriction	C. IV NaHCO₃
D. IV CaCl₂	E. IV albumin	F. Dialysis

15. A 60 y/o female complains of muscle weakness, fatigue, and polyuria for the past 3 week. P/E results are basically normal: HR = 80, BP = 120/80, T = 37.5°C. ECG shows U-wave and flattened T-wave. Blood test results: $[HCO_3^-]$ = 20, Na^+ = 130, Cl^- = 90, K^+ = 3.0 (mEq/L), increased renin level, and normal glucose concentration. What's the most likely Dx?

A. Conn syndrome   B. Bartter syndrome   C. Cushing syndrome

D. Type 1 RTA (renal tubular acidosis)   E. Type 4 RTA

16. A 65 y/o female has fatigue, weakness, constant left flank pain radiating to the groin, and blood in the urine twice in the past week. She has a history of recurrent UTIs with Klebsiella. P/E is unremarkable except for left flank pain upon percussion. Ultrasonography followed by IVP demonstrates a 5mm stone at the outlet of the left kidney. Urine analysis reveals that RBC, WBC, and protein are all (+), with alkaline pH. Apart from analgesia, what's the best next step?

A. Hydration with mild urinary acidification   B. Hydration with mild urinary alkalization

C. Anti-Klebsiella treatment   D. Shockwave lithotripsy

E. Percutaneous nephrolithotomy

17. A 60 y/o man presents with fatigue, weakness, discomfort of the left flank, and blood in the urine twice in the past month. P/E is unremarkable. Blood tests show Hb = 9.5 g/dL, total Ca = 13 mg/dL. Urine analysis reveals RBC (+) and protein (+). What's the best next step?

A. Plain X-ray   B. Ultrasonography   C. CT scan

D. IVP + cystoscopy   E. MRI

18. A 45 y/o man has fatigue, intermittent fever, headache, bilateral flank pain, and painful hematuria twice in a month. He has a 5-year history of smoking and alcohol use, and claims that his uncle died of a "similar disease." P/E finds T = 38.5°C, BP = 150/100 mmHg, and bilateral flank masses with pain upon percussion. Lab tests show WBC = 10,000/ul, Hb = 10.5 g/dL, and urinary RBC, WBC, protein, and esterase are all (+). The most likely Dx is

A. APKD   B. RCC   C. Simple renal cysts

D. Nephrolithiasis   E. Renal abscess

19. A 65 y/o man presents with urinary hesitancy, intermittent stream, and terminal dribbling and retention for the past 2 months. He smoked for 5 years before stopping 10 years ago. DRE (digital rectal exam) reveals a smoothly enlarged mass on the front wall without tenderness. Urine analysis shows protein (1+). What's the best next step?

A. Ultrasound-guided biopsy of the mass   B. PSA testing

C. Terazosin   D. Tamsulosin

E. Finasteride   F. Surgical resection.

20. A 72 y/o man presents with urinary hesitancy and retention, Wt loss, and back pain for the past 3 months. DRE reveals a firm nodule on the left side without tenderness, and an inflated bladder. 300 ml of urine is led out through a catheter. The best next step is

A. Bone Scint-scan   B. PSA + FNB   C. Orchiectomy

D. Radical prostectomy   E. Leuprolide + flutamide

21. A 60 y/o man presents with a 10-year history of alcohol use and smoking, as well as recurrent UTIs for the past 3 months. He complains of urinary frequency and seeing blood at the end of urination twice in the past month. P/E and CBC are mostly normal. Urine analysis confirms RBC and WBC in the urine. The best next step is

A. Cystoscopy   B. IVP   C. Ultrasound

D. MRI   E. CT scan

22. A 15 y/o boy accidentally finds a painless nodule on the right testicle, which is confirmed by ultrasonography. Blood PLAP is markedly increased. A radical orchiectomy is done. What's the most likely biopsy report?

A. Seminoma (germinoma)   B. Embryonic carcinoma   C. Choriocarcinoma

D. Nongerminal tumor   E. Dysgerminoma

23. A 60 y/o female presents with 2 months of minor urinary incontinence when sneezing during the day. She has given birth to five children throughout her lifetime. P/E reveals a cystocele. The Q-tip test is (+). Urine analysis shows protein (1+); no RBC or WBC. What's the best next treatment?

A. Urethropexy   B. Kegel exercise and estrogen replacement

C. Cholinergics   D. Anticholinergics   E. Etiologic treatment

24. A 65 y/o man presents with status epilepticus after progressive headache for the past 3 months. He has years of history of smoking, alcohol drinking, and 3-4 hour's daily use of cellular phone. P/E shows that his vital signs are about normal, his muscles are tender, and urine is dark. The best next step is to perform

A. ECG   B. CT scan of the head   C. serum CPK test

D. urine myoglobin test   E. dipstick urinalysis

25. A 66 y/o man presents with epigastric burning pain, fever, nausea, and vomiting for the past 3 months. His HIV is (+). He has an upper GI CT followed by endoscopy and bacterial culture, which shows Gram⁻ rods and Candida a. He is started on cyclosporine, gentamicin, vancomycin, and amphotericin B. On the third day, his BUN and creatinine levels are markedly elevated. The most likely cause of the acute kidney injury or tubular necrosis is

A. cyclosporine   B. gentamicin   C. vancomycin

D. amphotericin B   E. contrast media

Answers and Explanations

1. (E). The asthma and pneumonia with respiratory (Resp) compensation caused her respiratory alkalosis, and severe diarrhea caused her metabolic acidosis. Lab tests support 'E'. Normal (Nl) pH does not always mean normal (Nl) acid-base status.

2. (A). Like vigorous exercise and ischemia, a grand mal seizure causes lactate (Metabolic) acidosis with respiratory compensation. pH, P_{CO2} and HCO_3^- will all decrease, and P_{O2} will increase. For seizure-induced acidosis, most patients recover in 1 hour and no IV treatment (Tx) is needed.

3. (E). Respiratory alkalosis, metabolic acidosis, and metabolic alkalosis mixed, pH, P_{CO2} and P_{O2} may be normal (Nl). Tx should be toward the major causes and aided by O_2 supplement, IV saline, and monitoring of blood gases, pH and chemistry. $NaHCO_3$ is usually only given when pH < 7.20.

4. (C). This is Type 2 RTA, a defect of $KHCO_3$ reabsorption. Urine pH<5.3; serum K is low; urine K is high. Respiratory alkalosis is present here. Tx: Supply $KHCO_3$ +/- thiazide.

5. (D). This is Type 4 RTA due to aldosterone insufficiency, most common in CRF. Fludrocortisone is the best Tx to correct aldosterone deficiency, hyper-K, and hypo-Na. $NaHCO_3$ (when pH < 7.2) and K restriction are also good steps of Tx. 'A' and 'C' may worsen hypo-Na. It is too early for choice 'E'.

6. (B). The history is more typical of Wegener granulomatosis, a form of polyarteritis nodosa. 'D' has more diffuse pulmonary infiltrates and signs of renal failure. 'A' is more chronic and does not typically have hematuria or cANCA (+). "C and E" mostly have increased IgE and eosinophils in the blood, etc. TB skin test (+) only indicates a history of TB contact.

7. (D). A typical case of Goodpasture syndrome. 'C' usually has an URI 2-3 weeks prior to signs of hypertension, hematuria, and renal compromise. 'K' is an idiopathic form of severe glomerulonephritis characterized by abundant crescent formation, acute renal failure, and (+) pANCA without immune deposits.

8. (J). IgA nephropathy is the most common glomerulonephritis in adults; associated with infection, Henoch-Schonlein purpura, joint pain, and gross hematuria. Steroid Tx helps in acute flares.

9. (F). It's most likely membranous nephropathy, the most common form of adult glomerulonephropathy. It's associated with hepatitis B and C, syphilis, malaria, autoimmune disease, cancer, and drugs (gold, penicillamine); typically with low serum IgG, C_3, and anti-thrombin III. Membranoproliferative glomerulonephritis is a chronic glomerulonephritis that share mixed nephritic and nephrotic features and microscopic findings, with low serum C_3 and immune complex deposits.

10. (C). Typical post-infectious glomerulonephritis following a Strep-A infection. Biopsy usually shows lumpy-bumpy immune deposits, but these may not be necessary for Dx. Supportive Tx is adequate.

11. (A). Minimal change disease is the most common form of nephrotic syndrome in childhood. EM can show characteristic fusion of foot processes, but this is not necessary for Dx in most cases. Steroid Tx is very effective.

12. (I). Focal segmental glomerulosclerosis; renal biopsy will show segmental immune deposits. 'F' is the most common form in adults, associated with hepatitis B & C, SLE, drugs, etc; EM shows "spike and dome" deposits on the GBM; it is less likely with hematuria and ARF. "G and H" can have variable and similar presentations as 'I', but are less likely than 'I' with IVDA.

13. (D). Since she's at double risks for DVT and PE because of hypercoagulability secondary to urinary antithrombin III loss and pregnancy, patient needs long-term LMWH during her pregnancy. 'A' is the typical Tx for hepatitis B and C. "B, C, and E" are incorrect therapeutic strategies with pregnancy.

14. (D). This is a case of end-stage CRF, and all Tx options are potentially needed to correct the multiple disorders. Since her K is at a dangerously high level, IV $CaCl_2$ is the best initial Tx. ACE Inh is important to reduce mortality, but may worsen renal function when creatinine is > 3 and urine protein > (+++) with HTN. Dialysis is needed if the following are still present after the above Tx: acidosis, uremic syndrome, K > 6.5 mEq/L, etc.

15. (B). Bartter syndrome: Primary deficiency in NaCl reabsorption from Loop of Henle, causing high renin and aldosterone but Nl BP. 'A' is primary hyperaldosteronism, with serum hypo-K and hyper-Na, and increased BP. Type 1 RTA: deficiency in NH4Cl and H$^+$ secretion, with serum hypo-K but Nl or high NaCl. Type 4 RTA: aldosterone insufficiency, most common type in CRF, with high serum KCl but low Na.

16. (A). It's most likely a struvite stone, caused by UTIs with urease-producing organisms (Proteus, Staph., Pseudomonas, and Klebsiella) in highly alkaline urine. Because the stone size is < 6mm, 'A' is the best initial Tx. For stones > 0.6-2cm, "D or E" can be used. 'C' is better determined after culture and sensitivity testing of the urine.

17. (B). This is suspected RCC. Diagnostic steps: 1) If no mass is palpable, ultrasound is the first diagnostic test. 2) If P/E reveals a mass: CT can be the best initial exam. 3) IVP with cystoscopy is the most precise method to define the tumor (and stones, cysts). X-ray is a good initial tool for kidney stones. MRI is the best tool for most tumors but not for RCC.

18. (A). This is most likely APKD with a positive family history, flank pain with bilateral masses, hematuria, infections, and possible calculi. Esterase (+) indicates poly-WBC. U/S or CT scan confirms Dx. RCC is more likely with a single mass, older age and without family history. 'C' usually has milder symptoms, is unilateral, and has no family history. 'D' is probably part of the disease process here. 'E' would present with a history of exposure to a causative source, a unilateral mass, and higher fever and WBC.

19. (D). This is most likely moderate BPH, best treated with a new alpha-R blocker (tamsulosin) with high selectivity and least S/E. Terazosin is old and has more S/E. Finasteride (5-alpha-reductase Inh) is also effective in reducing blood flow and obstruction. Milder cases can be best managed by watchful waiting for shrinkage. Prostectomy is indicated after the above medications fail to alleviate symptoms. "A and B" are indicated when prostate cancer is suspected.

20. (E). This patient is > 70 y/a and has advanced prostate cancer with bone metastasis and urinary retention, therefore 'E' is the best initial Tx (GnRH agonist + androgen-R blocker). If it's milder, he may only need symptomatic Tx. All "A, B, C, and D" can be spared due to his old age but are indicated if he is < 70 y/a.

21. (A). Bladder cancer is highly suspected, and cystoscopy with biopsy is the best Dx means. IVP is perhaps the second best, together with CT, ultrasound or MRI, to determine the kidney lesions. Tx depends on staging.

22. (A). "A, B, and C" are Germ cell tumors (95%): Seminoma—Marker: placental alkaline phosphatase (PLAP); 'B'—alpha-FP markedly increased, beta-hCG increased in 50% of cases; 'C'—beta-hCG markedly increased. Nongerminal ('D') —Leydig-C, Sertoli-C, and gonadoblastoma; mostly with increased testosterone. Dysgerminoma ('E') —usually a type of ovarian tumor, with increased LDH, beta-hCG, and estrogen.

23. (B). This is typical of stress incontinence, the most common form of true urinary incontinence; best treated with Kegel exercises and estrogen replacement (> 50 y/a) female. If it fails, 'A' is indicated. 'C' is for hypotonic incontinence. 'D' is for hypertonic incontinence. 'E' is for irritative incontinence (infections, etc.).

24. (A). The patient is in status seizure with rhabdomyolysis—myoglobinuria most likely induced by an intracranial tumor. ECG is the best initial step here to detect the life-threatening hyperkalemia. Other options all need to be performed to confirm the diagnosis but hyperkalemia is a more risky and urgent issue in this patient.

25. (E). This patient most likely has acute tubular necrosis and AKI caused by the contrast media with the CT scan for infectious esophagitis. Cyclosporine, gentamicin, vancomycin, and amphotericin B are all nephrotoxic in certain extent, but they may need to take more than 5 days to result in renal failure rather than 2-3 days.

Chapter 8

DISEASES OF THE MUSCULOSKELETAL SYSTEM
AND CONNECTIVE TISSUE

PEARLS—Important Diagnostic Points for Chapter 8

1. Acute or chronic course

(1) Acute: Usually with a brief history of joint pain over 1-2 days, e.g., septic arthritis (see Chapter 1) and crystal-induced arthritis (gout and pseudogout).

(2) Chronic: History of joint pain over months and years [osteoarthritis (OA) and rheumatoid arthritis (RA)].

2. Joint distribution—Four basic patterns:

(1) Polyarticular symmetric: RA and SLE; may also be in Parv-B19 and hepatitis B infection.
(2) Monoarticular arthritis: OA, gout, and septic arthritis.
(3) Oligoarticular asymmetric: commonly with ankylosing spondylitis.
(4) Migratory arthropathy: seen in rheumatic fever, gonococcal arthritis, and Lyme disease.

3. Evidence of inflammation

(1) With inflammation: as in infectious arthritis, RA, SLE, gout & pseudogout, reactive arthritis, ankylosing spondylitis, etc; red, warm, erythematous joints; high ESR, the synovial fluid WBC count > 2000/uL (if purulent, WBC > 100,000/uL).

(2) Without inflammation: as in OA, osteoporosis, fibromyalgia, trauma, osteocondromatosis, osteocondritis dissecans, neuropathic arthropathy, hypertrophic osteoarthropathy, etc; normal ESR, the synovial fluid WBC count < 2000/uL.

4. Evidence of systemic manifestations

SLE: Involving the lungs (pleural effusions), kidneys (proteinuria and renal failure), CNS (vasculitis, strokes, and personality change), skin (malar rash with photosensitivity), and blood (hemolytic anemia and thrombocytopenia).

Sjogren syndrome: With keratoconjunctivitis, sicca (dry eyes and dry mouth), and parotid enlargement.

Systemic sclerosis: With skin sclerosis and Raynaud phenomenon.

5. Specific antibodies (Ab)

Anti-nuclear antibody: Highly sensitive for SLE.

Anti-ds-DNA (native DNA): Highly specific for SLE and lupus nephritis.

Specific Antibodies in MSK disease

Anti-SM: Also specific for SLE.

Anti-histone: Highly specific for drug-induced lupus (95% of cases).

Anti-Ro/SSA: Sensitive in neonatal lupus, Sjogren syndrome, and other connective diseases, but not specific.

Anti-LA/SSB: Highly specific for Sjogren syndrome.

Anticentromere: Highly specific for CREST syndrome.

Anti-RNP: 100% positive in mixed connective tissue disease (MCTD).

Antineutrophil cytoplasmic antibody (ANCA): Against certain proteins in the cytoplasm of neutrophils.

Cytoplasmic (c) ANCA (anti-proteinase-3 or anti-PR3 antibody) is seen in > 90% of patients with granulomatosis with polyangiitis (Wegener granulomatosis).

Perinuclear (p) ANCA (anti-myeloperoxidase antibody) is seen in > 60% of patients with microscopic polyangiitis or Churg-Strauss syndrome.

DEGENERATIVE AND CRYSTAL-INDUCED ARTHRITIS

Osteoarthritis (OA)

It's the most common chronic, degenerative joint disease characterized by **noninflammatory arthropathy** of the synovial joints, degeneration of the cartilage (due to wear and tear), and secondary bone hypertrophy. Major risk factors include age > 65, female gender, obesity, family history, and joint trauma (repeated occupational microtrauma and macrotrauma). Most cases are idiopathic. Some are secondary to other diseases (diabetes, gout, acromegaly, hemochromatosis, etc.).
[world: 740 handwritten above "age > 65"]

Essentials of diagnosis

1. Joint pain (monoarticular, insidious, deep, dull ache) and crepitation mainly involving weight-bearing joints (#1 is the knee; then the hip, and lumbar spine), and finger joints (**PIPs and DIPs**), **worsened with exercise and relieved by rest**; morning stiffness < 30 min; limited range of motion (late stage).

2. Joint lesions are asymmetric and monoarticular, and progressive slowly and irreversibly. Usually there are no systemic manifestations, erythema, warmth, or swelling. Other findings include sclerosis of subchondral bony end-plates adjacent to diseased cartilage, subchondral cysts, etc.

3. **Lab tests:** (1) **X-ray:** 1) Joint space narrowing; 2) **Osteophytes** (**Image 59**; in PIPs are **Bouchard's nodes**; in DIPs are **Heberden's nodes**). (2) Synovial fluid test is mostly normal (straw color, WBC < 2000/uL). All blood tests are normal. Abnormal results indicate possible complications. (3) MRI of the spine may be indicated if neurologic signs are found.

Treatment

—Aimed at reducing pain and maintaining mobility.

Osteoarthritis
— quadriceps strengthening exercises

1. **Supportive therapies**: They all help reduce weight and correct poor posture to decrease joint loading. Physical therapy and exercise programs are effective (swimming is the best). Advise patient to lose weight, rest, and avoid overuse of the joint.

2. **Palliative medicines**: A topical NSAID (**duloxetine or capsaicin gel**) should be initially used in most cases. NSAIDs can relieve symptoms but cannot stop the disease progression. If it's an inflammatory OA or with severe pain, a strong NSAID (**naproxen**) can be used. If NSAIDs are ineffective or intolerant, a cyclooxygenase-2 (COX-2) inhibitor (celecoxib or etoricoxib) is suggested. If the above treatment is still ineffective, intra-articular injection of corticosteroids is helpful (but should not be used frequently). Glucosamine and chondroitin may be variably helpful with OA.

3. Surgical joint replacement and arthroplasty: Reserved for advanced cases with poor life quality. It should be delayed as long as possible because a revision may be needed 10-15 years after the surgery.

Crystal-induced Arthropathies

It's a group of disease caused by microcrystal deposition in joints, by monosodium urate, Ca-pyrophosphate (CPPD), Ca-oxalate, and Ca-hydroxyapatite. Despite differences in crystal morphology, they have similar clinical presentations and can only be distinguished by synovial fluid analysis (**SFA**).

Gouty Arthritis

Gout is a kind of crystal-induced arthritis that occurs when uric acid builds up in blood and causes joint inflammation. Acute gout is a painful flare that typically affects one joint (#1 is the toe). Chronic gout is repeated episodes of painful inflammation, which may involve more than one joint.

Essentials of diagnosis

1. Typically a middle-aged man presents with acute monoarthritis. **The most common site is the first MTP joint and the first toe—podagra).** The first **acute episode** usually occurs as sudden, severe, excruciating pain of the big toe at night, with warmness, redness and tenderness, often after alcohol drinking, and wakes the patient from sleep. Fever is common and the gouty attack may resemble infectious arthritis or cellulitis, which requires arthrocentesis for differentiation. The joint pain can disappear spontaneously in a few days.

2. Precipitating factors include excessive alcohol ingestion, trauma, surgery, infection, steroid withdrawal, drugs (diuretics, anti-TB medicines), and serious disease.

3. **Chronic gout**: As gout becomes chronic, multiple joints may be involved, with possible deposition of urate crystals with foreign body reaction in soft tissues (**tophi**) and kidneys (uric acid **nephrolithiasis**). Long asymptomatic periods between attacks are commonly seen.

4. **Lab tests: SFA is the best diagnostic test, typically negatively birefringent crystals and monosodium urate are identified (+).** The serum uric acid during the acute attack may be normal or low, whereas many people with elevated serum uric acid levels never develop gout. Thus, the serum **uric acid level is not an accurate diagnostic test** for acute gouty arthritis.

Treatment

1. **Acute gout**: (1) **No.1 medicine is indomethacin or naproxen (a stronger NSAID), with dramatic therapeutic response.** (2) **Colchicine or glucocorticoids is the second best in acute gout flares and effective in preventing attacks.** (3) Intraarticular steroids is a good option for elderly patient who cannot tolerate NSAIDs or colchicine. The goal of therapy is to decrease inflammation and fluctuations in urate levels, and prevent erosions and joint destruction.

2. **Chronic gout—hypouricemic therapy**: To decrease urate levels for long-term stability. It is usually required for life in patients with recurrent gouty attacks not corrected by other treatment. **Probenecid and sulfinpyrazone** increase renal excretion of the urate and are used in the low-producers (> 80% of adults). **Allopurinol** is used in overproducers or patients with renal stones or failure. Monitoring the urate level is helpful in following the effects of hypouricemic treatment.

3. **Diet**: **Decrease alcohol** consumption (particularly beer), **high-purine foods** (such as meat and seafood), and weight. **Stop thiazides, aspirin, and niacin.**

Adverse effects of chronic treatment

Uricosuric agents: Hypersensitivity (rash, hemolysis, allergic interstitial nephritis).

Colchicine: May suppress WBC production.

Allopurinol: May cause epidermal necrolysis or Steven-Johnson syndrome.

Calcium Pyrophosphate Deposit Disease ("Pseudogout")

It's **CPP** crystal deposition (**CPPD**) in joints with preexisting damage in elderly patients, usually including **pseudogout, chondrocalcinosis, and pyrophosphate arthropathy**. It is almost always **accompanied by chondrocalcinosis,** which is the presence of Ca-containing salts in the affected articular cartilages.

Associated diseases or risk factors include "**4 Hs**": Hyper-PTH, Hyper-iron (hemochromatosis), Hypo-phosphate (PO4), and Hypo-Mg.

Essentials of diagnosis

1. Similar, acute, recurrent joint pain with warmness and welling as with gout. **The knee (and wrist) is the most common site** affected. The DIP and PIP are not affected. It may also be asymptomatic and chronic.

2. Diagnosis is confirmed by finding typical rectangular, rhomboid, and **positively birefringent crystals** on SFA. Uric acid levels are normal. X-ray may reveal linear radiodense deposits (calcification) in joint menisci or articular cartilage (chondrocalcinosis).

Treatment

Basically it's the same as for gout—**naproxen is the best initial treatment**. Intraarticular steroid is a good option for severe cases and elderly patients who cannot tolerate NSAIDs or colchicine. Low-dose **colchicine can prevent** subsequent attacks.

SERONEGATIVE ARTHRITIS

The seronegative arthritis family is differentiated from rheumatoid arthritis in that its RF is negative, more prevalent in males, sharing similar clinical features of arthritis, and associated with HLA B27 allele and possibly similar pathogenesis.

The common four seronegative arthropathies are summarized in Table 8-1 below.

Table 8-1: Summary of Seronegative Arthritis

Disease / Clinical features, diagnosis, and treatment
Ankylosing Spondylitis 1. It primarily affects the axial skeleton and peripheral joints (arthritis); male > female; starting around 30 y/a. 2. **Chronic low back pain + morning stiffness that worsen at rest and improve with activity**, with progressive limitation of back motion and chest expansion. 3. P/E shows positive **Schober test** (decreased spine flexibility). 4. Extra-joint: anterior uveitis (20%), aortic insufficiency (may cause CHF), and 3rd-degree cardiac A-V block. **Dx**: **X-ray** is the key means to show evidence of **sacroiliitis** (early) and eventual **fusing** of the sacroiliac joint and **bamboo spine** (late). **HLA B27 is (+)** and rheumatoid factor is (-). **Tx**: **Indomethacin or naproxen, COX-2 inhibitors (celecoxib, etoricoxib), or TNF inhibitors** (etanercept, adalimumab, infliximab) plus physical therapy and exercise can all alleviate symptoms. Most patients still have persistent symptoms for decades despite treatment.
Reactive Arthritis (Reiter Syndrome) 50-80% of cases are **HLA B27 (+)**. It usually occurs following (1) an STD in young men (by chlamydia, ureaplasma); (2) an inflammatory bowel disease (ulcerative colitis and Crohn disease); (3) a GI infection (**Enteropathic arthropathy**): caused by enteroinvasive Campylobacter (No.1), Shigella, or Salmonella. **Clinical features**: **Nongonococcal urethritis followed by conjunctivitis, oligoarthritis, and mucocutaneous disease** (keratoderma blennorrhagica, circinate balanitis, and oral or genital ulcers). Skin lesions of **pyoderma** can be characteristic of the enteropathic arthropathy. Symptoms may be more severe in HIV (+) patients. **Dx**: Based on clinical manifestations and exclusion of septic arthritis. **Tx**: **The same as for ankylosing spondylitis—NSAIDs** +/- sulfasalazine. Controlling the intestinal inflammation/infection and STD with related antibiotics usually eliminates the peripheral arthritis. The recovery is better with 3-4 weeks of antibiotics.
Psoriatic Arthritis (Image 60) 1. Psoriasis precedes onset of arthritis in 80% of cases. 2. It commonly involves the **distal interphalangeal joints** when associated with **psoriatic nail** disease (nail pitting, "oil spot", and onycholysis); may cause characteristic **sausage-shaped digits** and polyarthritis that resemble rheumatoid arthritis; ankylosis of the sacroiliac joints may occur. **Dx**: Based on clinical manifestations. **Tx**: NSAIDs +/- methotrexate or TNF inhibitors (if refractory).

AUTOIMMUNE CONNECTIVE TISSUE DISEASES

Rheumatoid Arthritis (RA)

It's a systemic autoimmune disease characterized by **chronic, destructive, symmetric, inflammatory arthritis and synovitis**. The intense joint inflammation can eventually destroy cartilage and cause bone erosions and joint deformity.

Etiology

Unknown. It may be associated with **HLA-DR4**, infection (mycoplasma, parvovirus), and smoking in a susceptible host. Female > male by 3 times, mostly at age 35-50.

Pathogenesis

1. Initiation phase of nonspecific inflammation.

2. Amplification phase resulting from T-cell activation.

3. Late stage of chronic inflammation and tissue injury. Symptoms of RA and other immune-mediated diseases will be alleviated with HIV infection due to low T-cell activities.

Essentials of diagnosis

1. 2/3 patients initially have systemic symptoms: Fatigue, weakness, anorexia, *↑ temp* and weight loss before the onset of the arthritis.

2. Typical joint presentations are insidious onset of morning stiffness for > 30 min along with *, improves w Activity* painful, warm, symmetric swelling of three joints—**wrists, MCPs, and PIPs** (not DIP; **Image 61**) for more than 6 weeks. Other joints (elbows, ankles, knees, shoulders) may also be involved.

3. Extraarticular manifestations: Some may have damage to the ligaments and tendons with *RA accels. osteoporosis* deformity, rheumatoid nodules (finger knuckles, elbow olecranon, and Achilles tendon, etc), Boutonniere deformity, Swan-neck deformity, Felty's syndrome, and Caplan syndrome. *Trigger finger, carpal tunnel sx., episcleritis*

4. **Lab tests**: **Rheumatoid factor (RF) is (+) in >75%** cases. RF is an IgM antibody against IgG Fc. ESR is high. Hb is low. **X-ray** shows soft tissue swelling (early), **joint erosions,** and space narrowing (late). *anti-CCP Ab is more specific*

Treatment

1. NSAIDs (**Naproxen**) are effective on inflammatory symptoms as the initial treatment, but are restricted due to its frequent GI side effects (S/E).

2. Start the disease-modifying antirheumatic drugs (**DMARDs**) early to add to or replace NSAIDs.

(1) **First-line medicines are methotrexate, chloroquine**, sulfasalazine, and azathioprine. Methotrexate is very effective in alleviating the inflammation and rheumatoid nodules.

Adverse effects: Hepatitis or hepatic fibrosis, pneumonitis, etc.; monitoring CBC and LFTs per 4-8 weeks. Hydroxychloroquine may cause retinopathy and thus requires regular eye exams.

RA

(2) Second-line DMARDs are COX-2 inhibitors (celecoxib and etoricoxib), rituximab (anti-CD20), and leflunomide. They have less toxicity and better tolerance for aged patients.

3. Other 2nd-line medicines include steroids and gold-salts. Gold may cause rash, mild WBC decrease, and nephritic syndrome. Routine renal, urinary and blood tests must be performed. Once itchy rash and proteinuria are found, gold-salts must be stopped.

Complications

More common with aggressive status of the disease: High titers of RF, diffuse rheumatoid nodules, early joint erosions, late age of onset, and certain subtypes of the HLA-DR4.

Juvenile Idiopathic Arthritis (JIA)   *chronic, inflamm, chronic joint pain, swelling, stiffness often worsen the Am*

Formerly called "**Juvenile rheumatoid arthritis**", it is a non-migratory rheumatoid arthritis occurring during childhood and lasting mostly for a few months. 95 percent of cases resolve by puberty. There are three subtypes. *enthesitis-related JIA : tenderness & swelling @ insertion point of achilles tendon into calcaneus*

RASH! Arthritis > 6weeks

1. **Systemic JIA**: High fever, joint pain (arthritis), erythematous or salmon-colored rashes or nodules, pericarditis, hepatosplenomegaly, and increased ESR, WBC, and platelet. It is probably an autoinflammatory disorder rather than an autoimmune disorder like other types of JIA.

Uveitis: intraocular inflamm. in pts w oligoarticular JIA. ANA = risk factor.

2. **Polyarticular type**: Multiple, inflamed, symmetric arthritis in small joints, resembling adult RA; with less systemic symptoms. *≥ 5 joints. within 6 months dz onset t. Symmetric involvement elbows, knees, wrists, ankles, most often. NO FEVER, RASH, or systemic sx in polyarticular.*

3. **Pauciarticular type**: Chronic arthritis usually involving a few big, weight-bearing joints.

(1) In ANA (+) female: Increased risk of iridocyclitis (may cause blindness without treatment).

(2) In HLA B27 (+) male: Increased risk of ankylosing spondylitis.

Diagnosis

Diagnosis is mainly based on clinical features and no specific tests are available. ESR and WBC are usually increased but RF is negative in 75 percent of cases. Thus, the diagnosis is sometimes difficult.

Treatment   *intraarticular corticosteroids tx JIpn & swelling from inflamm arthritis (JIA, psoriatic A)*

1. An NSAID or steroid is used initially. If not effective, methotrexate is given as a 2nd-line drug.

2. Joint strengthening exercise and monitoring for iridocyclitis are important steps, too.

Systemic Lupus Erythematosus (SLE)

SLE is a systemic disease in which multiple organs and tissues are damaged by pathogenic auto-antibodies and immune complexes. Clinical courses vary.

Etiology

SLE

Unknown; **90 percent of cases occur in females**. The abnormal immune response may depend on interactions between a susceptible host and environmental factors. UV-B light is a common inducing factor.

Essentials of diagnosis

1. **Skin (Image 62): Malar rash**, discoid rash, photosensitivity, and oral ulcers.

2. **Arthritis:** Similar to that of RA but is **non-erosive**.

3. **Serositis:** Pleuritis or pericarditis.

4. **Renal:** Proteinuria.

5. **Neuropsychological:** Seizures or psychosis.

6. **Hematologic:** Hemolytic anemia, leukopenia, and thrombocytopenia.

7. **Immunologic**: **Specific anti-ds DNA and anti-SM** (anti-histone, anti-SSA) antibodies (+). Anti-ANA (nuclear antibody) has high sensitivity but low specificity. Complement C3 and C4 are decreased; VDRL is false (+).

Differential diagnosis

Pregnancy with SLE:

Fertility rates are normal but **spontaneous abortions and still-births are increased, which may be associated with anti-phospholipid antibody and placental infarcts. This is treated with low-molecular weight heparin (LMWH),** and steroids may be used safely to suppress the SLE flare. All pregnant patients with lupus need to be screened for SSA or anti-Ro antibody, because they cross the placenta and can cause neonatal lupus.

Drug-induced lupus:

It's a limited form of lupus occurring with exposure to certain drugs, commonly including **procainamide, hydralazine, isoniazid, and methyldopa**. It primarily presents with a rash and anti-histone antibody without major organ-system involvement, and resolves after the offending drug is removed.

Treatment

1. Avoid sun exposure or use sunscreen as needed.

2. NSAIDs are used initially for mild arthritis. **Chloroquine** is very effective for the lupus skin rashes. **Steroids** are good for acute exacerbations with major organ involvement. **Pulse IV cytotoxics** (azathioprine or cyclophosphamide) are the best for refractory cases with renal damage.

Prognosis

SLE has a varied clinical course, ranging from a mild illness to a rapidly progressive disease. Clinical remission after appropriate therapy is common. Poor prognostic factors include renal disease (eg, diffuse proliferative glomerulonephritis), hypertension, male sex, younger or older age, antiphospholipid antibody (+), low socioeconomic status, black race, and high overall disease activity.

Systemic Sclerosis (Scleroderma, SSc)

It's a chronic multisystem disease characterized by progressive tissue fibrosis and thickening of the skin caused by excessive deposition of type I and III collagen. It usually manifests as "CREST" syndrome, but can also involve extensive visceral organs (GI, GU, kidneys, lungs, and CVS). It's more common in 35-50 y/o women.

Essentials of diagnosis

1. Skin: Typical **symmetric skin thickening in the face and sclerodactyly in distal extremities** (**Image 43**), and Raynaud phenomenon due to decreased terminal vessels and blood supply.

2. GI: Esophageal dysmotility and achalasia, hypomotility and distension of the small and large intestine with formation of large diverticula.

3. Lung: Pulmonary fibrosis with restrictive lung disease and Cor pulmonale, which is the #1 cause of death in SSc.

4. Kidney: Mainly the scleroderma renal crisis, leading to malignant hypertension and acute renal failure, which can be effectively treated with ACE-I.

5. Immune marker: Scl-70 antibody (anti-topoisomerase-1) is highly specific for SSc but lowly sensitive, and is associated a poor prognosis.

Differential diagnosis

CREST syndrome:

It's a limited form of scleroderma with symmetric skin thickening, along with "**C**alcinosis, **R**aynaud's phenomenon, **E**sophageal dysmotility, **S**clerodactyly, and **T**elangiectasias." It's associated with specific anti-centromere antibody (diagnostic mark) and has a better prognosis than SSc.

Treatment

Only symptomatic treatment is available; no cure. For acute flares, steroids are effective. Specific organ-based treatments include that for skin, Raynaud phenomenon (Ca-chanel blockers), renal, gastro-intestinal, pulmonary, musculoskeletal, cardiac, and genitourinary manifestations. Cyclophosphamide may be used in patients with severe or progressive lung fibrosis. D-penicillamine may alleviate pathologic changes of the skin. For renal hypertension, ACE-Inh is the drug of choice.

Mixed Connective Tissue Disease (MCTD)

—It's a mixed autoimmune connective tissue disease or syndrome that **includes features of SLE, scleroderma, and polymyositis.** It is further characterized by the uniform presence of high titers of autoantibody anti-U1 ribonucleoprotein (RNP) and previously termed antibody to extractable nuclear antigen (anti-ENA).

Essentials of diagnosis

Mixed CT dz

1. MCTD has mixed features of SLE, polymyositis, SSc, and RA together.

2. **Anti-RNP is almost 100% (+), especially with SSc** and primary pulmonary hypertension. Anti-ENA and RF are mostly positive.

3. The diagnosis of MCTD is often complicated by the sequential occurrence of the characteristic overlapping features, often over several years. There is no single set of universal diagnostic criteria.

Differential diagnosis

Adult Still's disease:

It holds mixed features of RA + SLE + SSc without specific antibodies.

Treatment

MCTD is **mainly treated for its arthritis** with these medications in order: NSAIDs, antimalarials, low-dose prednisone (<10 mg/day), methotrexate, and trial of TNF inhibitor or modafinil. MCTD can be significantly alleviated by immunosuppressive therapies but is still incurable. The efficiency is dependent on specific therapies for SLE, scleroderma, or/and polymyositis. Ca-blockers and other symptomatic treatment may be needed.

Sjogren Syndrome

It's a chronic autoimmune disease characterized by LC infiltration of the exocrine glands, resulting in dry mouth (xerostomia) and dry eyes. It primarily presents alone, but can also follow other autoimmune disease (RA, SLE, or primary biliary cirrhosis), or progress to systemic disease involving major organs (lungs, kidneys, or lymph nodes—malignant lymphoma).

Essentials of diagnosis

1. Patient usually presents with itchy dry eyes ("sandy feeling" due to decreased tear and corneal destruction), dry mouth, and difficulty swallowing food. Patient may also have more dental caries and parotid enlargement.

2. **Lab tests**: Schirmer test will show decreased tear production. Rose Bengal stain will show corneal ulcerations. Antibodies—mostly ANA and anti-Ro (SSA) are (+), but anti-La (SSB) (+) is more specific (with lower sensitivity).

Treatment

Symptomatic treatment is considered. Topical use of artificial saliva or pilocarpine (if no response) and artificial tears are helpful. Serious (rare) complications such as vasculitis and neurologic disease probably require immunosuppressive agents. No cure is available.

common in pts w SLE

@ Antibodies: Lupis anticoagulant → can cause false⊕ VDRL/RPR
anticardiolipin
anti - B2 glycoprotein

false ⊕ aPTT

Antiphospholipid (Antibody) Syndrome

Antiphospholipid (antibody) syndrome (**APS**), also known as **Hughes syndrome** or **lupus anticoagulant syndrome**, is an autoimmune disorder characterized by hypercoagulable state and arterial, venous or small vessel thromboembolism and/or recurrent spontaneous abortions in healthy women, with persistent antibodies against phospholipids or cardiolipins and other abnormalities.

Clinical features

1. Hypercoagulable state, with recurrent thromboses in either the venous or arterial circulation.

2. Pregnancy-related complications such as miscarriage or stillbirth (particularly after the first trimester), preterm delivery, or severe preeclampsia.

3. APS usually occurs as a primary autoimmune disease, particularly associated with SLE. Its cutaneous abnormalities include livedo reticularis (#1), splinter hemorrhages, cutaneous necrosis, superficial vein thrombosis, digital gangrene, skin ulcerations, and lesions resembling vasculitis.

4. Patient commonly has thrombocytopenia, elevated PTT, and false RPR (+).

Treatment

anti-phospholipid ABs bind phospholipids & prevent them from inducing coagulation.

Lifelong anticoagulation with <u>warfarin</u> is recommended for patients with serious complications and recurrent potentials. Patients with SLE are also treated with hydroxychloroquine.

Idiopathic Inflammatory Myopathies—Polymyositis and Dermatomyositis

Polymyositis is a progressive systemic connective tissue disease characterized by muscle inflammation and association of autoimmune antibodies. A third of patients have skin lesion—dermatomyositis.

Essentials of diagnosis

1. **Polymyositis:** Mostly in > 35 y/o females. Patient usually presents with progressive, symmetric, proximal muscle pain and weakness (shoulder and hip) —difficulty lifting objects, combing hair, and getting up.

2. **Dermatomyositis: Polymyositis plus skin** lesion—typical signs are the heliotrope rash (purple-lilac discoloration) over sun-exposed areas (face, eyelids, and hands), Gottron papules (red scaly patches over the knuckles—PIP and MIP), and calcinosis in the chest. 10% of cases may be **associated with common malignancies** (breast, lung, colon, or prostate).

3. **Lab tests: The most sensitive** test is muscle enzymes (**CPK** and aldolase), which increase many folds. EMG shows fibrillations. Anti-Jo-l (+) indicates the autoimmune nature of the disease. Diagnosis is confirmed by muscle biopsy, which will show inflammatory lymphocytes (LC) and muscle degeneration.

Differential diagnosis

Polymyalgia rheumatica, fibromyalgia, chronic fatigue syndrome, etc.

<u>**Myasthenia gravis and Eaton-Lambert syndrome:**</u>

Polymyositis / dermatomyositis
myasthenia but Eaton

Fluctuating course of muscle weakness in the order of eyes, limb, and face, which is reversible by use of cholinergic drugs; ocular muscles are usually spared in polymyositis.

Treatment

1. **Low-dose steroids** can be initially used in early stage, mild cases.
2. **High-dose steroids** are effective in improving severe polymyositis and dermatomyositis.
3. Unresponsive patients can be treated with immunosuppressive drugs such as cyclophosphamide (inclusion-body myositis may be resistant to it) and IVIG. Cancer monitoring for patients with dermatomyositis is recommended.

VASCULITIS SYNDROMES

Polymyalgia Rheumatica

PMR is an inflammatory syndrome of the muscles with pain or stiffness, usually in the neck, shoulders, and hips. Etiology is unknown.

Essentials of diagnosis

1. Most common in elderly females; 50% of cases **coexist with giant cell arteritis** and share the same HLA haplotypes and similar pathogenesis.
2. **Asymmetric muscle pain and stiffness in the shoulder and pelvic girdle areas**, often associated with fever, pallor, weight loss, and malaise. Patient typically complains of "unable to find a comfortable position."
3. **Lab tests**: **Marked increase in ESR;** anemia. Muscle biopsy is usually normal.

Treatment

Low-dose prednisone (5-20 mg/d) is the effective therapy. If symptoms are severe or giant cell arteritis is coexistent, high-dose prednisone is indicated.

Giant Cell Arteritis—Temporal Arteritis

It's a **subacute granulomatous inflammation of the large vessels**, including the aorta, external carotid (particularly the temporal artery), and vertebral arteries. The worst complication is blindness secondary to occlusion of the central retinal artery (a branch of the internal carotid artery). It's commonly coexistent with polymyalgia rheumatica (50%) and > 50 y/o women.

Essentials of diagnosis

1. Typically a woman over age 50 presents with new, uni-/bilateral headache associated with temporal tenderness, jaw claudication, scalp pain, symptoms of polymyalgia rheumatica, and transient or permanent visual loss.
2. **Lab tests:** ESR < 100. **Temporal artery biopsy confirms diagnosis** (inflammation in the media and adventitia with lymphocytes, plasma cells, and giant cells).

Differential diagnosis

Churg-Strauss syndrome, histocytosis X (see Chapter 3—Respiratory Diseases).

Treatment

1. Immediate **high-dose prednisone** (60 mg/d for one month) plus low-dose aspirin are recommended without waiting for the biopsy results.

2. Follow-ups of periodic eye examinations.

Henoch–Schönlein Purpura   *IgA-mediated leukocytoclastic vasculitis*

Henoch–Schönlein purpura (**HSP**), also known as **immunoglobulin A vasculitis, anaphylactoid purpura**, or **purpura rheumatica, is the most common form of systemic vasculitis in children** and is characterized by deposition *mesangial* of immune complexes containing the antibody IgA. The disease is mostly self-limited and the etiology is unknown.

Essentials of diagnosis

- Nonblanching, symmetric LE, back, buttcheeks.

1. HSP is often preceded by an URI (upper respiratory infection) in children, followed by palpable purpura (small hemorrhages, **Image 58**), joint pain (arthritis), abdominal pain, and renal involvement *—similar to IgA nephropathy p. 285* (hematuria or proteinuria).   *arthralgia*

2. Lab tests: Neither thrombocytopenia nor coagulopathy is present. Diagnosis is usually clinical and confirmed by skin or kidney biopsy when necessary. *Normal or ↑Cr.*

Treatment   *hydration + NSAIDs*

The disease usually resolves within several weeks and only symptomatic treatment is needed. Corticosteroids may be needed when severe (especially extrarenal) manifestations are present.
± hospitalization   *↠ nephrotic, HTN, and Acute Renal failure.*

Polyarteritis Nodosa

Polyarteritis nodosa (**PAN**) **is polyarteritis of the medium-sized arteries** mostly involving the nervous system, GI tract, and the kidney; the lungs are spared. It may be an immune complex-mediated hypersensitivity reaction. Some cases are **associated with hepatitis B or C, HIV, and drug reactions**.

Essentials of diagnosis

1. Depending on the arteries involved, clinical features include fever, weakness, abdominal pain, myalgias, arthralgias, hypertension (renin-mediated), livedo reticularis, mononeuritis multiplex, anemia, and weight loss.

2. Lab tests: Elevated acute phase reactants (ESR or C-reactive protein or both). Fecal occult blood and p-ANCA may be positive.

3. Diagnosis is confirmed by biopsy of involved tissue.

Differential diagnosis

Granulomatosis with polyangiitis: See below.

Hypersensitivity vasculitis:

It's a **small-vessel vasculitis in response to a drug (penicillin, sulfa medicines), infection**, or other stimuli. **Skin lesions are the main signs—painful palpable purpura**, macules, or vesicles commonly on lower extremities after the associated stimulus. Systemic symptoms may be present—fever, fatigue, and weight loss. **Diagnosis** is made by biopsy of tissue. **Treatment** of choice is withdrawal of the offending agent and **steroids**. Prognosis is usually good—spontaneous remission is common.

Treatment

1. **High-dose prednisone** is initially required. In patients with moderate to severe disease (renal insufficiency, GI, cardiac, or neurologic damage), both glucocorticoids and azathioprine or methotrexate (rather than cyclophosphamide) are used.

2. Hypertension should be treated with ACEI. Associated HBV or HCV should be treated with antiviral agents.

3. Prognosis is usually poor. Complications such as infarction and aneurysms may occur.

Granulomatosis with Polyangiitis (Wegener Granulomatosis)

It's a **granulomatous inflammation of the respiratory tract with characteristic necrotizing vasculitis of small and medium-sized vessels, a form of polyarteritis nodosa**. It's a rare disease with unknown etiology.

Essentials of diagnosis

1. **Manifestations of upper respiratory infection:** Allergic rhinitis, sinusitis, oral lesions, otitis media, or mastoiditis.

2. **Manifestations of lower respiratory infection/inflammation: Fever, cough, and hemoptysis;** CXR showing bilateral pulmonary lymph node infiltrations.

3. **Renal vascular lesions: Necrotic glomerulonephritis; hematuria**.

4. Systemic lesions in the skin, joint, and eyes.

5. **Lab tests: Hematuria, c-ANCA (+)**, and evidence of cell-mediated immunoreactions. Tissue biopsy is the gold standard for diagnosis.

Treatment

1. **High-dose steroids plus cytotoxics** (methotrexate, cyclophosphamide, or rituximab) are the effective therapy for immediate remission, necessary for the urgent nature of the disease.

2. **Prognosis**: Early diagnosis and treatment can significantly improve prognosis. Recurrence following remission may occur.

Microscopic Polyangiitis

Microscopic Polyangiitis (**MPA**) is a pauci-immune **nongranulomatous necrotizing vasculitis, the most common cause of pulmonary-renal syndrome** (more than Goodpasture disease), pulmonary alveolar hemorrhage and glomerulonephritis. It typically affects small- and medium-sized blood vessels (arteries, veins, and capillaries). It may also overlap both polyarteritis nodosa and granulomatosis with polyangiitis.

Essentials of diagnosis

1. **Similar manifestations as other polyangiitis**—upper and lower respiratory infection and inflammation (fever, cough, and hemoptysis); renal vascular lesions (hematuria).

2. Some systemic skin, joint, and muscle lesions may exist.

3. **Lab tests**: 75% of cases are associated with **p-ANCA (+)**; c-ANCA (PR3-ANCA) may also be positive (30%).

Differential diagnosis

Granulomatosis with polyangiitis:

More often associated with chronic destructive upper respiratory tract disease; with granulomatous inflammation that is absent in MPA.

Treatment

1. Because symptoms are urgent, **prednisone and cyclophosphamide** are usually needed to treat pulmonary hemorrhage and glomerulonephritis. **Rituximab** is similarly effective as cyclosphosmide in treating ANCA-associated vasculitis.

2. **Prognosis: Early diagnosis and treatment can significantly improve prognosis**. Recurrence following remission is about 30%.

Eosinophilic Granulomatosis with Polyangiitis (EGPA, Churg-Strauss Syndrome)

EGPA, formerly called the Churg-Strauss syndrome or **allergic granulomatosis and angiitis**, is a rare systemic granulomatous vasculitis and pulmonary-renal syndrome characterized by chronic rhinosinusitis, asthma, and prominent peripheral blood eosinophilia. The exact etiology of EGPA is unknown. It mainly affects small vessels (capillaries, venules, arterioles).

Essentials of diagnosis

1. Patients typically present with **asthma, pulmonary infiltrates (cough and hemoptysis), erythematous rashes, and significant eosinophilia**. Systemic vasculitis may result in fever, weight loss, and painful lesions on the skin, joint, muscle, and nerve.

2. **Lab tests: Eosinophilia** ($\geq$ 1500 cells/mL and/or > 10% eosinophils on differential leukocyte count) and **positive p-ANCA (50-80%)** helps confirm diagnosis. **Biopsy** is the most accurate test.

Treatment

Corticosteroids +/- cyclophosphamide can effectively alleviate symptoms. Rituximab may be tried in resistant cases.

Takayasu Arteritis

It is a rare vasculitis of the aortic arch and its major branches, which may lead to artery stenosis. It's most commonly seen in young Asian women.

Essentials of diagnosis

1. Systemic symptoms include fever, night sweats, malaise, arthralgias, fatigue, etc.
2. Chest pain and tenderness, and ischemic manifestations over affected vessels.
3. Absent pulse in carotid, radial, or ulnar arteries; with possible aortic regurgitation.
4. Diagnosis is made by arteriogram.
5. Severe complications include limb ischemia, aortic aneurysms or regurgitation, stroke, and secondary hypertension (due to renal artery stenosis). The presence or absence of these complications determines prognosis.

Treatment

1. Corticosteroids and anti-hypertensive therapies are initially used to help relieve symptoms. Methotrexate, azathioprine or anti-TNF agents may be used for severe cases.
2. Surgery or angioplasty may be required to recannulate stenosed arteries. Bypass grafting is sometimes necessary.

Thromboangiitis Obliterans (Buerger Disease)

It is a rare **inflammatory occlusive** disorder affecting the small and medium-size **arteries and veins in the arms and legs of predominantly young male smokers**. The disorder has been identified as an autoimmune response triggered when nicotine is present. Tobacco abuse is the major contributing risk factor (synergistic factor rather than the cause). Affected vessels can swell and become blocked with thrombi. This eventually damages or destroys skin tissues and may lead to infection and gangrene.

Essentials of diagnosis

1. Main clinical manifestations include **ischemic claudication**; cold, cyanotic, painful distal extremities; paresthesias of distal extremities; and ulceration of digits.
2. **Diagnosis is based on history of smoking or tobacco use; onset before the age of 50 years**; infrapopliteal arterial occlusive disease; upper limb involvement or phlebitis migrans; and **absence of atherosclerotic risk factors and specific serologic markers.**

Treatment

Cessation of all forms of tobacco ingestion is mandatory and the only way to reduce progression. The best therapeutic option for advanced peripheral artery disease in selected patients (E.g., rest pain, ischemic ulceration, gangrene) is revascularization (percutaneous or surgical). Otherwise, amputation of all or part of a limb may be necessary.

Behcet Syndrome (Disease)

Behçet syndrome is a rare **immune-mediated systemic vasculitis** characterized by recurrent oral aphthae and any of several systemic manifestations including genital aphthae, ocular disease, skin lesions, gastrointestinal disease, neurologic disease, vascular disease, and arthritis. By etiology, it may be an autoimmune inflammatory disorder, more common among **Asian and Middle Eastern people**.

Essentials of diagnosis
1. Recurrent, painful oral and genital ulcers.
2. Erythema nodosum-like lesions of the skin; a follicular rash; and the pathergy phenomenon (formation of a sterile pustule from minor trauma like a needle stick).
3. Ocular lesions leading to uveitis and blindness (by posterior uveitis);
4. Arthritis; CNS lesions mimicking multiple sclerosis (particularly though involvement of the brainstem).
5. Diagnosis is based on clinical findings because there are no special abnormal lab results.

Treatment
Colchicine is the initial treatment for pain and ulceration. Immunosuppression is the mainstay of therapy. Patient usually responds to initial corticosteroids. Doses are reduced gradually with azathioprine, cyclophosphamide, colchicine, or thalidomide.

Raynaud Phenomenon

Raynaud phenomenon (RP) is **a syndrome of paroxysmal digital ischemia**, most commonly caused by an **exaggerated vasoconstrictive response of digital arterioles to cold or emotional stress**. The phenomenon is characterized clinically by sharply demarcated color changes of the skin of the digits. The primary form mostly affects young women. The secondary form may affect males more with a later onset and association with another (autoimmune) disease. Etiology is unknown.

Essentials of diagnosis (Primary RP)
1. Initial phase—excessive vasoconstriction leading to sharply demarcated digital pallor or cyanosis; the subsequent (recovery) phase—caused by vasodilation leading to intense hyperemia and rubor. Thus, patient presents with paroxysmal bilateral digital pallor and cyanosis followed by rubor.
2. Symptoms are precipitated by cold or emotional stress, and relieved by warmth.
3. The primary form is benign; the secondary form can cause digital ulceration or gangrene.
4. Specific lab abnormalities are absent and diagnosis is clinical.

Treatment
1. Keeping the body warm.
2. Medications: **Ca-blockers** (nifedipine, amlodipine) are the **first-line** therapy. Other helpful medicines include angiotensin-converting enzyme inhibitors, prazosin, topical nitrates, etc.
3. Surgery: Sympathectomy may be considered cautiously if attacks are frequent and severe while medications fail to control symptoms.

Livedo Reticularis

Livedo reticularis (LR) is a common vascular condition characterized by a mottled, lace-like, purplish discoloration of the skin. It may be normal with cold-sensitivity, idiopathic, or secondary to a variety of pathological conditions associated with impaired circulation. LR is the most common cutaneous manifestation of antiphospholipid syndrome (APS).

Etiology
1. The condition may be **normal with cold-sensitivity, or idiopathic**.
2. Secondary to varieties of pathological conditions caused by swelling of the venules owing to obstruction of capillaries by microthrombi:

(1) Autoimmune vasculitis (livedoid vasculitis, polyarteritis nodosa, SLE, dermatomyositis, rheumatoid arthritis); Ehlers-Danlos syndrome, etc.

(2) Drugs (amantadine, etc.).

(3) Capillary obstructions (cryoglobulinemia, antiphospholipid syndrome, hyper-Ca, hematological disorders).

Diagnosis and differential diagnosis
Diagnosis of LR is based on a broad range of differential diagnosis associated with the above etiologies. The **characteristic mottled, lace-like, purplish discoloration of the skin (mostly on the legs; <u>Image 63</u>)** is usually aggravated by exposure to cold, and may predispose to stroke.

<u>Antiphospholipid (antibody) syndrome (APS):</u>
It is an autoimmune disorder characterized by hypercoagulable state and arterial, venous or small vessel thromboembolism and/or recurrent spontaneous abortions in healthy women, with persistent antibodies against phospholipids or cardiolipins and abnormalities such as elevated PTT, false RPR (+), etc. APS is particularly associated with SLE and LR.

Treatment
1. Identify and treat underlying secondary conditions.
2. Idiopathic livedo reticularis itself may improve with warming the legs, but once established the skin discoloration may become permanent.

PAIN SYNDROMES

Neck Pain

Clinical features
1. Most chronic neck pain is caused **by degenerative joint disease between C4 and C7**, with or without extremity pain and neurologic dysfunction, and more common in women around age 50.

NECK

2. There are several types of "**Axial neck pain syndromes**", including cervical strain, cervical spondylosis, cervical discogenic pain, cervical myofascial pain, whiplash injury, and diffuse skeletal hyperostosis. **Whiplash** is the most common type of traumatic injury to the neck.

3. Serious erosive disease of the atlantoaxial joint (C1-2) may lead to neurologic complications in patients with rheumatic arthritis and ankylosing spondylitis.

4. Diagnosis and differentiation can be difficult. **MRI should be the first-line imaging study in patients with progressive signs or symptoms of neurologic disease and with suspected infection or malignancy**. Electromyography (EMG) may help distinguish between peripheral nerve entrapment syndromes and cervical radiculopathy.

Treatment

Conservative management is proper for most cases: rest, analgesics, and physical therapy. Treat underlying cause.

Thoracic Outlet Syndrome

Thoracic outlet syndrome (**TOS**) is a syndrome involving **compression of the neurovascular structures supplying the upper extremity at the superior thoracic outlet** (just above the first rib and behind the clavicle). It can affect one or more of the brachial plexus and the subclavian artery (rarely the vein). The term TOS is not a specific diagnosis and the appropriate type of TOS, such as neurogenic **(nTOS), arterial (aTOS), or venous (vTOS) thoracic outlet syndrome should be used.**

Etiology

1. The most common causes include physical trauma from a car accident, repetitive injuries from a job such as frequent non-ergonomic use of a keyboard, sports-related activities, anatomical defects such as having an extra rib, and pregnancy.

FA 4
625 2. Other causes include abnormal compression from the clavicle, shoulder girdle on arm movement, or a Pancoast tumor in the progressive stages.

Essentials of diagnosis

1. It is mostly seen in **music players and traffic accidents**, causing neurovascular compression and compromised supply to the upper limbs. Patient feels uni-/bilateral "**needle sense**" and coldness of the local arm. Patient usually has normal inter-finger sensation and minimal muscle and pulse weakness.

2. Common orthopedic tests used are the Adson's test, the Costoclavicular Maneuver, and the "Hands-up" test or "EAST" test.

3. Careful examination and X-ray are required to differentially diagnose between the positional and static etiologies, first rib fixations, scalene muscle spasm, and a cervical rib or fibrous band.

Treatment

Adequate rest and physical therapy are helpful. Embolectomy, thrombolytic therapy, or anti-coagulation may be needed. Arterial TOS is nearly always associated with a correctable anatomic bony abnormality, and the recurrent rate of thromboembolism is high without decompression. Prognosis varies.

FA625
Pancoast Tumor: malig @ superior pulm
sulcus.
  —weakness, pain, paresthesias in hand
    from C8-T2 nerve root compression
  - shoulder pain
  - Horner syndrome
  ~ supraclavicular LAD

Subclavian Steal Syndrome

"**Subclavian steal**" describes retrograde blood flow in the vertebral artery associated with proximal ipsilateral subclavian artery stenosis or occlusion, usually to the origin of the vertebral artery. Symptoms, when they occur, are mainly **due to ischemia of the ipsilateral upper extremity**.

Essentials of diagnosis

"Subclavian steal" is frequently asymptomatic and may be discovered incidentally on ultrasonographic or angiographic examination for other indications. Symptoms may occur when ischemia of the ipsilateral upper extremity is significant. **Exercise-induced arm pain, fatigue, coolness, paresthesias,** or numbness occur in approximately one-third of patients, but ischemic and trophic changes are rare. **Significant pressure difference between the arms** may be associated with the symptoms. Less often, neurologic symptoms can be caused by vertebrobasilar ischemia of the brainstem, such as dizziness, vertigo, ataxia, diplopia, and syncope.

Treatment

1. Initial treatment includes early control of hypertension, hyperlipidemia and hyperglycemia, smoking cessation, therapeutic lifestyle changes, and antiplatelet therapy (aspirin).

2. Aggressive treatment for severe disease may include initial carotid artery endarterectomy (angioplasty and stenting) followed by open subclavian artery revascularization.

Fibromyalgia

It's a chronic **non-inflammatory musculoskeletal pain syndrome** with multiple tender points and weakness of the connective tissue. It's very common in **middle-aged women**, and perhaps associated with depression, anxiety, and IBS (irritable bowel syndrome).

Essentials of diagnosis

1. **Chronic multiple myalgias with more than 10 diffuse tender "trigger sites"** that reproduce the pain at palpation, together with body stiffness, aches, numbness, fatigue, and insomnia.

2. Objective signs of inflammation are absent and lab tests are normal. Diagnosis is based on clinical manifestations and by exclusion.

Differential diagnosis

Myofascial pain syndrome:

Less than 10 tender points or specific tender points.

Chronic fatigue syndrome:

(1) It may be associated with **EBV** or mycoplasma infections.

(2) Persistent fatigue, +/- low fever, pharyngitis, body aches, and depression.

(3) EEG shows non-restoring sleep (alpha- and delta-wave). It's diagnosed by excluding other similar disease.

(4) **Treatment**: 1) Psychological support. 2) Medicines: Antidepressants (TCAs, amytriptyline), tryptophan (increasing 5-HT and sleep), and/or anti-mycoplasma drugs may be helpful.

Treatment

Fibromyalgia

1. Supportive and physical therapy (stretching, heating, electrical nerve stimulation).

2. Medicines: Low-dose TCAs (**amytriptyline** or cyclobenzapine) are very effective, especially with coexisting depression. Other medications are **milnacipran** (inhibitor of the reuptake of 5-HT and NE) and **pregabalin** (analgesic and anticonvulsant). **NSAIDs are not effective** because the disease is non-inflammatory. Prognosis varies.

Carpal Tunnel Syndrome

It results from compression of the **median nerve within the tight confines of the carpal tunnel at the wrist**, causing pain and paresthesia in median nerve distribution. It's more common in people with **risk factors**: repeated wrist use (as with computer, music instrument), pregnancy, obesity, diabetes, wrist osteoarthritis/trauma, rheumatoid arthritis, acromegaly, hypothyroidism, amyloidosis, etc.

Essentials of diagnosis

1. **Thenar and wrist pain or tingling radiating up the arm and exacerbated by flexing the wrist**, and difficulty holding an ordinary object; usually worse at night.

2. **P/E**: (1) Weak grip and decreased thumb opposition with numb and tingling sense in the thumb and first-third digits. (2) Decreased 2-point sensation in the whole palm (except the radial part). (3) Possible thenar muscle weakness and atrophy.

3. Diagnosis is clinical, and can be confirmed by: (1) Abnormal **EMG or reduced neurological conduction (#1 reliable** test); or (2) **Phalen's sign (+)**: wrist flexing at 90° for 1 min causes numbness or pain (**highly specific but lowly sensitive**). Tinel's sign is lowly sensitive and specific, and only for reference. Tinel's sign (+): tapping on the wrist causes numbness/pain.

Treatment

1. Behavior modification of wrist motions (reduced use) is fundamental. The best initial treatment is to use wrist splints to immobilize the hand and relieve pressure.

2. Medicines: NSAIDs can reduce pain and inflammation. If it fails, focal steroids can be injected.

3. If symptoms persist, the effective therapy is surgical decompression or diversion of the transverse carpal ligament.

Complications

Permanent loss of sensation, strength, and fine motor skills of the hand can happen.

(Acute) Compartment Syndrome

It's defined as acutely increased pressure within a confined space that decreases the perfusion and functions of the nerve, muscle, and soft tissue. It mostly occurs in the forearm and anterior compartment of the lower leg secondary to trauma with fracture or muscle injury.

Essentials of diagnosis

Compartment syndrome

1. Typical pain out of proportion to the P/E findings: Obvious swelling after injury, severe pain with passive motion of the fingers and toes; **"5P" features—paresthesia, pallor, poikilothermia, paralysis, and pulselessness (late stage).**

2. **Diagnosis** is usually clinical and can be confirmed by measurement of the compartment pressures (mostly > 30 mmHg).

Treatment

1. **Immediately remove all external pressure** on the compartment—any dressing, splint, cast, or other restrictive covering. The limb should be kept level with the torso, not elevated or lowered. Analgesics should be given and supplementary oxygen provided. Hypotension should be treated.

2. **Urgent surgical fasciotomy** to decrease the pressure and increase the tissue perfusion.

Dupuytren Contracture

It is a relatively common, benign, slowly progressive fibroproliferative disease of the palmar fascia, a hand deformity that usually develops over years.

Clinical features

1. Initial fascial thickening is painless and often goes unnoticed. As the disorder progresses, nodules form on the palmar fascia, and the finger gradually loses its flexibility, with contractures that draw one or more fingers into flexion. It is the **hyperplasia of the palmar fascia that leads to nodule formation and contracture of the 4th and 5th fingers.** Patient typically loses the ability to extend the fingers and feels embarrassed about it.

2. Pathologically, Dupuytren contracture is characterized by fibroblastic proliferation and disorderly collagen deposition with fascial thickening. There is a genetic tendency and association with alcoholism, cirrhosis, and systemic fibrosing syndrome.

Treatment

1. The goals of treatment are to improve flexibility of the fingers and to evaluate the need for surgery. Initial treatment is focal **injection of glucocorticoids with triamcinolone, collagenase, or lidocaine.**

2. If the function is impaired, surgical correction (open fasciectomy) is indicated. All patients should receive posttreatment exercises of range of motion stretching, with or without night splinting. Prognosis varies.

Complex Regional Pain Syndrome

Formerly known as **"Reflex Sympathetic Dystrophy"**, it is defined as a disorder of the extremities characterized by **autonomic and vasomotor instability, regional pain that is disproportionate** in time or degree to the usual course of any known trauma or other lesion. The pain is not restricted to a specific nerve territory or dermatome and usually has a distal predominance of abnormal sensory, motor, sudomotor, vasomotor, and/or trophic findings. The disorder shows variable progression over time. Most cases are **secondary to a direct minor trauma.**

CRPS

Clinical features

The cardinal manifestations are burning pain localized to an arm (mostly) or leg, swelling, dystrophic changes in the muscle and overlying skin and nails, limited range of motion, sweating, and disturbances of color and temperature in the affected limb. X-ray may show osteopenia. Diagnosis is clinical.

Treatment

1. **Early mobilization and daily vitamin C** after injury can reduce the risk of developing this syndrome.

2. Early treatment of symptoms offers the best prognosis of recovery.

(1) For mild to moderate cases, a strong NSAID (naproxen), gabapentin, TCAs (amitriptyline or nortriptyline) or/and topical lidocaine cream can be effective.

(2) Severe cases (with edema): Oral prednisone for 2 weeks with tapering over 2 weeks is effective.

3. If persistent, the final effective treatment is sympathetic nerve-ganglion block. Prognosis varies.

LOW BACK PAIN (LBP)

It's a very common condition (80% of population over a lifetime) that may arise from paraspinous muscles (Mus), ligaments (Lig), facet joints, disk or neurologic roots. **Strains refer to muscle injury and sprains refer to ligament injury**. Diagnosis is based on clinical features and exclusion. Most cases relieve < 6 weeks without treatment. However, it's important to identify the underlying pathological causes and treat them accordingly.

Differentiation and management are summarized below.

I. Disk Herniation

Nucleus pulposus extrudes posteriorly mostly through the annulus fibrosis, resulting in neurologic root or cord compression, back pain, and sensory or motor deficiencies. **95% of cases occur in the lumbar region (L4-L5 or L5-S1 levels)**. The pain radiates to the posterior thigh, exacerbated by sneezing, coughing, or straining; relieved by recumbency (bed rest); characterized by **sciatica** (pain radiating down the leg in an L4-S3 distribution), with **straight leg raise (SLR) test positive** (pain going through the buttock and below the knee when the leg is raised above 60 degrees). A negative SLR test excludes herniation with 95% sensitivity. **MRI** is the most accurate means of diagnosis.

Levels of nerve root deficits:

T4: Loss of sensation below the nipples.

T10: Loss of sensation below the umbilicus.

L4 (L3-L4 herniation): Foot dorsiflexion, medial lower leg sensation, and patellar reflex (knee jerk).

L5 (L4-L5 herniation): Big toe dorsiflexion and foot dorsum sensation.

S1 (L3-L4 herniation): Plantar flexion or eversion of foot, Achilles reflex (ankle jerk), and outer foot sensation.

Low Back Pain – Disc Herniation

Large midline herniation may result in **cauda equina syndrome**—with motor/sensory deficits in the lower limbs and anal/saddle area, and urine/bowel incontinence, which **requires urgent decompression by laminectomy plus IV steroids**. If the pain is weaker while motion deficiency gets worse, it indicates worsened neurologic compression.

Treatment: (1) Bed rest, NSAIDs, local heat, physical therapy, and early motion. Most patients recover in 2-3 weeks. (2) With persistent or disabling symptoms, surgical disk removal is usually needed.

II. Compression of the Spinal Cord

A tumor or infection such as epidural abscess (mostly by Staph-aureus) may compress the spinal cord and cause emergency. Point tenderness at the spine with the vertebra percussion is highly suggestive of cord compression. Focal neurological deficits such as a sensory loss or hyperreflexia are usually found below the level of compression.

Treatment: Systemic glucocorticoids and chemotherapy for lymphoma; radiation for most solid malignancies; antibiotics (vancomycin, linezolid, or oxacillin) and steroids for epidural abscess. Surgical decompression is needed if those fail to alleviate symptoms.

III. Back Sprain or Strain

Patient usually presents with paraspinous muscular pain or spasm, history of injury or straining, and **normal X-ray**. Acute lumbar strain is very common. Sacroiliac sprain syndrome is caused by overextension, commonly seen in gymnastics. Idiopathic lumbosacral strain is usually diagnosed if other causes are excluded.

Treatment: (1) Rest for 2-3 days and early motion recovery; NSAIDs as the main treatment for both acute and chronic sprain/strain pain; local application of heat/warm baths; physical therapy.

(2) If symptoms persist after 4-6 weeks, a spinal cord MRI or CT with contrast is performed to examine compression.

IV. Spondylosis or Joint Degeneration

It is mostly caused by non-displaced stress or trauma/fracture of the inter-articular pars, spinal cord overextension, or joint degeneration. Lumbar is the most common site. Non-radiating LBP relieved by rest and worsened by exercise. X-ray may show sclerosis, lucency, or "Scotty dog" images.

V. Lumbar Spinal Stenosis

It's the idiopathic narrowing of the spinal canal due to degenerative joint disease, leading to compression of the cord and nerve roots. Back pain occurs when the back is in extension and the spinal cord presses backwards against the ligamentum flavum. Usually a patient over age 60 presents with back pain while walking or prolonged standing (**pseudoclaudication**), radiating into the buttocks and thighs bilaterally (with numbness and weakness), worsened with the hip extension ("downhill"), and alleviated with the hip flexion (sitting). **A differential point from claudication** is that the pedal pulses and the

Low Back — Lumbar Spinal
Pain   Stenosis

ankle or brachial index are normal. X-ray may show narrowed disk space and spinal canal. **MRI or CT** with contrast is the best means to confirm the spinal stenosis.

   Treatment: Weight loss and steroid injection into the lumbar epidural space improve many cases. Most patients still need surgical correction to dilate the spinal canal.

VI. Ankylosing Spondylitis (See <u>Table 8-1</u> and <u>Image 64</u>)

   Low back pain that improves with activity and worsens with rest. X-rays shows evidence of **sacroiliitis** (early), **fusing** of the sacroiliac (SI) joint(s), and **bamboo spine** (late). **HLA B27 is mostly (+)**.

VII. Neoplasms

   The most common spinal tumor is metastatic carcinoma (usually from the lungs, breast, prostate, GI, and GU). Multiple myeloma is rare. **Clinical features are gradually progressive back pain** (waist-level or middle back) that worsens at night and is unrelieved by rest in an elderly patient, with hyper-Ca, or risk factors of cancer, etc. **MRI or CT** with contrast is the best diagnostic means.

VIII. Other Causes for LBP

   Normal aging can cause LBP with decreased ankle reflex. Vertebral **osteomyelitis or compression fracture** may also have LBP with **point tenderness** over a specific vertebral body.

SPORTS MEDICINE — SPORTS INJURIES

Bursitis

   It's an inflammation of the bursae secondary to trauma, repetitive use, infection, or systemic diseases (gout, RA, osteoarthritis). Common sites are subacromial (subdeltoid, the No.1 site), olecranon, trochanteric, and prepatellar bursa. Infection can cause septic bursitis (more superficial bursa).

   Essentials of diagnosis

   1. History of trauma, repetitive use, or infection followed by localized tenderness, erythema, edema, and decreased ROM (range of motion). Diagnosis is clinical and aspiration analysis is only needed if septic bursitis is suspected.

   2. **Subacromial bursitis**: Common in athletes with repeated, improper use of the shoulder. Pain on overhead actions (arm abduction, flexion, or rotation) and limited shoulder movement. **Neer sign is (+)** (shoulder pain on **passive rotation** internally).

   3. **Olecranon bursitis**: Swelling and pain at point of elbow; spongy "bag of fluid" over the extensor surface of elbow.

   4. **Iliopsoas bursitis**: Overlies the capsule; an enlarging inguinal mass (to be differentiated from a hernia, hydrocele, and abscess).

Bursitis

5. **Trochanteric bursitis**: A common cause of lateral hip pain; with obvious pain on palpation of the greater trochanter.

6. **Ischial bursitis**: Inflamed bursa overlying the ischial tuberosity; with pain in the buttocks, especially when sitting and flexing the hip.

7. **Retrocalcaneal bursitis**: Between the calcaneus and the Achilles.

Treatment

1. **Combined therapies**: Immobilization (except for subacromial bursitis with risk of "frozen" shoulder) and rest; physical therapy—ice during acute phase; moist heat during chronic phase; exercise modification; NSAIDs as indicated.

2. **Intrabursal steroid** injection is saved for severe cases (pain), except for septic bursitis, which requires antibiotics for 7-10 days.

Differential diagnosis

Frozen shoulder:

(1) Glenohumoral joint stiffness causing limited motion of shoulder in all directions, passively and actively; no local warm, red, swollen, or tender signs.

(2) **Diagnosis**: Arthroscopy is confirmative, showing decrease in joint space and loss of normal auxiliary pouch.

(3) **Treatment:** NSAIDs, triamcinolone, focal injection of **steroid/lidocaine**, plus physical therapy.

Rotator Cuff Injury

I. Rotator cuff tear

It's the damage to the rotator cuff of the muscles, tendons, and the bursae around the shoulder leading to the inability to reflex or abduct the shoulder, due to acute or chronic trauma.

(1) Shoulder abduction decreases accompanied by pain with both passive and active arm lift to the shoulder level; drop arm sign is positive. The shoulder pain is worse at night when lying on the affected shoulder. Mild cases may only cause pain without dysfunction.

(2) **Diagnosis:** Based on clinical manifestations or confirmed by arthroscopy or MRI.

(3) **Diagnostic treatment: Lidocaine** injection **is not effective**.

Treatment

NSAIDs, rest and physical therapy are helpful. If ineffective, focal injection of steroids and surgery are indicated.

II. Rotator cuff tendinitis

See below.

Tendinopathy (Tendinitis and Tendinosis)

Tendinopathy is a clinical syndrome characterized by **inflammation, swelling, tendon thickening and pain** at tendinous insertions into the bone end due to overuse or occupational use. Common sites include the biceps, supraspinatus, wrist extensor, patellar, and Achilles tendons.

The common term tendinitis/tendonitis, which usually involves inflammatory injury, is confusing because inflammation is often not seen on histopathology. Tendinopathy is preferred to refer to acute and chronic pain associated with a tendon injury other than tendon tear or rupture. Tendinosis usually refers to chronic, degenerative change, mostly as overuse tendinopathy and with minimal inflammatory reaction.

Diagnosis and differentiation

Most cases are based on clinical manifestations.

1. **Rotator cuff tendinopathy and supraspinatus tendinopathy:**

(1) Shoulder abduction decreases; patient **cannot actively raise arm above the shoulder** level because of pain, which is usually on the lateral aspect of the shoulder but may be poorly localized and weaker than that of subacromial bursitis; drop arm sign is (+).

(2) It's commonly seen in elderly patients (degeneration of tendons) and in young patients with frequent overhand lifting or throwing.

(3) **Diagnostic treatment:** Focal injection of **steroid/lidocaine is effective**. Diagnosis is best initiated by ultrasound and may be confirmed by arthroscopy or MRI. Other helpful therapies include NSAIDs, rest, and physical therapy.

2. **Biciptal tedinitis:** Anterior shoulder pain and pain on flexion with forearm supinated and elbow extended (against resistance). Treatment: Rest, ice, tendon support, and NSAIDs.

3. **"Tennis elbow"** —**Lateral/extensional epicondylitis at the elbow:**

(1) Caused by inflammation or degeneration of the extensor tendons of the forearm due to excessive supination/pronation.

(2) Pain worsens with resisted dorsiflexion of the wrist.

(3) Treatment: Splinting the forearm (not the elbow) is the initial treatment.

4. **"Golfer elbow"** —**Medial (flexors of forearm) epicondylitis:**

(1) Caused by overuse of the flexor pronator muscle group.

(2) Pain distal to medial epicondyle; exacerbated by wrist flexion.

(3) Treatment: Rest, ice, tendon support, and NSAIDs. If pain persists > 6 months, surgery may be indicated.

5. **Achilles tendinopathy**

This can affect both competitive athletes and recreational people. Acute tendon pain generally develops when athletes abruptly increase their training intensity. Chronic tendon pain (> 3 months) may result from sustained stress, poor running mechanics, or improper footwear. Rupture occurs when a sudden shear stress is applied to an already weakened or degenerative tendon.

Treatment: Rest, ice, tendon support, and NSAIDs. For chronic midportion tendinopathy (> 3-month symptoms), a rehabilitation program is recommended to emphasize resistance exercise using heavy loads. Tendon rupture is treated with surgical repair.

Tendinopathy

6. **De Quervain tenosynovitis:**

In the chronic stage, it is also characterized by a lack of inflammation and widespread degenerative and fibrotic changes affecting the sheath and the tendon itself.

(1) Inflammation of the abductor pollicis longus and extensor pollicis brevis tendons.

(2) Commonly seen in postpartum women and similar patients due to repeated **baby-lifting**, causing wrist pain/tenderness on the radial side (especially with pinch gripping). Finkelstein sign is usually positive (pain produced by ulnarly deviating the wrist with clenched thumb).

(3) **Treatment:** 1) Combined therapies of rest, splinting or immobilization, physical therapy (heat and ice), exercise modification, and NSAIDs. 2) If the above treatment fails, focal injections of lidocaine and long-active steroid are used. Repetitive focal injections should be avoided due to risk of rupture.

MISCELLANEOUS DISEASES

Osteoporosis

It's a common metabolic disease of the bone characterized by **osteopenia (bone mass/volume reduction) with about normal bone mineralization**, which increases bone fragility and fracture risk. It mostly affects thin, postmenopausal, or White women, and elderly men. The basic mechanisms are failure to attain optimal bone mass before 30 y/a, or/and rate of bone resorption exceeds rate of bone formation after peak bone mass is attained.

Risk and precipitating factors

Female gender, estrogen depletion, smoking, long-term steroid or heparin therapies, immobilization, Vit-D deficiency, Cushing syndrome, hyperthyroidism, and male hypogonadism

Classification

1. **Primary osteoporosis: Type I** —excess loss of trabecular bone; common fractures of vertebral compression and Colles fracture; usually in 50-70 y/o women. **Type II** —equal loss of both cortical and trabecular bone; common fractures of femoral neck, proximal humerus, and pelvis; mostly seen in men and women over age 70.

2. **Secondary osteoporosis**: Resulted from an obvious cause—such as a risk or precipitating factor listed above.

Essentials of diagnosis

1. Long asymptomatic until a common fracture occurs after minor trauma, such as a **vertebral body compression fracture (No.1 common site)**, hip fracture, or distal radius fracture, usually in patients with above risk factors. Associated presentations include severe back pain, restricted spinal movement, height loss, and possible deformity (kyphosis, lumbar lordosis, and deformed limbs, etc.).

2. **DEXA** (dual-energy X-ray absorptiometry) scan is the No.1 diagnostic test, which may show **significant osteopenia** (after >30% bone density loss or compared with a healthy 30 y/o person). **Bone**

Osteo porosis

X-ray usually shows general **osteopenia +/- fractures (Image 65)**. Most lab tests are normal in osteoporosis except for secondary causes, which may show related deficits.

Treatment

—**Preventive treatment to inhibit bone resorption** is the mainstream.

1. **Cessation or reduction of smoking and alcohol intake**, weight-bearing exercises (stimulating bone formation) and Vit-D plus calcium supplement throughout adulthood help maintain bone density.

2. **Bisphosphonate** (Alendronate, risedronate) **and calcitonin** (intranasal) help increase bone density and decrease risk of fractures for most men and women.

3. **HRT** (hormone replacement therapy) plus alendronate is most effective in preventing and treating bone loss in perimenopausal women. **Raloxifene** is used as a substitute for estrogen to reduce LDL and the risk of breast cancer.

4. **Teriparatide** is an analogue of PTH that can stimulate new bone matrix formation.

Differential diagnosis

PEARLS—Vit-D deficiency and osteomalacia (**Image 65**):

Decreased bone mineralization and density while the bone mass:volume ratio is normal. **Lab tests: Low serum Ca and PO4 (phosphate), and high PTH** levels. Bone X-ray typically shows **"looser zones"**. **Treatment**: Ca + PO4 + Vit-D.

Paget Disease of Bone (PDB)

Also known as "**osteitis deformans**", PDB is a defective bone disease characterized by **abnormal osteoclasts and excessive bone resorption and remodeling** that results in deformities. It's often associated with **paramyxovirus** infection and genetic and environmental causes. Inheritance appears to be autosomal dominant with variable penetrance and with multiple genetic loci.

Essentials of diagnosis

1. Patient is commonly asymptomatic or with a history of paramyxovirus infection, which shows symmetric small joint pain and short morning stiffness (< 15 min).

2. Bone softening may lead to tibial bowing, kyphosis, and frequent fractures; remodeling can cause frontal bossing and decreased hearing (if severe).

3. **Lab tests: Increased alkaline phosphatase** (most common for asymptomatic cases) and urine hydroxyproline; serum Ca^{2+} and PO4 (phosphate) are normal.

Treatment

No treatment is necessary for asymptomatic patient. Treat symptomatic patient with high alkaline phosphatase levels with **alendronate (#1)** for long effects or calcitonin (#2) for short effects. Alendronate can be replaced by zoledronic acid in older patients.

Differential diagnosis

Osteitis fibrosa cystica:

osteitis fibrosis cystica

It's caused by **increased PTH**, leading to high serum Ca^{2+} and AKP (alkaline phosphatase). Low posterior bone X-ray usually shows diffuse bony rarefaction and disseminated focal osteolytic lesions.

Complications

Fractures, spinal cord compression, arthritis, deafness, cardiac failure, or osteosarcoma.

Langerhans Cell Histiocytosis

Langerhans cell histiocytosis **(LCH)**, formerly as "Histiocytosis X", is a rare chronic infiltrating disease mainly involving the bone (>50%), the skin (40%), and the lungs (10%, as interstitial pneumonia) caused by abnormal proliferation of histiocytes. It mostly occurs in children of 1-3 y/a.

Clinical features and diagnosis

1. Variants of disease **include eosinophilic granuloma** (localized to the bone, skin, or lung) **and two system forms—Letterer-Siwe disease and Hand-Schuller-Christian syndrome**.

2. Patients commonly presents with a localized bone pain, an eczematous rash in the axillae, inguinal folds, or genitalia regions, dyspnea, and nonproductive cough (especially with smoking). Other manifestations include spontaneous pneumothorax, lytic bone lesions, and diabetes insipidus.

3. **CXR typically shows a lytic, "punched out" appearance in the bone** and a honeycomb image in the lungs, and CT scan may reveal cystic lesions.

4. **Diagnosis** can be difficult. It's based on clinical manifestations and skin or bone biopsy. IHC staining for CD_{1a} and CD_{207} may be needed for confirmation.

Treatment

Treatment includes corticosteroids (prednisone +/- vinblastine for remissive control) and lung transplantation (may be curative). The prognosis and course are highly variable.

Scoliosis

It's defined as a lateral curvature of the spine of > 10 degrees mostly in the thoracic and/or lumbar spine, often with rotation of the vertebrae, and excessive kyphosis or lordosis. It's mostly idiopathic onset in early adolescence. It may also be congenital or associated with neuromuscular disease. It occurs more in female.

Essentials of diagnosis

1. The condition is mostly found out during P/E at school, which may also reveal possible vertebral and rib rotation deformities by a forward bending test.

2. Spine X-ray (anterior + posterior + full-length views) confirms the diagnosis.

Treatment

1. < 20° curvature: Observation.

2. 20-45° curvature: Spinal bracing (but it may not fully stop the progress).

Scoliosis

3. > 50° curvature: Surgical correction.

Complication

1. Hyperkyphosis: About 60% of cases.

2. Hypokyphosis: Less than 40% of cases. This may be associated with respiratory disorders (especially restrictive lung disease).

Duchenne Muscular Dystrophy (DMD)

DMD is a rare **X-linked** hereditary disease that results from a **dystrophin deficiency** (a cytoskeletal protein). It's the **most common and lethal muscular dystrophy** in male, usually starting at 2-6 y/a and dying by 20 y/a due to respiratory complications. It's always inherited from mother to son.

Essentials of diagnosis

1. Progressive fatigue, clumsiness, difficulty standing or walking, and waddling gait.

2. **P/E**: **Gower sign (+)**: pushing off with the hands when rising from the floor, indicating proximal muscle weakness; calf muscle pseudohypertrophy (due to fat increase); mental retardation.

3. **Lab tests**: **#1 diagnostic test presently is DNA analysis**, revealing dystrophin mutation (same for Becker muscular dystrophy). Second-line diagnostic test is muscle biopsy, showing negative dystrophin degeneration or regeneration of large muscle-fibers. Serum creatine kinase (CK) is elevated. EMG shows polyphasic waves.

Treatment

Glucocorticoids are the mainstay of treatment for DMD, which can improve muscular dystrophy and motor skills. **Prednisone and deflazacort** can be similarly effective. **Eteplirsen** is a new drug for DMD with confirmed dystrophin gene mutation. Supportive and physical therapy help maintain movements and prevent contractures. No cure is available for this disease presently.

Differential diagnosis

Becker muscular dystrophy (BMD):

This is the milder form of DMD and usually has a later onset, resulting from low or normal-level but abnormal dystrophin, and causes milder muscular dystrophy. Elevated serum CK, abnormalities on the ECG and skeletal muscle biopsy findings are similar in both DMD and BMD. However, the two may be distinguished by marked differences in dystrophin expression in skeletal muscle as detected by immunoblotting. Steroid treatment for BMD may not be as effective as for DMD.

Myotonic muscular dystrophy (MMD):

MMD type 1 and 2 are multisystem disorders characterized by skeletal muscle weakness and myotonia, cardiac conduction abnormalities, cataracts, testicular failure, hypogammaglobulinemia, impaired sleep and excessive daytime sleepiness, and insulin resistance. MMD-2 is a less severe adult disease whereas MMD-1 can be congenital, juvenile, and adult onset forms.

(1) **Autosomal dominant** inheritance: Significant family history; associated with cataract, diabetes, mental retardation, sick sinus syndrome, hypersomnolence, and frontal balding.

DMD

(2) **Distal muscular atrophy:** Limb wasting and dystrophy, with an upside-down 'V' face. Cardiac muscles may also be affected.

(3) **Myotonia:** Muscles fail to relax after forceful contraction.

(4) **EMG** shows myotonic discharges (resembling **"dive bombers"**).

(5) Treatment is symptomatic; no disease-modifying therapy is available.

ORTHOPEDIC NEOPLASMS

Osteosarcoma

It's also known as **osteogenic sarcoma**. It's the **most common primary** bone cancer (20%), mostly affecting children and young adults; the peak age is between 13 and 16. In adults it's mostly secondary to sarcomatous transformation of Paget disease of bone or some other benign bone lesions. It usually occurs in the distal femur, proximal tibia, and proximal humerus, and metastasizes to the lungs. Etiology is unknown. It's found that patients with **bilateral "white reflex eyes" have increased risk** for this disease.

Essentials of diagnosis

1. Progressive bone pain for months with a possible painful swelling or mass around the knee or a major joint. Systemic signs are rare in early stage.

2. **Lab diagnosis:** Alkaline phosphatase (**ALP**) is often increased. Bone **X-ray** typically shows a "**sunburst**" pattern of neoplastic bone (**Image 66**) or "**Codman triangle**", with periosteal new bone formation and inflammatory reaction, and osteolytic lesion. **MRI and biopsy** (required to show a malignant sarcomatous stroma) aid better in determination of the tumor extent, nature, and treatment plan. **Don't forget to order chest CT to check possible lung metastases.**

Differential diagnosis

Ewing sarcoma, giant cell tumor of the bone: See below.

Treatment

1. **Most localized diseases** are treated with adjuvant chemotherapy (methotrexate, doxorubicin, and cisplatin) plus limb-sparing **surgical removal** or amputation for large tumors. For older adults, cisplatin plus doxorubicin alone are suggested.

2. **Metastatic osteosarcoma** is treated with combined chemotherapy and surgery. Most patients have a poor prognosis, although long-term survival is possible in up to 50 percent of those with isolated pulmonary metastases.

General prognosis is still poor, with a 5-year survival rate of **60%**, despite obvious improvement in recent years.

Ewing Sarcoma (ES)

It is **a rare malignancy** that most often presents as an undifferentiated primary long bone tumor; less commonly, it arises in soft tissue. ES and peripheral primitive neuroectodermal tumors belong to **the Ewing sarcoma family of tumors** (EFT), sharing similar histologic characteristics and nonrandom chromosomal translocations [t(11;22)] and considered to be derived from a common cell of origin.

Essentials of diagnosis

1. Mostly ES presents with **localized pain and swelling, mostly in the midshaft of a long bone**, without systemic symptoms for a few weeks or months.

2. **X-ray shows lytic bone lesion with "onion skin" periosteal reaction**. CT scan better delineates the bone lesion and MRI the soft tissue. Only a biopsy can make a definite diagnosis.

Treatment

Treatment mostly begins with chemotherapy. Local control of tumors can be achieved by surgery, radiation therapy, or both.

Giant Cell Tumor of Bone

Also known as **osteoclastoma**, it is a **benign but locally aggressive** bone tumor that typically presents as a **lytic lesion** in the epiphyseal region of long bones in young adults, usually around the knee. The clinical course is unpredictable.

Essentials of diagnosis

1. It usually occurs in 20-40 y/o female, presenting with bone pain near the knee. Evidence shows a long bone tumor with mostly benign nature but with **local aggression and osteolytic lesion** composed of multinucleated giant cells and ovoid or spindle-shaped cells.

2. **Bone X-ray (Image 67)** often shows **"soap bubble"** sign in the epiphyseal end. Bone scan helps little.

Treatment

It is crucial to make **early diagnosis and treatment with an orthopedic surgery**—mainly intralesional curettage followed by filling of the cavity with bone cement. If surgery is inadequate, radiotherapy may be added. Local recurrence may be accompanied by **pulmonary metastases** (not highly malignant), which can be treated with targeted therapies, such as **denosumab, an RANKL inhibitor**. Screening of such patients with a chest CT is recommended.

Chapter 8: High-yield Questions (HYQ)

1-8: Match the following clinical scenarios with the most likely diagnosis (Dx).

A. Osteoarthritis (OA)	B. Rheumatoid arthritis	C. Rheumatic arthritis
D. SLE	E. Drug-induced lupus	F. Septic arthritis
G. Sjogren syndrome	H. Gout	I. Pseudogout
J. Ankylosing spondylitis	K. Systemic sclerosis	L. CREST syndrome
M. Mixed connective tissue disease (MCTD)		N. Polyarteritis nodosa
O. Giant cell arteritis	P. Polymyalgia	Q. Juvenile rheumatoid arthritis (JRA)
R. Reactive arthritis	S. Dermatomyositis	T. Antiphospholipid antibody syndrome

1. A 50 y/o woman complains of fever, headache, fatigue, and left knee pain for the past 3 days. Now she feels that the knee pain has lessened but there is new pain in the left toe. P/E finds T = 38.5°C and nodular rashes on the trunk; her knee and toe are red, swollen, and tender. CBC and serum urate are normal (Nl). ESR is elevated.

2. A 60 y/o farmer presents with intermittent right hand pain and fatigue for the past 3 months. He has brief morning stiffness in the hands, and his pain is worsened with activity and relieved by rest. Patient has a 5-year history of occasional smoking and alcohol use, but no chronic diseases. P/E finds swelling and tenderness of the PIP and DIP joints and the knees. Blood CBC and ESR are normal. X-ray shows joint space narrowing.

3. A 15 y/o girl presents with intermittent fever, bilateral hand pain, and fatigue for the past 2 months. She has more than 1 hour of morning stiffness and pain in the hands. The pain is only partially relieved by rest and NSAIDs. P/E finds symmetric swelling and tenderness of MCPs, PIPs, and the wrists. Lab tests reveal that WBC and ESR are mildly elevated, and ANA is (+) but RF is (-). X-ray shows soft tissue swelling.

4. A 45 y/o female presents with intermittent fever, fatigue, muscle weakness, chest pain and bilateral hand pain for the past 2 months. There is > 1 hour of morning stiffness and pain in the hands, and the patient has difficulty combing her hair. P/E finds low fever, multiple discoid rashes, symmetric swelling of the hands, and multiple tender points on both arms. Lab tests reveal that blood RBC, WBC, and platelets are mildly decreased; ANA, Anti-RNP, Anti-ds-DNA, RF, and VDRL are all (+). Urinary protein is (+). X-ray is normal.

5. A 25 y/o female presents with general fatigue and muscle weakness for the past 2 months. She has a history of pulmonary embolism during pregnancy 6 months ago, and has no children due to three spontaneous abortions. She denies any STD or other diseases. P/E results are mostly normal. Blood tests reveal elevated PTT and RPR (+).

6. A 30 y/o man presents with a 2-month history of fatigue, chest discomfort, decreased vision, low back pain, and morning stiffness that worsen at rest and improve with activity. P/E finds HR = 50/min, Schober test (+), and evidence of anterior uveitis. ECG reveals third-degree A-V block. X-ray shows evidence of sacroiliitis.

7. A 30 y/o female presents with 1 week of polyuria, dysuria, mucous in her urine, red eyes, and left knee pain. She is single and sexually active. P/E finds T = 38.5°C, bilateral congested conjunctiva, and swollen left knee with tenderness. Knee X-ray shows a soft tissue lesion. Analysis and culture of the joint fluid and urine reveal proteinuria without pathogens.

8. A 45 y/o female presents with a 2-month history of progressive bilateral muscle pain and weakness in her shoulders and hips, with difficulty lifting objects and arising from a seated position for the past week. P/E shows a purple rash over the face and red scaly patches over the PIP and MIP joints with tenderness. Serum CPK and creatinine are increased, and Anti-Jo-1 antibody is (+).

9. A 65 y/o man presents with a 3-month history of intermittent bilateral knee pain, which suddenly worsened for the past 3 days and has now disappeared. Symptoms were worsened with walking and alleviated with rest and NSAIDs. He has a 4-5-year history of smoking and alcohol use. P/E finds warm knees with mild tenderness. Serum chemistry reveals low Mg and phosphate, and normal uric acid. X-ray shows linear radiodense deposits in joint menisci. Synovial fluid analysis (SFA) has confirmed the Dx. What's the best next treatment?

A. Low-dose colchicine   B. Indomethacin   C. High-dose colchicine

D. Steroids   E. Ibuprofen   F. Allopurinol

10. A 60 y/o female presents with recurrent fatigue, chest discomfort, discoid rash on the face and arms, and morning stiffness and pain in both hands for the past 4 months. P/E results: T = 38°C, discoid rash on the face and both arms; warm, symmetric swelling of the joints of wrists, MCPs, and PIPs with tenderness but without deformation. Lab tests: mild pancytopenia, increased BUN:creatinine ratio, and proteinuria. CXR reveals a small amount of pleural liquid. Specific immunologic tests confirm the Dx. What's most effective treatment for this case?

A. Low-dose steroids   B. High-dose steroids   C. Azathioprine

D. Rituximab (anti-CD20)   E. NSAIDs   F. Chloroquine

11-16: Match the most likely diagnosis with the following clinical scenarios:

A. Polymyalgia Rheumatica (PMR)   B. Fibromyalgia
C. Myofascial pain syndrome   D. Chronic fatigue syndrome
E. Duchenne muscular mystrophy   F. Becker muscular dystrophy
G. Myotonic muscular dystrophy   H. Depressive disorder
I. Somatization disorder

11. A 40 y/o female presents with fatigue, insomnia, depressed mood, muscle weakness, stiffness, and multiple tender sites on the extremities for the past month. She has no history of chronic diseases and been unemployed for the past 3 months. P/E results: normal vital signs; in depressed and irritable mood; 5-6 tender sites on palpation on the arms and legs separately. CBC and ESR are normal. What's the most likely diagnosis from the above choices?

12. For Question 11, all the following therapies may be helpful EXCEPT:

A. psychological support   B. fluoxetine   C. tryptophan

D. anti-mycoplasma   E. NSAIDs   F. stretching and heating

13. A 40 y/o female complains of low fever, fatigue, insomnia, depressed mood, and muscle weakness and pain for the past month. She has no history of chronic diseases and been unemployed for the past 3 months. P/E results: normal vital signs; in depressed and irritable mood without suicidal ideas; various mild tenderness on palpation on

the extremities. CBC and ESR are normal. There are no other abnormal findings. What's the most likely diagnosis from the above Q11-16 choices?

14. A 50 y/o female complains of temporal headache, fever, neck stiffness, fatigue, insomnia, muscle pain and weakness on the left shoulder and right hip areas for the past month. She has no history of chronic diseases and been unemployed for the past 3 months. P/E results: normal vital signs; T = 38°C. There is tenderness on palpation of the left neck, shoulder, and right pelvic girdle areas. CBC is normal and ESR is 110. There are no other abnormal findings. What's the most likely diagnosis from the above Q11-16 choices?

15. What's the best treatment for the patient in Question 14?

A. Low-dose prednisone   B. High-dose prednisone

C. NSAIDs   D. Oxygen   E. Physical therapy

16. A 17 y/o boy presents with progressive fatigue, clumsiness, difficulty standing or walking, "pounding heart", decreased vision, and poor school scores for the past 3 months. His grandmother and father passed away due to similar conditions. P/E results: Stable vital signs, tachycardia, face-limb wasting and dystrophy, myotonia, and negative neurological signs. CBC is normal and CK is elevated. ECG reveals abnormalities. What's the most likely diagnosis from the above Q11-16 choices?

17. During routine P/E a 10 y/o girl is found to have lateral curvature and rotation of the spine during a forward bending test. Spinal X-ray (2-positional views) confirms 30° lateral curvature. The girl does not experience difficulty with daily activities. What's the best next step?

A. Observation   B. Spinal bracing   C. Surgical correction

D. Programmed exercise   E. Further examinations

18-21: Match the following clinical scenarios with the most likely diagnosis.

A. Malignancy   B. Spinal stenosis   C. Back sprain or strain

D. Ankylosing spondylitis   E. Spondylosis   F. Osteomyelitis

G. N-root L4 compression   H. N-root L5 compression   I. N-root S1 compression

18. A 60 y/o man is lifting a heavy object when he experiences sudden back pain. The pain is persistent, radiating to the posterior thigh, and is worsened by sneezing or coughing. History of chronic diseases is (-). P/E finds deficits in plantar flexion and sensation and decreased Achilles reflex. MRI confirms disk herniation.

19. A 60 y/o man is lifting a heavy object when he feels a sudden pain in the back. The pain radiates to the posterior thigh and exacerbated by sneezing or coughing. History of chronic diseases is (-). P/E finds defects in the big toe dorsiflexion and foot dorsum sensation. MRI confirms Dx.

20. A 60 y/o man falls off the stairs backwards and feels a sudden low back pain. The pain is dull, non-radiating, relieved by rest, and worsened by activities. He has history of diabetes for 6 years. P/E only finds tenderness over the lumbar area without neurologic deficits. X-ray shows images of lumbar sclerosis and lucency.

21. A 60 y/o man complains of insidious fever, cough, fatigue, and low back pain for the past 3 months, worsened after a fall off the stairs 3 days ago. P/E finds T = 38.5°C, swelling, and tenderness over the lumbar area. X-rays reveals pulmonary infiltration and pathologic lumbar fracture. Blood tests reveal anemia, leukocytosis, increased Ca, creatinine, IG, and urine acid.

22. A 50 y/o man presents with severe low back pain and loss of urine following a hip fall on a slope. His vital signs are stable. P/E finds motor and sensory deficits in the lower limbs and anal/ssaddle areas, but the back pain is alleviated now. The most appropriate next step is

A. urgent laminectomy   B. CT without contrast   C. NSAIDs

D. IV steroids   E. observation

23. A 47 y/o man presents with slowly progressive multiple joint pain, brief morning stiffness and mild deformation on both hands and feet for the past 3 months. His history is unremarkable except for occasional upper respiratory infections. P/E results: Mild joint deformation on both hands and feet; mild tibial bowing. Lab tests: Increased alkaline phosphatase and urine hydroxyproline; serum Ca^{2+} and phosphate are normal. X-ray shows uneven density changes on both tibia and feet. The most likely diagnosis is

A. osteoporosis   B. osteomalacia   C. Vit-D deficiency

D. Paget disease (Osteitis deformans)   E. osteitis fibrosa cystica

24. An 18 y/o boy presents with progressive pain around the right knee for the past month. He has no other symptoms except occasional headache. P/E shows a swelling with tenderness around the right knee. Lab tests reveal increased serum Ca, phosphate, and AKP. X-ray shows a focal osteolytic lesion beneath the knee with periosteal reaction. What's the most likely Dx?

A. Paget's disease of bone   B. Osteitis fibrosa cystica   C. Hyperparathyroidism

D. Giant cell tumour of bone E. Osteosarcoma

25. If a patient with rheumatoid arthritis presents with a swollen, red and painful calf, what's the best considerations of diagnosis and treatment?

Answers and Explanations

1. (C). Rheumatic fever includes fever, migratory arthritis, subcutaneous nodules, cardiac and CNS involvement.

2. (A). Most of the clinical features support OA, a degenerative, non-inflammatory arthropathy.

3. (Q). JRA—Pauciarticular type: Chronic symmetric arthritis with less systemic symptoms. RF is (-) over 75% of cases. In ANA (+) female: with increased risk of iridocyclitis. In HLA B27 (+) male: increased risk of ankylosing spondylitis.

4. (M). MCTD includes mixed features of SLE, polymyositis, SSc, and rheumatoid arthritis together, almost all cases with positive Anti-RNP, ANA, and RF. Anti-ds-DNA antibody (Ab) is specific for SLE, which involved the skin, chest, joint, and kidney, etc. False (+) VDRL may exist.

5. (T). "Lupus anticoagulant syndrome" is a hypercoagulable state associated with a group of antibodies that are directed against phospholipids or cardiolipins, causing abnormal tests such as elevated PTT and false (+) RPR and recurrent spontaneous abortions in healthy females.

6. (J). This is most likely a case of ankylosing spondylitis. Late X-rays may show "bamboo spin." HLA B27 is usually (+).

7. (R). This is most likely a Reiter syndrome. It usually occurs after a nongonococcal urethritis, causing a syndrome of conjunctivitis, arthritis, and mucocutaneous lesions (e.g., oral or genital ulcers). The other type occurs after an infectious diarrhea caused by enteroinvasive bacteria (Campylobacter, etc.).

8. (S). Dermatomyositis is polymyositis plus skin lesion—heliotrope rash, Gottron's papules, with or without cancer.

9. (A). It's most likely pseudogout, usually caused by CPPD crystal deposition in joints with preexisting damage in elderly patients. Dx is confirmed by positively birefringent crystals on SFA. Since now it's during a break, 'A' is the best to prevent frequent recurrences. 'B' is the best for acute gout or pseudogout attack; 'C' is the 2nd choice. "D and E" are not very effective. 'F' is for long-term effects (to decrease urate production).

10. (C). This is a typical SLE with multi-system impairs—skin rashes (discoid), arthritis (non-erosive), serositis, renal dysfunction, hematologic depression, etc. Specific Anti-ds DNA and anti-SM antibody are usually (+). All the above therapies are helpful but a pulse IV cytotoxic (azathioprine or cyclophosphamide) is the most effective for this refractory case. Rituximab (anti-CD20) is a cyclooxygenase-2 (COX-2) inhibitor.

11. (B). It's a typical case of fibromyalgia, with > 10 tender sites on the extremities. An extent of depression, insomnia may be present. Dx is clinical and by exclusion. Myofascial pain syndrome: <10 tender points or specific tender points. Chronic fatigue syndrome has persistent fatigue and is often associated with fever, pharyngitis, body aches, and depression.

12. (E). Fluoxetine is an antidepressant (SSRI). Tryptophan increases 5-HT in the brain and improves sleep. Anti-mycoplasma may also be helpful. No NSAIDs should be used for fibromyalgia because the disease is non-inflammatory.

13. (D). It's a typical case of chronic fatigue syndrome. It may be associated with EBV or mycoplasma infections; Dx is by excluding other similar disease. Depressive disorder has persistent depressed mood, fatigue, psychomotor agitation, feelings of worthlessness, +/- suicidal thoughts. Somatization disorder has many physical symptoms without medical explanations, and long, complicated medical history and psychosocial dysfunctions.

14. (A). PMR is an inflammatory syndrome of the muscles with pain or stiffness mostly in elderly females, usually asymmetric in the neck, shoulders, and hips. 50% of cases coexist with giant cell arteritis (with fever, anemia, etc.) and share the same HLA haplotypes. ESR is markedly elevated.

15. (B). Low-dose prednisone (5-20 mg/d) is very effective for typical PMR, but if giant cell arteritis is coexistent, high-dose prednisone should be given early to avoid blindness. NSAIDs are alleviative for general inflammatory pain. Oxygen is effective on cluster headache. Physical therapy may be helpful after the acute phase.

16. (G). MMD is autosomal dominant hereditary and associated with cataracts, diabetes, mental retardation, sick sinus syndrome, hypersomnolence, frontal balding, distal muscular atrophy (limb wasting and dystrophy), and myotonia. DMD is X-linked hereditary with similar symptoms. P/E typically shows Gower's sign (+) and calf

muscle pseudohypertrophy (due to fat increase), and intellectual disability. DNA analysis confirms Dx with evidence of dystrophin mutation. Becker muscular dystrophy is a milder form of DMD.

17. (B). Scoliosis is defined as a lateral curvature of the spine of > 10 degrees (mostly in the thoracic and/or lumbar). Treatment: (1) < 20° curvature: observation; (2) 20-45° curvature: spinal bracing; (3) > 50° curvature: surgical correction.

18. (I). A typical herniated disk. Levels of nerve root deficiencies should be remembered.

19. (H). A case of herniated disk compressing spinal nerve root L5. Remember L4 deficiency: Foot dorsiflexion, medial lower leg sensation and patellar reflex.

20. (E). Spondylosis or joint degeneration is caused by non-displaced stress or trauma/fracture of the inter-articular pars, spinal cord overextension, or joint degeneration. Lumbar is the most common site.

21. (A). It's most likely a multiple myeloma with lung infection. Bone marrow biopsy with > 10% plasma cells confirms the diagnosis. Osteomyelitis would only have signs of infection and local inflammation. Back sprain or strain: Paraspinous muscle pain or spasm and normal X-ray. Spinal stenosis: Neck pain +/- LBP radiating to the buttocks + numbness and weakness, worse with the hip extension or walking and alleviated with the hip flexion. MRI shows spinal stenosis best.

22. (D). This is a cauda equina syndrome caused by large midline herniation. It's an emergency requiring urgent decompression by IV steroids followed by laminectomy. That the pain is alleviating while motion deficiency gets worse indicates the neurologic compression may be getting worse.

23. (D). It's a typical Paget disease, a defective bone disease with excessive bone resorption and remodeling that results in deformities. It's often associated with paramyxovirus infection. The best medicine for symptomatic cases is alendronate. Osteoporosis is characterized by osteopenia (bone volume reduction) with normal bone mineralization. It usually causes compression/trauma fractures in thin postmenopausal patients. Vit-D deficiency and osteomalacia: decreased bone mineralization and density while bone volume is normal. Lab tests: Low serum Ca and phosphate, and high PTH level. Bone X-ray typically shows "looser zones". Treatment is Ca + phosphate + Vit-D.

24. (E). Osteosarcoma is the most common primary bone cancer (20%); alkaline phosphatase (ALP) is often increased; bone X-ray typically shows a "sunburst" pattern of neoplastic bone or "Codman's triangle". Giant cell tumor (osteoclastoma) is a benign but locally aggressive, osteolytic tumor; X-ray often shows "soap bubble" sign in the epiphyseal end.

25. Key: You should highly suspect ruptured Baker cyst (popliteal cyst) —the extension of inflamed synovium into the popliteal space. It may cause thrombophlebitis or a potentially life-threatening deep vein thrombosis (DVT). Initial diagnosis is confirmed by ultrasonography. A ruptured cyst is treated with rest, leg elevation, and injection of a corticosteroid into the knee. If symptoms get worse, a surgery may be needed, or blood gas is tested (if DVT is suspected).

Chapter 9

DISEASES OF THE NERVOUS SYSTEM

AND SPECIAL SENSES

NEUROLOGICAL TRAUMA AND INJURY

HEAD TRAUMA

1. **Head trauma with altered mental status or coma**: It first requires a CT scan (without contrast) to look for intracranial hematomas. If CT and neurologic signs are (-) within 24 hours, patients can go home and be watched closely by a family member during the next 24 hrs (to make sure no coma occurs again).

2. **Concussion**: It can be defined as trauma-induced brain dysfunction without structural injury on standard neuroimaging and as a type of mild traumatic brain injury. Most patients have no focal neurologic deficits, have normal CT scans, and good prognosis.

3. Contusion: There is occasionally focal neurologic deficit and CT scan may show ecchymoses.

4. **Penetrating head trauma**: It generally requires surgical repair of the damage.

5. **Open fractures**: Require wound closure. A depressed fracture needs to be treated in the operating room.

6. **Linear skull fractures**: Need observation only if they are closed without overlying wound. _mastoid or_

7. **Skull base fracture**: Signs are raccoon eyes, rhinorrhea, and otorrhea or ecchymosis behind the _postauricular (Battlesign)_ ear. Initial cervical spine x-rays or CT scan is necessary, especially with a prior history. The treatment guideline is **expectant therapy**. Antibiotic use is not indicated.

8. **Neurologic damage and deficits from trauma**—It can be caused by:

(1) The initial blow;

(2) The subsequent hematoma that displaces the midline structures;

(3) Secondarily increased ICP (intracranial pressure).

Therapeutic guidelines for head trauma

(1) No treatment is necessary for initial blow;

(2) Surgery can relieve secondary hematoma;

(3) Medical treatment can prevent or minimize the increase in ICP.

Acute Epidural Hematoma (EDH)

Clinical features and diagnosis

1. It occurs mostly in young patients, with modest trauma to the side of the head and **classic sequence of trauma—unconsciousness--lucid interval (asymptomatic)—coma again.**

2. Further development: Fixed dilated pupil mostly on the lesion side and contralateral hemiparesis with decerebrate posture (rigidity).

3. **CT is the best diagnostic tool**, typically showing a **biconvex lens-shaped hematoma (Image 68)**.

Treatment

Emergent craniotomy is crucial and curable.

Acute Subdural Hematoma (SDH)

SDH results from bleeding between the dura and the arachnoid membranes.

Clinical features and diagnosis

1. The trauma is much **bigger than EDH and patient usually older and sicker**, and the neurologic signs are more severe and mostly **with coma.**

2. **CT is the best diagnostic tool**, typically showing **a semilunar crescent-shaped hematoma (Image 69)**.

Treatment

1. Urgent surgical hematoma evacuation is necessary for most patients with acute SDH and the potential for recovery who have signs of brain herniation or elevated intracranial pressure (such as asymmetric or fixed and dilated pupils), evidence of neurologic deterioration, and clot thickness ⩾10 mm or midline brain shift ⩾ 5 mm on initial brain scan. All these usually indicate poor prognosis (with 40-60% mortality rate).

2. If there is no midline deviation and signs of neurologic deterioration, treatment is focused on prevention of further damage from subsequent elevated ICP. Monitor ICP, elevate the head, hyperventilate, and give necessary mannitol, furosemide and sedation. Avoid fluid overload or over-treating the ICP because this may reduce cerebral perfusion.

Chronic Subdural Hematoma (CSDH)

Clinical features and diagnosis

1. It mostly occurs in an **old patient +/- severe alcoholism**. Patient usually has a shrunken brain that is more vulnerable to minor trauma and tearing of the venous sinuses.

2. Neurologic signs appear over several days or weeks, and mental function deteriorates as hematoma forms.

3. **CT confirms the diagnosis by showing a semilunar, crescent-shaped lesion.**

Treatment

Chronic Subdural Hematoma

Surgical hematoma evacuation is necessary and curable for most patients. Those with midline brain shift have poor prognosis.

Diffuse Axonal Injury (DAI)

DAI is a common and devastating type of traumatic brain injury (TBI) with extensive lesions in white matter tracts. It's one of the major causes of unconsciousness and persistent vegetative state after head trauma. It occurs in about 50% cases of severe head trauma. Concussion may be a milder form of DAI.

Clinical features and diagnosis

1. Patient may only present with a coma after a severe trauma. Diagnosis can be difficult.

2. MRI scan (Image 70) usually shows typical diffuse blurring of the gray-white matter interface better than CT. If it's (-), newer studies such as diffusion tensor imaging (DTI) can demonstrate the degree of white matter fiber tract injury.

Treatment

Most patients with severe TBI require aggressive supportive therapies of maintaining oxygenation, ventilation, and blood pressure. It is recommended to use anticonvulsants to prevent early posttraumatic seizures and mannitol to prevent further damage from increased ICP. Surgery is generally not helpful and only indicated with hematoma. Prognosis is poor.

SPINAL CORD INJURY (SCI)

Traumatic spinal cord injury (TSCI) commonly affects young male adults as a consequence of motor vehicle accidents, falls, or violence. Most TSCI occurs with injury to the vertebral column, producing mechanical compression or distortion of the spinal cord with secondary injuries resulting from ischemic, inflammatory, etc. Most TSCI also involves injury to the brain, limbs, and/or viscera, which can obscure its presentations. About half of TSCIs involve the cervical spinal cord and produce quadriparesis or quadriplegia. Common types of SCI are listed below.

I. Complete Transection

Diagnosis is clear since no sensory or motor functions exist below the lesion level.

II. Hemisection (Brown-Sequard Syndrome)

It's mostly from a clean-cut injury (knife blade), with paralysis and loss of proprioception distal to the injury on the injury side, and loss of pain perception distal to the injury on the other side.

III. Anterior Cord Syndrome

Typically seen in burst fractures of the vertebral bodies; loss of motor function, pain, and temperature sensation on both sides distal to the injury, with preservation of vibratory and positional sense.

Spinal Cord Injury

IV. Central Cord Syndrome

It mostly occurs in the elderly with forced hyperextension of the neck (rear end collision). There is paralysis and burning pain in the upper extremities, with preservation of most functions in the lower extremities.

V. Posterior Cord Syndrome

It's a rare lesion of the posterior portion of the spinal cord characterized by differences in the extent of sensory and motor impairments below the level of the lesion. It is possible for it to present as Brown-Sequard syndrome. It can be caused by an interruption to the posterior spinal artery, injuries, neurosyphilis, etc.

Management of SCI

1. **All patients should start in the ICU with ABCDs** (airway, breathing, circulation, and disability), evaluation of the extent of injuries, and **immobilization** of the potentially injured spinal column.

2. All patients with suspected TSCI (with neck pain or neurologic deficits) should receive complete spinal imaging with **plain x-rays or helical CT scan**, and continued immobilization until imaging studies exclude an unstable spine injury.

3. Patients with abnormal screening imaging studies with suspected TSCI remains should have follow-up CT scans with fine cuts through the region of interest (based on localized pain and/or neurologic signs). **MRI can further accurately define the extent of TSCI** and should be performed on stable patients with TSCI as well as on suspected TSCI despite a normal CT scan.

4. Confirmed TSCI requires urgent neurosurgical evaluation and consultation to manage efforts at decompression and stabilization. Patients with TSCI should also receive prophylaxis to protect against deep venous thrombosis (DVT) and pulmonary embolism (PE).

5. **Steroid therapy: There is limited evidence that glucocorticoid therapy improves neurologic outcomes in patients with acute TSCI.** Thus, glucocorticoid therapy is not recommended in cases with clear risks associated with steroid use, such as penetrating injury, multisystem trauma, moderate to severe traumatic brain injury, and other comorbid conditions.

In other patients who present within 8 hours of isolated, nonpenetrating TSCI, administration of IV methylprednisolone may be considered with potential benefits and risks.

CEREBROVASCULAR DISEASES (STROKE)

FNDs

Stroke is the acute onset of focal neurologic deficits (Neurol-Def) resulting from disruption of cerebral circulation. It is generally classified into two major types: **ischemic and hemorrhagic stroke**. Approximately 80 percent of strokes are due to ischemic cerebral infarction and 20 percent due to brain hemorrhage.

Stroke

Risk factors for peripheral vascular diseases **are also for stroke**, such as **old age,** family history (Hx), hyperlipidemia, coronary artery disease (CAD), hypercoagulability, smoking, hypertension (HTN), diabetes (DM), alcohol and drug abuse, male gender, etc.

PEARLS—General Diagnostic Guidelines for Strokes

Diagnosis is based on history, physical examination (P/E), and imaging. Head CT scan is the best diagnostic means for hemorrhagic stroke and MRI is the best for embolic (ischemic) stroke.

Best consideration for an immediate head CT scan—for any suspicious space-occupying lesion:

1. **Focal neurologic deficits**, with or without confusion;

2. **Presentations of brain herniation or elevated intracranial pressure (ICP):** headache, vomiting, changed pupils, papilledema, seizures, etc.

ISCHEMIC STROKE

It is brain ischemia due to the **four common causes**:

(1) Arterial thrombosis (local blood clotting, No.1 cause);

(2) Arterial embolism (cardioembolism);

(3) Systemic hypoperfusion (shock);

(4) Venous thrombosis.

Deficits are mostly maximal at onset, but may also be "stuttering" sometimes. The brain generally gets up to 40% of systemic emboli. Large vessel (Vx) stroke includes carotid, vertebral, etc. Small vessel stroke includes lacunar, intracranial thrombosis, etc. See **Image 88**.

Important features: **Recurrent transient ischemic attacks (TIAs) in the same artery (A) distribution suggest large vessel stenosis. TIAs in different artery distributions suggest embolism.**

I. Large Vessel Stroke (Image 71)

Internal carotid artery (ICA) stroke: Commonly with cortical, cognitive, and visual field deficits, and with "stereotypic" symptoms (TIA presentations); may be maximal at onset or "stuttering".

Peripheral vascular diseases that lead to carotid stenosis also predispose to stenosis in the coronary arteries, the large arteries of the legs, renal arteries, etc. Therefore, **patients with carotid disease often have angina, claudication, and hypertension.**

Ischemic Stroke

II. Middle Cerebral Artery (MCA) Stroke

Typical signs are contralateral weakness, numbness in the face and arm, homonymous hemianopsia, +/- aphasia or hemineglect.

1. Dominant hemisphere: Mostly by the left MCA stroke with **aphasia**: expressive aphasia (**Broca's**) —inferior frontal; receptive aphasia (**Wernicke's**) —temporal lobe.

2. Nondominant: Right MCA stroke with **hemineglect** (patient may deny the stroke), construction apraxia, and anosognosia, as well as deficient sensory and motor functions of the opposite side.

Differentiation of aphasia (speech disorder)

1. Broca aphasia

It's a disorder in the production of language, unable to speak and write fluent language; comprehension is intact. "Broca = Broken speech" = motor aphasia. Patient is usually aware of his deficit and frustrated by it. It's frequently associated with face and arm hemiparesis, hemisensory loss, and oral apraxia. The lesion site is usually in the **Broca's area** in the **inferior frontal gyrus**, commonly seen after a left **superior MCA stroke**.

Treatment: Institute speech therapy, with variable outcomes depending on specific situations.

2. Wernicke aphasia   Wordy

It's a disorder in the comprehension of language, an expressive or fluent aphasia. Patient usually speaks **fluent, "nonsense"** language with impaired comprehension, and is not aware of his deficit. Hemiparesis is rarely seen. The lesion is commonly in the left **posterior superior temporal lobe (Sylvian fissure)**, usually secondary to a left **inferior MCA stroke**.

Treatment: Institute speech therapy, with variable outcomes.

III. Anterior Cerebral Artery Stroke

Typical deficits include contralateral leg paresis, foot drop, gait dysfunction, amnesia, and personality change.

IV. Posterior Cerebral Artery Stroke

Typical deficits include contralateral visual field deficits (homonymous hemianopsia, cortical blindness), memory deficiency, and reading deficits (dyslexia or alexia).

V. Basilar Artery Stroke

Typical deficits include: (1) Vertigo; (2) Unilateral facial paralysis; (3) Cerebellar signs, visual deficits, dysphagia, apnea, and coma.

VI. Vertebral Artery Occlusion

Typical deficits include symptoms and signs of cerebellar and brainstem dysfunction

Ischemic Stroke

VII. Posterior Inferior Cerebellar Artery infarction (Wallenberg syndrome) *FAB2 p.467*

It usually refers to infarction of the lateral medulla (part of the brain stem) and inferior cerebellum, causing ipsilateral ataxia, Horner's signs, face numbness (CN5), and decreased gag reflex (**CN9, 10, Image 72**); hiccoughs (nucleus solitarius), and contralateral body numbness (spinothalamic).

VIII. Lacunar Stroke *Pathoma p.182 .*

It refers to **small strokes (mostly lacunar infarcts) in the subcortical white matter as well as the basal ganglia (putamen, globus pallidus, thalamus, caudate) and pons.** It's usually caused by occlusion of a single penetrating branch of a large cerebral artery of the circle of Willis, the middle cerebral artery, and the basilar artery.

It usually includes a history of hyperlipidemia or hypertension, with an acute onset of limited, fluctuating neurologic deficits, but intact cognition. There are **five common types**:

1. Pure motor/hemiparesis: Impaired contralateral posterior limb of the internal capsule.

2. Pure hemisensory deficit: Impaired contralateral thalamus.

3. **Hemiballismus—"Dysarthria-clumsy hand syndrome"**: a violent, uncontrolled flinging motion of the limb plus dysarthria; impaired contralateral subthalamic nucleus.

4. Ataxic hemiparesis: Impaired pontine.

5. Sensorimotor stroke.

FAS1 p.458 →Transmits CL sensory info.

IX. Thalamus Stroke *PCA branch stroke*

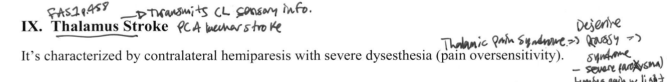

Thalamic Pain Syndrome => (Dejerine) => syndrome
- severe paroxysmal burning pain w light touch (allodynia)

It's characterized by contralateral hemiparesis with severe dysesthesia (pain oversensitivity).

XI. Transient Ischemic Attack (TIA)

It's defined as transient syncope and **neurologic deficits within 24 hours** (mostly < 1 hour). The risk factors **leading to TIA also predispose to CAD.** Most patients with TIA finally die from heart disease, not stroke. There are **three types of TIA:**

1. Embolic: Artery-artery or cardioaortic.

2. Large-vessel atherothrombotic.

3. Small-vessel atherothrombotic: due to low flow.

XI. Reversible Ischemic Neurologic Deficits (RIND)

It's defined as **ischemic neurologic deficits that recover in 1-7 days** (beyond 24 hours). It will be longer with a serious stroke. RIND is mostly caused **by atherothrombosis** and considered a minor ischemic stroke. RIND increases patient's risk of a subsequent major stroke. Other aspects are similar to

RIND

TIA. **Most patients with TIA or RIND finally die from ischemic heart disease, not stroke.** The best **preventive treatment is daily ingestion of low-dose aspirin (better with dipyridamole).**

PEARLS—Therapeutic Guidelines for Ischemic Stroke

1. **Control the risk factors**: Smoking, hypertension, diabetes, and CAD. Long-term BP control gives best benefit. For the first few days following the stroke, it's better to keep the BP at the high normal (Nl) end to avoid diminishing the perfusion pressure.

2. **Medicines**: Aspirin, ticlopidine, Aggrenox (aspirin + dipyramidole), and Plavix (clopidogrel) are all helpful. Warfarin can be added for recurrent emboli.

3. **Endarterectomy**: Indicated if **stenosis is > 60%,** ulcerated, or not responded to medications.

4. **TPAF** (Tissue plasminogen activating factor): With best effect if used within 3 hours of the onset of symptoms. The risk is intracranial bleeding. It reduces stroke disability if no bleeding by prior brain CT scan. **Contraindication**: Recent bleeding disease and uncontrolled hypertension.

HEMORRHAGIC STROKE   *disruption of cerebral circulation*

It's brain hemorrhage and associated neurologic deficits due to intracerebral hemorrhage (**ICH**) or subarachnoid hemorrhage (**SAH**). **Hypertension is the most common cause.** Incidence has been decreased due to stringent BP control. The duration is mostly less than 24 hours. Usually there are focal neurologic deficits in the anterior circulation—ipsilateral sensory, motor, or visual deficits. Posterior circulation deficits (vertebrobasilar) may appear as vertigo, diplopia, and dysarthria, etc.

FA469
Intracerebral Hemorrhage (ICH)

ICH is associated with a high mortality rate (about 50% at 30 days) and significant neurologic deficits for the survivors. Herniation and edema formation after ICH may lead to local injury and increase in intracerebral pressure.

Causes

1. **Hypertension is the most common cause, up to 50% of cases.** Sudden increase in BP can cause a deep vessel rupture within the brain parenchyma.

2. Ischemic stroke may convert to a hemorrhagic stroke.

3. Other causes: anticoagulant or antithrombolytic use, amyloid angiopathy, brain tumors, and arteriovenous malformations.

Locations

Basal ganglia (66%), pons, cerebellum, etc.

Diagnosis

1. CT scan makes 95% of ICH diagnosis.

2. Lab tests of coagulation panel and platelet count.

Complications

Intracerebral Hemorrhage ICH

Increased ICP, seizures, rebleeding, vasospasm, hydrocephalus, SIADH, etc.

Treatment

1. Admission to ICU for immediate care for ABCs.

2. BP reduction and monitoring.

3. ICP reduction: IV mannitol, etc.

Note: Surgical evacuation and steroids are not helpful in most cases.

I. Putamen Hemorrhage

It's the most common ICH, mostly from **lateral striate artery** and with internal capsule involved. About 40% of patients have histories of hypertension. Typical neurologic deficits include **hemiparesis, hemi-sensory loss, homonymous hemianopsia**, eyes deviating away from the paralysed side, stupor, and coma.

II. Pontine Hemorrhage

Typically, there is a history of hypertension, **fast coma, and paralysis** in a few min; **"pinpoint" pupils** reacting to light; decerebration rigidity; no horizontal eye movement.

III. Basal Ganglia Hemorrhage

Typically, there is a history of hypertension, **sudden coma; conjugated gaze deviated to the lesion** side; may have **nystagmus**.

IV. Subarachnoid Hemorrhage (SAH)

F♦469

It's most common with a berry aneurysm rupture, but can also be from arteriovenous malformation. Patient typically has **acute severe headache and neck stiffness** with an elder age and history of hypertension. It's commonly diagnosed by CT (better than MRI) or by spinal tap, rarely by arteriogram. <u>**Image 73**</u> **(CT)** shows the white center stretching into the side sulci due to the SAH.

Treatment: Clipping an unruptured aneurysm is low-risk compared with a ruptured aneurysm.

Prognosis: Poor with a ruptured aneurysm (with 75% death or disability), and with increased ischemic strokes from vasospasm after 3-5 days.

V. Cerebellar Hemorrhage

Patient usually has a history of hypertension or trauma, presenting with **ataxia, vomiting, occipital headache, gaze palsy,** and contralateral facial weakness; no hemiparesis. Early diagnosis and surgical decompression or evacuation are crucial to save life in cerebellar hemorrhage.

EPILEPSY

Seizure is the transient focal or general neurologic disturbance caused by abnormal discharge by cortical neurons. **Epilepsy** is the predisposition to recurrent, unprovoked seizures. First seizure should be evaluated for causes before treatment. More than 50% of patients with epilepsy have an **aura**. **EEG** is the most important diagnostic test for seizures. **Not all that seizes is epilepsy, and not all epilepsy seizes.** Many seizures are associated with other systemic diseases.

Classification of epilepsy

1. Idiopathic epilepsy: No identifiable causes; usually it's genetic, starting in childhood.

2. Secondary epilepsy: Usually secondary to structural lesions (stroke, tumor, trauma, etc.).

3. Generalized seizures: Arise from all areas of the brain at once.

4. Partial seizures: Arise from one focal area of the brain; it may or may not spread. It's the **most common type.**

Table 9-1: Etiologic Summary of Seizure by Age

Infant	2-10Y	Adolescent	18-35Y	35Y+
#1. Perinatal injury;	#1. Infection;	#1. Trauma;	#1. Trauma;	#1. Trauma;
Others: infection, metabolism, genetics	fever, trauma, idiopathic.	drug withdrawal, A-V malformation, idiopathic	alcohol, brain tumor	stroke, metabolism, alcohol, tumor.

Diagnostic guidelines

History and P/E are most important. EEG usually confirms diagnosis, but EEG negativity does not exclude it. A witness is good evidence of history in most cases. For complex partial seizure, brain MRI should be done. For prolonged seizure, EEG monitoring is needed.

I. Generalized Seizures

1. Tonic-clonic (Grand Mal)

It's mostly idiopathic, but can be developed from partial seizures. It begins with loss of consciousness and tonic extension of the back and limbs, followed by 1-2 min of repetitive, symmetric clonic movements, usually with postictal confusion. Secondary cyanosis, tongue biting, headache, incontinence, and muscle pain may occur.

Diagnosis

EEG usually shows 10-Hz discharges during the tonic phase and slow waves during the clonic phase. Serum **prolactin and cortisol** (in less extent) levels are **increased.**

Differential diagnosis

(1) **Pseudoseizure and focal seizures:** There is no serum prolactin increase.

(2) **Syncope:** Gradual progressive faintness and loss of consciousness, slow limb jerking, lasting > 15 sec, fast recovery to lucidity.

Treatment

Levetiracetam or fosphenytoin/phenytoin is the most effective medicine for tonic-clonic seizures in adults and lorazepam or phenobarbital in children. Valproate and lamotrigine (superior to topiramate) are the wide spectrum anti-convulsants commonly used in generalized seizures in both adults and children.

2. Absence (Petit Mal)

It mostly begins in childhood and subsides before adulthood, often with family history. Typical presentations are **a few seconds** of unnoticeable **impaired consciousness (staring** or daydreaming), followed by a brief **amnesia**, eye fluttering, or lip smacking. The episodes can occur abruptly many times a day and terminate without confusion.

Diagnosis: EEG shows 3-Hz spike and slow wave complexes.

Treatment: No.1 medicine is ethosuximide.

3. Myoclonic +/- atonic (Doose syndrome)

Brief bursts of "twitching" involving the face and arms and lasting 1-2 sec; more often in the morning and more common in adolescence.

Treatment: The effective drug is zonisamide or phenytoin. Clobazam can be the second choice.

4. Infantile spasm ("West syndrome")

It's a form of generalized epilepsy that usually begins < 6 months of life. It can be idiopathic or secondary to certain diseases such as perinatal infections, ischemic injury, PKU, etc. Prevalence is male > female and often with family history. Infants usually present with clusters of symmetric, tonic jerks of the head, limbs, and trunk. Most patients have arrest of psychomotor development and intellectual disability after the seizure onset.

Diagnosis: EEG typically shows **hypsarrhythmia.**

Treatment: Hormonal therapy with **ACTH** (No. 1) **or prednisone**, along with clonazepam or valproic is effective against the spasms, but not significantly on the long-term prognosis.

II. Partial (Focal) Seizures

1. **Simple partial**: Usually it's a focal motor twitching with a restricted distribution (e.g., foot or hand only); **no amnesia or unconsciousness.**

Treatment: Phenytoin in adults and valproate in children are effective.

2. **Complex partial**: 80% of cases involve **temporal lobe.** Patient usually presents with an aura or auditory or visual hallucinations, focal twitching or automatisms, and **post-seizure confusion or amnesia.** There are cases of "**partial seizure with secondary generalization**" -- complex partial plus tongue biting and bowel and bladder incontinence.

Note: The new classification may split partial seizures into "partial seizures with dyscognitive features" and "partial seizures without dyscognitive features".

Diagnosis: EEG shows aberrant discharges. Prolactin level is usually increased. A focal seizure may require MRI to rule out a mass.

Treatment: Carbamazepine or lamotrigine (with longer effects) is recommended. Intractable single temporal lobe seizures may be effectively treated by anterior temporal lobectomy without residual deficit.

III. Status Epilepticus

It consists of prolonged (>10min) or repetitive seizures without a return to baseline consciousness. It's a medical emergency because it carries 10-20% mortality.

Causes: anticonvulsant withdrawal or noncompliance, anoxic brain injury, alcohol intoxication or withdrawal, metabolic diseases (e.g., Hypo-Na), trauma, infection, etc.

Diagnosis: Etiologic diagnosis is usually deferred after the emergent treatment is done. EEG and CT are major diagnostic means; other tools include ABG, CBC, electrolytes, glucose, antiepileptic drug levels, toxicology screen, and renal/hepatic functions.

Treatment: 1. Maintenance of "ABC"—airway, breathing, and circulation. "IV dextrose + Vit-B1 + naloxone" is usually given for suspected alcohol/opioid intoxication.

2. IV **lorazepam or diazepam along with a loading dose of phenytoin or fosphenytoin** is the major therapy.

3. If seizures continue, IV loading dose of midazolam or phenobarbital for anesthesia, along with intubation and EEG monitoring.

PEARLS—Clinical Points for Antiepileptic Drugs

Monotherapy is preferable for less adverse effects (S/E) and better compliance.

Febrile seizure: Treated with oral or rectal **diazepam** to prevent subsequent seizures.

Valproic acid (VC): Effective on most seizures, migraines, and bipolar disorder; well tolerated. **Common S/E:** Weight gain, hair loss, and tremors; less common: hepatic or pancreatic toxicity; avoided in pregnancy. **Both VC and carbamazepine** have a low risk of teratogenicity, which is reduced with folate supply.

Enzyme-inducing AEDs (phenytoin, carbamazepine, phenobarbital, oxcarbazepine): With frequent interactions with warfarin, oral contraceptives, anti-cancer drugs, and anti-infective drugs.

HEADACHE   B+494

Most of the headaches are functional and history taking and physical examination are very important to initially identify the nature. If an ICH is suspected, CT scan is highly sensitive. If a non-bleeding lesion (brain tumor, aneurysm, infection/inflammation, etc.) is suspected, MRI scan is the most sensitive means of diagnosis.

Migraine Headache

It's considered an **inherited disorder**, probably an autosomal dominant trait with incomplete penetrance. **Etiology** includes genetics (> 70%), hormone disturbances (female > male by 3 times), stress, sleep disturbances, drugs, environmental triggers (weather), etc. Serotonin depletion plays a major role in the pathogenesis. NSAIDs are effective in about 50% of cases.

Clinical features and diagnosis

1. **Migraine headache without aura:** 80% of cases; "**common migraine**" or "sick headache." Headache may be bilateral, usually with nausea/vomiting and photophobia, and lasting for 2-24 hours. Patients usually immobilize themselves and avoid sound and light.

2. **Migraine headache with aura:** "**Classic migraine**", usually unilateral and with visual aura preceding the headache by 15-20 min, such as scintillating scotoma (flashing lights) or visual field cuts. The subsequent headache is variable in intensity and duration.

Treatment

1. **Acute attacks: NSAIDs** (naproxen, aspirin, ibuprofen, or diclofenac) should be first tried in mild cases. **Triptans** (**sumatriptan**, a highly-specific 5-HT1 receptor agonist) and **ergots** (dihydroxyergotamine-DHE) are highly effective in aborting migraine attacks. DHE (5-HT1 receptor agonist) is also effective in terminating the pain of migraines. Metoclopramide and prochloperazine (plus diphenhydramine) are effective for acute migraines with vomiting. Anti-emetics chlorpromazine may be needed sometimes. If none of the above medications work, it's probably not a migraine headache.

Adverse effects of triptans and ergots: Vascular contraction—be cautious in patient with suspected CAD, stroke, uncontrolled hypertension, use of MAOI, SSRI, or lithium.

2. **Prophylaxis:** (1) Avoid known triggers. (2) If headaches occur more than 2-3 times per month and affect work or quality of life, **daily use of beta-R blockers (No.1)**, **TCAs** (amitriptyline), Ca-blockers, valproic acid, or cyproheptadine. NSAIDs are effective for menstrual migraines.

Cluster Headache

It's rare and considered a variant of migraine headache by some, characterized by unilateral, centered over one eye, deep, burning/stabbing, intense pain, lasting 30-90 min. Most attacks are periodic ("clustering") and nocturnal in middle-aged men, accompanied by conjunctival and nasal congestion and
Lacrimation, rhinorrhea
can present w Horner Syndrome

Cluster HA

precipitated by alcohol or stress. It usually occurs episodically for 2-3 months (90% cases), with months to years of remissions.

Treatment

1. **Sumatriptan is the drug of choice, highly effective combined with 100% O$_2$. S/E:** Sumatriptan may cause retroperitoneal fibrosis after a few months of use.

2. Another therapy is dihydroxyergotamine, octreotide, or lidocaine (last).

3. **Prophylaxis:** It is very effective and is also important because the abortive medicine may be too late for the short-lived cluster headache. **Verapamil** taken daily is the drug of choice. Methysergide, ergotamine, lithium, and prednisone are alternative agents.

Tension Headache

It's characterized by diffuse, aching, "vicelike", and tight band-like distribution, most intense around the neck or back of the head, worsened throughout the day. It can be accompanied by tender posterior neck muscles, daily or episodic, and is often precipitated by anxiety, stress, or depression. Mild tension headache and migraine can be mutually confused.

Treatment

1. First try to find and stop the cause or trigger. Reduction of possible stress, depression or anxiety is important.

2. **NSAIDs combined with caffeine** are effective, standard therapies for mild to moderate headache. If severe, chlorpromazine or metoclopramide (plus diphenhydramine) can be used. Avoid medication overuse headache.

3. TCAs or muscle relaxants may be preventive.

NEUROCOGNITIVE DISORDERS

These include a syndrome of stupor or coma, delirium, dementia, and amnesia caused by general medical conditions or/and drug intoxication. They're more common in patients with debilitation or very young or old age. Broad cognitive mental disorders may include anxiety disorders, mood disorders, and psychotic disorders.

Clinical features

1. **Amnesia (especially recent memory), aphasia, apraxia** (unable to perform complex motor actions), **agnosia** (unable to recognize people or objects), or/and disturbances in general executive function (thinking, planning, and performing).

2. **P/E** may reveal evidence of impairment in CNS function, such as dyskinesia, incoordination, tremor, focal motor or sensory deficits, or substance withdrawal.

3. **EEG** may show generalized slowing of activity, fast-wave activity, or focal abnormalities. There may be abnormal neuroimaging findings.

Differential diagnosis

Separate dementia, delirium, substance intoxication or withdrawal, and psychotic disorders.

Therapeutic guidelines

1. Correction of underlying disorder is essential.

2. Frequent orientation, reassurance, and emotional support are helpful.

Amnestic Disorder

Also known as **amnesia**, it is characterized by **marked memory impairment in the absence of orientation disturbances and other cognitive diseases**.

Etiology

Alcohol may be the most common cause, often associated with bilateral damage to diencephalic and mediotemporal structures. Other causes include Vit-B1 deficiency, cerebrovascular diseases, hypoxia, local infection, surgery, head trauma, seizures, etc.

Essentials of diagnosis

1. **Recent memory loss**: It can be abrupt or gradual loss, **confabulation** as with "Korsakoff psychosis." Orientation is mostly normal.

2. History and P/E evidence of chronic alcohol abuse is usually present.

3. EEG may show abnormal, generalized slowing of activity or fast-wave activity.

Differential diagnosis

Dissociative amnesia:

It is a potentially reversible memory impairment that primarily **affects autobiographical memory** (disorientation to self). Patients mostly cannot recall important personal information, usually of a traumatic or stressful nature, but **can still learn new information** and recall selective things in the past.

Treatment

Correction of the underlying cause is essential. Empirically, IV Vit-B1 and glucose are the effective treatment for hypoglycemia- or alcohol-induced amnestic disorder.

DEMENTIA SYNDROMES

Dementia is not a specific disease, but a general term or condition to describe symptoms of impairment in memory, communication, and thinking in the absence of delirium. It's mostly secondary to CNS damage or a neurodegenerative disease. It is difficult to be diagnosed in early stage.

The major dementia syndromes include Alzheimer disease, vascular (multi-infarct) dementia, dementia with Lewy bodies, Parkinson disease with dementia, and frontotemporal dementia.

Differential diagnosis

1. **"Pseudodementia" —caused by depression, delirium or seizures:** Memory is improved with the improvement of depression, delirium, or seizure; very common in the elderly.

2. **Medications (toxicity):** Typical sensory deprivation (cataracts, hearing loss).

3. **Metabolic causes:** B12 deficiency, hypothyroidism.

4. **CNS Infections:** Neurosyphilis, HIV, Creutzfeldt-Jacob syndrome.

5. **Structural abnormalities:** Abnormal subdurals, normal pressure hydrocephalus (dementia + incontinence + gait apraxia).

6. **Dementia syndromes:** See below.

Alzheimer Disease (AD)

Etiology and pathogenesis

It's the most common type of dementia. Causes are unknown, possibly genetic predisposition along with environmental factors. Patients with chromosomes 21 and 14 deficiencies and homozygous **APOE4** (apolipoprotein E4) have a higher prevalence. Cholinergic neurons turn to be preferentially damaged by beta-amyloid (**A-beta**), causing **plaques of amyloid formed in the gray matter** (neurofibrillary tangles). **Trisomy 21 (Down syndrome)** precipitates A-beta after age 30-40 with similar pathology.

Essentials of diagnosis

1. **Recent memory loss in the 50's** is an early symptom. Long-term memory is spared until late stage, with slowly progressive cognitive deficits and neuropsychiatric symptoms, including disorientation, wandering, agitation, aggression, delusions, hallucinations, depression, apathy, disinhibition, paranoia, sleep disturbances, and impaired mobility.

2. Many elderly demented patients are socially sophisticated and able to "mask" their dementias until late stage, to be found out when they get into a hospital.

3. Neuropsychological testing can help distinguish dementia from depression. MRI or CT may reveal **brain atrophy** and rule out other causes. **Diagnosis is by exclusion and confirmed only by autopsy.**

4. **Hint:** If a patient complains of "a bad memory and possible AD," he may not have it; but if the family members agree the patient has a poor memory and the patient denies it, he may really have it.

Treatment

1. For patients with mild to moderate dementia, **the presently effective** medicine to slow the disease progression and improve symptoms is **acetylcholinesterase inhibitors—donepezil, rivastigmine,** or galantamine by increasing the Ach concentrations in CNS. **Vit-E** may also help slow the progress of dementia. **Memantine** (a N-methyl-D-aspartate receptor antagonist) may help with severe dementia.

2. Symptomatic and supportive therapies can be given to patients with significant neuropsychiatric dysfunctions.

Vascular (Multi-infarct) Dementia (VaD)

It's the **second common form of dementia**, usually caused by a cerebrovascular disease or **cortical stroke**, and with similar risk factors as for stroke (hypertension, hyperlipidemia, diabetes, smoking, old age, etc.). **Binswanger dementia** is characterized by a subcortical vascular disease along with dementia and hypertension.

Essentials of diagnosis

1. Abrupt stroke-associated focal neurologic deficiencies (sensory, motor, language, vital sign changes) followed by dementia, which is usually milder than with AD.

2. CT or MRI reveals evidence of old cortical infarctions or extensive white matter lesions secondary to chronic ischemia.

3. There are no uniform diagnostic criteria for VaD. Evidence of prominent neurologic dysfunction, risk factors and history of stroke, and a high Hachinski Ischemic Score should suggest VaD rather than AD.

Treatment

Treatment is the same as for stroke (control of blood pressure, lipid levels, etc.), plus **donepezil and memantine for dementia** (including preventive effect for AD).

Dementia with Lewy Bodies (DLB)

DLB, also called **Lewy body dementia**, is the **second most common form of degenerative dementia** after Alzheimer disease, especially in older adults. DLB is **characterized by deficits in attention and visuospatial function, fluctuating cognition, and spontaneous motor features of Parkinsonism**. The pathologic feature is **diffuse Lewy bodies—abnormal deposits of protein α-synuclein in the brain—far more than in "Parkinson disease with dementia"**.

Essentials of diagnosis

1. Usually an older patient presents with deficits in attention and visuospatial function; fluctuating cognition; recurrent visual hallucinations; rapid eye movement sleep disorder, and spontaneous motor features of Parkinsonism. Other associated symptoms include repeated falls, syncope, autonomic dysfunction, neuroleptic sensitivity, delusions, and depression.

2. The **diagnosis is made primarily by clinical criteria based on suspicion and specific collection of cardinal features**, which may not be volunteered by patients or caregivers. Radiologic features may be helpful but are not required.

Treatment

1. Nonpharmacologic, behavioral therapies are preferred over medications due to many adverse effects.

2. **Rivastigmine, donepezil and memantine** can ameliorate cognitive and behavioral symptoms. Low-dose atypical neuroleptic agent (e.g., quetiapine) may be added for persistent symptoms. **Levodopa** is indicated for disabling Parkinsonism.

Frontotemporal Dementia (FTD; Pick Disease)

It's a rare, progressive form of dementia characterized by prominent changes in social behavior, personality, or aphasia, accompanied by degeneration and **atrophy of the frontal and/or temporal lobes**, and pathologic mark of **"Pick bodies"** (intraneuronal round inclusions). FTD includes behavioral variant type (most common) and three forms of primary progressive aphasia.

Essentials of diagnosis

1. Early presentations are significant personality changes, dementia, followed by speech and social disturbances, inattentiveness, and extrapyramidal signs.

2. Diagnosis is usually made by the clinical features and frontotemporal atrophy shown by MRI.

Treatment

Symptomatic and supportive treatment only: paroxetine (SSRI), trazodone, or quetiapine for neurobehavioral symptoms; exercise program, speech therapy, or behavioral modification techniques.

Creutzfeldt-Jakob Disease (CJD)

CJD is a **prion** disease, a rare form of dementia, and one of the transmissible spongiform encephalopathies. It's characterized by abnormal accumulation of the prion protein (protease-resistant), spongy degeneration, neuronal loss, and astrocytic proliferation in the brain. Most patients die within a year of symptomatic onset.

Essentials of diagnosis

1. Subacute (weeks-months of course), progressive memory loss, pyramidal signs, extrapyramidal signs (hypokinesia, cerebellar dysfunctions), myoclonus, and behavioral abnormalities.

2. Lab tests: EEG shows periodic sharp waves. MRI with DWI (diffuse-weighted imaging) may reveal abnormal cortex and basal ganglia. CSF is usually normal, but positive protein 14-3-3 is helpful in diagnosis. Definite diagnosis is only made by brain biopsy or autopsy.

Treatment

Symptomatic treatment only; no effective therapy is available currently. Death usually occurs within one year of onset of symptoms.

Normal Pressure Hydrocephalus (NPH)

It's a potentially **treatable form of dementia** probably due to impaired CSF outflow in the brain.

Essentials of diagnosis

1. **Classic triad**: dementia, gait disturbance ("shuffling gait"), and urinary incontinence. There are generally no signs of elevated ICP and headaches.

2. Diagnosis is mostly made by clinical features and LP (lumbar puncture), which will usually show normal or mildly elevated CSF-P (pressure), and will improve symptoms. CT or MRI may reveal ventricular enlargement out of proportion to sulcal atrophy.

Treatment

1. Repeated spinal taps to remove large-volume CSF is the initial helpful therapy.

2. The preferred treatment is ventricular shunting, although variances and complications are common and potentially severe, which require vigilance in the follow-up.

Elevated Intracranial Pressure (EICP)

EICP is a potentially devastating complication secondary to intracranial trauma, tumor, infection, venous outflow impairment, hydrocephalus, or hepatic encephalopathy, etc.

I. Acute EICP

Essentials of diagnosis

1. Typical symptoms include **nausea, headache, agitation, amnesia, and visual deficiency;** severe cases may also have confusion, ataxia, spasticity, seizure, and coma.

2. P/E may find papilledema (irregular blurred disc margin with tortuous vessels).

3. CT/MRI may show ventricular enlargement or shrinking. **LP confirms elevated ICP** (> 500 mmH$_2$O).

Treatment

1. Intubation/hyperventilation (fast effect).

2. Anticonvulsants.

3. Osmotic diuretics (mannitol +/- furosemide). Be cautious with an LP if a tumor or other space-occupying lesion is present.

II. Chronic EICP

Similar etiologies and diagnostic points as above.

Treatment

Short-term use of corticosteroids may be effective against vasogenic edema but not against cytotoxic edema. **Decompressive craniectomy** may help lower ICP and improve brain tissue oxygenation.

Idiopathic Intracranial Hypertension (IIH)

Formerly known as **pseudotumor cerebri or benign intracranial hypertension**, it is a neurological disorder characterized by increased intracranial in the absence of a tumor or other diseases. It's mostly a self-limited ICP increase with some neurologic deficits. However, up to 25% of cases are associated with **loss of vision**, and **persistent headache** is also a source of lost quality of life.

Risk factors include obesity, long-term use of oral contraceptive (OCP), tetracycline, etc.

Essentials of diagnosis

1. Most patients have typical **pulsatile nausea/vomiting, headache, tinnitus, agitation, amnesia, visual deficiency,** and shoulder pain. P/E may find **CN$_6$ palsy, papilledema**, etc.

2. (1) **No.1 diagnostic test: LP-CSF assay** usually shows elevated CSF pressure > 500 mmH$_2$O with normal contents. Note that CSF pressure for most obese patients may be > baseline but < 300 mmH$_2$O.

(2) No.2 test: MRI or cerebrovasography should be done to exclude thrombo-embolism and artery-vein deformity; MRI may reveal ventricular enlargement or shrinking.

Treatment

1. **Acute**: Acetazolamide or topiramate is helpful; if resistant, adding furosemide may provide an additional benefit. Prolonged use of corticosteroids is not recommended.

2. **Chronic**: Weight reduction is helpful. Short-term use of corticosteroids and serial lumbar punctures are recommended in patients with rapidly progressive symptoms waiting for definitive surgical therapy.

3. For patients with **progressive symptoms and visual loss**: Optic nerve fenestration or lumbo-peritoneal shunting is performed.

CENTRAL NERVOUS MYELINOPATHIES

CASI p492

Multiple Sclerosis (MS)

Etiology and pathogenesis ↑ Risk w/ Vit D def, USA/europe cold climate, ↓ sunexposure, smoking

It's currently considered an **autoimmune demyelinating disease of the CNS**. Genetic predisposition along with environmental triggers may be the etiology. If one of the homozygotic twins has the disease, the other twin may have 40% chances of developing MS. Risk is higher in more northerly people and White people. Plaques of MS are glyptic lesions in the white matter clustering around the lateral ventricles, spinal cord, brain stem, and cerebellum.

Essentials of diagnosis

Multiple Sclerosis

Vit. D def = ↑ risk

Lateral rectus palsy

1. Typically with "**disseminated lesions in time and space**": More than one area of the **CNS white matter** involved in more than one attack. History and P/E usually reveal evidence of optic neuritis, intranuclear ophthalmoplegia, hemiataxia, hemisensory deficit, hemiparesis, or trigeminal neuralgia.

- cerebellar sx: ataxia, diplopia.

well-demarcated

2. **Lab tests:** (1) **MRI is most sensitive** (> 90%) for white matter disease), showing multiple plaques *of demyel.* *periventricular* in a callosal and pericallosal white matter distribution (**Image 75**). (2) **CSF: Oligoclonal bands** are the pathologic features. (3) Evoked potentials involve visual, auditory, and brainstem origins.

3. **Diagnosis:** In most cases, history, P/E, and MRI scan can establish the accurate diagnosis.

4. Relapsing forms: Occasional attacks followed by near-recovery. Gradual deficits may develop.

Treatment

1. **Primary or acute attack**: Monthly IV-pulse **high-dose steroids** can shorten the attack duration and delay the secondary attack.

2. **Symptomatic treatment**: Baclofen/Zanaflex for spasticity; carbamazepine for pain; amitriptyline for depression with fatigue; cholinergics for urinary retention; anticholinergics for urinary incontinence.

3. **For secondary or worsening relapsing cases: Monthly IV-pulse immunosuppressants** (methotrexate, cyclophosphamide, etc.), IVIG, and plasmapheresis can be helpful. Cladribine and mitoxantrone may delay progression.

4. **For prophylaxis and relapse reduction: Immunomodulators** (interferon-β1a, interferon- β1b, or Copolymer-1) may be helpful.

Differential diagnosis

Other Myelinopathies: Vit-B_{12} deficiency, Vit-E deficiency, abetalipoproteinemia, syringomyelia, adrenoleukodystrophy, Tabes dorsalis, etc.

Differential diagnosis

Other Myelinopathies: Vit-B_{12} deficiency, Vit-E deficiency, abetalipoproteinemia, syringomyelia, adrenoleukodystrophy, Tabes dorsalis, etc.

Central Pontine Myelinosis (Osmotic Demyelination Syndrome, ODS)

It's the **destruction of the myelin sheaths in the central pons** and can cause a flaccid quadriplegia, bulbar dysfunctioning, coma, and death. It usually follows a rapid or over-correction of severe hyponatremia. **Prognosis is poor**.

Essentials of diagnosis

1. The clinical manifestations are typically delayed for 2-6 days after overly rapid elevation of the serum sodium, including dysarthria, dysphagia, paraparesis or quadriparesis, behavioral disturbances, movement disorders (increased muscle tone, horizontal gaze paralysis, facial weakness), seizures, confusion, disorientation, and coma. Severely affected patients may become "locked in" —patients are awake but are unable to move or verbally communicate. Some symptoms of the ODS are reversible and some are not.

Central Pontine Myelinosis (Ref: p.442)

2. An **MRI scan** of the brain will show a serious symmetric demyelination in the central pons.

Differential diagnosis

"Locked-in syndrome":

It is usually caused by basilar artery thrombosis and can also be caused by severe OSD. The patient is awake and alert, but unable to verbally communicate or move except vertical eye movements.

Treatment

1. The key is to prevent severe damage by early monitoring, evaluation, and gradual correction of hyponatremia in patients with risks. For patients with hyponatremia, the serum sodium should be raised by less than 6 to 8 mEq/L in any 24-hour period to prevent ODS.

2. For patients who have developed myelinolysis, treatment is supportive only.

PERIPHERAL NEUROPATHIES

Most peripheral neuropathies are **demyelinating** as opposed to axonal. In neurologic conduction studies, the demyelinating disease will show slowed velocity but normal amplitude (strength), whereas the axonal disease will show diminished amplitude. Common types are below.

1. **Sensory neuropathy**: Numbness or burning pain.

2. **Motor neuropathy**: Weakness and atrophy.

3. **Autonomic neuropathy**: Vasomotor disturbances, impotence, and arrhythmia.

4. **Mononeuropathy**: Only one nerve involved, often seen in compressed lesion (Carpal tunnel syndrome, sciatica, etc.).

5. **Mononeuritis multiplex**: Vasculitis causes interruption of blood supply to individual nerves in a random pattern; often seen in polyarteritis nodosa, lupus, etc.

6. **Polyneuropathy**: Usually sensory or motor. Stocking or glove distribution is most common. The **No.1 cause is diabetes; No.2 is alcohol**. Primary treatment is etiologic. Neurologic pain is best treated with **gabapentin**.

Guillain-Barre Syndrome (GBS)

GBS is an acute demyelinating disease of the peripheral nerve, and inflammatory polyradiculopathy. It may be associated with Campylobacter infection, antibody against peripheral myelin, and focal segmental demyelination in the peripheral nerves and motor nerves. It often follows a vaccine or viral infection.

Rx rarely provoke GBS

Essentials of diagnosis

GBS

1. **Recent history of viral infection, immunization,** or diarrhea, **followed by ascending paralysis** (distal weakness first), gait disturbances, symptoms of the cranial nerves, and respiratory depression.

2. **P/E**: Limb weakness, **areflexia, and normal sensory function.**

3. **Lab diagnosis**: CSF—increased protein (> 55 mg/dL) without matched pleocytosis (**"Protein-cell dissociation"**). EMG and neurologic conduct tests—showing evidence of diffuse demyelination.

Treatment *If hemodynamically stable, do PFTs, spirometry. FVC & neg inspiratory force monitor resp. muscle strength.*

-↓ in FVC indicates impending resp failure warrants endotrach intubation.

The option of treatment is rapid IV administration of plasmapheresis or immunoglobulin (IG). Note that steroids are not helpful and IVIG is contraindicated with IgA deficiency.

-also, resp distress, HR & BP instability, or widened pulse pressure are indications for GBS intubation.

Prognosis: Gradual, full recovery can be obtained in up to one year. Permanent partial dysfunction may occur in about 35% of cases.

Myasthenia Gravis (MG)

It's an autoimmune neuromuscular disease with antibodies against the postsynaptic neuro-muscular (N-M) junction, which can saturate 80% of the receptors and cause neuro-muscular weakness. There are increased B cells in lymphoid organs and thymus. It mostly occurs before 40 y/a and female > male by about three times.

Essentials of diagnosis

1. Typically fluctuating course of muscle weakness in the order of eyes, limb, and face.

2. Rapid reversal of symptoms after use of cholinergic drugs (IV edrophonium test); evidence of antibodies to Ach-receptor (binding, blocking, modulating).

3. EMG (Electromyogram): Diminished amplitude of the compound muscle action potential to repetitive stimulation.

4. Ocular myasthenia: Common variant; manifested only by diplopia and ptosis.

Differential diagnosis

Eaton-Lambert syndrome:

It's due to **presynaptic blockade** of the N-M junction. Repetitive neuro-stimulation causes an increment of the muscle response, especially after a brief rest (the opposite of MG). It's often associated with small cell lung carcinoma.

Botulism toxin:

It's usually from a GI infection, also due to a presynaptic blockade of the neuromuscular junction, causing muscular weakness or paralysis.

Treatment

1. **Oral cholinergics or anticholinesterase agents have slow and long effects. Plasmapheresis or IVIG has fast reversal of weakness. Steroids or immunosuppressants are used for severe cases.**

2. **Thymectomy is the last powerful treatment** for MG but may take months to work.

Complications

Myasthenic crisis: It's a state of severe myasthenia in which the patient has the risk of respiratory failure secondary to weakness, infections, and over-treatment, etc. **Immediate intubation and plasmapheresis plus IVIG are required therapies.**

CENTRAL NERVOUS MOVEMENT DISORDERS

Parkinson Disease (PD)

PD is an **idiopathic movement disorder of the central nervous system**. It usually occurs after 50 y/a. In pathology, it's **mainly due to dopamine (DA) depletion in the striatum-substantia niagra.**

Essentials of diagnosis

1. Patient typically presents with "Parkinsonism" —**resting tremor**, rigidity, akinesia (poverty of movement), and **masked facial expression**. The **gait** is slow, rigid, and **shuffling**. The handwriting is micrographic. If there is co-existing autonomic instability, it's **Shy-Drager syndrome**.

2. **Pathologic marks**: (1) **Lewy bodies** (eosinophilic intranuclear inclusion/protein bodies), which accounts for the potential dementia expressed as "**Parkinson disease with dementia**"; (2) **hypertonic-hypokinetic syndrome**.

Differential diagnosis

Parkinsonian syndromes:

These include Wilson disease, Huntington disease, Shy-Drager syndrome, Creutzfeldt-Jacob disease, drug-induced Parkinsonism (neuroleptics, metoclopramide), and toxin-induced Parkinsonism (CO, cyanide). Compared to PD, these syndromes start at younger ages, progress fast, and lack of response to levodopa.

Shy-Dragger syndrome:

A neurologic degenerative syndrome, including: (1) Parkinsonism; (2) Autonomic neurologic dysfunction (BP decrease, incontinence, impotence, sweating, tearing); (3) Wide-spread neurologic signs (cerebellar, pyramidal, lower motor neurons, etc.). Symptomatic treatment only; no cure presently.

Treatment

1. **Levodopa/Carbidopa**: It's the first line of medicines for a long term. S/E: Potential damage to the striatonigral pathway.

2. **Dopamine-receptor (R) agonists**: Bromocriptine and pramipexole (but not pergolide or cabergoline) are a useful group of drugs that may be employed either as monotherapy in early PD or in combination with other drugs in more advanced disease. These have better effects in young patients.

3. MAO-B inhibitor (selegiline) and SSRIs (sertraline): Good options for PD with depression.

Parkinson Disease

4. **Parkinson disease with dementia**: Anticholinergics (**donepezil, rivastigmine**) and/or memantine may improve both Parkinsonian symptoms and dementia.

5. Surgery: Includes pallidotomy, thalamotomy, or stimulation. It's chosen only when all medicines fail, with limited success.

General adverse effects of anti-PD medicines: Potential confusion, insomnia, or dyskinesia.

Huntington Disease

It's a rare autosomal dominant disease involving **striatum-caudate neuro-degeneration and diminished GABA.** It's associated with multiple abnormal triple CAG repeats on chromosome 4. Death eventually occurs within 20 years of diagnosis. Symptomatic treatment only; no cure is available.

Essentials of diagnosis

1. Usually starts at 35-40 y/a, with gradual **chorea,** continuous **personality and behavior changes** (irritable, moody and anti-social), progressive **dementia**, and impaired **mobility**.

2. **Diagnosis** is based on clinical features and **chromosome analysis**. Head CT or MRI will reveal enlarged ventricles with cortical atrophy.

Treatment

1. Initial therapies include supportive care and **tetrabenazine**. If tetrabenazine is not effective, an **atypical neuroleptic** (olanzapine, risperidone, or aripiprazole) is suggested. If it's not effective, a **typical neuroleptic** (haloperidol and fluphenazine) is given.

2. Symptomatic treatment may also be needed: TCAs or SSRIs for depression; lithium for chronic moodiness; reserpine for unwanted movements. Genetic counselling for offsprings is important.

Amyotrophic Lateral Sclerosis (ALS)

ALS is a movement disease characterized by a sporadic, chronic, progressive amyotrophic lateral sclerosis, **degeneration of the corticospinal tracts**, and **loss of motor neurons** in the spinal cord, brainstem, and motor cortex. Etiology is unknown. It eventually progresses to respiratory failure and death.

Essentials of diagnosis   Sometimes
vworld: no confirm lab tests, but mild ↑CK due to denervation or hypermetabolism of atrophied muscles. "brisk"

1. **Mixed upper motor neuron signs** (spasticity, increased DTRs) and **lower motor neuron signs** (flaccid paralysis, loss of DTRs). It's usually associated with **Bulbar** involvement (tongue fasciculations and atrophy). Sensory and bladder functions are usually normal.

2. **EMG**: Widespread fasciculations and fibrillations in all four limbs and the tongue.

Differential diagnosis

Cervical stenosis: It can show upper motor neuron or lower motor neuron signs below the foramen magnum, but no bulbar signs (tongue fasciculations).

Amyotrophic Lateral Sclerosis

Syringomyelia: A cavitation or cyst in the central portion of the spinal cord, usually in the C7-T2 area. The cyst first involves the crossing spinothalamic fibers, thus causing the initial sensory loss in the hands and shoulder blades.

Others: Guillain-Barre syndrome, Polio, benign fascinations, hypo/hyper-parathyroidism, and demyelinating disease.

Treatment

1. **Riluzole is the only drug to modify disease and reduce mortality.** It may slow the progression by reducing presynaptic glutamate release.

2. Supportive care, patient education, and strict prevention of respiratory infection.

Friedreich Ataxia   *AR . loss of fxn trinucleotide repeat GAA in frataxin gene*

It's a rare autosomal recessive syndrome of the CNS in early teenagers, characterized by degeneration of the dorsal columns, spinocerebellar tracts, and corticospinal tracts. Patient is progressively disabled by the 20's, and only supportive treatment is available currently.   *↓ descending voluntary movement of CL limbs*

Clinical features and diagnosis

1. Spinal cerebellar ataxia—ataxia with arthralgia. *dysarthria,*

2. Scoliosis (80%) or feet deformity (75% with "Clubfoot").

3. Cardiomyopathy or hypertrophy (90%). *(Mort. due to arrhythmia, CHF, etc)*

4. Dorsal column deficiency—areflexia, *↓ DTRs*

5) Diabetes Mellitus *↓ vibration & proprioception*

INTRACRANIAL NEOPLASMS

General clinical features of brain tumors

1. Usually found in about 2% of all people by autopsy. Common brain tumors signs are **mass effect**, cerebral edema, elevated ICP, and ventricle obstruction. Patient mostly presents with persistent headache, nausea, vomiting, lethargy, seizures, neuro-deficits, memory decrease, and mood or personality changes.

2. Primary tumors rarely spread beyond the CNS. **Adult** tumors are mostly **supratentorial**, whereas **childhood** tumors are mainly **infratentorial**. **Metastatic tumors are more common** than primary ones, often from the **lung, breast**, kidney, GIT, and melanoma, and tend to be more **invasive** and destructive (causing necrosis).

3. **MRI is the best means of diagnosis.** CT with contrast or biopsy is also good. Biopsy is necessary for confirmation.

PEARLS—Table 9-2: **Summary of Primary Intracranial Neoplasms**

Tumor / Clinical features, diagnosis, and treatment

Glioblastoma (Grade IV or high-grade astrocytoma, Image 77)

1. **The most common and aggressive primary brain tumor in adults.** Usually the malignant high-grade gliomas are divided into anaplastic gliomas and glioblastoma. 2. It mainly presents with progressive headache, vomiting, and signs of increased ICP (papilledema, changed pupils, etc.). MRI with biopsy is diagnostic. 3. **Progress is rapid and prognosis is poor** (<1y after Dx). **Tx:** Surgical **resection** plus postoperative radiation therapy and **temozolomide.**

Astrocytoma

1. It belongs to **low-grade glioma** and is the **#1 common brain tumor in children** and mostly as **diffuse astrocytomas in the cerebellum.** 2. Chronic headache, vomiting, increased ICP, new seizures, ataxia, +/- CN5 and CN7 deficits (**Image 87**). 3. Slow, protracted progress and better prognosis. **Tx:** Resection plus radiation +/- chemotherapy.

Meningioma

1. **#1 benign tumor in CNS.** It mostly originates from dura mater or arachnoid. Incidence increases with age. 2. Chronic headache +/- focal findings. 3. Growing slowly and good prognosis. **Tx:** Observation, resection +/- radiation.

Medulloblastoma

1. **#1 common malignant brain tumor in children.** 2. It arises from the **cerebellum vermis and 4th ventricle.** 3. Increased ICP and progressive headache + vomiting. 4. Highly malignant and may occupy subarachnoid space; poor prognosis. **Tx:** Combined modality therapy, including surgery, craniospinal radiation therapy, and chemotherapy (sensitive) is the standard management.

Acoustic neuroma   CN8: SNHL, ↓ balance

NF2, next page

1. **Vestibular schwannoma, neurofibroma II.** 2. **Typical ipsilateral hearing loss, tinnitus,** vertigo, CN7 deficits, and cerebellum dysfunction. **Tx:** Resection +/- radiation.

Craniopharyngioma (Image 78).

1. **#1 supratentorial tumor in children.** 2. Above sella turcica, pressing optic chiasm (bitemporal heteronymous hemianopsia), 3rd-ventricle hydrocephaly, papilledema, polyuria (DI), decreased GH and thyroid hormone (short stature). 3. Pathology: **90% with calcification**; may have "cyst of machine oil." **Tx:** Resection +/- radiation.

Pituitary adenoma

1. It may have some similar symptoms as craniopharyngioma, but more common in **female** and mostly with **prolactinoma, high prolactin, GH, and ACTH.** 2. **Rarely calcified. Tx:** 1. For prolactinoma, dopamine agonists (cabergoline) can decrease tumor size and alleviate symptoms. 2. Adenectomy for recalcitrant tumor.

Ependymoma

1. Mostly in children, rare, arising from ependyma of the 4th ventricle or spinal cord. 2. May cause obstruction, hydrocephalus, increased ICP, headache, vomiting, neck stiffness, etc. **Tx:** Resection.

Brain-stem glioma

1. Uncommon posterior fossa tumor in children. 2. Usually with **personality changes, decreased memory** and school scores, and brain-stem dysfunctions. 3. Pathology: (1) anaplastic astrocytoma; (2) low-grade focal glioma. **Tx:** For newly diagnosed focal glioma, surgical resection can be considered if excessive surgery can be avoided. For unresectable tumor, limited radiation plus chemotherapy +/- steroids are considered.

Optic glioma

NF1

1. Rare, associated with **neurofibromatosis** and chiasmal tumor. 2. **Proptosis, visual deficiencies**, papilledema, disc-pallor, or optic nerve atrophy. **Tx:** It should be delayed until progress of the disease. Treatment may include surgery, radiotherapy, or/and chemotherapy.

MISCELLANEOUS DISORDERS

Vitamin Deficiency and Associated Neurologic Disorders

PEARLS **Table 9-3: Neurologic Disorders Associated with Vitamin (Vit) Deficiency**

Vit-deficiency & disorder / Clinical features, diagnosis, and treatment
Vit-B$_1$ (thiamine) deficiency
I. Wernicke encephalopathy (WE): It's an **acute** neurologic disorder caused **by thiamine deficiency. 1. Risk factors**: Alcoholics, starvation, hyperemesis, renal dialysis, AIDS, and high-dose glucose IV. **2. Features: Classic triad—(1) encephalopathy** (disorientation and confusion); **(2) ataxia** (symmetric polyneuropathy, cerebellar and vestibular dysfunction); **(3) ophthalmoplegia** (nystagmus, conjugate-gaze palsy, and lateral rectus palsy). **Tx:** Symptoms will be **reversed rapidly after IV Vit-B$_1$** (Vit-B$_1$ before glucose to avoid worsening of symptoms).   **II. Korsakoff syndrome (KS):** It's a **late**, neuropsychiatric manifestation of **WE. 1. Same risk factors and clinical triad as for WE. 2. Marked anterograde and retrograde amnesia, confabulation**, and horizontal nystagmus, which are **irreversible**. Alcoholic cerebellar degeneration occurs after 10 years of alcohol abuse.
Vit-B$_{12}$ deficiency--Pernicious anemia; degeneration of the posterior and lateral columns of the spinal cord
1. **Risk factors:** Strict vegetarians and gastric or ileal resection. 2. **Features: Gradual, progressive, symmetric paresthesia, stocking/glove- sensory deficits, spasticity**, paraplegia, leg stiffness, weakness, bowel and bladder dysfunction, and dementia. 3. **Lab tests** show pancytopenia with oval macrocytic RBC and hypersegmented WBC. **Tx:** Vit-B$_{12}$ **IM** or large-dose PO.
Folic acid deficiency--pernicious anemia
1. **Risk factors:** Alcoholics; diet lack of green vegetables. 2. **Features:** Symptoms of anemia, irritability, weakness, dementia, and personality changes; **no neurologic deficiency**. 3. **Lab tests** show pancytopenia with oval macrocytic RBC and hypersegmented WBC. **Tx:** Reversible with early diet supplementation of folic acid.

[handwritten notes in top margin:]
AD.
NF2: Bl acoustic schwannomas (SNHL), juvenile cataracts, meningiomas, ependymomas.
NF2 gene on chr 22. Cutaneous tumors or skin plaques
dx:-audiogram,
-ophthalmic eval
Brain/spine MRI

Neurocutaneous Diseases

Summarized in Table 9-4 below.

Table 9-4: Summary of Neurocutaneous Diseases

Disease / Clinical features, diagnosis, and treatment
Neurofibromatosis—Von Recklinghausen disease (VRD) *NF1*
1. **Autosomal dominant inheritance**, 100% penetrance; variable clinical expression. The gene locus is chromosome-17 defective in Type I and chromosome-22 defective in type II. 2. Higher risk of other tumors such as pheochromocytoma, neuroblastoma, and optic nerve glioma. **Type I ("Classic"):** (1) **Family history**; (2) **> 5 cafe-au-lait spots** > 1.5cm in diameter; (3) **Neurofibromas**; (4) **Lisch nodules** (Iris hamartomas, Image 120), best seen by a slit lamp exam; (5) Higher risk of **optic glioma**. **Type II**: Associated with bilateral **acoustic neuromas** in the cerebellopontine angle. Early presentations include ipsilateral tinnitus, hemiataxia, vertigo, hearing loss, and CN8 weakness. **Tx:** Mostly symptomatic. Regular check-up of BP, vision, and neurologic functions for patients risky of CNS tumors. Genetic counselling is helpful.
Tuberous sclerosis complex (TSC)
1. **An autosomal dominant** genetic disorder with a variety of benign tumors in multiple organs; with chromosome-9 defect. 2. **Clinical features**: (1) Typical **calcified** nodules around the **lateral ventricle**. (2) May have intellectual disability, seizures (including infantile spasms), or associate cardiac rhabdomyomas or renal tumors. 3. **Differential diagnosis**: TORCH infections often cause **intracerebral calcification**, not lateral ventricle calcification. **Tx:** Mostly symptomatic.
Arnold-Chiari Malformation
Type I: Cerebellar tonsil drops down, pressing the foramen magnum. Mostly asymptomatic, but can compress and obstruct the 4th ventricle, causing hydrocephalus and death. **Type II**: Small posterior fossa, syringomyelia, meningocele, and early death.
Von Hippel-Lindau (VHL) syndrome
An autosomal dominant syndrome manifested by a variety of benign and malignant tumors. **Most patients have hemangioblastoma plus retina-angiomas, or/and renal cell carcinoma**, showing ataxia, visual deficits, and increased erythropoietin and RBC. **Dx:** Testing of VHL gene. **Tx:** Based on conditions of tumors.

VERTIGO AND DISEQUILIBRIUM

Vertigo is an abnormal sensation of motion. It can occur in the absence of motion or when a motion is sensed inaccurately. Spinning vertigo is usually of inner ear origin.

Disequilibrium is a sensation of impending fall or of the need to obtain external assistance for proper locomotion. Vertigo and disequilibrium are common symptoms in neurologic disorders.

Vertigo

Common causes of disequilibrium are summarized in Table 9-5 below.

Table 9-5: Common Causes of Disequilibrium

A: Peripheral vestibular disease:
Drug intoxication (alcohol, aminoglycoside, salicylates), BPPV, Meniere disease, acute peripheral vestibulopathy, acoustic neuropathy, otosclerosis, and cerebellopontine-angle tumor.
B. Central ataxia:
Drug intoxication (alcohol, BZ, barbiturates, anticonvulsants, hallucinogens), Wernicke encephalopathy, CNS inflammation (virus, bacteria), cerebellar hemorrhage or degeneration, vertebrobasilar ischemia or infarction, posterior fossa masses, MS, ataxia-telangiectasia, Wilson disease, CJD, and Friedreich ataxia.

Positional Vertigo

It's a common condition that can be caused by both central (E.g., brainstem or cerebellum) and peripheral (e.g., canalithiasis) vestibular lesions. Central positional nystagmus is usually static (as the head is kept in the provoking position), whereas peripheral vestibular nystagmus is transient and more common.

I. Benign Paroxysmal Positional Vertigo (BPPV)

It results from a dislodged otolith that causes disturbances in the semicircular canals. It's a common form of peripheral (end-organ) vertigo. Recent trauma is the most common cause.

Essentials of diagnosis

1. **Transient, episodic vertigo** (< 1 min), nystagmus, nausea, and vomiting with specific **head postures**, and exacerbated by changes in position.

2. **Habituation of vertigo or nystagmus** (decreased with repeated motion tests).

Treatment

Physical therapy--particle repositioning maneuvers (The Epley and Semont maneuvers) is effective. Self-treatment by home exercises is also helpful.

II. Static Positional Vertigo

It's the nystagmus that persists as long as the provocative position is maintained occurs with static positional vertigo. The main differential diagnosis of positional downbeat nystagmus is the anterior canal form of BPPV. Alcohol can also induce a static positional vertigo with horizontal nystagmus. Treatment should target underlying cause.

Meniere Disease (Endolymphatic Hydrops)

It's a form of **chronic peripheral or labyrinthine vertigo** that results from distention of the endolymphatic compartment of the inner ear and disrupted drainage of the endolymph. It's mostly idiopathic, but can be due to trauma of the head or inner ear membrane. It has also been associated with tertiary syphilis.

Essentials of diagnosis

1. Usually > 40 y/a, episodic vertigo, tinnitus, nausea, and bilateral hearing loss, lasting from hours to days. Recurring over years may lead to permanent hearing loss.

2. Audiometry shows fluctuating hearing loss with low frequency and pure tone.

Differential diagnosis

Acoustic neuroma:

Patient may have similar vertigo and hearing loss, along with deficiencies of **CN_7 and corneal reflex** (as oppose to Meniere disease).

Labyrinthitis:

Most patients present with "acute labyrinthine vertigo and nystagmus" **without hearing loss**, tinnitus, or brain stem dysfunction, but associated with viral infection and inflammation. It's usually self-limited.

Others: BPPV, hypothyroidism, and aminoglycoside or furosemide toxicity.

Treatment

1. Initially treat with **limiting intake of salt, caffeine, nicotine, and alcohol; use acetazolamide.**

2. For acute attack: Antihistamines, antiemetics, +/- diazepam.

3. For refractory cases: Surgical decompression (endolymphatic mastoid shunt) is the last resort.

Essential Tremor

Previously known as **benign essential tremor**, it is a neurologic movement disorder characterized by involuntary fine rhythmic tremor of a body part, primarily the head and upper limbs. It may be associated with **autosomal dominant** inheritance and alcoholism.

Essentials of diagnosis

1. Patient usually has a **family history** and history of alcohol drinking, and presents with head and upper limbs tremor, especially when reaching out for something. Finger-nose test is usually (+), whereas the legs are mostly (-).

2. Diagnosis by clinical features and excluding other diseases.

Differential diagnosis

Acute intermittent porphyria: Abdominal pain, headache, tremor, dizziness, confusion, and hallucination. Urine porphobilinogen test (+) is necessary for differentiation.

Treatment

Essential Tremor

The most effective medication is beta-R blocker propranolol +/- primidone. Primidone is anti-convulsive (by transforming to phenobarbital) but may precipitate acute porphyria.

HEARING DISORDERS

There are two types of hearing loss—conductive and sensorineural hearing loss, summarized below.

PEARLS—Table 9-6: Summary of Hearing Losses

Disease / Causes, clinical features, diagnosis, and treatment
Conductive hearing loss
Cause: Lesions in the external (cerumen/ear wax, inflammation), tympanic membrane (perforation), or middle ear (inflammation, effusion, otosclerosis—bony fusion of the stapes the oval window). **Otosclerosis**: 1. Autosomal dominant and variable inheritance; the **No.1 common conduct hearing loss**; 30+ y/a onset; family history (+). 2. Hearing loss typically for low frequency sound; loud noise can be heard. 3. Osseous dyscrasia limited to temporal bone; stapedial reflex deficiency. 4. Weber test: sound lateralizes to the affected side.
Tx: Treat underlying cause. 1. Cerumen impaction is best treated by irrigation after several days of softening with carbamide peroxide or triethanolamine. 2. Hearing aids for most patients. 3. Tympanoplasty for recalcitrant chronic otitis media; stapedectomy for severe otosclerosis.
Sensorineural hearing loss
Cause: Lesions in the cochlea or cranial nerve 8 (CN_8) —presbyacusis (most common), noise, drugs, infection, injury, CNS cause, Meniere disease, etc. **Presbyacusis:** Senile sensory hearing loss, typically for **high frequency sound** (rings, child's voice, female voice, and loud noise); tinnitus may be present. Weber test: sound lateralizes to the unaffected side.
Tx: Treat underlying cause. 1. **Acute sensorineural hearing loss**: A 10-14-day course of high-dose prednisone can be tried, plus antiviral agents if virus is suspected. 2. **Presbyacusis**: Hearing aids; cochlear implants to transducer sounds to stimulate CN_8.

fixation of the stapes

OPHTHALMOLOGY—VISUAL DISORDERS

Glaucoma

Glaucoma is one of the most important causes of blindness worldwide. It's characterized by increased intraocular pressure (IOP), damage to the optic nerve, and irreversible vision loss. The pathogenesis is not fully understood. Ischemia may play a major role in leading to atrophy of the optic disc ("**disc cupping**", **Image 150**).

GLAUCOMA

I. Open-angle Glaucoma   ~ gradual loss of peripheral vision →tunnel vision

It's the **most common type of glaucoma**, accounting for 90% of cases and mostly bilateral.

Etiology and pathogenesis

The basic pathology is gradual **IOP** increase due to the trabecular meshwork disorder and drainage obstruction, causing progressive vision loss from peripheral to central areas.

Risk Factors: older age (> 40), family history, diabetes, myopia, intraocular trauma or inflammation, steroid medications, and the Black race.

Essentials of diagnosis

1. Over 40 y/a, frequent lens changes due to progressively decreased vision (early with perinasal field, often at darkness), gradual headache, and painless increase in IOP. It may take years before diagnosis. Fundoscopy usually shows cupping of the optic disc. Gonioscopy is used to visualize the anterior chamber and help to determine the cause of glaucoma.

2. **Lab tests**: (1) Tonometry may be normal or increase (The borderline is approximately 20).

(2) If the IOP is normal, then a vision test is done, which may show **peripheral field vision decrease (early stage)**. Central field vision testing is important to evaluate the stage—positive result indicates advanced stage.

Treatment

1. Prevention is the most important treatment: (1) All > 40 y/a should have eye exam per 3-5 years; (2) Patients with risks need annual exam.

2. Topical medications: In most cases, IOP can be controlled by a **topical beta-R blocker** (timolol or betaxolol eyedrop, to decrease aqueous humor production), **or pilocarpine** (to increase aqueous outflow). If failed, a carbonic anhydrase inhibitor (acetazolamide) is used.

3. If all medicines fail, laser trabeculoplasty is performed to improve aqueous drainage.

II. Closed-angle Glaucoma

It's an urgent condition caused by an acute closure of a **narrow anterior chamber angle** (usually unilateral), mostly seen in older Asian patients. Common causes include **pupil dilation** (by prolonged stay in darkness, medicines, stress), anterior uveitis, and the lens dislocation. Hyperopia is a risk factor.

Essentials of diagnosis

Sudden, severe, painful, red eyes and blurred vision, commonly with headache, nausea, vomiting, hard eyeballs, dilated pupils (non-reactive to light), steamy cornea, and **elevated IOP**. Fundoscopy reveals increased cup:disk ratio.

Treatment

1. **Lower IOP:** (1) Focal drops of timolol, apraclonidine, or/and pilocarpine; (2) Oral or IV acetazolamide or mannitol if the IOP is too high.

2. **Laser iridotomy is a curative treatment**.

Age-related Macular Degeneration

Age-related macular degeneration (AMD) is the **No.1 cause of permanent, bilateral visual loss in the elderly (> age 65),** characterized by <u>central vision</u> loss and peripheral vision reservation. Risk factors include advanced age, female gender, <u>smoking</u>, hypertentsion, diabetes, and family history.

Essentials of diagnosis

1. **Atrophic macular degeneration ("Dry AMD"):** Gradual painless central vision deficiency (with blurred vision), the more common type. Peripheral vision and eye moving are usually normal. *Multiple sores in macular region.*

2. **Exudative macular degeneration ("Wet AMD"):** Less common but more rapid and severe *new blood vessels, may* painless central vision loss (due to leakage of serous fluid into the retina followed by neovasculization). *leak, bleed & scar the retina*

3. **Fundoscopy (Image 151):** It shows pigmentary or hemorrhagic lesion in the macular region -- central scotomata, line distortion, and **drusen** form (yellowish-white deposits).

Treatment

1. **"Dry AMD":** Age-Related Eye Disease Study 2 (AREDS2) is recommended because it contains high-dose Vit-A and Vit-C, Vit-E, lutein, and zeaxanthin in lieu of beta-carotene (for risk of lung cancer). Quit smoking.

2. **"Wet AMD":** (1) The best initial therapy for foveal lesion and neovasculization is **VEGF inhibitors** such as **bevacizumab or ranibizumab,** which are injected into the vitreous chamber and can effectively slow down progression. (2) **Laser photocoagulation** may delay central vision loss in exudative macular degeneration and proliferative retinopathy. However, the effect is limited.

aorta→R or L common carotid a. →internal carotid → ophthalmic →retinal
supplies
—inner retina
— choroids
— anterior globe

Retinal Vascular Occlusion

I. Central Retinal Artery Occlusion

Abrupt, painless unilateral blindness. Pupils are sluggishly reactive to light. **Fundoscopy (Image 152)** usually shows retinal swelling, **cherry-red spot** on the fovea, and **pale artery** and optic disc **(ischemic area).** It's an ocular emergency. *Amaurosis fugax*

Treatment
& hi-flo oxygen
1. Early stage: 1st try **ocular massage** to get through the thrombosis. *—dislodges the embolus to a point further down the arterial circulation & improves retinal perfusion*
2. If not effective, use **thrombolytics within 8 hours** of onset, along with acetazolamide or mannitol to decrease IOP; or transfer to an ophthalmologist. Without immediate treatment, retinal infarction and permanent blindness may occur.

II. Central Retinal Vein Occlusion

Rapid (but slower than artery) **painless vision loss. Fundoscopy (Images 153)** usually reveals **retinal hemorrhage, cotton wool spots and fundus edema.** It's often idiopathic in elderly patients, leading to glaucoma and macular disease.

CRVO

Treatment

1. **If patient has macular edema**: **VEGF inhibitors** are the first-line therapy and **dexamethasone** the second-line.

2. **If patient has neovascularization**: **Laser photocoagulation** is recommended.

3. If patient has neither macular edema nor neovascularization: Observation and follow-ups.

Retinal Detachment

Sudden onset of **painless blurred vision** in one eye *unilaterally* that progressively gets worse, described by the patient as "like a curtain coming down in front of my eye." It usually occurs spontaneously but can happen after **trauma or surgery**.

Risk factors

History of eye trauma, severe myopia (eye shape change), diabetic retinopathy, and cataract extraction in elderly patients.

Diagnosis—Fundoscopy (Image 154) retina hanging in the vitreous

Gray-cloudy or **dark-red retina debris** hanging in the vitreous humor.

Treatment

1. Posterior vitreous or rhegmatogenous detachment: Most patients may not have any retinal breaks or tears and only need monitoring and education.

2. Retinal hole or tear without detachment: Clearly benefit from laser retinopexy or cryoretinopexy.

3. Symptomatic patients with a full-thickness retinal break and a small retinal detachment can be treated with delimiting laser photocoagulation or cryoretinopexy barrier.

Optic Neuritis

It's an acute **inflammatory demyelinating** injury to the optic nerve. An acute case typically shows **monocular peripheral visual loss with painful eye** movement that evolves over hours to days. Chronic signs include an **afferent pupillary defect and central scotoma**, **color desaturation**, and optic atrophy. These signs often persist despite visual recovery. Optic neuritis is more common in patients with multiple sclerosis (MS), recurrent history, and in young women.

Treatment

Target improving vision and preventing or ameliorating the development of MS. Corticosteroids +/- IVIG can be considered in an acute case. Chronic immunomodulatory therapy such as beta interferon or glatiramer acetate can be used in high-risk patients for MS.

Uveitis

It can be **infectious or noninfectious** inflammation as anterior, intermediate, or posterior uveitis depending on the leukocyte location in the chamber. It's characterized by **painful eyes, blurred vision, hazy cornea with pus,** smaller pupils, and decreased light reflex. It can be associated with infections, HLA-B27, juvenile rheumatoid arthritis (JRA), etc. **Slit lamp exam:** Pre-aqueous flare and cells (+).

Treatment

Target underlying cause through an ophthalmologist.

Myopia

Objects at **far distance cannot be seen clearly** and have to be moved closer and closer. In astigmatism, the refractive errors in the horizontal and vertical axes differ. In the vision exam, use atropine/cycloplegic drops for accurate results (same for hyperopia).

Treatment

Minus or concave lenses are used for correction. **Excimer laser** is now the most widely used surgical treatment.

Hyperopia

Patient **cannot see objects clearly either at infinity or at close distance** because of the decreased accommodation. It's often associated with fatigue and headache, and in children with family history.

Treatment

Convex or plus lenses are used for correction.

Presbyopia

The **natural loss** of accommodative capacity **with age,** usually called "**Elderly hyperopia**". Patient often complains, "I have to read at arm's length."

Treatment

Correction with **plus lenses** for near work.

Amblyopia

Namely **"weak vision"**, developed in early childhood. **Strabismus is the No.1 cause.** If not corrected in time, vision loss may occur.

Treatment

Continuous **covering of the good eye** and using the weak eye.

Cataract

FA 465

It refers to opacifications of the natural lens of the eye, usually bilateral. Senile cataract is the most common type and cause. Other causes: smoking, congenital (rubella or CMV infection, galactosemia, etc.), trauma, prolonged UV light exposure, diabetes, Wilson disease, and steroid use.

Diagnosis

1. Painless blurred vision, progressive over months or years.

2. Eye exam reveals lens opacities.

Treatment

Surgical removal of the cataract and implantation of an artificial lens is the effective therapy.

Chapter 9: High-yield Questions (HYQ)

Q1-5: Match the following clinical scenarios with the most likely results of CSF assay.

	Pressure (mmH2O)	Protein (mg/dL)	Glucose (mg/dL)	RBC per uL	WBC per mm^3	γ-globulin protein %
A.	280	150	66	800	15	13
B.	150	200	88	0	8	11
C.	130	70	70	0	8	18
D.	220	90	20	5	120	12
E.	250	100	60	10	70	14
F.	120	44	75	0	5	8
G.	380	35	70	0	2	6

1. A 70 y/o female is brought to the ER for a generalized convulsion followed by coma. Three days ago she had fever, cough, nausea, headache, and blurred vision. Head CT and MRI scans are unremarkable.

2. A 30 y/o man is brought to ER for a generalized convulsion followed by coma. He has had fever, cough, nausea, headache, blurred vision, and mood and behavior changes for the past 5 days. Drug screening results are (-). Head CT is (-), and MRI reveals unilateral changes on the left side.

3. A 20 y/o man has had fever, cough, and headache for the past week followed by progressive bilateral weakness of the ankles, legs, and arms, and difficulty breathing. P/E shows decreased limb sensation and reflexes.

4. A 35 y/o female presents with gradual, intermittent eye pain, blurred vision, slurred speech, clumsy limb movement, and bed-wetting for the past month. Her symptoms come and go but progress slowly. P/E finds rapid speech and poor limb movements. Babinski signs are (+) bilaterally.

5. A 30 y/o over-weight female presents with fatigue, headache, dizziness, and blurred vision for the past 10 days. She has no history of fever or drug use in the past few months. Vital signs are normal (Nl). P/E reveals papilledema but no hemorrhage. Neurologic signs are normal. CT is (-).

6. A 30 y/o man is hit over the head with a blunt tool. He has a scalp laceration, and skull x-rays show a linear skull fracture. He is conscious. His vital signs are normal and neurologic signs are (-). The most appropriate treatment (Tx) is

A. supportive Tx   B. repair of skull fractures   C. laceration cleaning and closing   D. observation in hospital for 24 hours   E. antibiotics

7. A 20 y/o female is hit by a car, unconscious for a few min, and brought to the ER lucidly. She has minor bruises and lacerations, and can speak normally, but cannot recall the accident. His vital signs are normal and neurologic signs are (-). What's the most appropriate next step?

A. Head CT scan   B. Observation for 24 hours by family members at home
C. Observation for 24 hours in ER   D. Head MRI
E. Supportive Tx

8. A 20 y/o man is hit by a car and brought to the ER in coma. P/E finds HR = 100/min, BP = 90/65 mmHg, with ecchymosis around both eyes and behind both ears and clear fluid dripping out of his nose and ears. What's the most appropriate next step?

A. Immediate IV fluid and surgery   B. Head CT
C. Prophylactic antibiotics   D. Cervical spine CT
E. Observation for 24 hours in ER

9. A 30 y/o man hits the right side of his head in a high-speed car collision and is in a coma in the ER. His vital signs are stable. P/E reveals contralateral hemiparesis. CT scan shows a small crescent-shaped hematoma on the right and deviation of the midline structures to the left. What's the most appropriate next step?

A. Supportive Tx and observation   B. Cervical spine CT
C. Craniotomy   D. Hyperventilation, mannitol, and furosemide
E. Anti-bleeding Tx

10. A 30 y/o man is involved in a high-speed car collision. He experienced a brief coma at the site, regained consciousness temporally and is now brought to the ER in a deep coma, with a fixed and dilated left pupil and contralateral hemiparesis. What's the most appropriate next step?

A. Head CT   B. Cervical spine CT   C. Craniotomy
D. Hyperventilation, mannitol, and furosemide   E. Supportive Tx

11. A 30 y/o man is involved in a high-speed car collision and is in deep coma, with bilateral fixed and dilated pupils in the ER. CT and MRI reveal diffuse blurring of the gray-white mass interface and multiple small punctate hemorrhages, but no displacement of the midline structures. What's the best next step?

A. Supportive Tx and ICP monitoring   B. Anti-bleeding Tx

C. Craniotomy   D. Hyperventilation, mannitol, and furosemide

E. IV steroids

12. A 20 y/o man is shot in the upper part of the neck. The entrance and exit wounds are all above the level of the mandible angle. There is a steady trickle of blood from both wounds that does not stop with local pressure. The patient is irritable but vital signs are stable. What's the most appropriate next step?

A. Continuous local pressure   B. Neck CT or MRI   C. Surgical exploration

D. Angiography   E. Supportive Tx

13. An 18 y/o man is hit by a blunt pole on both sides of the neck and face and comes to the ER with multiple facial lacerations and persistent pain. His vital signs are stable. Neck exam reveals multiple tender points and limitation of movement. Neurologic exam is normal. What's the most appropriate next step?

A. Repair of the facial lacerations   B. Neck CT scan   C. Surgical exploration of the neck

D. Neck X-ray   E. Observation and support

14. A 20 y/o man suffers a burst fracture of the vertebral bodies in a motor vehicle collision. He has lost motor function and pain-temperature perception on both sides distal to the injury, while maintaining good sense of vibration and position. What type of spinal cord injury does he have?

A. Lateral cord injury   B. Brown-Sequard syndrome   C. Anterior cord syndrome

D. Central cord syndrome   E. Posterior cord syndrome

15. During a fight, a 17 y/o boy gets shot in the back, just to the left of midline. He has paralysis and loss of proprioception distal to the injury on the left side, and loss of pain sensation distal to the injury on the right side. What type of spinal cord injury does he have?

A. Lateral cord injury   B. Brown-Sequard syndrome   C. Anterior cord syndrome

D. Central cord syndrome   E. Posterior cord syndrome

16. During a major car collision with sudden braking, a 70 y/o man hyperextends his neck. He develops paralysis and burning pain down both upper extremities while preserving motor function in his legs. What type of spinal cord injury does he have?

A. Lateral cord injury   B. Brown-Sequard syndrome   C. Anterior cord syndrome

D. Central cord syndrome   E. Posterior cord syndrome

17-21: Match the following clinical scenarios with the most likely site of stroke.

A. SAH   B. Cerebellum   C. Pontine

D. Putamen   E. Basal ganglia   F. Cerebral cortex

G. Cerebral white matter   H. Brain stem   I. Ventricular

17. A 70 y/o man is brought to the ER for a generalized convulsion followed by coma. He drank alcohol and fell 5 hours ago, followed by acute nausea, vomiting, and severe headache. P/E finds neck stiffness. Vital signs are stable except BP = 160/110 mmHg. CT is ordered. CSF results are as in choice 'A' of the above table.

18. A 20 y/o athlete falls in a 100-meter running race and is brought to the ER. He presents with vomiting and right occipital headache. P/E finds ataxia, gaze palsy, and left facial weakness. No hemiparesis is found.

19. A 70 y/o man fell down the stairs and hit the right side of his head. 4 hours later he is brought to the ER in a coma. He has a 5-year history of hypertension and alcoholism. P/E reveals nystagmus and conjugated gaze deviated to the right side. His vital signs are stable.

20. A 70 y/o man fell down the stairs and hit the right side of his head. 4 hours later he is brought to the ER in a stupor. He has a 5-year history of hypertension and alcoholism. P/E reveals paralysis and sensory loss of the left limbs and eyes deviated away from the paralyzed side. His vital signs are stable.

21. A 70 y/o man fell down the stairs and hit the right side of his head. 10 min later he is brought to the ER in a deep coma. He has a 5-year history of hypertension and alcoholism. P/E finds "pinpoint" pupils reactive to light, bilateral limb paralysis with rigidity, and no horizontal eye movement. His vital signs are stable.

22. A 60 y/o man fell at home and is brought to the ER. He has a 10-year history of hypertension and smoking. Vital signs are stable. P/E shows weakness and numbness on the right face and arm, eyes deviated to the right side, and a left visual field deficit. He can relate what happened before the fall in stuttering words. The most likely injured artery is

A. L. anterior cerebral artery   B. L. posterior cerebral artery   C. L. basilar artery

D. L. posterior inferior cerebral artery   E. L. middle cerebral artery (MCA)

23. A 60 y/o man awakes from a nap and cannot move his right leg. He has a 10-year history of hypertension and smoking. In the ER, his vital signs are stable. P/E shows weakness and numbness of the right foot and a clumsy gait. He cannot recall what happened before taking the nap. The most likely stroke is

A. L. anterior cerebral artery   B. L. posterior cerebral artery   C. L. basilar artery

D. lacunar   E. L. middle cerebral artery (MCA)

24. A 10 y/o boy is brought to the clinic by his mother for "weird daydreams and failing grades." His school teacher reports that for the past 2 months he was often inattentive in class and occasionally stared at the ceiling and smacked his lips for < 1 min. During these spells, he stopped what he was doing and gave no response when his name was called. He never fell or wet his pants. This condition is best treated with

A. carbamazepine   B. phenytoin   C. haloperidol

D. valproic acid   E. ethosuximide

25. A 28 y/o man is brought to the clinic for "strange behavior." He is recently unemployed, and now has changes in mood and irrational behavior (such as discarding his favorite books and collections). His wife notices that he occasionally has 2-3 min spells in which he is unresponsive and remains motionless. A physician gave him an antipsychotic but this only made the spells worse. He sometimes complains of smelling an unpleasant odor. This condition is best treated with

A. carbamazepine   B. phenytoin   C. haloperidol

D. valproic acid   E. ethosuximide

26. A 49 y/o female complains of throbbing headache three times for the past mo. She describes it as bilateral and periorbital, with nausea and vomiting, lasting for 2-3 hours, and alleviated with naproxen. Her sister has had similar symptoms before. She has no fever or vision/memory loss but has a mild headache at this time. P/E shows normal results. The best next step is

A. amitriptyline   B. sumatriptan   C. propranolol
D. 100% oxygen   E. head MRI scan

27. A 49 y/o female complains of fever and headache over the past 2 days. She describes it as bilateral forehead and periorbital pain with tearing, accompanied with blurred vision, nausea and vomiting. It lasts most of the day without alleviation by naproxen. P/E finds T = 39°C, soft neck, bilateral orbital edema, and decreased vision. CBC reveals elevated WBC. Head CT scan is normal. The best next step is

A. CSF analysis   B. taking blood for culture and sensitivity
C. IV ceftriaxone   D. 100% oxygen   E. IV oxacillin + ceftazidime

28-33: Match the following clinical scenarios with the most likely diagnosis.

A. Pseudodementia   B. vascular dementia   C. B12 deficiency
D. Diffuse Lewy Body disease E. Parkinson disease   F. Normal pressure hydrocephalus
G. Multiple sclerosis   H. Hepatolenticular disease I. Locked-in syndrome
J. Pseudotumor cerebri   K. Pituitary adenoma   L. Alzheimer disease
M. Glioblastoma   N. Acoustic neuroma   O. Craniopharyngioma
P. Brain stem glioma   Q. Astrocytoma   R. Meniere disease

28. A 40 y/o female complains of intermittent eye pain and decreased vision on the right side for the past 3 months, during which she was generally healthy and practicing a vegetarian lifestyle. P/E reveals slurred speech, ocular dysmetria, decreased vision acuity, and poor bilateral hand and foot coordination. EEG is normal.

29. A 50 y/o man complains of decreased memory, fatigue, and mood changes for the past two months. He said he generally felt well before he lost his job 3-month ago, and is now worried about getting Alzheimer disease. He feels better after taking prescribed medicine for 2 weeks, but he has now run out of it. Neuropsychological testing reveals decreased recent memory, slow speech and movement, and irritable mood. MRI is unremarkable.

30. A 55 y/o man presents with 3-month of progressive memory loss, tremor, and difficult walking. He has no history of chronic diseases or medicine use. Neuropsychological testing reveals flat mood, decreased memory, difficult speech, rigid limb movement, and tremor upon sitting. MRI is normal.

31. A 55 y/o obese female complains of decreased memory, slowed speech, "shuffling gait", and urinary incontinence for the past months. She denies any history of fever, headaches, chronic diseases, or medicine use. Neuropsychological testing reveals flat mood, decreased memory, slowed but logic speech, and gait ataxia. CSF pressure = 180 mmH$_2$O and biochemistry is normal. MRI shows mild ventricular enlargement.

32. A 15 y/o boy complains of progressive headache, decreased vision, cold intolerance, and increased urinary frequency for the past 3 months. He has a short stature and worsening school scores. Neurologic exams reveal papilledema and bitemporal heteronymous hemianopsia. Serum growth hormone and T4 are decreased. MRI shows a calcified mass above sella turcica.

33. A 50 y/o female complains of continuous dizziness, tinnitus, and hearing loss for the past 2 months. She denies fever or headache. P/E reveals impaired facial expressions and an absent corneal reflex.

34. A 15 y/o boy complains of chronic headache that has bothered him since 3 months ago. He has used prescribed analgesics frequently but the headache seems unchanged, with occasional nausea, vomiting, convulsion, and difficulty running in balance. He has no history of drug abuse. CBC and P/E results are unremarkable. Head MRI reveals a 2-cm mass near the cerebellum vermis.

35. A 15 y/o girl presents with progressive headache, decreased vision, and increased breast size for the past 3 months. P/E confirms that she has a taller stature and larger breasts than normal for her age. Neurologic exams reveal no other deficiencies except for papilledema and bitemporal heteronymous hemianopsia. Serum prolactin and GH are increased. MRI reveals a 2-cm mass above sella turcica.

36. A 15 y/o boy presents with progressive headache, decreased memory and school scores, and frequent mood tantrums and rule violations that started 3 months ago. Neurologic exams reveal increased sensation of pain and temperature. Blood tests are normal. MRI reveals a 2-cm mass in the posterior fossa.

37. A 35 y/o female complains of gradual hearing decrease since she was pregnant 3 months ago. She has no fever, nausea, vomiting, headache, dizziness, or tinnitus. She recalls that her aunt has a similar history. Audiometry finds she has low-frequency hearing loss. The stapedial reflex is abnormal but the sensory hearing is normal. There are no other abnormal findings. What's the most likely diagnosis?

A. Labyrinthitis	B. Otosclerosis	C. Hereditary hearing loss
D. Presbyacusis	E. Meniere disease	

38-41 (Ophthalmology): Match the following clinical scenarios with the most likely diagnosis.

A. Open-angle glaucoma	B. Closed-angle glaucoma	C. Macular degeneration
D. Central retinal artery occlusion	E. Central retinal vein occlusion	F. Retinal detachment
G. Optic neuritis	H. Cataract	I. Amblyopia
J. Presbyopia	K. Myopia	L. Hyperopia

38. A 60 y/o female presents with 3 months of gradual, painless visual decrease for both nearby and distant objects. She has a 10-year history of diabetes for which she's taken oral hypoglycemics. She has no myopia, hyperopia, or other diseases. P/E finds decreased central vision but normal peripheral vision. Fundoscopy reveals pigmentary lesion in the macular region. IOP is normal. Fasting serum glucose is 150 mg/dL.

39. A 60 y/o female complains of a rapid, painless visual loss in the left eye for the past 3 days. She has a 10-year history of diabetes for which she has taken oral hypoglycemics. She denies history of other chronic diseases. P/E finds significantly decreased central and peripheral vision in the left eye, with normal movement. Fundoscopy reveals retinal hemorrhage, cotton wool spots, and edematous fundus. IOP is Nl. Fasting serum glucose is 150 mg/dL.

40. A 60 y/o man presents with a sudden, painless blurred vision in the left eye that is progressively worse, "like a piece of thin cloth in front of the eye." He has a 10-year history of severe myopia and had cataract extraction 6 months ago. Fundoscopy reveals dark-red debris hanging in the vitreous humor. IOP is elevated.

41. A 60 y/o man presents with headache, nausea, and a suddenly blurred vision with pain in the left eye that is progressively worse. He has a 10-year history of severe myopia. P/E finds bilateral red eyes with hard eyeballs, steamy cornea, dilated pupils non-reactive to light, and increased IOP. Fundoscopy reveals increased cup:disc ratio.

Answers and Explanations

1. (D). The patient most likely has bacterial meningitis: with increased ICP (and manifestations), milky CSF, protein and WBC but decreased glucose.

2. (E). The patient most likely has viral encephalitis: with increased ICP and its manifestations, changes in cognition and behavior, cloudy CSF, increased protein and WBC but normal (Nl) glucose.

3. (B). Typical Guillain-Barre syndrome (GBS): with thick, yellow CSF, very high protein but low WBC.

4. (C). The patient most likely has multiple sclerosis: with clear CSF, high IgG (> 15% protein), mildly increased protein and WBC, but Nl opening pressure and glucose.

5. (G). This is most likely pseudotumor cerebri due to idiopathic elevated ICP, mostly in obese, pregnant female, or in patients over-taking vitamins. There is very high ICP but the rest of the CSF indexes are Nl. The high ICP does not increase the risk of brain herniation before or during gradual spinal taps.

6. (C). Closed skull fractures without overlying wounds or symptoms require no repairs ('A'). Otherwise surgery is usually required.

7. (A). Anyone with head trauma and loss of consciousness needs a CT scan to exclude ICH. If the CT and the neurological exam are Nl, do 'B'. 'C' is for patients with suspected ICH. 'D' is best for ischemic stroke or tumor.

8. (B). This is a case of typical basal skull fractures. 'B' is the first choice because the patient is in coma with suspected ICH; then 'D' because it's severe head trauma; then 'A' if there is ICH together. Usually the CSF leak will stop by itself. Prophylactic antibiotics may not decrease the risk of meningitis.

9. (B). It's a severe subdural hematoma. First do 'B' to exclude spinal cord injury, then 'C' (decompression). 'D' (also decompression) should replace 'C' if the trauma is less severe and no midline shift or neurologic signs.

10. (A). Follow the order of 'A', 'B', 'C', and 'D' in this case. It's most likely an acute subdural hematoma because it's major head trauma; CT scan will show semi-lunar, crescent-shaped hematoma. It could be an acute epidural hematoma if it's less severe.

11. (D). The MRI reveals typical diffuse axonal injury (DAI). Surgery has little benefit and prognosis is poor. 'D' first plus 'A' and 'B' may prevent further injury by decreased ICP and improving brain perfusion.

12. (D). This is a very high-level neck injury without tracheal or esophageal involvement. Vascular injuries are the major concern. Angiography is both for Dx and potential Tx with embolization. Surgery is difficult for this case, but will be a good choice for a lower-level neck injury.

13. (D). This is a case of neck injury from blunt trauma with potential cervical spine injury (persistent local pain). First get anteroposterior (AP) and lateral X-ray films of the cervical spine (including T1). If it's (-) but still suspicious to you, a CT scan should be followed.

14. (C). A typical case of anterior cord syndrome.

15. (B). A typical case of spinal cord hemisection.

16. (D). A typical case of central cord syndrome. X-rays and CT scans are good to exam cervical bones. MRI is better to exam the spinal cord. Early high-dose corticosteroids after a spinal cord injury may have limited protective effects.

17. (A). SAH typically has acute severe headache and neck stiffness in an elderly patient with hypertension (HTN). #1 cause is berry aneurysm rupture; also from artery-vein (A-V) malformation. It's commonly diagnosed by CT and can also be proved by spinal tap.

18. (B). Typical cerebellar hemorrhage. Early Dx and surgical decompression are crucial to save life.

19. (E). Typical basal ganglia hemorrhage.

20. (D). Typical putamen hemorrhage, the most common type of ICH; mostly from lateral striate artery with internal capsule involvement.

21. (C). Typical pontine hemorrhage. Grasp all of the above differential diagnoses well.

22. (E). L-MCA stroke: contralateral weakness, numbness in the face and arm, homonymous hemianopsia, plus expressive (Broca's) aphasia (for dominant hemisphere; nondominant: hemineglect). 'D' has ipsilateral ataxia, Horner's signs, face numbness, decreased gag reflex, contralateral body numbness, etc.

23. (A). Anterior cerebral artery stroke: contralateral leg paresis, foot drop, gait dysfunction, amnesia, or personality change. 'B' has contralateral visual field deficits, memory deficiency, and reading deficiency. 'C' has vertigo, unilateral facial paralysis, cerebellar signs, visual deficits, dysphagia, apnea, or coma. Lacunar stroke usually has pure hemiparesis/sensory deficiencies, or dysarthria (hemiballismus).

24. (E). Ethosuximide is used generalized absence seizures (Petit Mal). Carbamazepine is the #1 common drug for complex partial seizures. Phenytoin is the #1 medicine for simple partial seizures and all generalized seizures except Petit Mal. Haloperidol is a strong medicine for psychomotor status and schizophrenia. Valproic acid is a secondary drug for most seizures with mood disorders.

25. (A). Carbamazepine is the #1 medicine for complex partial seizures. Phenytoin is the #1 drug for simple partial and all generalized seizures except Petit Mal. 'E' is best for absence seizure.

26. (C). This is a typical migraine without aura and with family history. Triptans and ergots are first line Tx for acute attack. Since this patient had three times of headaches in one month, a beta-R blocker is the best Tx (prophylaxis). 'A' is more suitable for a migraine with depression and fatigue. 'C' is for cluster headache. MRI is indicated if a mass is suspected (progressive symptoms but no family history).

27. (B). This is most likely cavernous sinus thrombosis without CNS involvement, and the best choice here is 'B' followed by 'E'. CSF, CT, and MRI may help with CNS involvement. 'C' is good for Gonococcal/Meningococcal meningitis. 'D' is good for cluster headache.

28. (G). This is most likely MS. B12 deficiency has macrocytic anemia and similar but progressive neurologic deficits and usually occurs after > 1 year of a strict vegan diet or in those with a B12–exhausting disease without sufficient vitamin intake. 'B' usually has 'Binswanger dementia', with vascular risk factors and history of cortical strokes.

29. (A). Pseudodementia is characterized by recent memory loss and improvement after proper antidepressant use; very common in the elderly and in patients with excess stress in their lives. AD usually shows gradual, progressive dementia with brain atrophy by MRI, without clear causes.

30. (D). Diffuse Lewy body disease: Dementia + Parkinson symptoms.

31. (F). Normal pressure hydrocephalus triad: dementia + incontinence + gait apraxia. 'J' is a benign increase in ICP with pulsatile headache and neuro-visual deficits. Risk factors include obesity and prolonged OCP use.

32. (O). Craniopharyngioma is a common supratentorial tumor in children, pressing on the optic chiasm and causing visual deficits and decreased ADH, GH, and thyroid hormone. Optic glioma is also a chiasmal tumor with similar symptoms, associated with neurofibromatosis and rarely calcified.

33. (N). Most likely it's an acoustic neuroma. Resection is the cure. Meniere disease: Episodic vertigo and tinnitus associated with nausea, vomiting, and bilateral hearing loss, but no CN7 deficiency.

34. (Q). Astrocytoma is the #1 common primary tumor in children and mostly in the cerebellum, with chronic headache, increased ICP, new seizure, ataxia, etc; with slow progress. Medulloblastoma is the #2 common CNS tumor in children, arising from the cerebellum vermis and 4th ventricle and progressing rapidly. Glioblastoma is the No.1 primary CNS cancer in adults, with rapidly progressive headache and increased ICP.

35. (K). Most likely it's a pituitary adenoma together with prolactinoma, with increased prolactin, GH, and ACTH; rarely calcified. Resection is the cure.

36. (P). Most likely it's a case of brain-stem glioma, a common posterior fossa tumor in children, affecting memory, personality, and some other brain-stem functions.

37. (B). Otosclerosis is the most common conduct hearing loss in adults with variable inheritance. 'C' is both autosomal dominant and recessive, with sensory hearing loss in adults. 'D' is primarily senile sensory hearing loss, typically for high frequency sound. Tx is hearing aids for most of these hearing losses. Labyrinthitis—acute vertigo and nystagmus following URI; usually no hearing loss or tinnitus; self-limited.

38. (C). Typical atrophic macular degeneration. Exudative macular degeneration can cause rapid and severe painless central vision loss.

39. (E). Hypertension and diabetes are common risk factors for this condition. Central retinal artery occlusion would have more abrupt, painless unilateral blindness. Fundoscopy often shows retinal swelling, cherry-red spot on the fovea, and pale artery and optic disc. Refer to a specialist ASAP.

40. (F). Typical retinal detachment. Tx is emergent surgery to close the retinal tears by an expert.

41. (B). Closed-angle glaucoma is caused by an acute closure of a narrow anterior chamber angle. Tx is lowering IOP and laser iridotomy immediately. Open-angle glaucoma is the most common glaucoma, primarily with gradual IOP increased and peripheral visual loss. Please review other diseases of the eyes.

Chapter 10

DISEASES OF THE SKIN AND SUBCUTANEOUS TISSUE

COMMON TERMINOLOGY AND LESIONS IN DERMATOLOGY

The skin consists of layers of epidermis, dermis, and subcutaneous tissue. Common dermatological terms and lesions are summarized in Table 10-1.

PEARLS—**Table 10-1:　Common Dermatological Terms and Lesions**

Lesion / Definition
Vesicle: A tiny, raised lesion with fluid inside (< 0.5mm).
Bulla: A large vesicle (> 5mm).
Macule: A flat, nonpalpable area with different color from surrounding skin.
Papule: A small, raised, solid lesion with distinct borders (< 5mm).
Plaque: A large-diameter, broad-based papule.
Patch: A small lesion with distinct borders and different color/structure from the surrounding skin (> 1cm)
"Ash leaf" spot: A depigmented macule on the trunk; an early pathologic marker of tuberous sclerosis.
Cyst: An epithelial-lined sac containing fluid or semi-fluid material.
Wheal/hive: Localized edema after vascular leakage, mostly disappears in a few hours.
Erosion: A superficial depression of localized skin resulting from the epidermal loss.
Ulcer: A deeper local depression resulting from destruction of the epidermis and upper dermis.
Scale: A thin piece of the outermost layer of skin resembling a fish scale; dry shedding of stratum corneum in flakes.
Scar: A mark left after a surface injury/trauma has healed, usually on the dermis layer.
Crust: "Scab": Dried blood, pus, or skin fluids on the surface of the skin.
Lichenification: Thickening of the skin with accentuation of normal skin markings; usually a result of chronic scratching or rubbing.
Shagreen patch: A thickened, yellowish plaque in the lumbosacral area with a "pig skin" texture.
Sebaceous adenomata: An oil-producing, solitary, yellow nodule on the face or scalp (hamartoma).
Phakoma: A retinal astrocytoma (mulberry lesion).

DERMATOLOGIC INFECTIONS

VIRAL INFECTIONS

Molluscum Contagiosum

It is a **poxvirus** infection most common in **young children and immunodeficient** patients. It is contracted by direct physical or sexual contact.

Essentials of diagnosis

1. A young patient presents with one or several small, oval, **fleshy, shiny, waxy, painless papules** on the face, trunk, or extremities for children (**Image 23**) and genital area for adults. Larger lesions are often on the face in immunodeficient patients.

2. **Diagnosis**: Based on the above clinical features, plus **KOH smear** or Giemsa/Wright's stain showing characteristic large intracytoplasmic inclusion bodies or molluscum bodies.

Treatment

Cryotherapy or TCA for local destruction is effective. In many patients, particularly children, lesions often resolve spontaneously over months to years without treatment.

Common Warts (Verruca Vulgaris)

Common warts are the most common **HPV** infection of different types, spread by direct contact, and occur on skin, mucous membranes, and other epithelia. Though most are benign, some subtypes (especially **16, 18, and 31**) can cause hyperproliferation of infected cells and squamous cancer (SCC, cervix cancer).

Essentials of diagnosis

1. Common warts are mostly **on the hands**. In young adults, **genital warts** are also common, typically showing **cauliflower-like papules or nodules** with velvety or white color on the genitoanal area (**condyloma acuminate, Image 27**).

2. Infant laryngeal warts: Usually transmitted by mothers with genital HPV infection. The latency period can be as long as months to years.

3. Diagnosis is clinical. **Acetowhitening** specifically aids in visualizing mucosal lesions.

Treatment

1. Many warts eventually spontaneously resolve without treatment. The main therapy is to destruct the local tissue by cryotherapy, curettage, TCA, podophyllin, imiquimod, or 5-FU.

2. Cervical HPV infection must be monitored by cytology for evidence of cancer.

Herpes Simplex

It is a recurrent, painful vesicular lesion of the mucocutaneous surfaces caused by two types of HSV. **HSV-1** usually generates **oral lesions, and HSV-2** produces **genital lesions**. Both are very prevalent in the general population and passed by direct contact. The virus remains in local nerves and spreads through epidermal cells, forming giant cells and causing local inflammation as erythema and swelling.

Essentials of diagnosis

1. **HSV-1 (Image 30):** It typically causes lesions of the oropharynx in infants and children, presenting with severe, widespread, painful vesicles and erosive vesicular gingivostomatitis.

2. **HSV-2 (Image 29):** It typically causes lesions of the genitalia in adults, presenting with bilateral, erosive, painful vesicular lesions on the genitoanal area, with possible edema and lymph node (LN) enlargements. Initial infection may not be noticed by the patient.

3. Both viruses can cause either type of lesions. Primary lesions are usually longer and more severe than recurrences. Manifestations vary by types and stages.

(1) Recurrent oral herpes: Commonly as "cold sore" (a cluster of crusted vesicles with an erythema base), often triggered by sun and fever.

(2) Recurrent genital herpes: Usually as a unilateral cluster of blisters on an erythema base, less painful than the primary herpes.

(3) Disseminated HSV: Usually occurs in immunocompromised patients and pregnant women, and may result in encephalitis, meningitis, keratitis, chorioretinitis, esophagitis, and pneumonitis.

(4) Neonatal HSV: Transmitted from mother at delivery; associated with congenital malformations, intrauterine growth retardation, chorioamnionitis, and even neonatal death.

4. **Diagnosis:** By clinical manifestations and **Tzanck smear**—Wright staining, showing **multinucleated giant cells**; **VZV** can also show these cells, and thus HSV culture (taking 2-3 days) or fluorescent antibody staining or ELISA (fast) may be needed for differential diagnosis.

5. **In immunodeficient or AIDS** patient, the HSV lesion can **persist** > 1 month even with anti-HSV therapy, which is oppositely a signal of immunodeficiency or AIDS.

Treatment

1. **Acyclovir** is the correct therapy—PO for most patients and IV for severe or immunodeficient patients. Topical acyclovir ointment (7-10 days) is only effective in reducing the duration of lesion but not in decreasing the recurrence as by PO.

2. Valacyclovir and famciclovir have better bioavailability. Foscarnet can be reserved for resistant cases in immunocompromised patients.

Differential diagnosis

Dermatitis herpetiformis (Image 79):

Pruritic papules or vesicles over extensive surfaces (elbow, knee, etc), with scaling, bleeding, and GI symptoms (malabsorption); **anti-endomysial antibody (+)**; associated with **celiac sprue** and increased risk of lymphoma (decreased by gluten-free diets). **Treatment:** No.1 choice is **dapsone**.

Eczema herpeticum:

It is locally superimposed on healing **atopic dermatitis** lesions after exposure to **HSV**, presenting with fever and vesicles. **Treatment:** Give **acyclovir** immediately, especially for infants (with life risk).

Varicella and Herpes Zoster

VZV is one of eight herpes viruses known to infect humans. It commonly causes two different diseases—primary infection as **chicken-pox (varicella) in children** and adults and recurrent infection as **herpes zoster (shingles) in adults**. VZV infections are transmitted by respiratory droplets or direct contact, with 10-20 day's incubation period, contagious 24 hours before the lesion erupts, and lasting until lesions have crusted.

Essentials of diagnosis

I. Varicella (Chickenpox, Image 80):   Tx: oral acyclovir

1. A general prodrome of fever, malaise, headache, and myalgia followed by pruritic rash in crops over 1-3 days, changing from red macules to centrally grouped vesicles (like **"dewdrops"**), then crusting over. All stages of rash can be present over the body but rarely on the palms and soles. WBC is usually normal or slightly depressed.

2. In adults, it causes a more severe infection called chicken-pox with systemic complications (pneumonia, encephalitis, etc.).

II. Herpes Zoster (Image 81):

1. Recurrent VZV lesions crop up along a specific nerve's **dermatomal distribution**, presenting with intense local pain followed by erythematous, segmented, grouped vesicles/blisters +/- scars.

2. Symptoms can be more severe in immunodeficient and older patients, with prolonged post-herpetic neuralgia.

Treatment

1. In most children: Usually self-limited and only supportive care is needed.

2. In adults and immunodeficient children: Systemic acyclovir and analgesics are necessary.

Prevention

A varicella vaccine is routinely given to infants, children and > 60 y/o adults.

BACTERIAL INFECTIONS

Impetigo

It's a superficial, pustular skin infection mostly in children, with honey-colored oozing, crusting, ulceration (ecthyma), and draining of the lesions. The commonest organisms are **Staphylococcal aureus ("S. aureus or Staph-A", bullous impetigo) and Group-A Streptococcus (Strep-A, non-bullous),** transmitted by direct contact.

Essentials of diagnosis

1. A superficial pustular lesion commonly seen on the face and limbs (**Image 82**). It may follow skin trauma. The lesion usually begins as maculopapules and rapidly progresses to vesiculo-papules or bulla. Without treatment, it can progress to lymphangitis, furunculosis, cellulites, SSSS, etc.

2. Bullous impetigo can be complicated by staphylococcal scalded skin syndrome (SSSS), and non-bullous Strep-A lesion by acute glomerulonephritis. Diagnosis is clinical.

Treatment

1. Topical mupirocin or bacitracin is adequate for mild lesions. *oral clindomycin*

2. Oral **anti-Staph penicillin** (PCN: oxacillin, cloxacillin, dicloxacillin) is necessary for severe cases. Clarithromycin or azithromycin is for penicillin-allergic patients.

Cellulitis

It's a deep, focal infection of the skin, subcutaneous tissue, or muscle. It's most commonly caused by **Group-A Strep** or **Staph-aureus** from a local skin lesion or systemic infection. Virulent cellulitis is often caused by community-acquired methicillin-resistant Staph-aureus (MRSA). **Risk factors** include diabetes, IV drug use, venous stasis, and immunodeficient state.

Essentials of diagnosis

1. Patient usually presents with a localized, warm, red, edematous, tender lesion on the skin; may be accompanied with high fever, chills, and tachycardia, etc.

2. **Erysipelas (Image 83)** is a **superficial form of cellulitis**, characterized by the above lesion confined to the dermis and lymphatics with a sharply-demarcated border, mostly on the face and limbs. Fever and chills may or may not be present. Rate of recurrence is high.

3. Wound culture and sensitivity (C/S) is helpful in diagnosis and treatment with sensitive antibiotics, especially in case of MRSA.

Treatment

7-10 day's antibiotics against Strep-A and Staph-aureus, PO for mild cases and IV for severe ones (with systemic toxicity or metabolic disease).

Differential diagnosis

Necrotizing fasciitis:

It is a rare, rapidly spreading infection of the fascia of deep muscle and deep layers of skin, easily spreading across the fascial plane within the subcutaneous tissue. It's mostly caused by Group-A Strep, S. aureus, and/or anaerobe Clostridium perfringens, and more common in patients with immunosuppression or chronic systemic diseases, or after trauma or surgery. It usually presents with purplish discolor of skin with **necrotization/gangrene of deep tissues**, swelling, severe tenderness (early) or cutaneous anesthesia (late), crepitus, and systemic toxicity (fever, malaise, etc). It may rapidly progress to sepsis, toxic shock syndrome, and multi-organ failure. **Treatment**: (1) IV fluid, high oxygen flow, and broad-spectrum antibiotics (such as vancomycin plus gentamycin). (2) Rapid surgical exploration and excision of necrotized tissue is a crucial therapy.

Thrombophlebitis:

Limb pain, systemic symptoms, along with palpable, indurated, cordlike, and tender subcutaneous vein segments. Treat as for DVT.

Other differential diagnosis: abscess, contact dermatitis, urticarial hives, and osteomyelitis.

Folliculitis

Also known as "**hot tub rash**", it is a common infection and inflammation of the hair follicle that can occur anywhere on the skin except the palms and soles. It's mostly caused by **S. aureus, Strep** or Gram⁻ bacterial (**Pseudomonas**) infections, and occasionally by yeast (Candida or Pityrosporum ovale), or mechanical factors from ingrown hair (more common with curly hair).

Essentials of diagnosis

1. **One or more tiny pustule(s) at the hair follicle** opening with a penetrating hair (**Image 84**), usually starting as a trivial lesion and developing into a **furuncle** or abscess with deeper infection.

2. Furuncles can **become larger and more painful or pruritic**, and involve adjacent follicles to form a **carbuncle**, especially in patients with chronic disease, diabetes, or immunosuppression.

Treatment

1. Mild cases only need topical antibiotics (clindamycin, macrolides, doxycycline, TMP-SMX); severe cases require systemic antibiotics (vancomycin, linezolid) and longer treatment for resistant patients with diabetes or immunosuppression. Antiparasitic agents, such as permethrin and oral ivermectin, can be effective for demodex folliculitis.

2. Prolonged and large lesions require incision, drainage of pus, and culture to rule out MRSA. Patient should keep the skin dry and clean, and avoid shaving with ingrown hairs.

Pilonidal Cyst

Also known as a pilonidal abscess or sinus, it is a cyst or abscess near the natal cleft of the buttocks that often contains hair and skin debris. Possible **causes** include ingrown hair, excessive sweating, and repetitive local injuries, leading to folliculitis, abscess, or Bacteroides infection locally.

Risk factors include middle-aged, obese male, sedentary lifestyle, and deep hairy natal clefts.

Essentials of diagnosis

A warm, tender, fluctuant and indurate abscess at the natal cleft; may be accompanied with purulent drainage or cellulitis; may develop into multiple cysts and perianal fistulas. Rule out perirectal and anal abscess.

Treatment

1. Incision and drainage of the abscess under local anesthesia, followed by sterile packing of the wound. Follow-up is needed.

2. Antibiotics are only used when cellulitis exists, with both aerobic and anaerobic coverage.

3. Educate patients to keep good local hygiene and shaving to prevent recurrence.

Acne Vulgaris

It's a common disease of the hair follicle associated sebaceous gland among adolescents, usually self-limited. The main etiology includes endogenous **androgen**-stimulation of sebaceous glands, follicular plugging or comedo formation, and infection and inflammation caused by **Propionibacterium acnes**.

Essentials of diagnosis

1. There are **two types of lesions**:

(1) **Non-inflammatory comedo (Image 85)**: The initial stage of lesion; can be numerous closed comedones (whiteheads) or open comedones (blackheads). Comedo may be associated with use of medicines (steroids, lithium) or cosmetics (topical occlusion). Closed comedones can progress to inflammatory lesions. **Epidermoid cysts** can develop along the eyebrows and by the ears.

(2) **Inflammatory**: Include papules, pustules, nodules, and cysts. **A scar** usually develops after the inflammation heals; repeated picking and healing produce larger scarring.

2. Acne mostly develops at **puberty** and persists for a few years. **Males** usually have **more severe** cystic acne and females tend to have cyclic flares and fewer comedones with menstruation.

Treatment

1. Topical **tretinoin (Retin-A) and benzoyl** are first-line treatment for mild lesion. Oral taking is for multiple or recurrent lesions. Isotretinoin (accutane) is highly efficient but teratogenic; also with transient hyperlipidemia, liver enzymes and depression.

2. Oral **clindamycin or erythromycin** is effective for moderate lesions (with inflammation). **Tetracycline** may be needed for months for severe disease.

Differential diagnosis

Rosacea (Acneiform, Image 86):

Also known as **adult acne or acne rosacea**, it is a similar chronic skin condition with unknown etiology. It may be associated with alcohol, spicy food, and sunlight exposure. Typically, a middle-aged patient presents with erythema, papules, pustules, red nose, flushing face, teleangiopathy, or rhinophyma (with alcohol drinking). **Treatment:** (1) Topical metronidazole, **tretinoin, or benzoyl** for most cases. (2) Systemic doxycycline or erythromycin for severe disease.

Felon

It's a **bacterial** infection of the closed volar space of fingertip pulp, causing abscess and intense pain. **Staph-aureus is the most common** cause. Gram⁻ bacteria can be the cause in immunosuppressed patients. It's commonly seen in **gardeners.**

Diagnosis: Marked throbbing pain, tension, and edema of the fingertip pulp, usually after an injury.

Treatment: Incision and drainage plus antibiotics against Staph-aureus +/- Gram⁻ bacteria.

Differential diagnosis

<u>Sporotrichosis</u>:

It's the most common **"Gardener's lesion",** a chronic **fungal** infection of the hands and arms. Symptoms include a small, painless, red lump that develops at the site of injury and infection, and eventually turns into an ulcer. Fungal lymphadenopathy may occur. The ulcers will not heal if untreated (with **itraconazole**) and may remain ulcerated for years.

FUNGAL INFECTIONS

Dermatophyte Infections

It's a superficial infection caused by a dermatophyte fungus (Microsporum, Trichophyton or Epidermophyton) that invades and lives in dead tissue of skin and appendages (nails, hair, and stratum corneum). **Risk factors** include chronic diseases, diabetes, peripheral vascular diseases, immunodepression, and pets (a reservoir for Microsporum).

Essentials of diagnosis

1. Tinea corporis: Papulosquamous annular lesions of the body, with scaly, pruritic eruption and a raised, irregular border, expanding peripherally and clearing centrally.

2. Tinea pedis/manuum: Presents as flaking, itching, macerated, and scaling borders (interdigital space) of the foot (**"Athlete's foot"**), or as thickened, scaly soles.

3. Tinea capitis ("ringworm"): Small, scaly, semibald, greyish patches on the scalp with broken lustreless hair, and similar to seborrheic dermatitis. Scaly, erythematous plaque on scalp => patchy alopecia.

4. Tinea cruris ("jock itch"): Chronic, ringed lesion on the groin, usually sparing the scrotum but co-existing with Tinea pedis.

5. Tinea unguium: Thickened and lustreless nails.

6. Tinea barbae: Lesion on the face.

Diagnostic guidelines: Above clinical features plus 10% KOH smear **showing mold hyphae.**

Treatment *PO griseofulvin terbinafine . Selenium Sulfide or Ketoconazole shampoo.*

1. Oral terbinafine or itraconazole is necessary for **Tinea capitis**, corporis, and unguium.

2. Topical miconazole, clotrimazole, or ketoconazole is for Tinea cruris, pedis, and corporis.

Tinea (Pityriasis) Versicolor

A fungal infection caused by **Pityrosporum** orbiculare (**Malassezia** furfur), a yeast as part of the normal skin flora (mostly asymptomatic). **Risk factors** include immunodepression, Cushing syndrome, and humid conditions.

Essentials of diagnosis

1. It's characterized by **multiple scaly patches of lesions that vary in color** from white to brown, from **hypopigmented to hyperpigmented**, and tend to coalesce. Lesions usually occur on the chest, neck, face or back (**Image 87**).

2. Diagnosis is usually clinical, and can be confirmed by 10% KOH smear of the scale showing a "**spaghetti with meatballs**" pattern of hyphae and spores.

Treatment

Topical selenium sulfide or ketoconazole for 7 days, or oral itraconazole if the lesion is large and severe.

Seborrheic Dermatitis

Also known as seborrhea, seborrheic eczema, dandruff, or cradle cap (infant), it is a common, relapsing, mild dermatitis. It usually affects the sebaceous-gland-rich areas of skin, such as scalp, face, and torso. It may be caused by **Pityrosporum** ovale, a normal yeast in sebum and hair follicles under special conditions.

Essentials of diagnosis

1. Rash varies with ages. In infants: Severe, red diaper rash with yellow scale, erosions, and blisters. On the scalp is often a thick crust ("cradle cap").

2. In adults: Typically presents with **scaly, flaky, itchy, red patches around the ears, eyebrows, nasolabial fold, midchest, and scalp**; more localized (**Image 88**).

3. Immunodeficient patients: May develop an overlapping syndrome (severe seborrheic dermatitis, psoriasis, arthritis, and Reiter syndrome).

Treatment

Antifungal shampoos is recommended—selenium sulfide 2.5%, ketoconazole 2%, or ciclopirox 1%. Nonmedical shampoos may not be helpful.

Candidiasis

It's a yeast infection caused by candida albicans, usually in patients with immunodepression and involving focal skin and mucous membranes. Systemic infection may occur under very weak immunity. **Risk factors** include prolonged systemic use of antibiotics, steroids, or cytotoxics, obesity, diabetes, pregnancy, debilitating disease, and AIDS.

Essentials of diagnosis

1. **Oral candidiasis (<u>thrush; Image 32</u>):** White patches of exudates on the tongue or buccal mucosa.

2. **Vulvovaginitis:** White or yellowish virginal discharge with inflammation of the vaginal wall and vulva; more common in patients with diabetes or pregnancy.

3. **Intertriginous infection:** Well-demarcated, erythematous, exudative, itchy patches; may be with small pustules; usually occurs in the axilla, umbilicus, groin, gluteal folds.

4. **Candidal paronychia:** Red, painful swelling around the nail.

Diagnosis: Based on the above clinical features plus **10% KOH** preparation to visualize fungi.

Treatment

1. Topical nystatin or ketoconazole/miconazole for mild cases.

2. Oral fluconazole for moderate systemic infection (including candida paronychia). Amphotericin is strong and toxic, and only used for serious cases.

PARASITIC INFECTIONS

Scabies

It's a parasitic skin infection by Sarcoptes scabiei (a tiny arthropod itch mite), spread by direct skin contact and characterized by superficial burrows, intense pruritus, and secondary infections.

Essentials of diagnosis

1. Marked **pruritus, erythematous and excoriated papules, and burrows (<u>Image 89</u>)**, commonly found on flexural surfaces of finger webs, wrists, elbows, axillary folds, breast areola, and the genital areas.

2. **Diagnosis**: Based on clinical features plus visualizing the mite in scrapings [scrape] with mineral oil under the microscope (sometimes the mite may not be seen).

Treatment

Both patients and contacts should be treated with **<u>permethrin</u>** [topical 5%] **or <u>lindane (Kwell)</u>** for several times. Oral ivermectin is also effective. Anti-histamine drugs should be given for pruritus > 1 week.

Prevention: decontaminating linens via hot water washings of clothing & bedding

Pinworm enterobis:
FAS1 p.143, FAS2 p.429

Pediculosis (Lice)

It's a skin infestation by lice that can live in different parts of the body, and is spread by body contact or sharing clothes/bed covers mostly in unsanitary persons.

There are **three common sites**:   *direct visual: Nits, lice*

(1) **Head lice**—pediculus humanus capitis, living on the scalp and laying eggs attached to hair;

(2) **Body lice**—pediculus humanus corporis, living in clothing;

(3) **Pubic lice**—living on pubic hair. They secrete local toxins and cause pruritus.

Essentials of diagnosis

1. Itching and excoriations in unsanitary persons; may or may not have secondary bacterial infection.

2. Diagnosis is made by direct exam of the scalp, axilla, pubic area, and clothes for the lice.

Treatment   *don't cut the hair.*

1. Wash the head and body frequently, and sterilize the clothes and bed covers fully.

2. Treatment of choice is **permethrin**. Lindane is less used due to its toxicity and resistance by lice.

path 203

IMMUNE-MEDIATED SKIN DISEASES

Angioedema

It's an abrupt swelling of the face, eyes, tongue, or/and airway typically associated with minor physical trauma. While it's often idiopathic, it can be due to a hereditary deficiency of C_1 esterase inhibitor.

Essentials of diagnosis

1. **Abrupt swelling of the face, eyes, or/and tongue with stridor** following minor physical trauma or without a clear reason. **Pruritus and urticaria are absent**. See **Image 90**.

2. The best test is for decreased C_2 and C_4 levels in the complement pathway and deficiency of C_1 esterase inhibitor.

Treatment

1. Immediate airway protection is performed first. Effective therapies include glucocorticoids, antihistamines, epinephrine (if severe), IV fresh frozen plasma (FFP), or/and C_1 inhibitor.

2. Long-term treatment with androgens (danazol or stanazol) if helpful. Hereditary angioedema does not respond to glucosteroid therapy.

Urticaria (Hives)

It's both a clinical condition and disease as a **type I hypersensitivity** reaction, characterized by abrupt superficial edema in a localized skin area, resulting from the release of vasoactive substances (histamine, prostaglandins, etc.) from mast cells. It's mostly acute and caused by a **drug, food (gluten), virus, insect bite, or physical condition (such as cold, pressure, or vibration)**. Chronic form is often idiopathic and can last over weeks to months.

Essentials of diagnosis

1. Severity can vary from a few itchy pumps to life-threatening anaphylaxis. Typical lesion is a **reddish/blanching, elevated papule/plaque (wheal) with variable sizes (Image 91)**, spreading widely but lasting only a few hours.

2. Severe allergic cases frequently show extra-skin presentations: fever, asthma, tongue and joint swelling, angioedema, and GI symptoms. Some forms of urticaria (especially with joint/kidney disease) are associated with neutrophilic vasculitis and hypocomplementemia.

3. Diagnosis is clinical, and causes are not always clear.

Treatment

1. Systemic antihistamines (hydroxyzine or diphenhydramine plus steroids if severe) are usually necessary. Topical drugs are not effective.

2. Leukotriene receptor antagonists (monteleukast or zafirlukast) can be helpful.

Differential diagnosis

Drug Reaction/Eruption:

It can cause **all four forms of hypersensitivity** reactions and present as any form of urticaria, vasculitis, purpura, lupus, blisters, or lichenoid lesions. It usually occurs 7-14 days after exposure, and is widespread, symmetric, pruritic, and short-lived (1-2 weeks). Fixed drug eruptions are usually reddish papules and occur in the same area with the same agent exposure. **Rare but severe complications or reactions** include erythroderma and toxic epidermal necrosis (**TEN**). **Treatment:** Stop the offending drug and treat with antihistamines and specific support.

Atopic Dermatitis
Eczematous

It's considered an **autosomal dominant** inherited allergic dermatitis, characterized by **erythema, lichenified plaques**, and **white dermatographism**. 30-50% of cases are associated with autosomal dominant ichthyosis vulgaris.

Essentials of diagnosis

1. It usually starts in childhood, and the child presents with dry, itchy, scaly patches, and plaques with red edema, blisters, crusting, and **white dermatographism** mostly in flexural areas (**Image 92**). In adults, it can be chronic skin thickening and scaling on any surface.

2. Triggers include stress, dry skin, foods (eggs, peanuts, milk, seafood, etc), air-allergens (dust, pollen, and mites), weather, etc. Associated diseases include allergic rhinitis, asthma, and cellulitis.

Atopic Eczematous Dermatitis

3. Diagnosis is clinical. Elevated IgE is helpful.

Treatment

1. Topical steroid +/- tacrolimus, tepid compression or oral anti-histamine agents.

2. Methotrexate can be used for severe cases. If no response, biopsy is needed to rule out malignancy.

Differential diagnosis

Ichthyosis vulgaris (Image 115):

It's a dermatosis without clear etiology, with **autosomal dominant** trends. The skin is normal at birth, and gradually grows dry, rough, and scaly mostly over the limb extensor surfaces (except the face and diaper area). It's usually worst in the winter, like "**lizard skin**". Diagnosis is clinical and treatment is skin ointment.

Contact Dermatitis

It's a **type IV cell-mediated hypersensitivity** reaction that develops from contact with an allergen previously exposed to (sensitized), with activated macrophages and T cells involved.

Common allergens include poison oak/ivy, nickel, detergents, perfumes, and cosmetics. It's more prevalent among adults.

Essentials of diagnosis

1. Itchy, erythematous, weepy, crusted patches; vesicles or plaques **grouped in linear arrays or geometric shapes** (e.g., **poison ivy**, **Image 93**).

2. Types: According to the appearing time of symptoms after exposure, it can be divided into acute (< 48 hours), subacute (in 1 week) and chronic type (> 1 week).

3. **Diagnosis**: Based on clinical impression. A **patch test** can help identify the causative allergen after the acute treatment, if necessary.

Treatment

1. For mild lesions: Cool compression and topical steroid are adequate.

2. For severe cases: Systemic steroids, anti-histamine agents and IV fluid are usually needed to relieve symptoms.

Psoriasis

It's a chronic, non-contagious, autoimmune dermatosis characterized by **erythematous patches and silvery scales** due to dermal inflammation and epidermal hyperplasia. Vulgaris (guttate) is the most common type among others. It may be associated with seronegative arthritis and polygenic factors, and more common in young patients.

Essentials of diagnosis

1. Typical psoriatic lesion is a round, **sharply bordered erythematous patch with silver scales**; mostly on extensor surfaces (elbow, knee, scalp, nail, etc.) and gradually enlarging from small patches. Lesions can be provoked by local irritation, trauma, infection, or drugs (such as a beta-blocker, ACE-I, and lithium).

Psoriasis

2. **Psoriatic arthritis (Image 60)**: Usually it's present in the hands as "**sausage fingers**" and in the lumbosacral region with "**oil spots**". HLA-B27 is mostly (+).

3. Psoriatic nails: With typical pitting, nail plate lifting, and onycholysis.

4. Pustular psoriasis: Less common. It can be localized on the palms and soles, or widespread. It may cause life-threatening metabolic disorder and serum protein loss.

5. **Diagnosis**: Based on clinical features. Auspitz sign (capillary bleeding when scale is scraped) is helpful and biopsy may be needed to rule out malignancy.

Treatment

1. Topical steroids and UV light are commonly used, along with keratolytic agents, tar, or anthralin. Methotrexate is effective for severe cases, and retinoids are effective for pustular psoriasis. Systemic steroids should be avoided, because dosing off may induce psoriatic flares.

2. Psoriatic arthritis: NSAID should be first tried. If it's ineffective, methotrexate is given. TNF-alpha inhibitor is an effective new medicine.

Erythema Nodosum

It's a panniculitis (fat cell inflammation) characterized by painful erythematous nodules under the skin on the lower legs. It can be triggered by infection (Strep, TB, Coccidioides, etc.), drug reaction (sulfonamides, OCPs, etc.), or chronic inflammatory diseases (ulcerative colitis, Crohn disease).

Essentials of diagnosis

1. **Tender, erythematous nodules on the lower legs**, slowly spreading and turning brown or gray (**Image 94**); may be accompanied with malaise, fever, joint pain, and local swelling.

2. Diagnosis is based on clinical features.

Treatment

Remove the causative factors and treat underlying disease. Use NSAIDs with caution because they can be both therapeutic and causative.

Path 206

Erythema Multiforme

It's a **type IV hypersensitivity reaction** caused by many triggers and characterized by **an annular, pruritic cutaneous reaction**. Those triggers include **HSV infection (#1)**, medications, mycoplasma, or idiopathic causes.

Essentials of diagnosis

1. History of recurrent labial HSV infections or drug use.

2. Typical lesions are **multiple target-like, centrally clear, erythematous macules** on the skin (**Image 95**) and mucous membranes, progressing to blisters or erosions.

3. Minor form is usually localized to the skin, whereas severe form can develop Stevens-Johnson syndrome or toxic epidermal necrolysis. Diagnosis is clinical.

Differential diagnosis

Erythema Toxicum (Urticaria Neonatorum, Image 96):

Erythema Multiforme

An autoimmune rash in newborns, with typical small, red, white or yellow, papules or pustules on an erythematous base; usually appear after the 1st day of life and resolve within 2 weeks. The pustules are benign lesions full of eosinophils if scraped for examination. The infant generally looks well otherwise.

Stevens–Johnson syndrome: See TEN below.

Treatment

Symptomatic treatment is adequate for mild cases (antihistamines, etc.). Acyclovir is needed for HSV infection and burn care for severe cases. Systemic steroids have limited effects.

Toxic Epidermal Necrolysis (TEN) and Stevens–Johnson Syndrome (SJS)

TEN is a rare but **serious, life-threatening hypersensitivity reaction** with severe erythroderma and epidermal necrosis, mostly induced by certain medications in adults. The main drugs that can cause it include sulfonamides, phenytoin, carbamazepine, and allopurinol. Infections and cancers may also induce the condition, though rarely.

Stevens–Johnson syndrome (SJS, Image 97) is a **milder form of TEN, characterized by widespread erythematous maculopapular rash. Both diseases can be mistaken for erythema multiforme**, which is more often a hypersensitivity reaction to an infection (mostly by HSV, sometimes by a medication) and is relatively benign. **IVIG (not steroids)** may be effective.

Essentials of diagnosis

1. Usually there is a history of medication use and maculopapular rash, followed by **widespread erythema and shedding of large sheets of skin**, and eroded or hemorrhagic mucous membranes of the eyes, mouth and genitals, etc. Systemic symptoms may exist.

2. **Biopsy shows full-thickness damage of the epidermis**, which is different from SSSS below.

Treatment

Treatment should include maintenance of fluid and electrolyte balance, skin coverage, and preventive antibiotics, the same as treating complications of burns (thermo-instability, electrolyte imbalance, secondary infection, etc.). **IVIG (not steroids)** may be helpful. The mortality risk is high.

Differential diagnosis

Staph scalded-skin syndrome (SSSS, Image 98):

Also known as **pemphigus neonatorum or Ritter disease,** it is characterized by severe, widespread shedding of sheets of skin caused by the epidermolytic exotoxins of **S. aureus** in both children (more) and adults. The widespread blisters with fluid and thin wall can easily rupture and be positive for **Nikolsky's sign**. Biopsy shows **superficial damage** of the epidermis only. Antibiotics (oxacillin or nafcillin) can kill the Staph that produces the toxin but not reverse the disease.

Warfarin-induced skin necrosis:

Painful skin lesion followed by bulla and skin necrosis on breasts, abdomen, thigh, or the hip a few weeks after warfarin use. **Treatment**: Stop warfarin, use heparin for maintenance, and Vit-K against warfarin.

Path 204

Pemphigus Vulgaris

Pemphigus is a rare group of blistering **autoimmune diseases** that affect the skin and mucous membranes in the middle-aged people. It's characterized by an intraepidermal blister that develops widespread painful erosions of the skin and mucous membranes. The anti-desmoglein IgG causes keratinocyte adherence and stimulates proteinases and complement in the cells, resulting in inflammation and cellular separation. The original cause is unknown.

Essentials of diagnosis

1. Usually presents with **erosions, crusting, and weeping** involving the skin and mucous membrane (**Image 99**), and secondary infections.
2. **Diagnosis**: **Nikolsky's sign (+)** (producing a blister by rubbing adjacent skin); skin biopsy shows **acantholysis**. Immunofluorescence or ELISA can confirm specific **anti-desmoglein IgG**.

Treatment

1. Treat skin lesion with burn care.
2. High-dose IV steroids and fluid are necessary even with adverse effects. Anti-metabolites (azathioprine) can replace steroids with severe adverse effects afterwards.

Bullous Pemphigoid

It's a **chronic, autoimmune, subepidermal, blistering** skin disease, characterized by blisters and separation at the epidermal basement membrane, and mostly seen in elder patients. It involves anti-pemphigoid IgG and C_3 deposited at the dermal-epidermal junction. Antigen-antibody complexes activate complement and eosinophils, resulting in inflammation and separation of the basement membrane. The blisters are relatively firm, and epidermis and mucous membranes are usually normal.

Essentials of diagnosis

1. Patient usually presents with a history of urticarial lesions, followed by stable blisters arising on erythematous skin (it is basically **urticaria plus erythematous blisters**, **Image 100**). Nikolsky's sign is (-). Mucous membranes are rarely involved.
2. Diagnosis is clinical. Skin biopsy shows subepidermal blister with eosinophil infiltration.

Treatment

Early use of topical steroids can help prevent blister formation. Systemic steroids to inhibit inflammatory lesions are necessary in most cases.

Pityriasis Rosea

It's an **idiopathic, self-limited cutaneous eruption** usually seen in children and women. It may or may not be associated with an infection.

Essentials of diagnosis

Pityriasis Rosea

Patient may have a history of URI, followed by an itchy, diffuse eruption of round-oval erythematous papules and plaques covered with a fine white scale mostly on the trunk. The pathognomonic sign is a **"herald patch"** (a solitary patch 2-6 cm in diameter preceding the rest of the rash) followed by smaller satellite rash (**Image 101**).

Differential diagnosis

Secondary syphilis, psoriasis, cutaneous T-cell lymphoma (parapsoriasis), etc.

Treatment

This disorder is self-limited. Pruritus may be relieved by a topical steroid or talc. Strong sunlight or UVB treatment may hasten its healing.

FA52 296, Path66

Kawasaki Disease (Mucocutaneous Lymph Node Syndrome)

It's a rare, **self-limited, acute inflammation of the blood vessels, skin, membranes, and lymph nodes in children** with unknown etiology. Without treatment, the mortality rate may reach 1%.

Essentials of diagnosis

usually, never give kids w/ viral dz aspirin bc => Reye syndrome

1. Patient may have a brief history of **viral infection followed by a persistent high fever** that is not very responsive to common NSAIDs (acetaminophen or ibuprofen).

2. Typical presentations also include **painful** red swelling of the skin, membranes, conjunctiva, and lymph nodes (may be > 1.5 cm); **cracked or bleeding lips, strawberry tongue**; multi-form, purple rash on the trunk, palms, and soles (rarely on face) that progresses to **desquamation**. See **Image 36**. Diagnosis is clinical.   *Sterile pyuria*

Treatment

in this case ASA OK - inhibits TXA2 => ↓ Thrombus formation.

Early, high-dose IVIG (< 24 hours) plus aspirin (special recommendation in children) are highly effective and important to prevent coronary artery aneurysms (the No.1 common complication); steroids are ineffective. Supportive care in hospital is also important. If aspirin is a life-long need, Flu-vaccination can be used together.

DYSPLASIAS AND NEOPLASIAS

Path 206

Seborrheic Keratosis

Also known as **"senile wart"**, it is **the most common benign skin tumor that originates in keratinocytes**, mostly after 40 y/a. The etiology is unknown. Sometimes, they may erupt abruptly in a large number and cause a paraneoplastic syndrome by tumor-releasing epidermal growth factors. There is no major harm except for a cosmetic issue.

Essentials of diagnosis

Seb Ker

1. Typically as multiple **exophytic, waxy, brown papules, nodules, and plaques**, with obvious follicle openings (**Image 102**). Lesions can become smoother and redder after irritation or trauma.

2. Diagnosis is by clinical impression. Biopsy is rarely needed but will show hyperplasia of benign, basaloid epidermal cells.

Differential diagnosis

Seborrheic dermatitis, actinic keratosis, lentigo, basal cell carcinoma, and squamous cell carcinoma.

Treatment

Curettage or cryotherapy is the cure.

Actinic Keratosis

It's also called "solar keratosis" or "senile keratosis". It is a premalignant condition of squamous cell carcinoma (SCC) in situ. Without treatment, it carries 20% risk of slow progression to SCC. It's mainly caused by sunlight overexposure and more common in fair-skinned, older people.

Essentials of diagnosis   sandpaper-like scale

1. Typical lesion is an **erythematous, thick, scaly, crusty, and sharply demarcated patch of skin**, mostly on sun-exposed areas (particularly face, neck and arms; **Image 103**). Early lesions may be difficult to visualize but easier to find by palpation.

2. Diagnosis is clinical. Biopsy may only be needed when the lesion is thick and large (to exclude SCC), and will show intraepidermal atypia over a sun-damaged dermis.

Differential diagnosis

Bowen disease (Image 104):

It's another form of SCC in situ, an early stage or intraepidermal form of SCC; may be due to solar damage, arsenic, immunosuppression, or viral infection (HPV). It's typically a gradually enlarging, well-demarcated erythematous plaque with an irregular border and surface crusting or scaling on sun exposed areas of the skin, mostly in an elder female. Biopsy shows atypical squamous cell proliferation through the epidermis.

Treatment: Cryotherapy or topical imiquimod or 5-FU can destroy the lesion effectively. If cancer is suspected, biopsy is done followed by excision or curettage. Use of sun protection is recommended.

Path 207
Basal Cell Carcinoma (BCC)

BCC is the **most common type of skin cancer**, usually on sun-exposed area (face, neck, and head). It grows slowly and locally, rarely metastasizes (Met), but can cause significant local destruction and disfigurement. The incidence of trunk-BCC seems increasing.

Risk factors include chronic sun (**UV light**) exposure (#1 factor), arsenic exposure, and inherited BCC nevus syndrome.

Essentials of diagnosis

1. BCC can appear as several forms: **nodular (No.1 common, fleshy nodule with "pearl" surface, Image 105**), ulcerated, superficial, sclerosing, pigmented BCC, and BCC nevus syndrome, with various degrees of pigmentation, ulceration, depth of growth, and translucent surface.

2. **Diagnosis is confirmed by biopsy**—will show islands of proliferating epithelium that resembles the basal layer of the epidermis.

Differential diagnosis

Melanoma, hypopigmented nevi, psoriasis, and Paget disease, etc.

Treatment

Any of the following treatment to remove the tumor can have > 95% cure rate: excision, curettage, electric cautery, deep cryotherapy, Mohs surgery (with the best cure rate), and superficial radiation.

path 207

Squamous Cell Carcinoma (SCC)

SCC is a form of squamous epithelium carcinoma that may occur in many different organs, including the skin, mouth, esophagus, prostate, lungs, vagina, cervix, etc. SCC of the skin is **the No.2 common skin cancer**, with local destruction and a deadly metastatic potential. It's mostly in elder patients with **history of actinic keratosis or chronic sun/UV light exposure (#1 risk factor)**. Other risk factors include chemical carcinogens, radiation exposure, and chronic draining infection or lesion.

Essentials of diagnosis

1. Patient usually presents with an **irregular plaque with surface scaling, erosion, or ulceration** on sun exposed areas of the skin, which can be in various forms of lesions—**nodular (No.1 common, Image 106)**, exophytic, verrucous SCC, and SCC with cutaneous horn.

2. **Diagnosis is confirmed and graded by biopsy**: Will show intraepidermal atypical keratinocytes, with malignant epidermal cells penetrating the basement.

Treatment

Mohs surgery or aggressive surgical excision is necessary and the best therapy for most tumors, plus radiation or chemotherapy for those with a high metastatic potential.

Differential diagnosis

Keratoacanthoma (Image 107):

It's a relatively common, low-grade malignancy that originates in the pilosebaceous glands and closely resembles SCC, or considered a "**well-differentiated SCC.**" It occurs on the site of sun exposure, a firm, flesh-colored "volcano" nodule of about 1 cm^2, with a sharp rising edge and kerato-debris in the crater center. The size may increase rapidly in 3-4 months then decrease spontaneously. It's usually **difficult to be distinguished from SCC clinically**, except by histology showing benign features—well-differentiated intraepidermal atypical keratinocytes.

Table 10-2: Comparison of Basal Cell Carcinoma and Squamous Cell Carcinoma

Basal Cell Carcinoma (BCC, Image 105)

Nodular: No.1 common type, as nodular, pearly tumor with telangiectasias, and frequent ulceration.

Superficial: Usually appears as a flat patch on the trunk, with occasional bleeding or peeling; may have arsenic association.

Ulcerated: Usually crusted with bleeding and healing over.

Sclerosing: Appears as a spontaneously scarred tumor.

Pigmented: Due to secondary proliferation of melanocytes in the tumor; most common in the Black population.

BCC nevus syndrome: An autosomal dominant inherited disease, presenting with multiple BCCs from childhood, along with CNS tumors, frontal bossing, and jaw cysts.

Squamous Cell Carcinoma (SCC, Image 106)

Nodular: No.1 common, a thick nodule or papule tumor, frequently with central ulceration.

SCC with horn: The above nodular SCC with a hyperkeratotic growth on top.

Exophytic: A red, friable nodule tumor often with bleeding and usually arising from Bowen disease.

Verrucous: A low-grade SCC resembling a wart, usually on mucous membranes and plantar surfaces.

Melanoma ^(Path 208)

It is the **most malignant tumor of the skin** originated from melanocytes (which produce melanin), one of the less common types but **causes the majority (75%) of skin cancer related deaths**. Morbidity is increased around the world. **Risk factors** include intense **sun (UV light) exposure** on congenital melanocytic or dysplastic nevi (multiple or at young ages), immunodeficiency, familial atypical mole, and melanoma syndrome, etc.

Essentials of diagnosis

1. History of intense sun exposure, with **pruritus** as an early sign, and a typically pigmented nodule with **"ABCD" features: A**symmetric, **B**order and **C**olor irregularity, and **D**iameter > 6 mm (**Image 108**). Presenting forms are summarized in the table below.

2. The tumor initially grows horizontally and intraepidermally, showing a flat lentigo maligna or melanoma in situ; later it grows vertically into the dermal layer. It can metastasize to nearby skin, regional lymph nodes (LN), or distant organs.

3. **Diagnosis:** Clinical features plus **biopsy** of the suspicious tumor following **Clark's levels and TNM staging.**

Table 10-3: Forms of Presentation of Melanoma

Forms / Clinical features
Nodular: Rapidly, vertically growing reddish-brown nodule with ulceration or bleeding.
Superficial: Prolonged superficial spreading and confined to the epidermis, possibly early diagnosis. It usually presents on the legs or trunk of young adults.
Lentigo maligna: It arises in a lentigo maligna and develops a nodule with ulceration; mostly on the face with sun-damage.
Acral lentiginous: Slowly spreading, pigmented patch starting on the hands and feet; more common among Asians and Black populations.
Amelanotic: A lesion without obvious pigmentation; very difficult for diagnosis.

Table 10-4: Clark's Levels and Staging of Melanoma

Clark's Levels
Level I: Depth within the epidermis; 5-year survival rate: 99%.
Level II: Into the papillary dermis; 5-year survival rate: 95%.
Level III: Filling the papillary dermis; 5-year survival rate: 90%.
Level IV: Into the reticular dermis; 5-year survival rate: 65%.
Level V: To subcutaneous fat; 5-year survival rate: 25%.
TNM Staging
I: Primary skin melanoma; 5-year survival rate: 70%.
II: Local and regional Met; 5-year survival rate: 30%.
III: Distant metastasis; 5-year survival rate is almost '0'.

Treatment

1. Tumor confined to the skin should be treated by surgical excision with adequate margins. Mohs surgery has a relatively high cure rate. Lymph node dissection is helpful for staging but not for survival increase. Chemotherapy or radiation may only have limited effects.

2. Prognosis depends on the tumor thickness, depth, type of melanoma, location of lesion, and status of metastasis. Malignant melanoma has the special potential to relapse and metastasize to distant organs after several years. Therefore, patient follow-up is very important. When there is distant metastasis, melanoma is generally considered incurable. The five-year survival rate is less than 10%.

Differential diagnosis

Atypical mole (Image 109):

Also known as **dysplastic nevus**, dysplastic melanocytic nevus, it is pigmented mole-like lesion on sun-exposed areas, mostly 0.5-1 cm in diameter and larger than an ordinary mole, with irregular borders and colors and a flat shape. They can be multiple and may not change much for a few months. Pathological results are **between nevi and malignant melanoma**. Individuals with it are at **higher risk for developing melanomas** (especially with multiple moles), and thus regular photographic monitoring is necessary. **Early treatment of excision and biopsy** is recommended if they look complex, grow larger, or change in color, shape, or other features (itching, oozing, etc.).

Xeroderma pigmentosum (XP)

XP is an autosomal recessive **genetic disorder of DNA repair** in which the ability to repair damage caused by UV light is deficient. The most frequent defect is **mutations in the CDKN2A** tumor suppressor gene. There are multiple types. It is more common in Japanese people. Due to the forced avoidance of sunlight, young patients are often referred as **"Children of the Night"**.

Clinical features and diagnosis (Image 110)

1. Typical manifestations include **numerous, sun-sensitive, rough-surfaced growths (solar keratosis**—scaly, dry skin, irregular dark spots on the skin) with freckling (early age); sun-sensitive painful eyes, spidery blood vessels, and corneal ulcerations; with hair growth on chest and legs.

2. **Multiple types of BCC and other skin malignancies (SCC, melanoma) frequently occur at a young age in those with XP.**

Treatment

The most obvious and important part of treatment is avoiding exposure to sunlight, as well as close clinical surveillance and education regarding melanoma risk-reducing behaviors. Keratoses can also be treated using cryotherapy or fluorouracil.

Prognosis

Fewer than 40% of individuals with the disease survive beyond the age of 20. Metastatic melanoma and SCC are the two most common causes of death with XP.

Kaposi Sarcoma (KS)

It's a rare malignant tumor originated from lymphatic endothelium and vascular proliferation, but generally not considered a true sarcoma. It's associated with **HIV and HHV-8** (a HSV), which is also called KS-associated-herpesvirus (KSHV). It occurs particularly with chronic immunodeficiencies or AIDS (also known as an AIDS defining illnesses). There are several clinical types.

Clinical types and diagnosis

1. Epidemic HIV-associated KS: Aggressive form of KS; it's the most common HIV-associated malignancy and decrease due to the application of "Highly active anti-retroviral (anti-HIV) therapy" (HAART).

2. Endemic or African KS: Mostly among Africans and immunodeficient patients.

3. Classic variant KS: It typically manifests as multiple red-purple nodules and surrounding pink-red macules, or multicentric vascular macules and coalescent papules and plaques on the upper trunk, face, oral mucosa, and lower limbs (**Image 31**).

4. **Diagnosis** is by clinical impression and **confirmed by a tissue biopsy**, which shows spindle cells and viral protein LANA in the cells. If clinically indicated, internal imaging should be done.

Treatment

KS is not curable, and thus the main treatment is **palliative only,** based on the four subtypes and the state of the disease. No surgery is effective or recommended. Antiretroviral therapy may induce regression of the HIV-associated KS for some patients. Local tumors can be treated with cryotherapy or radiation; widespread lesions are treated with chemotherapy (paclitaxel, anthracyclines, or interferon-alpha). Prognosis is poor.

Cutaneous T-Cell Lymphoma (Mycosis Fungoides)

It's a rare, slow, progressive proliferation of T-cells rather than fungal infection. It may be associated with chronic exposure to irritating chemicals and immunostimulation leading to T-helper cells gathering in the epidermis. Male > Female.

Clinical features and diagnosis (Image 111)

1. Stage I (early lesion, plaque): A pruritic, palpable, patchy, psoriatic plaque on the skin.
2. Stage II (nodules): Confluent, multicentric, reddish-brown nodules on the skin.
3. Stage III (tumors): May involve systemic lymph nodes and internal organs (liver, spleen, etc.)
4. **Diagnosis** is clinical and confirmed by **biopsy,** showing the typical **cerebriform lymphocytes (Sezary or Lutzner cells)**.

Differential diagnosis

Early lesions are hard to be differentiated from **dermatitis**, therefore histology is necessary for any chronic dermatitis resistant to decent treatment.

Treatment

Stage I: Topical steroids, retinoids, chemotherapy, or PUVA.
Stage II: Systemic retinoids, interferon, monoclonal antibody, or chemotherapy.
Stage III: Systemic chemotherapy mainly.

MISCELLANEOUS SKIN DISORDERS

Ischemic Skin Lesions

Summarized in Table 10-5.

Table 10-5: Comparison of Ischemic Skin Lesions

Lesion / Clinical features, diagnosis, and treatment
Gangrene Necrosis of body tissue, often with anaerobic infection. There are three subtypes: 1. **Dry gangrene**: Caused by lack of blood flow to tissue, commonly from atherosclerosis. Risk factors: DM, vascular disease, smoking, etc. Early signs are dull pain, cold, pale flesh; later the tissue (like the toe) turns bluish/black, dry, and shriveled. Diagnosis is clinical. 2. **Wet gangrene**: Due to ischemia plus bacterial infection (mostly skin flora). The tissue becomes swollen, bruised, or blistered with pus. Diagnosis is clinical. 3. **Gas gangrene**: Caused by anaerobic Clostridium perfringens infection, usually at a site of recent injury or surgery. Swelling around the injured skin, with pallor, dark redness, and crepitus. The bacteria are gas-producing and very destructive, causing an ER case. **Treatment**: 1. Surgical debridement and necessary amputation is the major treatment; antibiotics are an adjuvant to surgery. 2. Gas gangrene should be treated with hyperbaric O_2, which is toxic to the anaerobic C. perfringens. Early preventive treatment for susceptible injury (especially foot) is highly important.
Decubitus Ulcer Ischemic necrosis resulted from continuous pressure on a skin area that causes compromised microcirculation to it. 1. Ulcers are commonly seen in long bedridden patient (#1 Risk factor). Other risk factors: Lack of mobility, skin area with bone prominence or lack of fat, urine/stool incontinence, etc. 2. Ulcers are graded by three degrees/phases: (1) persistent redness; (2) ulceration; (3) destruction of structures beneath the skin (muscle, fat). Diagnosis is by clinical impression. **Treatment: 1. Prevention is the best Tx**—frequently and routinely moving bedridden patient and using special beds (distributing pressure). 2. A mild ulcer is treated with routine wound care (hydrocolloid dressings, etc). 3. A severe ulcer requires surgical debridement.

Differentiations of Miscellaneous Skin Lesions

Summarized in Table 10-6.

PEARLS—Table 10-6: Summary of Miscellaneous Skin Lesions

Disease / Clinical features, diagnosis, and treatment
Lichen Planus (Image 113) A chronic intensely pruritic skin condition without clear etiology. 1. **Violaceous, flat-topped, polygonal papules;** may have **Wickham striae** (white stripes) and ulceration. 2. Lesions often appear initially on the genital areas or the trauma site. Most lesions resolve spontaneously in ½-1 year, whereas the oral lesions can be longer. 3. **Dx:** Histology reveals a "**lichenoid pattern**" (typical T-cell band at the dermal-epidermal junction with basal layer damage). **Tx:** Mild lesions: topical steroids and tretinoin gel. Severe lesions: systemic steroids can be added.

Lichen Simplex Chronicus (also "scratch dermatitis" or "neurodermatitis")

Itching, scratching, cyclic dermatitis.

Tx: Topical steroids.

Acanthosis Nigricans (Image 114)

1. A condition of **hyperkeratotic and hyperpigmented** skin with **velvety** appearance, usually in the **intertriginous zones** (nape of the neck, auxiliary and genital regions). 2. It may be **associated with diabetes** and obesity (especially inherited with insulin resistance) **in young** adults, and underlying **adenocarcinoma** (GIT mostly) **in elder patients**. 3. **Dx:** Clinical.

Tx: 1. Topical steroids or retinoid. 2. Weight reduction and exercise.

Leukoplakia

A focal, whitish, painless patch/plaque with clinical uncertainty. Usually it's found on the mouth mucosa, vulva and with granular texture that is hard to be removed. It's associated with smoking, alcohol, Vit-A or Vit-B deficiency, and risk of transferring to SCC. Treat original disease.

Hairy Leukoplakia

A hairy, whitish, painless patch mostly caused by EBV, usually localized on the lateral tongue of immunodeficient patient (such as AIDS; **Image 33**).

Tx: Treat EBV and original disease.

Chapter 10: High-yield Questions (HYQ)

1-6: Match the following clinical scenarios with the most likely cause.

A. HPV	B. HSV-1	C. HSV-2
D. VZV	E. Poxvirus	F. EBV
G. HIV	H. Vitamin deficiencies	I. Anti-endomysial antibody (Ab)

1. A 10 y/o girl presents with a 3-day's fever and multiple painful vesicles on the perianal area, following a healed skin rash of dry, scaly, and itchy patches on the same area a month ago. There is no evidence of local trauma, abuse, or other abnormal findings.

2. A 9 y/o girl presented with fever, malaise, and headache 3 days ago followed by pruritic vesicles in crops with crusting today. The rash is present all over the body except the palms and soles. Her immunization history is uncertain. CBC is normal (Nl).

3. A 30 y/o man presents with a 3-day's pruritic, erythematous papules, and vesicles over extensive surfaces of the elbows and knees with scaling and petechiae. He has a history of chronic diarrhea for the past 3 months. He is otherwise fine. CBC, stool and urine analysis are mostly normal.

4. A 20 y/o female presents with several oval, fleshy, shiny, waxy, painless papules on the genital area for the past month. She is sexually active for a year. KOH smear of the tissue reveals large intracytoplasmic inclusion bodies. There are no other abnormal findings.

5. A 20 y/o female presents with several cauliflower-like, pruritic papules and nodules with gray-white color on the genital area for the past month. She is sexually active for a year. There are no other abnormal findings. Acetowhitening test confirms the diagnosis.

6. A 25 y/o man presents with fever, fatigue, weight loss and a hairy, whitish, painless patch on the lateral tongue for the past month. He has a history of homosexual behavior for several years. Physical examination (P/E) finds multiple lymph node (LN) enlargements. CBC reveals WBC < 1000/uL with predominant lymphocytes (LC).

7-13: Match the following clinical scenarios with the best initial treatment.

A. steroid	B. oral oxacillin	C. vancomycin and gentamycin
D. oral metronidazole	E. tretinoin	F. systemic doxycycline
G. permethrin or lindane	H. incision and drainage	I. incision and drainage plus oxacillin
J. oral itraconazole	K. oral azithromycin	L. topical selenium sulfide or ketoconazole

7. A 60 y/o man presents with a 3-day's high fever, headache, and painful left foot with purplish discolor of the skin with marked swelling and tenderness. He also has tachycardia and hypotension. Blood glucose and WBC are elevated, with predominant neutrophils and bands. IV fluid is started.

8. A 10 y/o boy is found with a superficial, pustular bulla on the nose, with yellowish crusting. It's been there for the past 3 days and he feels generally well except for mild fever and local pain.

9. A 60 y/o man presents with a 5-day history of 1-2 cm pruritic pustule at the hair follicle of the head, with warmness and tenderness. He's been on oral cloxacillin along with topical ketoconazole for the past 5 days and the pustule seems still the same. He is otherwise feeling well.

10. A 60 y/o woman fond of trimming roses in the yard had an injury on a right finger 5 days ago. She now presents with a mildly painful red lump and ulcer on the finger. P/E finds moderate fever and swollen lymph nodes under the right armpit. CBC is normal.

11. A 40 y/o man complains of redness and pimples on the nose, cheeks, and forehead for the past month, especially after alcohol drinking. He has a history of smoking and alcohol drinking for several yrs. P/E finds facial erythema, papules, pustules, and flushing, and red nose and rhinophyma. There are no other abnormal findings.

12. A 50 y/o man presents with a month of small, itching, scaly, greyish patches on the scalp with broken lustreless hair and a semibald head. He drinks alcohol and has diabetes for the past 10 years. There are no other abnormal findings.

13. A 50 y/o man presents with a month of multiple itching scaling patches of lesions on the chest with varied colors from white to brown and hypopigmented to hyperpigmented. He drinks alcohol and has diabetes with a 10-year's history. There are no other abnormal findings.

14-20: Match the following clinical scenarios with the most likely diagnosis.

A. Ichthyosis vulgaris	B. Kawasaki disease	C. Atopic dermatitis
D. Urticaria (hives)	E. Toxic epidermal necrolysis	F. Staphylococcal scalded skin syndrome
G. Bullous pemphigoid	H. Pemphigus vulgaris	I. Erythema multiforme
J. Erythema nodosum	K. Contact dermatitis	L. Psoriasis

14. A 7 y/o boy presents with a month of dry, scaly, itchy, erythematous patches with blisters and whitening changes with local pressure in flexural areas of both elbows. He recalls that he had a seasonal rhinitis before this skin rash. There are no other abnormal findings.

15. A 5 y/o boy has gradually progressed dry, rough, scaly skin over the limb extensor surfaces for the past few months, and it's worse in the winter. His uncle has a similar history. There are no other abnormal findings.

16. A 45 y/o woman has recovered from a joint pain with aspirin treatment. Now she finds an itchy, reddish, blanching, elevated plaque on the arm, spreading widely and recovering mostly in a few hours, accompanied with mild wheezes. There are no other abnormal findings.

17. A 20 y/o woman presents with multiple target-like, centrally clear, erythematous, erosive, itchy macules on the palm, sole and perianal areas. She admits that she is sexually active and had multiple painful, erosive, erythematous vesicles on the labia twice for the past 3 months. She denies other symptoms and recent drug use.

18. A 25 y/o Asian woman presents with fever, congested conjunctiva, cracked lips, strawberry-like tongue, and painful, erythematous swelling of the extensive skin, membranes, and lymph nodes. She denies any history of recent drug use and other diseases. Vital signs are stable.

19. A 30 y/o man had a major seizure attack with aspirated pneumonia and has been controlled with antibiotics and anti-seizure agents for the past 3 days. Yesterday he found multiple red itchy rashes on the chest. Today he is

found with fever, tachycardia, hypotension, widespread erythema, erosion, and shedding of large sheets of skin over the body. WBCs are elevated.

20. A 40 y/o man has chronic asthma under medical control. Now he presents with painful, erythematous, erosive, crusting rashes with some pustules involving the skin and mucous membrane. P/E also finds that rubbing adjacent skin produces blisters. WBCs are elevated and other results are suspended.

21-26: Match the following clinical scenarios with the most likely diagnosis.

A. Seborrheic keratosis   B. Acanthosis nigricans   C. Actinic keratosis

D. Keratoacanthoma   E. Squamous cell carcinoma (SCC)

F. Basal cell carcinoma (BCC)   G. Melanoma   H. Cutaneous T cell lymphoma

I. Kaposi sarcoma (KS)   J. Bowen disease   K. Paget disease

L. Lentigo

21. A 60 y/o man presents with a palpable, erythematous, sharply demarcated lesion on the forehead, with some scaly and crusting changes over the past year. He likes outdoor activities all the times. Biopsy shows intraepidermal atypia over a partially damaged dermis.

22. A 60 y/o woman presents with a gradually enlarging, well demarcated erythematous plaque with an irregular border and surface crusting or scaling on the left lower leg for the past month. She likes outdoor activities for years. Biopsy shows atypical squamous cell proliferation through the epidermis.

23. A 62 y/o man presents with fatigue, darkening skin, abdominal distension, weight loss, and black stools for the past 2 months. He has a history of smoking and alcohol drinking for 10 years. P/E finds hyperkeratotic and hyperpigmented skin with velvety appearance in the nape of the neck, axillary, and inguinal regions. Lab tests reveal anemia and FOBT (+).

24. A 50 y/o man presents with a 4-mm nodule on the neck that started 3 months ago, with gradual, mixed changes of pigmentation, erythema, ulceration, and smooth appearance. The size is about the same now as he noticed before. He likes outdoor activities all the times. Biopsy shows islands of proliferating epithelium resembling the epidermis.

25. A 55 y/o man presents with a 6-mm nodule on the neck that began 3 months ago, with gradual, mixed changes of pigmentation, erythema, ulceration, and irregular appearance. The size was about 4-mm 3 months ago as he noticed. He likes outdoor activities all the times. Biopsy shows malignant cell proliferation invading the epidermis.

26. A 55 y/o man presents with a 6-mm firm nodule on the forehead that started 3 months ago, with flesh color, "volcano"-shape, and kerato-debris in the center. The size was about 4-mm 3 months ago as he noticed. He has longed enjoyed outdoor activities. Biopsy reveals relatively well-differentiated, atypical intraepidermal keratinocytes.

Answers and Explanations

1. (C). Eczema herpeticum is a locally superimposed lesion on healing atopic dermatitis lesions after exposure to HSV, presenting with fever and vesicles. HSV-1 is usually associated with severe, erosive, vesicular gingivostomatitis. Treat with acyclovir ASAP.

2. (D). A varicella case caused by VZV. Recurrent VZV infection causes zoster, showing typical dermatomal distribution.

3. (I). Dermatitis herpetiformis is associated with celiac sprue, anti-endomysial antibody, and increased risk of lymphoma. Treatment is dapsone.

4. (E). A molluscum contagiosum caused by poxvirus through sexual contact. Treatment is cryotherapy or TCA.

5. (A). Common warts are the No.1 common HPV infections over the body and spread by direct contact. Though most are benign, some subtypes (16, 18, or 31) can cause SCC. Treatment is cryotherapy or TCA.

6. (F). Hairy leukoplakia is mostly caused by E-B virus in immunodeficient patients, such as possible AIDS in this case. Confirm or exclude AIDS, and treat EBV and original disease.

7. (C). This is most likely necrotizing fasciitis caused by Strep-A or Staph-aureus and/or anaerobics after trauma or surgery. Treatment is IV fluid, high oxygen flow and broad-spectrum antibiotics to cover all the above mixed pathogens before culture/sensitivity confirmation.

8. (B). Impetigo is a common skin infection in children, usually caused by Staph-aureus (bullous impetigo) or Strep-A (non-bullous). 'B' is adequate for this case. 'K' is for PCN-allergic cases.

9. (H). It's a case of folliculitis developing into a furuncle or abscess; usually caused by Staph, Strep or Candida. After proper treatment, prolonged and large lesions require incision, drainage of pus, and culture to rule out MRSA.

10. (J). Sporotrichosis is the No.1 common "Gardener's lesion", a chronic fungal infection of the hands and arms. The ulcers do not heal unless treated (with itraconazole). Felon is another similar lesion usually caused by Staph-aureus and with marked throbbing pain but rarely lymphadenopathy.

11. (E). Rosacea (Acneiform) is also known as "adult acne", similar to acne vulgaris in treatment with 'E' or topical metronidazole.

12. (J). Tinea capitis is similar to seborrheic dermatitis in some extent, and best treated with oral itraconazole. Other Tinea types can be treated with topical agents.

13. (L). Tinea versicolor is caused by yeast M. furfur and characterized by multiple patches with different colors. KOH smear will show a typical "spaghetti with meatballs" pattern. Treatment for this mild case is 'L'.

14. (C). A common case of atopic dermatitis, treated with topical steroid +/- tacrolimus, etc. Contact dermatitis has typical itchy erythematous vesicles or plaques grouped in geometric shapes.

15. (A). Also known as "lizard skin." It seems to be associated with atopic dermatitis of autosomal dominant inheritance. Diagnosis is clinical and treatment is skin ointment. Psoriasis is a dermatosis characterized by sharply bordered erythematous patches and silvery scales; treat with topical steroids and UV light.

16. (D). This is an aspirin-induced hives, a type I hypersensitivity reaction; treat with oral antihistamines.

17. (I). It's an annular, pruritic cutaneous reaction mostly by recurrent HSV infection. Erythema nodosum is a panniculitis triggered by infection, drug reaction, or chronic inflammatory diseases.

18. (B). Kawasaki disease is an acute inflammatory syndrome of the skin, membranes and LN with unknown etiology. Treatment is aspirin and IVIG.

19. (E). Most likely a TEN induced by phenytoin, carbamazepine, or sulfonamides. It's a rare but serious drug reaction. Biopsy shows full-thickness damage of the epidermis, which is different from staphylococcal scalded skin syndrome (superficial damage). Warfarin may also induce similar skin bulla and necrosis after weeks of use.

20. (H). Pemphigus vulgaris--an intraepidermal blister. It's diagnosed and differentiated from bullous pemphigoid by Nikolsky's sign (+) and anti-desmoglein antibody (+). Skin biopsy will show acantholysis, whereas in pemphigoid it will show subepidermal blister with eosinophil-rich infiltrate. Both are treated with high-dose systemic steroids.

21. (C). Actinic keratosis is a precursor of SCC, evolving slowly and confirmed by biopsy.

22. (J). It's also called "Early SCC." Typical SCC biopsy will show malignant epidermal cells penetrating the basement. Treatment for Bowen disease is cryotherapy or topical 5-FU, and aggressive surgery for SCC.

23. (B). This is often associated with diabetes in young adults and GIT adenocarcinoma in older patients—most likely colon cancer in this patient.

24. (F). BCC is the No.1 common skin cancer mostly caused by solar UV light exposure, slowly growing and rarely metastasizes. It can appear as nodular (No.1), ulcerated, superficial, sclerosing, pigmented form, etc.

25. (G). Melanoma is the most lethal skin cancer, mostly caused by sun exposure. It can present as nodular, superficial, lentigo maligna, acral lentiginous, or amelanotic form. Aggressive surgical excision is the treatment for this stage I, level I malignancy.

26. (D). It's often difficult to be differentiated from SCC clinically, and only by histology to show the benign feature of well-differentiated atypical keratinocytes.

Chapter 11

GYNECOLOGY

AMENORRHEA AND RELATED DISORDERS

Amenorrhea is defined as the absence of menstruation.

Primary amenorrhea: absence of menstruation and lack of secondary sexual characteristics by age 14. The absence of menses alone by age 16 is called "**isolated primary amenorrhea**".

Secondary amenorrhea: absence of menses for 3 cycles or 6 months with prior normal menses.

Etiology

1. **Primary amenorrhea**: Gonadal agenesis or failure (Turner syndrome), androgen insensitivity syndrome, mullerian duct defect (Def), hypopituitary failure, constitutional development delay, etc.

2. **Secondary amenorrhea: pregnancy (No.1 cause)**, hyper-/hypo-thyroidism, hypo-thalamic/pituitary failure (Sheehan or Kallmann syndrome), polycystic ovarian syndrome, premature menopause, hyperprolactinemia, anorexia nervosa, etc.

Diagnostic Steps

Think of the defect or cause at three levels: (1) Uterus or ovaries; (2) genital tract; (3) pituitary, hypothalamus, or CNS. Start evaluations as for secondary amenorrhea. Testosterone, LH: FSH levels and karyotype can help with diagnosis.
   1. **Beta-hCG test** is always the first consideration for most patients of reproductive ages.
   P/E for outflow tract defects: May reveal absent uterus or vagina.
   2. **Prolactin test**: Increased prolactin leads to decreased FSH and LH. Common causes are pituitary tumor, hypothyroidism, and dopamine-antagonists (phenothiazines, etc.). The diagnostic means is TSH testing and CT/MRI scan of the pituitary.
   3. **Progestin challenge**: (1) If withdrawal bleeding occurs after 5-day's progesterone (test '+'), the patient has normal estrogen and outflow tract, and thus anovulation is the diagnosis.
   (2) If the test is (-) —no bleeding, the estrogen-progestin challenge test is performed.
   4. **Estrogen-progestin challenge test:** (1) If withdrawal bleeding occurs, the cause is at the follicle or the hypothalamus-pituitary axis. (2) If there is no bleeding, Asherman syndrome is the diagnosis (endometrial fibrosis, commonly caused by IUD or D&C).
   5. **Gonadotropins (FSH/LH) tests**: (1) If the levels are low, meaning central GnRH is low, consider hypothalamic/pituitary dysfunction (Sheehan syndrome, pituitary tumor, etc.).
   (2) If FSH/LH is high, meaning the estrogen is low, consider gonadal failure (Turner syndrome, gonadal agenesis, or 17-hydroxylase deficiency).

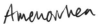

Treatment

Treat underlying cause.

Table 11-1: Differentiation and Management of Amenorrhea

Phenotype, Clinical features, diagnosis, and treatment

Breasts and uterus both present

Diagnosis (Dx) is based on secondary amenorrhea, testosterone level, LH:FSH ratio, and chromosome analysis. **Luteal phase deficiency:** It's commonly seen in polycystic ovarian syndrome (**POS**) or ovarian dysfunction. Basal body temperature (BBT) is abnormal, short menstrual cycles, low mid-luteal progesterone, high LH:FSH ratio, and history of spontaneous abortions. Dx is best confirmed by endometrial biopsy, showing maturity lag > 2 days.

  Tx: (1) Vaginal supply of progesterone. (2) Give clomiphene or beta-hCG, which can increase FSH and LH levels, and lead to ovulation.

Breasts present, uterus absent (by ultrasonography)

  1. Mullerian agenesis: Genetically females (46, XX) with normal secondary sexual characteristics, pubic or axillary hair, and testosterone, but absence of the Mullerian duct derivatives (fallopian tubes, uterus, cervix, and upper vagina). **Tx**: Surgical elongation of the vagina for satisfactory sexual life.

  2. Androgen insensitivity (testicular feminization): Genetically male (46, XY) but no androgen-R function—the body does not respond to the high levels of androgens present. Testicular Mullerian inhibition factor is present. Patients show female breasts and external genitalia (by estrogen from the testes) but no or scant pubic/axillary hair, with internal Wolffian duct structures atrophy (no fallopian tubes, uterus and vagina). Patient is brought up as girl, and diagnosed when primary amenorrhea is noted (16 y/a). **Tx:** (1) Remove the testes by 20 y/a to avoid testicular cancer. (2) Long-term estrogen replacement.

Breasts absent, uterus present

  1. Gonadal dysgenesis (Turner syndrome): (45, X), lack of two X chromosomes leading to deficient ovarian follicles (streak gonads). FSH levels are elevated because of lack of estrogen (feedback). There are no secondary sexual characteristics. **Tx**: Estrogen and progesterone replacement for development of the secondary sexual characteristics.

  2. Hypothalamic-pituitary failure: Lack of FSH, FH, sex hormones, and secondary sexual characteristics but with a uterus. **Kallmann syndrome** is the genetic failure of the hypothalamus to produce GnRH and may also have anosmia and color blindness. **Tx**: Estrogen and progesterone replacement for development of the secondary sexual characteristics (along with pulsatile GnRH for ovulation).

Hypothalamic-pituitary Dysfunction

  Causes include stress, anxiety, anorexia nervosa, excessive exercise, etc. Manifestations vary. Other disorders may be involved apart from amenorrhea.

  Tx: Treat underlying cause.

Ectopic Pregnancy

A pregnancy in which implantation has occurred outside of the uterine cavity. The most common location is oviduct (95% in distal ampulla). Risk factors include a history of PID (#1), prior ectopic pregnancy, tubal or pelvic surgery, and DES or IUD use.

Essentials of diagnosis

1. **Triad:** (1) Amenorrhea; (2) Unilateral lower abdominal pain; (3) Spotting vaginal bleeding (1-2 weeks after LMP).

2. Other possible findings: Generalized abdominal pain and tenderness, a pelvic mass, and orthostatic hypotension (if ruptured).

Diagnostic steps

1. First test beta-hCG for any suspected patient.
2. If it's (+) but < 1500 mIU/mL), perform transvaginal ultrasound or repeat beta-hCG in 24 hours.
3. If the patient has the "triad" with orthostatic hypotension, fast culdocentesis can be done first, which may reveal > 5 mL of nonclotting blood.
4. Definitive diagnosis is made by laparoscopy or laparotomy.

Treatment

—Determined by the results of serial beta-hCG and ultrasound studies.

1. Patient with stable, unruptured fallopian tube pregnancy, falling hCG, and < 3.5cm mass can be managed expectantly for spontaneous course.
2. Cases with stable beta-hCG, unruptured ectopic pregnancy, < 6 week's gestation, and < 3.5cm mass can be treated with methotrexate.
3. All other cases must be treated with surgery—laparoscopy (if stable) or laparotomy (if unstable) to perform unilateral salpingostomy (#1 choice), salpingectomy (tube rupture), or salpingo-oophorectomy.
4. Most patients should receive RhoGAM.

Complication

Fetal loss, hemorrhagic shock and death, future ectopic pregnancy, infertility, and Rh sensitivity.

Differential diagnosis of lower abdominal pain

1. Surgical conditions: Appendicitis, abdominal abscess, twisted/ruptured ovary cyst, endometriosis, and intestinal obstruction.
2. Pregnancy (+) conditions: Ectopic pregnancy, threatened abortion, incomplete abortion, and hydatidiform mole.

Premenstrual Syndrome (PMS)

Clinical features and diagnosis

Pre Menstrual Syndrome

PMS includes a wide range of physical and emotional conditions, including fluid retention (bloating, breast tenderness, and edema), autonomic symptoms (insomnia, fatigue, and heart pounding), musculoskeletal pains, or emotional symptoms (crying, anxiety, depression, and mood swings).

Diagnosis is made by review of patient's diary of the above symptoms for three menstrual cycles.

Treatment

Fluoxetine (a SSRI), progesterone, spironolactone, or/and Vit-B6 may help.

Menopause

It's defined as the permanent cessation of menstruation secondary to ovarian degradation and resistance to gonadotropins. The average age of menopause is 50 y/a. Age < 40 is considered premature menopause, which is mostly due to idiopathic premature ovarian failure; age between 40 and 50 is early menopause, which is often associated with smoking, alcohol, and chronic diseases. Due to lower protective estrogen, menopausal females have more risks of developing osteoporosis and heart disease.

Essentials of diagnosis

1. Irregular menses (decrease, increase or menorrhagia), hot flashes (due to vasomotor instability), sweats, mood changes, depression, sleep disturbances, lower libido, dyspareunia (due to vaginal atrophy), urinary irritation, etc.

2. **P/E** reveals vaginal dryness and genital tract atrophy. **Lab tests**: low estrogen; high FSH.

3. **Diagnosis** is made with the above presentations and no menses for one year.

Treatment

1. Hormone replacement therapy (HRT): This can relieve some symptoms and reduce risk of osteoporosis and cardiovascular diseases. If the patient still has a uterus, opposed progesterone/estrogen should be used. If the patient has no uterus, unopposed estrogen is used.

2. Non-hormone therapy: Ca, P2, and Vit-D can alleviate osteoporosis but no other symptoms.

Complication

Atrophic vaginitis, osteoporosis, cardiovascular diseases (MI, stroke), etc.

ABNORMAL UTERINE-VAGINAL HEMORRHAGE

Prepubertal Vaginal Bleeding

It refers to vaginal bleeding before puberty, mostly < 10 y/a. The most common cause is **foreign body**, followed by trauma, early menses, etc.

Precocious puberty refers to development of secondary sexual characteristics and accelerated growth before age 8 in girls and age 9 in boys. Cases of precocious puberty are increasing nowadays probably because people turn to ingest more foods containing steroids. It is more common in girls than in boys.

Abnormal Uterine Bleeding

It includes (1) Menstrual flow lasting > 8 days; (2) A menstrual interval < 21 days; (3) Total blood loss per menstrual cycle > 80 mL.

Common causes

Dysfunctional uterine bleeding and bleeding caused by ectopic pregnancy, threatened abortion, adenomyosis, endometriosis, uterine polyps, and cervical or endometrial cancer.

Diagnostic tests

1. **Beta-hCG (#1 test,** to rule out pregnancy), CBC, endocrine factors (TSH, prolactin, FSH/LH).

2. D&C for uterine lesions, ultrasound for mass, and Pap smear or biopsy for cancer.

Differential diagnosis

DUB and anovulation, pregnancy and its complications, anatomic defects, etc.

Treatment

Treat underlying cause.

Dysfunctional Uterine Bleeding (DUB)

It includes menorrhagia (excessive menses), metrorrhagia (irregularity), menometrorrhagia (irregular and excessive menses), polymenorrhea (frequency-increased menses), and oligomenorrhea (scanty menses). It's mostly due to functional hormonal imbalance, and the **No.1 common cause** is **anovulatory cycles**, which is caused by **unopposed estrogen**. Continuous stimulation of the endometrium without secretory phase leads to estrogen breakthrough bleeding.

Essentials of diagnosis

1. History of irregular, non-cramping menstrual bleeding, and normal beta-**hCG** and anatomic exams.

2. Cervical mucus will be clear and thin or watery. A basal-body temperature (BBT) chart lacks a mid-cycle temperature rise. An endometrial biopsy will show proliferative endometrium.

Treatment

1. < 30 y/a: OCP or cyclic progestin, or IV estrogen if heavy.

2. > 35 y/a: Endometrial biopsy is performed first, and patient is treated accordingly.

3. Severe, uncontrollable uterine bleeding may require D&C with endometrial ablation, vaginal packing, uterine artery ligation, or hysterectomy (as the last resort).

Endometriosis

It refers to the existence of endometrial glands and stroma outside the uterus. It's a benign condition, not a premalignancy. The etiology is unknown and may be due to retrograde menstruation. The **most common site is the ovary**; the second is the cul-de-sac. It bleeds monthly and can create adnexal enlargements called endometriomas or chocolate cysts.

Essentials of diagnosis

1. Typical history of dysmenorrhea, painful defecation (dyschezia), painful intercourse (dyspareunia), chronic abdominal pain, abnormal bleeding, and infertility. Pregnancy will alleviate symptoms because of amenorrhea.

2. P/E usually reveals pelvic tenderness, uterosacral ligament nodularity, a fixed, retroverted uterus, or tender and enlarged adnexa.

3. **Lab tests**: CA-125 may be elevated. WBC and ESR are normal. Ultrasound may show an endometrioma. Definite diagnosis is made by **laparoscopic biopsy** of endometriotic nodules or cysts ("chocolate cysts" or "powder-burns" lesions).

Differential diagnosis

PID, pelvic adhesion, ectopic pregnancy, adnexal torsion, endometrioma, appendicitis, amenorrhea.

Treatment

1. Medications: After initial NSAIDs, the **best choice is GnRH analog (leuprolide)** for 3-6 months, **or OCPs** if patient is young and does not expect pregnancy. This is to mimic the atrophic changes of pregnancy.

2. Surgery: Conservative—laparoscopic ablation of visible endometriosis for patients who expect pregnancy; aggressive—total abdominal hysterectomy for severe, recurrent disease and infertility. Estrogen replacement is required with bilateral salpingo-oophorectomy.

3. Annual gynecologic examination is necessary.

Adenomyosis

Ectopic endometrial glands and stroma are located within the myometrium of the uterine wall, commonly diffusely involved. If the lesion is focal and surrounded by a pseudocapsule, it's called adenomyoma.

Essentials of diagnosis

1. Most patients are **asymptomatic**. Common symptoms are secondary dysmenorrhea, menorrhagia, and anemia.

2. **Pelvic exam**: Most of the diagnosis is made clinically by finding a diffusely enlarged, symmetric, tender uterus in the absence of pregnancy. Tenderness is usually immediately before and during menses. Definite diagnosis is made by surgical biopsy.

3. **Imaging**: Ultrasound usually shows a diffusely enlarged uterus with cystic areas found within the myometrial wall.

Adenomyosis

Treatment

Hysterectomy is the definitive therapy for patients with significant symptoms because no medication is satisfactory.

GYNECOLOGIC INFECTIONS

Pelvic Inflammatory Disease (PID)

Ascending

It refers to infections involving the fallopian tubes, uterus, ovaries, or ligaments of the uterus; usually follows cervical or vaginal infections. The most common pathogens are **Chlamydia and Gonococcus**. Others include Mycoplasma, anaerobic or Gram⁻ bacteria. Risk factors include unprotected or over-frequent sexual intercourse, multiple sexual partners, early-age intercourse, and intrauterine devices (IUD) use. Females are more vulnerable from male infections. Use of oral contraceptive pills (OCP) and barrier contraception is protective from PID.

Essentials of diagnosis

1. History of low fever and abdominal or pelvic pain on palpation of the cervix, uterus, or adnexa. **Cervical/adnexa tenderness** on motion is the best sign for diagnosis, along with cervix discharge.

2. **Lab tests**: WBCs $> 10 \times 10^3$/uL. Beta-hCG test, discharge culture on **Thayer-Martin** for Gonococcus and Gram stain should be done. **Laparoscopy** is the definitive means of diagnosis. Pelvic ultrasound can help exclude other disease, such as an ovarian cyst, tumor, abscess, etc.

Differential diagnosis

Ectopic pregnancy, endometriosis, ovarian cyst (bleeding, twist) or tumor, UTI, appendicitis, and diverticulitis.

Treatment

1. Mild: Outpatient is treated with a single dose of ceftriaxone *IM* (for Gonococcus) along with azithromycin or 7-day doxycycline (for Chlamydia), or 2-week ofloxacin along with metronidazole (for the anaerobic).

2. Severe (high levels of WBCs, T $> 39°$C): Inpatient is treated with cefoxitin (or cefotetan) IV along with azithromycin or doxycycline PO. *—if severe, has N/V, pregnant, or can't tolerate PO.* *Cefoxitin + Doxy IV. backup regimen for allergies or Preg: clinda + gentamycin*

3. Chronic PID (with abscess): Treat with ampicillin + gentamicin + metronidazole + clindamycin for > 72 hours.

Complication

Infertility and ectopic pregnancy are common.

Vaginitis

Normally the vagina contains mixed bacterial flora in an acidic environment (pH 3.5-4.5), which is maintained by lactobacilli. Any factors that increase the vaginal pH value (such as drugs, diseases, frequent sexual activities) can cause overgrowth of other bacterial species and infection. Common pathogens include chlamydia, bacteria, fungi, and protozoan, and should be treated accordingly (Table 11-2).

PEARLS—Table 11-2: Etiologic Comparison of Vaginitis

Variable	Bacteria	Chlamydia	Trichomonas	Fungi
Incidence	High; anaerobic, Gardnerella as #1; may be an STD	High, #1 STD	May coexist with bacteria or be an STD	Candida is #1; not an STD, more common in immunodeficient patients
Symptoms and signs	Homogeneous, grayish, watery discharge with fishy/stale odor; burning vagina	Painless, yellow, mucopurulent discharge	Profuse, yellow-green, malodorous, frothy discharge; strawberry petechiae in upper vagina/cervix	Itchy, thick, white, cottage or cheese-like discharge; no odor; excoriated erythema on the anterior vaginal wall
Saline smear	Clue-cells (epithelial cells with bacteria) plus WBCs	Many WBCs without bacteria	Motile trichomonads (flagellated, larger than WBCs)	(-)
KOH prep	Whiff test (+) (fishy smell)	(-)	Whiff test (+/-)	Pseudohyphae
Vaginal pH	> 4.5	> 4.5	> 4.5	Normal (< 4.5)
Treatment	Metronidazole, oral or vaginal, 7 days; if pregnant: clindamycin. Treat partner if it recurs.	Azithromycin 1-day or doxycycline 7 days.	Oral metronidazole to both patient and partner; if pregnant: metronidazole cream or clindamycin cream.	Topical antifungals (nystatin, miconazole).

Cervicitis

It's the inflammation of the uterine cervix, usually coexists with vulvovaginitis. The prevalence is > 80% among sexually active females.

Etiology
1. Infection: Common pathogens are Chlamydia, Gonococcus, Trichomonas, HSV, and HPV.
2. Others: Trauma, malignancy, radiation, etc.

Essentials of diagnosis
1. Most patients are asymptomatic. Yellow-green mucopurulent discharge from the cervix indicates bacterial or trichomonas infection.

Cervicitis

2. A pelvic exam usually reveals redness of the cervix, evidence of discharge, and cervical motion tenderness.

3. Lab tests: Discharge inspection under a microscope may prove candidiasis, bacteria, or trichomoniasis. Special tests may be performed for suspected Chlamydia or Gonococcus. Pap smear for cytology may be needed for patients with cancer risks.

Treatment

Based on etiology (See "PID") —similar antibiotics for PID are used to cover Gonococcus, Chlamydia, and the anaerobic.

GYNECOLOGIC NEOPLASMS

Most of the gynecologic tumors are benign. Common gynecologic malignancies include **breast (most common)**, endometrial, ovarian, cervical, and vulvar cancers.

UTERINE NEOPLASMS

Endometrial Carcinoma

It is malignant proliferation of glandular and stromal elements of the endometrium, mostly from atypical complex endometrial hyperplasia. It's the #2 most common gynecologic malignancy after breast cancer, occurring in 1% of women and mostly around 60 y/a.

Pathologic types

Type I—Endometrioid (adenocarcinoma): > 80%, associated with unopposed estrogen use or stimulation and atypical hyperplasia. It's low-grade, superficial, and prognosis-favorable, with typical abnormally postmenopausal bleeding. **Risk factors:** Obesity, diabetes, hypertension, nulliparity, late menopause, and polycystic ovarian syndrome (POS).

Type II—Serous: < 20%, mostly associated with p53 mutation but not estrogen, with endometrial intraepithelial cancer as the precursor lesion. It's a high-grade tumor, with deep invasion and poor prognosis but no typical manifestations.

Essentials of diagnosis

1. **The most common symptom** is abnormally heavy **postmenopausal bleeding** (+/- enlarged uterus), which must be evaluated with an endometrial sampling.

2. **Hysteroscopy and ultrasound**: These can help diagnose cervical or endometrial cancer, polyps, and leiomyoma.

3. **Staging**: By surgery and pathologic report.

Treatment

Endometrial Carcinoma

1. Stage I—Age-dependent: Premenopausal patients—high-dose progestin; postmenopausal patients—hysterectomy and bilateral salpingo-oophorectomy (TAH-BSO), plus pelvic and para-aortic lymphadenectomy plus peritoneal washing. Add chemotherapy for serous cancer.

2. Chemotherapy (cisplatin + doxorubicin) or radiation: Used for intermediate-risk or high-risk cancer with poor prognosis by pathologic report (advanced stage, metastasis, recurrent cancer, and poor differentiation).

Differential diagnosis of postmenopausal bleeding

Vaginal or **endometrial atrophy:** Most common, to be treated with estrogen and progesterone replacement; hormone replacement therapy (**HRT**).

Prevention

Postmenopausal patients taking estrogen replacement therapy must also take progestins to lower the risk of endometrial cancer by unopposed estrogen. Similarly, patients with anovulatory disease (such as POS) should also take progestin.

Uterine Leiomyoma (Fibroids)

It is a benign smooth muscle growth of the myometrium, the No.1 common benign uterine tumor. It can develop from intramural, submucous, and subserosal locations. Tumor sizes are various depending on the reproductive life stage (estrogen and its receptor level).

Essentials of diagnosis

1. Most leiomyomas are **small, slow growing, and asymptomatic**. Some may have longer, **heavier menses**, and secondary anemia and dysmenorrhea.

2. **Changes in size**: When estrogen level is high (as in pregnancy), it can grow fast and big enough to cause pelvic pressure symptoms (bloating, constipation, etc.). When the estrogen level is as low as in postmenopause, myomas will shrink.

3. **Pelvic exam**: Mostly reveals an enlarged, firm, asymmetric, nontender uterus ("lumpy-bumpy") in the absence of pregnancy, to make the **clinical diagnosis**. Definite diagnosis is made by surgical histology.

4. **Imaging: Ultrasound or MRI** can show large intramural or subserosal myomas. **Hysteroscopy** can help visualize submucous myomas directly.

Treatment

1. **Observation**: Most leiomyomas will regress after menopause, and thus can be observed with regular pelvic examinations.

2. **Medications for bleeding**: Progesterone or danazol can slow or stop bleeding. GnRH analogs (leuprolide) can reduce the myoma size.

3. **Surgery** for persistent bleeding and anemia: Myomectomy is for childbearing-age patients and total hysterectomy for post-childbearing patients. Emergent surgery is for torsion of a pedunculated myoma.

degenerating uterine leiomyoma:
- rapid growth during pregnancy from ↑ estrogen ↑ progesterone
- myometrial blood flow shifts to fetus ↓ placenta, thus ↓ fibroids outgrow their blood supply.

- This leads to fibroid infarction and necrosis
- uterine cotractions from cytokines, Prostaglandin inflam release
fundal tenderness, tender uterus 442
leukocytosis from inflam cytokines

CERVICAL NEOPLASIA

Cervical Dysplasia

It's a premalignant lesion of the cervix, usually asymptomatic. Some lesions will spontaneously regress, others remain static, and only a minority progress to cancer after 8-10 years.

Etiology

HPV 16 and 18 (more risk), and 31, 33, 35, and 58 are the common HPV types associated with cancerous lesions of the cervix, whereas HPV 6 and 11 are associated with benign condyloma acuminata.

<u>**Risk factors for cervical dysplasia and carcinoma**</u>

Early-age menarche/sexual activity, multiple male sex partners (with associated viruses), STDs, **HPV** and other infections, smoking, family history, OCP use, immunosuppression, and lower-income status.

<u>**PEARLS: Screening for cervical carcinoma**</u> (updated by USPSTF)

Women 21 to 65 (Pap smear) or 30-65 (in combo with HPV testing):

The best test is cytology—**Pap smear is started at age 21** (regardless of sexual activities) and repeated every 3 years thereafter until age 30 (as long as results are normal). Between ages 30 and 65, patients should be screened every 5 years with cytology and HPV testing.

Cervical intraepithelial neoplasia (CIN) and Bethesda classification system of cervical lesions

1. Normal (Nl);
2. Inflammatory;
3. Atypical squamous cells of undetermined significance (ASCUS);
4. CIN1 —Mild dysplasia or low-grade squamous intraepithelial lesion (LSIL);
5. CIN2 —Moderate dysplasia or high-grade squamous intraepithelial lesion (HSIL);
6. CIN3 —Severe dysplasia to carcinoma in situ;
7. Carcinoma. The commonest site for cervical dysplasia/cancer is the transformation zone (T-zone).

Essentials of diagnosis

It is mostly asymptomatic and found out by screening test.

Lab tests:

(1) (+) **Pap smear** or colposcopy (with cervical dysplasia): Must be followed with cone biopsy, which will reveal either CIN (LSIL or HSIL) or invasive cervical cancer.

(2) **Colposcopy:** This is usually done after an abnormal Pap smear, and can significantly expand positive results of the cervix lesions. It is also frequently **followed by an endocervical curettage and ectocervical biopsy** to rule out endocervical lesions.

(3) **Cone biopsy:** Indications include 1) Pap smear results worse than the histology (suggesting the site of abnormal Pap smear cells was not biopsied), 2) abnormal endocervical curettage histology, 3) an endocervical canal lesion, and 4) a biopsy showing microinvasive carcinoma of the cervix.

Complications: Cervical stenosis; incompetent cervix (often caused by deep cone biopsies).

Cervical Dysplasia

Treatment—based on pathologic results:

1. **CIN1-2**: Excision or ablation of the transformation zone are equally effective for patient with a satisfactory colposcopy and without suggestion of microinvasive disease.

2. **CIN2-3**: Laser or LEEP (loop electrodiathermy excision procedure) is the preferred therapy for recurrent CIN2 and CIN3.

3. **Follow-Ups**: Patient treated with premalignant lesions should have Pap smears every 4-6 months for the next 2 years.

Differential diagnosis

ASCUS (Atypical squamous cell of undetermined significance) Pap smear:

It accounts for < 5% of cytology results; usually by benign causes from HPV infection, inflammation or atrophic lesions. About 10% of patients with ASCUS Pap smears may have a premalignant lesion. PEARLS: ASCUS management: (1) First perform HPV testing. If (+), colposcopy with cytology is done (because of higher risk of cancer). (2) If HPV is not found, repeat the Pap smear/cytology at 4-6 months. (3) If follow-up results are certainly (-) in 4-6 months, further routine follow-up is performed 4-6 months for 2 years until there have been three consecutive normal smears, at which time routine screening can be resumed. (4) If the repeated Pap smear is ASCUS again, then colposcopy with biopsy is indicated. (5) If follow-up is uncertain or unreliable, it's safer to proceed directly to colposcopy with biopsy.

Cervical Carcinoma

Cervical neoplasia that has penetrated through the basement membrane is defined as invasive cervical carcinoma (**ICC**). **Etiology, risk factors, and screening points are the same as for "Cervical Dysplasia"**. It's the 3rd most common gynecologic cancer with an average of 45 y/a.

Essentials of diagnosis

1. Usually it is asymptomatic and found out by Pap smear. The most common symptom is **postcoital vaginal bleeding**. Others include irregular vaginal bleeding, vaginal discharge, and pelvic pain, etc.

2. P/E may reveal cervical discharge or ulceration, pelvic mass, or fistulas.

3. **Lab tests: Cone biopsy** is the initial diagnostic test, **mostly** showing **SCC**.

4. **Metastatic workup**: Starts following the diagnosis of ICC, including CXR, pelvic exam, IV pyelogram, cystoscopy, and sigmoidoscopy.

5. **Staging**: ICC is the **only** gynecologic cancer staged **clinically**, based on pelvic exam mainly, or adding IV pyelogram if lymph nodes (LNs) are involved. It is not staged by CT/MRI or surgery as for most cancers.

Treatment

1. **Early stage**: Modified radical hysterectomy with pelvic lymphadenectomy.

2. **Late or advanced stage**: This includes metastasis to lymph nodes, tumor > 4cm, with positive margins, or with poor differentiation. Treat with radical hysterectomy along with radiation and with or without chemotherapy (cisplatin). Distant metastasis should be treated with chemotherapy mainly. **Uremia is the #1 cause of death** in the end stage.

Cervical Carcinoma

3. **Follow-Up**: Colposcopy and cytology should be repeated at 4-6 month intervals for 2 years after treatment. For CIN1, cytology or HPV DNA testing should be done at 12 months. If testing is normal, routine cytological screening can be resumed.

Prevention--beneficial for reduced mortality

1. **Minimize risk factors** (see above). **HPV vaccination** is given to all females between ages 9-26.

2. **Screening**: Start Pap smear at age 21 and repeat the test every 2 to 3 years until the age of 65 (with normal results). 85% cases of fatal cervical cancers have never had a Pap smear.

OVARIAN MASSES

Most ovarian masses are benign and summarized in the table below.

Table 11-3: Summary of Ovarian Masses

Disease / Clinical features, diagnosis, and treatment
<u>Simple cyst</u> **#1 common** ovary mass in the reproductive age is a physiologic cyst (**luteal or follicular cyst**). It's fluid-filled and functional. **Tx:** Mostly managed expectantly. Laparoscopy or surgery indications: Cyst > 7 cm or prior use of steroids, which may be a non-functional cyst.
<u>Complex mass</u> **#2 common** ovary mass in the reproductive age is a **dermoid cyst** (or benign teratoma). Others include endometrioma, tuboovarian abscess, and ovarian cancer. **1. Benign teratoma**: Non-functional cystic tumors; can contain tissues from all three germ layers. The commonest histology is ectodermal skin appendages (hair, sebaceous glands), as well as GI and thyroid tissue. If the thyroid tissue > 50% of the dermoid, it's called struma ovarii. **Dx:** Beta-hCG test helps rule out pregnancy. Ultrasound helps rule out a functional cyst; examine both sides. **Tx:** Surgery by laparoscopy or laparotomy. (1) Cystectomy to preserve ovarian function in the reproductive age. (2) If it's not feasible, oophorectomy is done. **2. Ovarian torsion:** Sudden onset of severe lower abdominal pain; P/E finds an adnexal mass with tenderness. **Tx:** (1) Laparoscopy or laparotomy to un-twist the ovary, and observe the ovary shortly in the operating room to assure revitalization; then cystectomy can be performed to save the ovary. (2) If the ovary is necrotic, then a unilateral salpingo-oophorectomy is performed. **Follow-up:** Routine exam 4 weeks after the surgery and then yearly to exclude malignancy.
<u>Prepubertal adnexal mass</u> Usually it's non-functional and abnormal. Suspected **germ cell tumors** should be evaluated by obtaining related tumor markers (see **Table 11-4**), and ultrasound. **Tx:** A suspected adnexal mass should be removed by surgery. <u>**Polycystic ovary syndrome:**</u> See Table 11-6 below.

OVARIAN NEOPLASMS

Ovarian tumors are common and **most of them are benign. However, the malignancy is the No.1 cause of death from female genital cancers, which mostly results from bowel obstruction**.

Ovarian Carcinoma

Most ovarian carcinomas (> 90%) are classified as "**epithelial**" arising from the surface of the ovary. Symptoms are usually insignificant early and later on may include GI discomfort, bloating, early satiety, **pelvic pressure and pain**, constipation, and frequent urination (late). They can be easily confused with other illnesses. **Pelvic examination, serum CA-125, and ultrasound are mainstays of diagnosis.**

Risk factors

Family history of ovarian or breast cancer, nulliparity, infertility, delayed childbearing, BRCA1 gene mutation (45% of risk), BRCA2 mutation (25% risk). Lynch II syndrome and hereditary nonpolyposis colorectal cancer (HNPCC) are associated with higher risk of colon, endometrium, ovary, and breast cancer. OCP use and pregnancy are with lower risk.

Classifications and clinical features of ovarian neoplasms are summarized in **Table 11-4** below.

PEARLS—**Table 11-4: Summary of Ovarian Neoplasms**

Tumor / Clinical features, diagnosis, and treatment
I. Epithelial carcinoma
Also known as <u>surface epithelial-stromal tumor</u> (including serous, endometrioid, and mucinous tumor)**,** it is the **#1 common** ovary tumor (mostly **malignant, especially endometrioid tumor**). **Tumor markers**: Increased CA-125, CEA. It's usually asymptomatic until late stage (late diagnosis). Patient may present with abdominal bloating or distention (the most common symptom) and pelvic pain, early satiety, constipation, frequent urination, vaginal bleeding, and systemic symptoms. P/E may reveal a palpable abdominal/adnexal mass and ascites. **Tx: Cisplatin first; if resistant, paclitaxel or bevacizumab.**
II. Germ cell tumors
They can be cancerous or non-cancerous tumors; in the ovary or testis). **Markers:** Increased LDH, beta-hCG, +/- AFP. Commonest in young females; grows rapidly and gives early symptom compared to the epithelial cancer. #1 symptom is sudden lower abdominal pain, along with local compression. **Tx: Surgery, surveillance and radiation (sensitive) or cisplatin-based chemotherapy.** **(1) <u>Germinomatous or seminomatous</u>:** Germinoma; dysgerminoma; seminoma. **Germinoma:** 10% with high hCG. **Dysgerminoma: Malignant.** Abnormal gonads (due to gonadal dysgenesis and androgen insensitivity syndrome) have a high risk. **Markers:** Increased serum **LDH**, beta-hCG, estrogen, and **Ca.** **(2) <u>Non-germinomatous or non-seminomatous</u>:** **Embryonal carcinoma:** Pure tumors do not secrete hCG and AFP. **Choriocarcinoma: Marker:** Increased hCG (100%). **Endodermal sinus tumor:** Marker: **Increased AFP (100%).**

Ovarian Neoplasms

Teratoma: Mature teratoma, dermoid cyst, immature teratoma, and malignant teratoma. **Malignant teratoma**: Young female, irregular, firm adnexal mass. Some tumors secrete AFP.
III. Sex cord/Gonadal stromal tumor
Including estrogen-producing granulosa cell tumor and virilizing Sertoli-Leydig cell tumor or arrhenoblastoma, accounts for 8% of ovarian cancers. **Tx:** Surgery followed by surveillance and chemotherapy. **Granulosa cell tumor: Marker**: Increased **inhibin and estrogen**. 80% is benign (20% malignant). **Sertoli-Leydig cell tumor (arrhenoblastoma, androblastoma; androma):** A rare, generally benign (75%) tumor of the ovary or testis. **Markers**: Markedly increased **testosterone and estrogen**, causing **virilization and amenorrhea** in female or feminism in male. FSH and LH are decreased. *unilateral solid adnexal mass*
IV. General guidelines for treatment (Tx) and prevention of ovarian neoplasms
Teatment: 1. TAH/BSO (total abdominal hysterectomy and bilateral salpingo-oophorectomy) and surgical staging (peritoneal and diaphragmatic biopsies, cytology, pelvic and para-aortic lymph node excision, and omentectomy). 2. All patients require postoperative chemotherapy (cisplatin, paclitaxel). 3. Radiation Tx is mostly effective with germ cell tumors. 4. Follow-up: Per 3-months, with pelvic exam and tumor marker tests. **Prognosis:** Most cases are poor due to late diagnosis, recurrence, and spread after Tx. **Screening:** Not recommended by the USPSTF since 2012 for lack of mortality benefits. **Prophylactic oophorectomy** is recommended for high-risk women (especially **BRCA1 mutation**) by age 35 or childbearing is complete. OCP use may lower the risk of ovarian cancer.

BREAST DISEASES

Benign Breast Diseases

Common benign breast diseases are summarized in the table below.

Table 11-5: Benign Breast Diseases

Disease / Clinical features, diagnosis, and treatment
Fibrocystic disease
1. **Most common**, at ages 20-50. 2. Hormone changes cause breast tissue change and cyclic bilateral breast engorgement and pain, with nodules and fluctuation. **Tx**: 1. FNA (fine needle aspiration): if fluid is clear, no biopsy but observation is needed for 4 weeks (with breast support, OCP or expectant resolve); otherwise a biopsy is done. 2. If FNA is negative but the cyst recurs, an open biopsy is performed. 3. If severe: danazol, bromocriptine, tamoxifen, or surgery.
Fibroadenoma
1. Stimulated by estrogen, increased in childbearing age, and decreased after menopause. 2. 20% of cases are with multiple lesions. 3. Patient is mostly in the 20's, presenting with a firm, smooth, mobile, painless mass. **Tx**: Surgical excision and biopsy.

Benign Breast Dz

Intraductal papilloma
Usually < 40 y/a, serous or bloody discharge, recurring; **mammography is usually negative because the tumor is too small**.   **Tx**: Lactogram-guided resection and biopsy.

Breast Cancer

Presently, **breast cancer is the most common malignancy and the second cause of death from cancer in women**. The incidence is up significantly after 50 y/a, up to 12% in the US.

Risk factors

1. **Age > 50.**
2. Family history of breast cancer in 1st-degree relatives.
3. Personal history of breast cancer.
4. History of benign breast disease with atypia.
5. Others: Nulliparity, early menarche, late menopause, 1st pregnancy > 35 y/a, and tumor markers.

Essentials of diagnosis

1. **History:** Most cases are asymptomatic and a lump is often found during physical examination (P/E) or mammography. Patient may present with a breast lump, infection or nipple discharge. Bloody discharge is most often from an intraductal papilloma.

2. **Physical examination (P/E):** May reveal a firm, immobile, painless lump usually in the upper outer quadrant of the breast in early stage. Late-stage signs include skin redness, edema, ulceration, nodularity, and fixed axillary lymph nodes (LN), which is associated with poor prognosis.

3. **Mammography (Image 116):** It should always be performed for a suspicious lesion and regular screening starting at the age of 50. It can detect the tumor 2 years earlier than clinical palpation, usually showing increased density with microcalcifications and irregular borders. If results are indecisive, pressured mammography or ultrasound followed by fine needle aspiration (**FNA**) is performed. If the FNA is still negative, core or excision biopsy is done.

Insensitive mammography conditions include (1) young age (breast too dense); (2) breast-feeding (too much milk); (3) intraductal papilloma (too small).

4. **Ultrasonography:** It's usually indicated when the lesion is painful or variable in size with menstruation. It can help determine if it's cystic or solid. If it's cystic (benign), clinical follow-up or biopsy may be performed; if solid, biopsy should be performed.

5. **Biopsy:** (1) **FNA** is usually the best initial biopsy. The false positive rate is < 2% but false negative rate is about 10%.

(2) **Core needle biopsy** takes a larger sample of the breast, causing some deformity but can be tested for estrogen receptors (ER), progesterone receptors (PR), and HER 2/neu (an abnormal ER). ER and PR testing is routine for all patients; if either one is (+), hormonal therapy is indicated.

Breast Cancer

(3) **Open surgical biopsy** is the most accurate and reliable means of diagnosis, which allows frozen sections followed by immediate resection of cancer. An **excisional biopsy** should replace FNA for these situations—cellular bloody cyst fluid on aspiration; bloody nipple discharge +/- mass; suspicious mass still present upon fluid aspiration; skin edema and erythema (suggesting inflammatory breast cancer).

(4) **Lymph node (LN) biopsy**: Sentinel node biopsy is routinely done in all patients at the time of lumpectomy or mastectomy. If it's negative, there is no need for axillary lymph node dissection.

6. **Types:**

(1) **Carcinoma in situ (CIS):** It can be **ductal carcinoma (DCIS, most common type), Paget disease of the breast** (__Image 117,__ **nipple CIS,** typically with redness, itching, burning, and erosion of the nipple), or lobular carcinoma (LCIS).

(2) **Bilateral breast cancer**: It mostly presents as **lobular** carcinoma.

(3) **Inflammatory breast cancer: Highly malignant and invasive**, poor prognosis. It usually presents with local orange-peel skin, ulceration, inflammation, and LN metastasis.

7. **Stages:** Stage I: tumor size < 2 cm; Stage II: tumor size 2-5 cm; Stage III: axillary LN metastasis (Met); Stage IV: distant metastasis.

8. **Tumor markers:** For recurrent breast cancer—CA15-3, CA27-29; BRCA1 and BRCA2 mutations—only about 10% of cases, not used for screening; indicating higher risk of breast and ovary cancers. BRCA-guided management has not shown a reduced mortality yet.

Differential diagnosis

Mammary dysplasia, fibroadenoma, fibrocystic disease, papilloma, mastitis, and fat necrosis.

Treatment

It depends on the type and stage of the cancer. **#1 factor for the prognosis is LMN**—poor outcome with ipsilateral axillary LN metastasis and fixation.

1. **Intraductal papilloma**: Galactogram-guided resection.

2. **CIS:** (1) DCIS can be treated with surgical resection plus radiation (without LN dissection), and follow-ups.

(2) LCIS should be treated with bilateral mastectomy plus radiation and close follow-ups because of the risk of invasion of both breasts.

3. **Invasive cancer:** It can also be ductal (worse prognosis) or lobular. Staging must be done based on size, LN status, and metastasis.

(1) Small, localized tumor: lumpectomy + axillary LN dissection + radiation.

(2) Big tumor +/- metastasis: mastectomy + axillary LN dissection + radiation +/- chemotherapy.

4. **Treatment by ER, PR and Her 2/neu status:**

(1) ER or PR (+) and LN (-): use an ER blocker (**tamoxifen or raloxifene**) or better an aromatase inhibitor (**anastrazole**). This status has better prognosis.

(2) ER or PR (+) and LN (+): chemotherapy for premenopausal; tamoxifen for the postmenopausal.

(3) ER and PR (-): chemotherapy only; with poorer prognosis.

Breast Cancer TX:

(4) **Her 2/neu (+)**: anti-Her 2/neu antibody—**trastuzumab** is preferred regardless of the ER status, which reduces the cancer recurrence. It's important to repeat HER2 testing upon diagnosis of metastatic breast cancer.

5. **Metastasis** to a local nodule (lung, brain), even ER (+): Surgical resection is the first choice, followed by adjuvant chemo- or hormone therapy +/- local radiation. Combined chemotherapy is the mainstay of treatment for late-stage patients.

6. Breast cancer with pregnancy: Treat it as for most breast cancers (modified mastectomy), but delay chemotherapy until after the 1st trimester), and no radiation used.

PEARLS—**Prevention and screening—beneficial for reduced mortality!**

1. Clinical breast exam every 2-3 years until 50 y/a then annually can be a health evaluation for breast diseases (not a strict cancer screening). Monthly breast self-exam may not give much benefit.

2. Annual mammography screening starts in all women > 50 y/a (till 74 y/a), and earlier with positive family history or personal breast injury.

3. Use of prophylactic ER blockers may lower the incidence of breast cancer in high-risk patient but may increase the risk of uterine cancer. Thus it's a personal decision.

4. Women at high risk for breast cancer (lifetime risk ≥ 20%) should be referred for genetic counseling to determine the likelihood of a BRCA mutation and to decide on management options.

MISCELLANEOUS DISORDERS

Pelvic Relaxation

Uterine prolapse and urinary incontinence are commonly seen in childbearing and elder women. For urinary incontinence, see "Chapter 7 UROGENITAL DISEASES".

Uterine Prolapse

The most common cause of uterine prolapse is trauma during childbirth, in particular multiple or difficult births. The mechanical trauma of childbirth and long-term heavy-object lifting damages the supporting ligaments of the pelvic retroperitoneum in the pelvis that support the pelvic viscera. About 50% of women who have had children develop some form of pelvic organ prolapse in their lifetime. It is more common as women get older and go through menopause.

Diagnosis

Diagnosis is usually made by observation at the time of pelvic exam. The prolapsed vagina, rectum, and uterus are easily visualized as the patient increase intra-abdominal pressure by straining.

Treatment

Effective treatment is surgical hysterectomy or a uterus-sparing sacrohysteropexy.

Hirsutism and Virilization

1. Hirsutism   *hyperandrogenism: acne, hirsutism*

Hirsutism is defined as excessive male-pattern hair growth in a female on the upper lip, chin, chest, abdomen, back, and proximal extremities, usually accompanied with acne, menstrual disorders, etc.

2. Virilization

Virilization is hirsutism plus other masculinizing signs in a female—clitorimegaly, deepening voice, increasing muscle mass, and male body contours.

PEARLS—Table 11-6: Differential Diagnosis of Hirsutism

Disease / Clinical features, diagnosis, and treatment
Polycystic ovarian syndrome (PCOS, Stein-Leventhal syndrome)   **Triad:** Hirsutism (hyperandrogenism), amenorrhea/oligomenorrhea, and infertility (#1 cause in women); plus obesity, treatment-resistant acne, and mild virilization from adolescence on. P/E and ultrasound may help find bilateral ovarian masses. **Lab tests:** High levels of **LH:FSH (>3)**, estrogen, **androstenedione, and DHEAS**; low progesterone.   **Tx:** 1. **Weight reduction** is highly cost-effective. 2. Expecting pregnancy: **clomiphene** to induce ovulation (may cause multiple pregnancies). 3. Not expecting pregnancy: **OCP** to suppress pituitary LH secretion. 4. **If resistant** to the therapy: dexamethasone androgen-suppression test to find out rare disorders. **Screen for type 2 diabetes.**
Adrenal tumor   Virilization and markedly **elevated** dehydroepiandrosterone sulfate (**DHEAS**), which is produced only in the adrenal glands. Testosterone is normal.   **Dx:** CT or MRI will show an abdominal mass, plus surgical biopsy.   **Tx:** Surgical removal of tumor.
Ovarian tumor (Sertoli-Leydig cell tumor, hilus cell tumor, arrhenoblastoma)   Rapid virilization and markedly **elevated testosterone**, which is produced by both the ovary and the adrenal glands. DHEAS is normal.   **Dx:** P/E and ultrasound will reveal an adnexal mass, confirmed by a surgical biopsy.   **Tx:** Surgical resection.
Congenital adrenal hyperplasia *- virilization in 46,XX*   **(1) 21-Hydroxyolase deficiency:** **#1 common cause.** Decreased cortisol and aldosterone (**hypo-Na, hyper-K, and low BP**), increased 17-OH progesterone, ACTH, and DHEAS, along with **virilization**. Onset is in early ages.   **Tx:** Continuous cortisol replacement.   **(2) 11-hydroxylase deficiency:** **Hyper-Na, hypo-K, hypertension**, and increased 17-OH progesterone **(markedly)** and DHEAS (mildly). Usually late-onset, with evident **hirsutism** but insignificant virilization. Irregular menses and precocious puberty are common.   **Tx:** Continuous cortisol replacement, which may cease the androgenic signs and restore ovulatory cycles.

5-α-reductase def: ↓ T:DHT ratio

Infertility

It's defined as inability for a childbearing-age couple to achieve pregnancy after 12 months of regular, normal sexual intercourse. The incidence is about 10% for all couples.

Etiology

1. Male: Accounting for 30-40% of cases; mostly due to sperm abnormalities. Common causes are varicocele, testicular injury or infection (epididymitis or mumps orchitis), medicines (steroids, cimetidine, spironolactone), primary testicular failure, and complications of thyroid or liver diseases.

2. Female: (1) Pelvic/peritoneal factors: 30%, endometriosis as #1, then tubal/uterine abnormalities, STD, abortions; (2) Ovulation deficiency: endocrine or psychosocial disorders; (3) Cervical deficiency.

Diagnostic steps

1. Male:

(1) Semen analysis is done first; if **the sperm count is low (the most common cause)**, then hormone study is done.

(2) If FSH and LH are high and testosterone is low, it's primary testicular failure; if all three are low, it's secondary testicular failure.

2. Female:

(1) Postcoital test is done first to assess cervical mucus.

(2) Daily basal body temperature (BBT) can verify ovulation: BBT decreases at menses and increases after LH and progesterone surge. Endometrial biopsy confirms diagnosis.

(3) Serum FSH, LH, progesterone, and prolactin tests can rule out endocrine diseases.

(4) Hysterosalpingogram can rule out tubal/uterine abnormalities.

Treatment

1. Male: Intrauterine insemination; donor insemination; in vitro fertilization (IVF), etc.

2. Female: Clomiphene (induce ovulation); GNRH analogs (with fibroids and endometriosis); tubal/uterine surgery; IVF, etc.

CONTRACEPTION

Namely birth control, it prevents pregnancy by interfering with the normal process of ovulation, fertilization, or implantation. There are varieties of birth controls that act at different points in the process.

Table 11-7: Common Contraceptive Methods

Method / Advantage and adverse effect (S/E)
Postpartum   (1) **Lactation**: Associated with temporary anovulation; contraceptive use may be deferred for 3 months.   (2) **Minipill**: Suppresses LH and ovulation, with the best effect during lactation because it contains only progesterone (not affects milk production). **Adverse (Side) effects (S/E)**: Vaginal bleeding, breast tenderness, galactorrhea, weight gain, mood changes, hair loss, acne.
OCPs   Suppress ovulation by inhibiting FSH/LH; interfering with implantation by changing the consistency of cervical mucus. **#1 choice is loestrin** (with lowest estrogen). Combined estrogen-progesterone can be the choice for primary dysmenorrhea in teenagers. **S/E**: Nausea, headache, benign breast changes, acne, hypertension, hepatic adenoma, mood changes, and increased DVT risk (but possibly decreased risk of PID and ovarian/endometrial cancers).
Levonorgestrel (Norplant)   Progestin-only subdermal implant; inhibiting ovulation by suppression of LH peak; effective for 5 years.   **S/E:** Same as that of other progesterones; difficult to remove.
Postcoital "morning-after" pill   Estrogen or estrogen-progesterone to suppress ovulation or implantation of fertilized ovum, taken within 72 hours of unprotected sex (2 tablets immediately followed by another 2 tablets in 12 hours). Failure rate is only 1%.   **S/E:** Nausea; malformation if pregnancy occur; increased risk of vaginal clear-cell cancer (after long estrogen use).
IUD   Prevent implantation by producing a local sterile inflammatory reaction in the endometrium. **S/E**: Increased vaginal bleeding, uterine infection/perforation, PID, and ectopic pregnancy.
Barrier methods (diaphragm, condom, sponge)   Physical blockade of sperm into the uterine cavity; effective in contraception and protective against STDs, PID, and cervical cancer. S/E is rare.

Chapter 11: High-yield Questions (HYQ)

1-5: Match the following clinical scenarios with the most likely diagnosis (Dx).

A. Ovarian dysfunction

B. Mullerian agenesis

C. Testicular feminization

D. Gonadal dysgenesis

E. Kallmann syndrome

F. Hypothalamic-pituitary dysfunction

G. Polycystic ovarian syndrome (POS)

H. Ovarian tumor

1. A 16 y/o girl complains of never having a menstruation. P/E finds a short figure and no significant secondary sex characteristics (breast, pubic and axillary hair). She also has deficiencies in color differentiation and olfactory sensation. Ultrasonography shows small ovaries and uterus. Serum FSH, LH, estrogen and progesterone are all low.

2. A 16 y/o girl complains of never having a menstruation. P/E finds a short figure and no significant secondary sex characteristics. Ultrasonography shows small ovaries and uterus. Serum FSH is high, and estrogen and progesterone are very low.

3. A 20 y/o girl complains of amenorrhea for the past 3 months. Pregnancy test is (-). P/E finds about normal secondary sex characteristics. Her basal body temperature (BBT) monitoring mostly shows T = 37.5°C, and she usually has short menstrual cycles. Ultrasonography shows normal uterus and ovaries. Serum estrogen is normal, progesterone is low, and LH:FSH ratio is high.

4. A 16 y/o girl complains of never having a menstruation. P/E finds normal secondary sex characteristics. Ultrasonography shows absence of the fallopian tubes and uterus. Serum testosterone is normal, estrogen is low, and FSH is high.

5. A 16 y/o girl comes to the physician because she has never had a menstruation yet. P/E finds development of female breasts and external genitalia, but no pubic and axillary hair. Ultrasonography shows absence of the fallopian tubes and uterus. Serum testosterone is high and estrogen is low.

6. A 20 y/o female is brought to the clinic for cough, vomiting and non-cramping, heavy vaginal bleeding for the past 2 days. Her LMP was 6 weeks ago. She looks pale with a weak voice. P/E finds T = 37.5°C, HR = 100 bpm, and BP = 80/60 mmHg. Her fundal height is 2 fingers below the umbilicus. Pelvic exams are not done because of the severe bleeding. Lab tests show Hb = 10 g/dL, WBC = 5,000/uL, and β-hCG is 200, 000 mIU/mL. Abdominal ultrasound shows "snowstorm" image. What's the best treatment along with IV fluid?

A. IV oxytocin + estrogen

B. Oxytocin + blood transfusion

C. D&C

D. Chemotherapy

E. Hysterectomy

7. A 17 y/o girl is brought to the clinic for irregular, non-cramping, heavy vaginal bleeding for the past 7 days. She looks pale with a weak voice. P/E finds T = 37.7°C, HR = 100 bpm, and BP = 90/60 mmHg. Pelvic exams are normal. Lab tests show Hb = 10g/dL, WBC = 10000/uL, and β-hCG (-). What's the best next step besides IV fluid?

A. Blood transfusion + antibiotics

B. D&C

C. IV estrogen

D. Cyclic progestin

E. Endometrial biopsy

8. A 38 y/o woman complains of intolerable periodic lower abdominal pain during menses for the past 3 months. She's been married for the past 10 years and no pregnancy with regular sexual life, which is often bothered

by the abdominal pain. She denies chronic diseases. P/E finds a diffusely enlarged, tender uterus. Routine tests of the blood, urine, and stool are mostly normal except anemia. What's the most appropriate next step?

A. Pregnancy test   B. Laparoscopy plus biopsy   C. Leuprolide for 3-6 months

D. Ultrasound   E. Hysterectomy

9. The above patient is negative for pregnancy test. Laparoscopy plus biopsy is done and reveals diffuse endometrial glands and stroma located within the myometrium of the uterine wall. Now what's the best next step?

A. OCP for 3-6 months   B. D&C   C. Leuprolide for 3-6 months

D. Total abdominal hysterectomy and salpingo-oophorectomy (TAH/BSO)

E. Hysterectomy

10-14: Match the following clinical scenarios with the most likely cause.

A. Gardnerella   B. Chlamydia   C. Trichomonas

D. Candida   E. Gonococcus   F. HSV-2

G. HPV6 or 11   H. HPV16 or 18   I. Mixed pathogens

J. Endometrial atrophy   K. Endometrial cancer   L. OCP use

10. A 25 y/o woman comes to the physician for abnormal, painless vaginal discharge. She admits having "a couple of boy-friends" for the past 2 years and not always used condoms. Pelvic exams show yellow-green, mucopurulent discharge from the cervix. Saline smear reveals many WBCs without bacteria.

11. A 26 y/o woman comes to the physician for intolerable, burning vaginal discharge. She admits having "a couple of boy-friends" for the past 2 years and not always used condoms. Pelvic exams show malodorous, profuse, grayish, yellowish, frothy discharge from the vagina, with petechiae in the cervix. Saline smear shows epithelial cells with numerous bacteria, WBCs, and flagellated pathogens. KOH (Whiff) test is (+).

12. A 70 y/o woman comes to the physician for abnormal, itchy vaginal discharge. She admits "frequently catching cold" for the past year. Pelvic exams show thick, white, odorless, cottage-like discharge from the vagina, with erythema on the anterior wall. KOH test is in suspension. Saline smear is (-) and pH < 4.5 (Nl).

13. A 36 y/o woman comes to the physician for fatigue, weight loss, chronic, nonproductive coughs, and intermittent vaginal bleeding for 3 months. She admits having "a couple of boy-friends" for the past 5 years and never used condoms, with three abortions in the past year. The bleeding occurs mostly after sexual intercourse. Pelvic exams show painless erythema with scant malodorous discharge in the vagina, and a mass over the Os with irregular margin. CBC shows Hb = 10 g/dL and WBC = 1000/uL.

14. A 60 y/o woman presents with fatigue and heavy, irregular vaginal bleeding for the past week. She occasionally uses OCP, smokes and drinks alcohol for several years. Pelvic exams reveal mild vaginal atrophy without discharge. CBC shows Hb = 10 g/dL and WBC = 8000/uL.

15-19: Match the following clinical scenarios with the most likely type of ovarian tumors.

A. Epithelial   B. Germ cell (embryonal, choriocarcinoma)

C. Dysgerminoma   D. Endodermal sinus   E. Granulosa cell

F. Malignant teratoma   G. S-Leydig cell   H. Arrhenoblastoma

I. Endometrioid   J. Adrenal tumor

15. A 45 y/o woman complains of gradually increased hair on the upper lip, chest, and proximal extremities, and deepening voice. P/E finds clitorimegaly. Blood tests show markedly elevated DHEAS and normal testosterone.

16. A 25 y/o woman complains of progressive fatigue, abdominal distention and pain, constipation, and irregular vaginal bleeding for the past 2 months. She has moderate vaginal bleeding today. P/E finds an irregular, firm adnexal mass. Lab tests reveal markedly elevated β-hCG and AFP.

17. A 25 y/o woman complains of progressive fatigue, abdominal bloating and distention, constipation, and irregular vaginal bleeding for 2 months. Pregnancy test is (-). P/E finds an adnexal mass. Ultrasonography shows evidence of fluid. Lab tests reveal increased AFP, CA-125, and CEA.

18. A 45 y/o woman complains of gradual fatigue, abdominal bloating and distention, and irregular menses for the past 2 months. Pregnancy test is (-). P/E finds a small adnexal mass. Lab tests reveal increased inhibin and estrogen.

19. A 45 y/o woman complains of rapidly increased hair on the upper lip, chest and proximal extremities, and deepening voice. P/E finds clitorimegaly and a lower abdominal mass. Blood tests show markedly elevated testosterone and estrogen, and normal DHEAS.

20. A 16 y/o girl presents with a firm, mobile, rubbery mass measuring 5 cm in diameter in her right breast. She noticed the mass a year ago when it measured only 1-2 cm. What is the most appropriate diagnosis and treatment?

A. Cystosarcoma phyllodes, radical resection   B. Giant juvenile fibroadenoma, cosmetic resection
C. Adenocarcinoma, radical surgery   D. Abnormal breast development, referral
E. Fibroadenoma, observation

21. A 30 y/o woman from a small village presents with a firm, mobile, rubbery mass in the right breast that has been there for the past 5 years. It has grown slowly to its present size of 6x7 cm². No evidence of local invasion or palpable lymph node is found. What's the most likely diagnosis?

A. Cystosarcoma phyllodes   B. Giant juvenile fibroadenoma
C. Adenocarcinoma   D. Abnormal breast development
E. Fibrocystic breast disease

22. A 48 y/o woman has her yearly mammogram performed and is found to have "a cluster of micro-calcifications." There is no history of breast cancer in her family or relatives. She has two children and generally feels well. The best next step is

A. follow-up exam in 3 months   B. reassurance because 80% of the cases are benign
C. fine needle aspiration (FNA)   D. surgical removal of the "cluster" with biopsy
E. radiotherapy

23. A 40 y/o woman has a 7-year history of tenderness and multiple lumps on both breasts. Their sizes seem to change at different times in the menstrual cycle. For the past month, she's had a persistent, firm, round mass on the left breast measuring 2.5 cm in diameter. There is no family history of other diseases. What's the most likely Dx?

A. Cystosarcoma phyllodes   B. Fibrocystic disease   C. Adenocarcinoma
D. Fibroadenoma   E. Polycystic disease

24. A 50 y/o woman presents with a firm and mobile 2 cm mass in the left breast for the past 2 months. There is no history of breast cancer in her family and relatives. She is generally well. The best next step is

A. re-examination in 3 months   B. mammography   C. FNA (core biopsy)

D. excisional biopsy   E. radiotherapy

25. A 51 y/o woman presents with a firm, 3 cm mass with unclear borders in the upper left breast, mobile from the chest wall but not mobile within the breast. The skin overlying the mass is retracted. The most likely Dx is:

A. cystosarcoma phyllodes   B. fibrocystic disease   C. adenocarcinoma
D. fibroadenoma   E. Paget disease of breast

26. A 58 y/o woman presents with a fast-growing, firm, 3.5 cm mass under the right nipple. "The most common type of breast cancer" is diagnosed from a core biopsy. P/E shows axillary lymph nodes (-). The mammography reveals no other lesions. What's the best treatment for this patient?

A. Lumpectomy   B. Modified radical mastectomy (MRM)
C. Radical mastectomy   D. Radiotherapy
E. Chemotherapy

27. A 55 y/o woman presents with fatigability and a hard, mobile, about 1.5 cm mass in her left axilla that she accidentally found. P/E confirms this mass as an enlarged lymph node without tenderness; her breasts and other lymph nodes are (-). T = 38°C. She denies any history of pregnancy or other medical conditions. What's the most likely diagnosis?

A. Lymphoma   B. Lymph node (LN) infection   C. Breast cancer with metastasises
D. Lymph node hyperplasia   E. Lymph node TB

28. A 47 y/o woman presents with a fast-growing, 2-cm mass in the left breast with local invasion. A lumpectomy and axillary lymph node dissection were performed, with a pathology report of clear surgical margins, positive estrogen receptor (ER+), and metastatic cancer in 5/10 axillary lymph nodes. What's the best next Tx?

A. Chemotherapy   B. Tamoxifen   C. Radiotherapy
D. Follow-up exam in 3 mo   E. Radical surgery

Answers and Explanations

1. (E). It's a genetic disease (mostly 46, XX); due to the failure of the hypothalamic production of GnRH. Treatment (Tx) is estrogen and progesterone replacement plus GnRH.

2. (D). It's most likely Turner syndrome, and genetic studies will confirm female genotype (45, X). Tx is estrogen and progesterone replacement for development of the secondary sexual characteristics.

3. (A). Luteal phase deficiency. Tx is progesterone or clomiphene/hCG to induce ovulation. POS may have similar symptoms but can be diagnosed by ultrasound.

4. (B). It's genetically female (46, XX), but with defects in the development of Mullerian duct derivatives. Tx is surgical elongation of the vagina for sexual satisfaction.

5. (C). Androgen insensitivity: genetically male (46, XY), but no androgen-R function, with internal Wolffian duct structures atrophy. Tx: (1) Remove the testes by 20 y/a. (2) Long-term estrogen replacement.

6. (E). It's most likely a malignant GTD (choriocarcinoma) with unstable vital signs and possible metastasis to the lungs (CXR or CT is needed for Dx). Urgent hysterectomy (with biopsy) plus chemotherapy and hCG monitoring are the most effective Tx. D&C can be chosen for a benign, complete mole.

7. (C). It's a severe dysfunctional uterine bleeding (DUB) in a young patient (#1 cause is anovulation). IV estrogen is the best initial Tx. If it fails, transfusion, D&C plus vaginal packing or uterine artery ligation may be necessary. 'D' is for most mild to moderate DUB. 'E' is for > 35 y/o DUB.

8. (A). Pregnancy must always be excluded first in a reproductive-age female with amenorrhea, especially with an enlarged uterus. Then 'B' is the best step to confirm adenomyosis (most likely) and exclude endometriosis (less likely, with endometrial glands outside the uterus). Ultrasound may also help.

9. (E). Hysterectomy is the definitive and adequate Tx, since pregnancy is no longer the major concern for the patient, and the ovaries should be reserved. Medicines are good for initial Tx of endometriosis; if failed, 'D' is the radical therapy as the last resort.

10. (B). Chlamydial cervicitis and vaginitis are the #1 common STD in a sexually active, unmarried woman. Tx is azithromycin once or doxycycline for 7 days.

11. (I). Mixed pathogens here include the commonest Gardnerella and Trichomonas. Best Tx is metronidazole to both patient and sexual partner.

12. (D). It's the #1 common vaginitis in immunodeficient or elder patients, not a STD. Tx is topical antifungals.

13. (H). This patient most likely has cervical cancer (associated with HPV16, 18 infections), with potential immunodeficient or AIDS. HPV6 and HPV11 are associated with condyloma acuminata, and HSV2 is associated with painful erythema around the vagina.

14. (J). Endometrial atrophy is more common than cancer, but endometrial or cervical cancer is also likely for her age and history, therefore hysteroscopy with endometrial sampling is the best next step to do. After cancer is excluded, estrogen and progesterone replacement can be the first Tx.

15. (J) It's most likely an adrenal tumor. Dx: CT or MRI will show an abdominal mass. Tx is surgical removal.

16. (F). It's most likely a teratoma; perform Ultrasound confirmation followed by surgery.

17. (A). Epithelial tumor is the #1 common ovarian cancer. Primary Tx is TAH/BSO.

18. (E). Granulosa cell tumor; 80% is benign.

19. (G). Leydig cell cancer. Tx is adnexectomy.

20. (B). It's most likely a benign tumor. Incidence of breast cancer for a female < 20 y/a is extremely low.

21. (A). It's a rare cystosarcoma phyllodes. Core or incisional biopsy followed by free resection is the best Tx.

22. (C). Although 80% of the microcalcifications are benign, because of her age it's important to exclude malignancy with a FNA for core biopsy before making other choices.

23. (B). Cystic mastitis or mammary dysplasia. First perform a mammogram to see if there are other lesions. FNA is therapeutic; if bloody fluid is found, cytology is done. Biopsy may not be necessary if the masses change with menstruation.

24. (B). It can be a benign or malignant tumor, and thus a mammogram is started to make sure there are no other tumors in the breasts. Then a core biopsy or excisional biopsy is followed. If the core biopsy is negative, excisional biopsy is still necessary to rule out cancer.

25. (C). It's most probably an adenocarcinoma. Start with a mammogram to determine the number of tumors, and then perform FNA with biopsy to confirm Dx before making Tx choices.

26. (B). Infiltrating ductal carcinoma. MRM includes axillary dissection. 'A' is only used for a very small tumor located where most of the breast tissue can be spared. 'C' is outdated and no longer used. 'D' is not needed when the whole breast is removed.

27. (C). 'C' is more likely given her age and lack of a history of breast-feeding. She needs a mammogram followed by LN biopsy. 'A' is more likely if it's a younger patient.

28. (A). Tx for breast cancer with estrogen receptor ER (+): (1) ER (+) and LN (+): chemotherapy for premenopausal patients and those with distant, blood-borne metastasis; ER blocker (tamoxifen) for postmenopausal patients. (2) ER (+) and LN (-): an ER blocker is the best Tx, and it has a better prognosis.

Chapter 12

OBSTETRICS

PHYSIOLOGY OF NORMAL PREGNANCY

Menstrual Cycle and Hormonal Changes in Order

1. FSH peak (Day 3-4); 2. Estrogen peak (Day 10); 3. LH peak (Day 12-13); 4. Ovulation (Day 14); 5. Progesterone peak (Day 21); 6. Menstruation (Day 28).

Table 12-1: Summary of Hormones in Pregnancy

Hormone / Sources and Functions
Estrogen **Source**: Ovary (estradiol), placenta (estriol), blood, and testes. **Function**: 1. Follicle growth. 2. Endometrial proliferation and increase (Incr) in myometrial excitability. 3. Genital and breast development. 4. Fat deposit and hepatic synthesis of transport proteins. 5. Positive feedback on LH (surge), and negative feedback inhibition (Inh) of FSH.
Progesterone **Source**: Corpus luteum, placenta, adrenal cortex, and testes. **Function**: 1. Stimulation of endometrial glandular secretions and spiral artery development. 2. Inhibition of myometrial excitability and maintenance of pregnancy. 3. Producing thick cervical mucus and preventing sperm entry into the uterus. 4. Increasing body temperature (by 0.5 degree). 5. Feedback inhibition of gonadotropins (LH, FSH).
Human Chorionic Gonadotropin (β-hCG) **Source**: Trophoblast of placenta. **Function**: 1. Acts like LH to maintain the corpus luteum and progesterone for the first trimester because it's not susceptible to feedback inhibition by estrogen and progesterone. In the second and 3rd trimester, the placenta makes its own estrogen and progesterone so that the corpus luteum degenerates. 2. Used to detect pregnancy because it appears in the urine 8 days after successful fertilization, and doubles every 2 days during early pregnancy. 3. A markedly high level of hCG at < 20 week's gestation indicates molar pregnancy, whereas a low level of hCG may indicates ectopic pregnancy, threatened abortion, or missed abortion.
Human Placental Lactogen Chemically it is similar to anterior pituitary growth hormone and prolactin. Low levels may indicate threatened abortion, or IUGR.

Table 12-2: Physiologic Changes during Pregnancy

Organ/system   Physiologic Changes and Signs during Pregnancy
Vagina: 1. Increased blood flow leading to a typical **violet color (Chadwick's sign)**. 2. Thick acidic secretions.
Cervix: 1. Highly vascular, softening, and cyanotic. 2. Thick mucus clots in the cervical os expelled at labor "**bloody show**"). 3. Cervical mucus appears granular or crystallized with beading under the microscope (**"ferning"**) in response to progesterone. 4. Tissue at the os is friable and easily bleeds upon contact.
Uterus: 1. Uterus softening after 6 weeks (Ladin sign). 2. Palpable above the **pubic symphysis at 12 weeks**. 3. Irregular painless contractions (Braxton Hicks) occur during pregnancy and may become frequent and rhythmic in the late 3rd trimester ("**false labor**").
Breasts: 1. **Colostrum** can be seen at 3-4 months. 2. At birth, abrupt progesterone decrease makes prolactin act unopposed in favor of breast feeding.
Respiratory: **Progesterone stimulates the respiratory system: tidal volume and ventilation/min increase by 30-40%**; total lung capacity and residual volume are decreased, resulting in increased alveolar and arterial PO_2 and decreased the PCO_2. **Respiratory rate is normal**.
Cardiovascular: 1. **Cardiac output increases by 50%** (due to HR and stroke volume increase), with normal systolic murmur and S1 split. 2. **Vascular dilation** (by progesterone and PG) causing mild BP decreased before 24 weeks and normal by 40 weeks.
Hematologic: 1. Blood volume increased 40-50%, with **increased plasma, WBCs, and RBCs but slightly decreased Hb** level due to the hypervolemia (**physiologic anemia**). 2. Risk of hypercoagulable **DVT** in the puerperium **(pulmonary embolism as the #1 cause of postpartum death),** and Fe-deficiency anemia if Hb <11 g/dL.
Endocrine: 1. **Increased total and free cortisol** (by the placenta and the fetal adrenal gland). 2. Estrogen increases thyroid-binding globulin; **total and bound T3 and T4 are increased**, but active unbound T3 and T4 are normal. 3. Human placental lactogen **(HPL): Increased lipolysis and free fatty acids; risk of postprandial hyperglycemia and gestational diabetes** (or worsening).
Gastrointestinal: 1. **Nausea/vomiting and acid reflux**, resolves by 14-16 weeks (after the beta-hCG peak). 2. **Constipation**. 3. Increased biliary cholesterol (Chol) saturation and risk of **gallstones**.
Renal: 1. Renal plasma flow and **GFR increase** by 40-50%, and **BUN-creatinine decreases** by 25%. 2. Physiologic hydronephrosis caused by renal dilation and compression by the ureter; increased **risk of pyelonephritis** and asymptomatic bacteriuria.
Musculoskeletal: Increased motility of pubic, sacroiliac, and sacrococcygeal joints.
Skin: 1. Increased estrogen causes **cirrhosis-like** spider angiomas, palmar erythema, and striae (breast, abdomen, etc.). 2. **Hyperpigmentation** over the abdomen (**linear nigra**), face (**melasma**), nipples, and perineum (by melanocyte-stimulating hormone).

Basic Concepts of Pregnancy

Pregnancy Duration and Dating

1. **Menstrual dating**: This is mostly determined to be 280 days or 40 weeks from the LMP. It's more easily identified than conception dating (266 days or 38 weeks postconception). It is based on 28-day menstrual cycle in which ovulation occurs on day 14 after LMP starts.

2. **Basal body temperature (BBT)**: Increased by the effect of progesterone from the corpus luteum that formed after ovulation. The accuracy of BBT is ± 1 week.

3. **Fetal heart tones**: First heard by Doppler stethoscope at 10-12 weeks.

4. **Uterine fundal height**: After 20 weeks, measurement in cm from pubic symphysis to top of fundus approximates gestational week.

5. **Ultrasound dating**: The accuracy is ± 5 days at < 12 weeks GA, and ± 7 days at 12-18 weeks.

6. **Nagele's rule:** Estimation of the due date of delivery by taking the LMP--subtracting 3 months (or adding 9 months) and adding 7 days to the LPM. E.g., if a woman's LMP is May 1, her estimated delivery date is Feb. 8 next year.

Pregnancy tests: It can be done by an OTC-kit (over-the-counter) and lab serum tests for beta (β)-hCG. Beta-hCG is produced by the placenta and peaks at 100×10^3 mIU/mL by 10 weeks of gestation, decreased throughout the 2nd trimester, and staying flat in the 3rd trimester. Beta-hCG levels double about every 48 hr during early pregnancy.

Diagnosis of pregnancy: Usually it's made by presumptive signs of amenorrhea, nausea, vomiting, breast tenderness, Incr skin pigmentation and striae, etc, confirmed by a (+) pregnancy test.

Developmental age (DA): The number of weeks and days since fertilization.

Gestational age (GA): The number of weeks and days measured from the last menstrual period (LMP). GA can be determined by LMP, fundal height, quickening (at 17-18th week), fetal heart tones (at 10th week via Doppler), or ultrasound (U/S).

Gravity: The number of times of pregnancies.

Parity: The number of pregnancies resulted in a birth beyond 20 weeks GA or a baby over 500g.

Trimester Breakdown

First trimester: fertilization until the 12 weeks (DA) or 14 weeks (GA).

Second trimester: 12 (DA) or 14 (GA) weeks until the 24 weeks (DA) or 26 weeks (GA).

Third trimester: 24 (DA) or 26 (GA) weeks until delivery.

Term Lengths

Pre-viable: fetus born before 24 weeks.

Preterm: fetus born between 25 and 37 weeks.

Term: fetus born between 38 and 42 weeks.

Postterm: fetus born after 42 weeks.

PRENATAL DIAGNOSIS, CARE, AND SURVEILLANCE

PRENATAL DIAGNOSTIC TESTING

MSAFP Testing

Maternal serum AFP is produced by the fetus and mainly found in the amniotic fluid, with small amount crossing the placenta into mother's serum and should be tested at 16-18 weeks of gestation.

Common causes of **high AFP**: **GA error** (#1 common), neural tube defect (anencephaly or spina bifida), abdominal wall defect, placental abruption, multiple gestation, and fetal death.

Major cause of **low AFP**: **Down syndrome**; amniocentesis for karyotyping is recommended.

Triple Screen of AFP, Beta-hCG, and Estriol

It's usually done at the 16th week to screen for Down syndrome (trisomy 21), trisomy 18, and neural tube defect.

Down syndrome: beta-hCG is high; AFP and estriol are low.

Trisomy 18: All three tests are low.

If the screen is abnormal or the patient's age is over 35 at the time of delivery, ultrasound or amniocentesis is performed for confirmation.

Quad Screen: Triple screen + inhibin A

Both beta-hCG and inhibin A are high in Down syndrome. All four tests are **low in trisomy 18**.

Amniocentesis

It refers to ultrasound-guided, trans-abdominal needle aspiration of amniotic fluid (cells) to evaluate fetal genetic abnormalities, blood typing and lung maturity. Sensitivity for Down syndrome is about 65%. Risks are maternal hemorrhage (1%) and fetal loss (0.5%).

Indications

1. At 15-20 weeks of GA: To detect fetal chromosomal abnormalities when triple or quad screen is abnormal, or over 35 y/a with risk factors.

2. After 20 weeks of GA: To get fetal blood type or detect fetal hemolysis in Rh-sensitized pregnancy.

3. In the 3rd trimester (after 34 weeks of GA): To evaluate fetal lung maturity (lecithin/sphingomyelin ratio is over 2.5, or phosphatidylglycerol is normal).

Chorionic Villous Sampling (CVS)

It refers to ultrasound-guided transcervical or trans-abdominal aspiration of placental (chorionic) tissue for fetal karyotyping.

Advantages: It can be performed as early as 9-12 weeks of GA and with similar accuracy as that of amniocentesis.

Disadvantages: Rates of pregnancy loss and failure to detect neural tube defect are higher than with amniocentesis.

Percutaneous Umbilical Blood Sampling (PUBS)

It refers to ultrasound-guided trans-abdominal aspiration of fetal blood from the umbilical vein. It is performed after 20 weeks usually for fetal infection, Rh blood typing, blood transfusion, hemolysis, and karyotyping. Pregnancy loss rate is 1 to 2%.

Ultrasonography (U/S)

A noninvasive imaging method usually used for guidance of invasive prenatal diagnosis procedures, with limited obstetric indications (fetal structural anomalies, best done at 18-20 weeks of GA). For GA dating, the accuracy is + 5 days at < 12 weeks of GA, and + 7 days at 12-18 weeks. Adverse fetal effects are rare.

Table 12-3: Causes of Various Fundal Sizes (Diagnosed by ultrasonography)

Fundus smaller than dates
Fetus: IUGR, fetal death;
Oligoamniosis: 4-quad AFI < 5cm;
Placenta: molar pregnancy.
Fundus larger than dates
Fetus: multiple or macrosomia;
Polyhydramnios: 4-quad > 20 cm: diabetes, TE fistula, duodenal atresia, spina bifida, or anencephaly;
Uterus: leiomyoma;
Placenta: texture.

PRENATAL CARE AND NUTRITION

These are very important to prevent, diagnose and treat the adverse conditions early.

Table 12-4: Important Standard Prenatal Care

Category / Recommendation
Nutrition
Patient needs additional 100-300 kcal/d during pregnancy and 500 kcal/d during breast-feeding. **Folic acid**: 0.4 mg/d, required to decrease neural tube defect (3 months before pregnancy). **Iron**: 30 mg/d elemental iron (325 mg Fe-sulfate) in the later half of pregnancy. Demand is increased by both the mother and fetus. Most other vitamins can be met by normal diet. Vit-A is potentially teratogenic and thus should not be ingested).
Weight gain: Expected to be an average **gain of 25-35** lbs during pregnancy with a BMI of 20-26.
Exercise: 30 min of moderate daily exercise.
Prenatal visits: Week 0-28: every 4 weeks; Week 29-36: every 2 weeks; Week 36-birth: every week.
Prenatal lab tests
1st visit: 1. **Blood**: CBC, ABO type, Rh factor, and antibody screen. 2. **Infectious disease**: Urinalysis (UA) and culture, cervical chlamydia and gonorrhea (PCR or culture), syphilis screen (VDRL/RPR), HBsAg, rubella antibody titer, PPD, HIV (patient with risk). 3. **Mix**: Pap smear, glucose challenge test (patient with family history or diabetes risks), Sickle cell test preparation.
15-20 weeks: Maternal serum alpha-fetoprotein (**MSAFP**) or squad screen (MSAFP, estriol, beta-hCG and inhibin A). Offer amniocentesis to patients > 35 y/a. 18-20 weeks: ultrasound (U/S) to determine GA (best time), amniotic fluid volume, fetal anatomy, and placental location.
26-28 weeks: Repeat hematocrit and Rh Ab; give **RhoGAM** if the mother is Rh (-) and father is (+) or unknown. **Diabetes screen**: 1. **Glucose tests** or everyone: urine glucose test first; if (+), 1h (50g) glucose tolerance test (GTT) followed. 2. **Patients with risks** (with obesity, back pain, > 35 y/a, and family history): **1-hour GTT** can be done for the first visit.
32-36 weeks: 1. **Step-B** (swab) screen; if (+) without symptoms, give ampicillin during labor to prevent the newborn infection. 2. Repeat hematocrit, and cervical chlamydia, gonorrhea, PRP, HIV tests in high-risk patients.

Antepartum Fetal Surveillance

Antepartum fetal tests are highly accurate in confirming fetal well-being, but relatively less in predicting fetal risks. Common reasons for fetal testing include decreased fetal movements, postdates, diabetes, chronic hypertension, and IUGR. All these conditions increase the risk of antepartum fetal death.

Fetal Heart Rate (FHR) Monitoring

This is the most commonly used obstetric procedure during the labor (for > 85% of cases).

Recommended indications

1. Patients without complications: FHR tracing checked per 30 min in the first stage of labor and per 15 min in the second stage.

2. Patients with complications: FHR tracing checked per 15 min in the first stage of labor and per 5 min in the second stage.

Table 12-5: Changes and Causes of Fetal Heart Rate (FHR)

Type	Description	Causes
Bradycardia	Baseline FHR < 110bpm.	Congenital heart defects; severe hypoxia (secondary to uterine hyperstimulation or cord prolapse).
Tachycardia	Baseline FHR > 160bpm.	Hypoxia; anemia; maternal fever.
Acceleration	A visually apparent increase in FHR from the most recent baseline: onset to peak < 30sec.	Fetal movements.
Early deceleration	An apparent, gradual decrease in FHR with return to baseline: onset to nadir > 30sec.	**Normal head compression** from the uterine contraction.
Late deceleration	An apparent, gradual decrease in FHR (onset to nadir > 30sec), with return to baseline whose onset, nadir, and recovery occur after the start, peak, and end of uterine-contraction, respectively.	Uteroplacental insufficiency and **fetal hypoxia/stress. P.472**
Variable deceleration	An abrupt decrease (onset to nadir <30sec) in FHR below baseline, lasting 15sec to 2min	Umbilical **cord compression** (#1 cause is oligohydramnios).

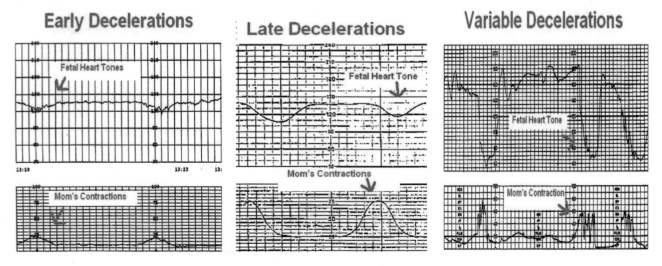

Figure 12-1, 2, 3: Fetal Heart Rate (FHR) Monitoring: early, late, and variable decelerations

(Courtesy of www.registerednursern.com)

Fetal Movement Assessment

It's the number of fetal movements per hour assessed by the mother, with 10 movements in 20 min as the average. If the mother reports decreased fetal movements, you should perform the tests below.

Nonstress Test (NST)

For this test, the fetal heart rate is monitored by an external Doppler along with a tocodynamometer to detect uterine contractions. Acoustic stimulation can be used for faster results. **Normal response ("Reactive")** is two accelerations of > 15 bpm above baseline for > 15 sec.

"**Nonreactive NST**" (+): Diagnosed when any criteria for the above reactivity are not met: either the number of accelerations in 20 min or the amplitude/duration of the acceleration. 80% of nonreactive nonstress tests are false (+), meaning the fetus is not hypoxemic, but due to GA < 32 weeks, fetal sleeping, or maternal sedative use. If NST is persistently nonreactive, then a biophysical profile is performed.

Contraction Stress Test (CST) *done during maternal contraction. don't induce contraction CTX to assess baby*

An electronic fetal monitor tracing performed in the lateral recumbent position. **FHR determines** the reactivity and is monitored during spontaneous or induced contractions. Nipple stimulation or oxytocin can be used for induction.

1. **CST (+)**: Presence of late decelerations associated with > 50% contractions in 10 min. It's worrisome for the fetus and an indication for delivery.

2. **CST (-)**: No late decelerations or significant variable decelerations in 10 min and for > three contractions. Highly predictive of fetal well-being combined with a normal NST.

3. "**Equivocal**": Intermittent late decelerations, or significant variable decelerations. Close follow-ups are recommended.

Contraindications: PROM, placenta previa, preterm labor, and history of uterine surgery.

Biophysical Profile (BPP)

It measures five components of fetal well-being: NST, amniotic fluid index (AFI), fetal gross body movements, fetal extremity tone, and fetal breathing. All are assessed using obstetric ultrasound except NST. Scores for each component are 0 or 2, with maximum scores of 10.

1. **Score of 8-10**: Highly reassuring of fetal well-being. **Treatment**: Repeat the test weekly.

2. **Score of 4-6**: Worrisome. **Treatment**: Delivery if the fetus is 36 weeks or more, or repeat the biophysical profile in 12-24 hours if < 36 weeks.

3. **Score of 0-2**: Highly worrisome and predictive of fetal hypoxia (low false positives). **Treatment:** It requires **urgent delivery regardless of GA**.

Modified BPP (mBPP)

It includes only the nonstress test and amniotic fluid volume. Its predictive value is almost as high as a complete BPP.

Umbilical Artery Doppler Velocimetry

It's only beneficial for suspected **IUGR**, showing reduced diastolic flow in the umbilical artery.

NORMAL LABOR

Definition: Labor is a process with regular uterine contractions and progressive effacement and dilation of the cervix, resulting in delivery of the fetus and expulsion of the placenta. Contractions occur at least every 5 min lasting 30 sec.

Types of Pelvic Shapes

Gynecoid shape: The classic female pelvis and found in 50% of women. This pelvis is spacious for the fetal head to pass through. Other pelvic shapes (Android, anthropoid, platypelloid shape) all are variably difficult for normal delivery.

Fetal Orientation in Uterus

Lie: Orientation of the long axis of the fetus to the long axis of the uterus. The most common lie is longitudinal.
Presentation: Portion of the fetus overlying the pelvic inlet. The most common one is cephalic.
Position: Relationship of a definite fetal part to the maternal bony pelvis. The commonest position is occiput anterior.
Attitude: Usually refers to the position of fetal body and limbs, commonly as vertex.
Station: Degree of descending, recorded as number of cm above (as "-") or below (as "+") the ischial spine. E.g., if the station is "3+", it's low enough for vacuum/forceps-aided delivery; if the station is "3-", it's too high for the assisted delivery.

Obstetric Examination

Leopold's maneuvers: Used to determine fetal lie (longitudinal or transverse) and fetal presentation (breech or cephalic); with limitation.

Cardinal Movements of Labor

1. Engagement: the presenting part moving below the plane of the pelvic inlet.
2. Descent: the presenting part down through the curve of the birth canal.

Cardinal Movements of Labor

3. Flexion: placement of the fetal chin on the thorax. These first 3 steps occur simultaneously.
4. Internal rotation: rotation of the fetal head in the mid pelvis from transverse to anterior- posterior.
5. Extension: the fetal chin moving away from the thorax.
6. External rotation: rotation of the fetal head outside the mother.
7. Expulsion: delivery of the fetal shoulders and body.

Stages of Labor

Table 12-6: Labor Stages, Arrest, and Management

Stage: Start—End	Duration	Duration	Arrest and Treatment
First	Primiparous	Multi-	
Latent: Labor onset to Os 3-4cm dilation	6-11 hrs	4-8 hrs	Causes of arrest: No.1 is over-anesthesia; hypo-/hypertonic uterine contraction. Tx: Observation; IV fluid (to wash out anesthetics).
Active: Os 3-4 to full 10cm or Os > 1cm/hr	4 hrs +/-	2-3 hrs	Causes of arrest: #1 is to cephalopelvic disproportion (big fetal size, abnormal fetal orientation or birth canal); hypotonic contract. Tx: Prepare for C-section.
Second Full Os dilation to	< 2 hrs	< 1 hrs	Baby undergoes all cardinal movements of labor. Causes of arrest: hypotonic contraction. Tx: Oxytocin IV and forceps or vacuum extractor delivery.
Third Delivery of baby to delivery of placenta	< 0.5 hrs	< 0.5 hrs	Placenta separates and uterus contracts. Causes of arrest: No.1 is atonic uterine contraction and retaining placenta. Tx: It may require manual placental removal or hysterectomy (with severe bleeding).

ABNORMAL LABOR

In general, abnormal labor is the result of problems with one of the 3 Ps:
(1) Passenger [infant size, fetal presentation (occiput anterior, posterior, or transverse)];
(2) Pelvis or passage (size, shape, and adequacy of the pelvis);
(3) Power (uterine contractility)

Dystocia

It's defined as slow, abnormally protracted progression or arrest of labor, which is the most common indication for C-section. Risk factors are chorioamnionitis, occiput posterior position, giant baby, and nulliparity. It's usually not diagnosed until adequate labor has been tried. Dystocia is determined by labor stages and summarized in "Table 12-6".

Fetal Malpresentation

It refers to any presentation other than vertex, such as breech, chin to chest, head close to birth canal, and occiput anterior.

Risk factors: Prematurity, prior breech delivery, poly- or oligohydramnios, multiple gestations, uterine or fetal anomalies, placenta previa, and PROM, etc.

Breech Presentation: The most common type and accounts for 3% of all deliveries; involving presentation of the fetal lower limbs or buttocks into the maternal pelvis.

Breech subtypes

1. Frank breech: 50-75%, thighs flexed and knees extended.
2. Footling breech: 20%, 1-2 legs extended below the buttocks.
3. Complete breech: 5-10%, thighs and knees are both flexed.

Management

1. Follow-ups: Most malpresentations (75%) will change to vertex spontaneously by week 38.
2. External cephalic version: If the fetus has not reverted spontaneously by 37-38 weeks, externally manipulate the gravid abdominal to turn the fetus (from transverse lie or breech presentation) to vertex. Be prepared for 60% of success rate and C-section if failed.
3. Breech vaginal delivery: Can only be tried when delivery is imminent and C-section is prepared. Contraindications include cord prolapse and head entrapment.
4. Elective C-section: Practiced in many hospitals with varied outcomes.

Premature Rupture of Membranes (PROM)

Rupture of the fetal membranes prior to the onset of labor at term or preterm.

Risk factors: No.1 common factor is **ascending infection** from the lower genital tract. Others are local membrane defects and smoking.

Essentials of diagnosis

1. Typically a sudden gush of copious vaginal fluid. On external examination, clear fluid is flowing out of the vagina. Ultrasound confirms oligohydramnios.
2. Diagnosis is confirmed by speculum exam:
(1) Pooling (+): clear amniotic fluid seen in the posterior vaginal fornix;
(2) Nitrazine (+): the fluid turns pH-sensitive paper blue;
(3) Fern (+): the fluid displays a ferning pattern after air-dried on a microscope glass slide. → Fetal tachycardia
3. **Chorioamnionitis** is diagnosed clinically with: (1) maternal fever and uterine tenderness; (2) (baseline >160/min) confirmed PROM in the absence of an URI or UTI.

Treatment

1. If uterine contractions occur, tocolysis is contraindicated. If chorioamnionitis is present, obtain cervical cultures, start broad-spectrum IV antibiotics, and initiate prompt delivery.
2. Without infection, treatment is based on GA.
(1) Before viability (< 24 weeks), outcome is dismal; either placing patient at bed rest or labor trial.

PROM TX

(2) With preterm viability (24-35 weeks), conservative treatment. Hospitalize the patient at bed rest, IM inject steroid to enhance fetal lung maturity if < 32 weeks, obtain cervical cultures, and start a 7-day prophylactic ampicillin.

(3) At term (> 36 weeks +/-), prompt delivery. If vaginal delivery is chosen, oxytocin can be used; otherwise, C-section is performed.

Preterm Labor

Preterm delivery is the most common cause of perinatal morbidity and mortality, occupying 8-10% of pregnancies. Preterm contractions may not mean preterm labor.

Braxton-Hicks Contractions

These are **sporadic uterine contractions without cervical dilation occurring during the 3rd trimester**. If they become regular, the cervix should be examined—if the cervix is open, it is preterm labor before 37 weeks. **Beginning at 37 weeks, the cervix should be examined at every visit**.

Three criteria for preterm labor (must be met for diagnosis)

1. GA: > 20 weeks but < 37 weeks.
2. Uterine contractions: > three contractions in 30 min.
3. Cervical Os change: serial Os dilation in progression or a single dilation of > 2 cm.

Treatment

1. Rule out contraindications for tocolysis, and initiate IV isotonic fluids with $MgSO_4$.
2. Obtain cervical and urine cultures, followed by IV antibiotics (PCN for Strep-B prophylaxis).
3. Maternal IM betamethasone to accelerate fetal lung maturity (by stimulating type 2 pneumocyte surfactant production).

Cesarean Section (C-Section)

It's a procedure in which the fetus is delivered through incisions in the maternal anterior abdominal and uterine walls. The overall C-section rate is > 20%. **Risk factors**: Maternal mortality and complications (hemorrhage, infection, visceral injury, DVT, etc) are higher than with vaginal delivery. Successful vaginal delivery rate can be up to 80% if patients with C-section history are carefully selected.

Indications for C-section

1. Maternal and fetal factors: **Cephalopelvic disproportion (No.1 common reason)**, placenta previa/abruption, failed operative vaginal delivery, or post-term pregnancy.

2. Maternal factors: Active herpes infection, prior classical C-section (vertical incision increasing the risk of uterine rupture with vaginal delivery), cervical cancer, or maternal trauma/death.

3. Fetal factors: Fetal distress, cord compression, fetal malposition (transverse lie, posterior chin, shoulder presentation, etc.), or erythroblastosis fetalis (Rh incompatibility).

Episiotomy

Also known as perineotomy, it is a surgically planned incision on the perineum and the posterior vaginal wall to expand the vaginal opening during second stage of labor. It is performed in approximately 30% vaginal births. Commonly used types are median and mediolateral cuts. Routine episiotomy is not recommended because it has not shown reduction of pelvic floor damage or shoulder dystocia at labor; rather, it lengthens the recovery time—longer than natural perineum tear. Complications include extended injury to anal sphincter (3rd degree) and rectum (4th degree), bleeding, infection, and dyspareunia.

Intrauterine Resuscitation Measures for Fetal Hypoxia

uterine tachysystole=>
↑interrupt utero-
placental flow
=> LATE
DECELERATION
=> fetal
hypoxemia
+
acidemia

1. Decrease uterine over-contractions: Stop any IV oxytocin infusion, or give terbutaline SC to enhance intervillous placental blood flow.

2. Augment IV fluid volume: IV infusion of 500 mL of bolus N.S. (normal saline) rapidly to enhance uteroplacental infusion.

3. Supply high-flow oxygen: Increased maternal oxygen to the placenta.

4. Change position: Changing from the supine position decreases inferior vena cava (IVC) compression and enhances cardiac return, thus cardiac output to the placenta. Turning from side to side may relieve possible umbilical cord compression.

5. Vaginal exam: Perform a digital vaginal exam to rule out possible prolapsed cord.

6. Scalp stimulation: Perform a digital scalp stimulation observing for accelerations, which would be reassuring of fetal condition.

PEARLS—Indications for Antibiotic Use in Labor

1. History of a neonate with Group-B Strep infection.
2. Urine Strep-B test (+): IV antibiotics 30 min before and after delivery.
3. Membrane rupture > 18 hours.
4. Preterm labor < 34 weeks GA.
5. T > 38ºC.

MEDICAL COMPLICATIONS OF PREGNANCY

Gestational and Chronic Hypertension (HTN)

I. Gestational hypertension

An idiopathic hypertension that develops > 20 weeks GA, usually with mild proteinuria and similar complications to those of preeclampsia. About 1/3 of cases can develop preeclampsia.

II. Chronic hypertension

Hypertension present prior to conception or at < 20 weeks GA. About 1/3 of cases can go to preeclampsia, with similar complications as for preeclampsia.

Gestrtional & chronic HTN

Differential diagnosis

1. Transient hypertension in pregnancy: BP >140/90 mmHg shortly but not sustained, returning to baseline after a transient period of observation or rest. No proteinuria.

2. Preeclampsia: Always needs to be ruled out (see below).

Treatment

Monitor BP closely and treat with appropriate anti- hypertensive medicines (methyldopa or labetalol). Avoid ACE-I (causing fetal defects and uterine ischemia) or diuretics (lowering plasma volume).

Preeclampsia and Eclampsia *- vasoconstriction everywhere*

Eclampsia is an acute and life-threatening complication of pregnancy associated with pregnancy-induced hypertension and seizures not related to brain conditions. It's summarized in the table below.

PEARLS **Table 12-7: Summary of Preeclampsia and Eclampsia**

Stage	Clinical features	Management
Preeclampsia	**Mild:** BP > 140/90 twice with 6-hrs apart. Renal: proteinuria >300 mg/24hrs or 1-2(+) on dipsticks. **Severe:** BP >160/110 twice with 6-hrs apart. Renal: proteinuria > 5 g/24hrs or 3-4 (+) on dipsticks, or oliguria (< 500 ml/24hrs). CNS: headache, somnolence, blurred vision, hyper-reflexes, and clonus. GI: epigastric pain. **HELLP syndrome:** Hemolysis, Elevated Liver enzymes, and Low Platelets. **Complications**: Prematurity, placental abruption, stillbirth, seizure, DIC, ICH, or maternal death.	1. If it's close to term or symptoms worsen, induce labor with IV oxytocin, PG, or amniotomy. 2. If it's far from term, bed rest and expectant Tx. 1. BP control: labetalol +/- hydralazine (keep <160/90-110 to maintain fetal blood flow. 2. Deliver by induction or C-sect if patient is stable. 3. Seizure prophylaxis: MgSO$_4$ IV drip extended for 24hr postpartum. 4. With toxic signs of MgSO$_4$ (respiratory and DTR suppression); treat with Ca-gluconate.
Eclampsia	**Typical preceding triad: headache, visual changes, and epigastric pain**; severe seizures may occur if not controlled with anticonvulsants. **Complication:** Stroke, hypoxic encephalopathy, aspiration pneumonia, or fetal/maternal death.	1. **"ABC" + O$_2$.** 2. **Seizure control: IV MgSO$_4$;** if it recurs, IV diazepam. 3. BP control: labetalol +/- hydralazine. 4. Limit and monitor fluids (in/out by Foley); monitor MgSO$_4$ toxicity and fetal status. 5. Start delivery if patient is stable with seizures controlled. 6. Postpartum: Same as that for the preeclampsia. Most seizures occur < 48hrs postpartum.

HELLP Syndrome

It's a syndrome characterized by **hemolysis (with anemia), elevated liver enzymes (LFTs), and low platelets**. It occurs in 5-10% of preeclamptic patients and more often in multigravidas than primigravidas.

Differential diagnosis
It may be confused with TTP and hemolytic uremic syndrome; hypertension may not always be present.

Treatment
Prompt delivery at any GA. Maternal steroid use may enhance postpartum recovery.

Complication
DIC, placental abruption, fetal demise, hepatic rupture, or ascites.

Gestational Diabetes Mellitus (GDM)—Important!

It is defined as the failure of a pregnant female to maintain fasting or post-challenge glucose levels in the normal pregnant range, before or after a standard 2-hour 75g glucose tolerance test (GTT) or 3-hour 100g GTT. The prevalence is about 2-3%. It's mainly caused by the diabetogenic effect of human placental lactogen, placental insulinase, cortisol, and progesterone.

Risk factors
Obesity, > 35 y/a, family history, back pain, and fetal macrosomia. If the fetus is larger for GA, the mother should be suspected of GDM.

PEARLS—Screening for GDM
1. **Glucose tests** for everyone: urinary glucose test first; if it's (+), 1-hr 50g GTT is followed (normal value < 140 mg/dL).

2. **Patient with any risk factor (see above): 1-hour 50g GTT, 2-hour 75g GTT, or 3-hour 100g GTT** can be performed for the first visit.

3. For most **patients at 26-28th weeks**, a urinary dipstick test for glucose is done first; if it's (+), a fasting urine or plasma glucose test is performed.

PEARLS—Diagnosis of GMD (Any standard below)
1. Fasting plasma glucose > 126 mg/dL (7 mmol/L) or HbA1C > 6.5%: Overt diabetes.
2. 2-hour 75g GTT plasma glucose $\geq$ 200 mg/dL (11.1 mmol/L).
3. Any two of the standards below met in the 3-hour 100g GTT (most widely used in the US):
1-hour > 180 mg/dL (10 mmol/L);
2-hour > 155 mg/dL (8.6 mmol/L);
3-hour > 140 mg/dL (7.8 mmol/L).
If only one value is abnormal in the 3-hour GTT, "impaired GTT" is diagnosed.

Treatment
1. Strict diabetic diet.
2. If diabetes cannot be controlled by diet alone, regular/NPH insulin is needed. Oral hypoglycemics should not be used (to avoid fetal hypoglycemia).
3. Ultrasonography is used to evaluate fetal growth.

Pregestational Diabetes

It's the condition that diabetes exists prior to pregnancy. Poorly controlled diabetes (best indicated by HbA1C > 10) is associated with increased risk of congenital malformation and maternal morbidity during labor and delivery.

Maternal treatment

1. Routine prenatal screening and care (including nutritional counseling).

2. Strict glucose control (80-100 mg/dL) to minimize fetal defects. Use insulin when needed instead of oral hypoglycemics.

3. Regular renal, cardiac, and ophthalmologic exams to evaluate the extent of end-organ damage.

Fetal treatment

1. **16-20 weeks**: Ultrasound to determine fetal age, size and AFI for macrosomia, polyhydramnios and IUGR, etc.

2. **20-22 weeks**: Echocardiogram to assess cardiac anomalies.

3. **3rd trimester**: Close fetal monitoring (NST, BPP, etc). Hospitalize the patient at 32-36th weeks if maternal diabetes cannot be controlled well.

Delivery

1. Early delivery is indicated with poor maternal glucose control, preeclampsia, or macrosomia, or with evidence of fetal lung maturity.

2. C-section is appropriate for fetal weight > 4000g.

3. Continuous postpartum glucose monitoring, because the insulin demand is decreased rapidly after delivery.

Complication

1. **Maternal:** DKA (type I) or HHNK (type II), preeclampsia or eclampsia, cephalopelvic disproportion, preterm labor.

2. **Fetal:** Macrosomia, cardiac, renal or neural tube defect, secondary hypoglycemia, hypocalcemia, hyperbilirubinemia, polycythemia, IUGR, RDS, etc.

OBSTETRICAL COMPLICATIONS OF PREGNANCY

Table 12-8: Summary of Obstetric Complications of Pregnancy

Complications / Causes, diagnosis (Dx), and treatment (Tx)
Antepartum hemorrhage, Abortion, IUGR, Uterine rupture, Hydatidiform mole: See below.
Fetal macrosomia
Birth weight > 90th percentile; commonly secondary to gestational diabetes. **Dx**: Weighing the newborn at birth (prenatal Dx is not precise). **Tx**: C-section planned for expected fetal weight (EFW) > 5kg (or > 4.5kg with maternal diabetes). **Complication**: Increased risk of shoulder dystocia and secondary brachial plexus injury and Erb-Duchenne palsy.

Oligohydramnios

AFI < 5cm on ultrasound. **Cause**: fetal UT abnormalities (renal agenesis, GU obstruction), **Pulmonary hypoplasia**, PROM, uteroplacental insufficiency.

Dx: May be asymptomatic; fetal distress or IUGR; summary of amniotic fluid pocket in all four abdominal quadrants, with the common error in GA ruled out.

Tx: Further evaluation for causes. **Complication**: 40% increase in perinatal deaths; musculoskeletal abnormalities, cord compression, and IUGR.

Polyhydramnios

AFI > 20cm on ultrasound. **Cause**: Normal pregnancy, fetal chromosomal abnormalities, maternal diabetes, multiple gestation, isoimmunisation, cystic lung abnormality, fetal anomalies (anencephaly, tracheo-esophageal fistula, duodenal atresia, etc), and twin-twin transfusion syndrome.

Dx: Perform ultrasound for fetal abnormalities, glucose for diabetes, and Rh screening.

Tx: Based on etiology. **Complication**: Preterm labor, fetal malpresentation, cord prolapse, etc.

Ectopic pregnancy

Usually tubal, but can also be abdominal, ovarian, or cervical; often associated with a PID history.

Dx: 1. Abdominal pain and vaginal bleeding/spotting. 2. Serial beta-hCG testing (single hCG may be +/-), combined with vaginal ultrasound.

Tx: 1. Medications (methotrexate) for small, unruptured tubal pregnancy. 2. Most other cases—surgery: salpingectomy (by laparoscopy or laparotomy). **Complication**: Tubal rupture or hemoperitonium (emergency).

Rh isoimmunization FAS/ P.382

Fetal RBCs leak into the maternal circulation, inducing anti-Rh IgG antibody that can cross the placenta and cause hemolysis of fetal Rh RBCs ("**erythroblastosis fetalis**").

Dx: Sensitized Rh (-) mothers with titers > 1:16 should be monitored closely with serial ultrasound and amniocentesis for evidence of hemolysis.

Tx: If severe, give intrauterine blood transfusion and induce preterm labor (with prior steroid if fetal lung is not mature). **Prophylaxis**: 1. At 28 week's GA, if the mother is Rh (-) and father is Rh (+) or unknown, give RhoGAM. 2. Post-partum RhoGAM if the baby is Rh (+). 3. Rh (-) mother should have RhoGAM if she has a history of abortion, ectopic pregnancy, vaginal bleeding, amniocentesis, placenta previa, or placental abruption.

Multiple gestations

Accounting for about 3% of live births, increased with assisted reproductive tech.

Dx: 1. Rapid increase in uterine size, maternal weight, hCG, HPL and MSAFP for GA, and palpation of > 3 large fetal parts. 2. Ultrasound confirms Dx.

Tx: 1. Antepartum fetal monitoring for IUGR. 2. Selective fetal termination. **Complication**: Increased risk of maternal preeclampsia, placental abruption, postpartum bleeding, fetal IUGR, preterm PROM and labor, cerebral palsy, and twin-to-twin transfusion syndrome.

Prolapsed umbilical cord

It's an obstetric emergency because fetal oxygenation will be jeopardized by the compressed cord, with potential fetal death.

Tx: Do not hold the cord or try to push it back into the uterus. Place patient in knee-chest position, elevate the presenting part, avoid palpating the cord, and perform an immediate **C-section**.

Antepartum Hemorrhage

It's defined as any bleeding after 20 weeks of gestation, occurring in 3-4% of pregnancies. The most common causes are **placental abruption and placenta previa**; others include abnormal placentation, ruptured uterus, genital tract lesion, and trauma. Bleeding before 20 weeks of gestation refers to threatened abortion.

Table 12-9: Comparison of Placenta Previa and Placental Abruption

Comparison	Placenta previa	Placental abruption
Pathophysiology	Abnormal placental implantation: **Total:** Placenta covers the cervical Os. **Marginal:** Placenta extends to Os margin. **Low-lying:** Placenta is close to the Os.	Premature separation of normally implanted placenta.
Risk factors	Prior C-sections or placenta previa (5%), multiple (grand) gestations, or advanced maternal age. Incidence is 1/200.	Hypertension, abdominal/pelvic trauma, smoking, drug abuse, previous abruption, or rapid uterine decompression. Incidence is 1/100.
Clinical features and diagnosis (Dx)	**Painless, bright vaginal bleeding**, mostly stopped in 1-2 hrs without fetal distress and with very few uterine contractions. **Dx:** Transabdominal/vaginal ultrasound, with > 95% sensitivity.	**Painful, dark, non-stop vaginal bleeding;** abdominal pain, uterine hypertonicity, and fetal distress. **Dx:** Mainly on clinical features; ultrasound sensitivity is only 50%. Retroplacental clot found helps rule out placenta previa.
Treatment	1. **No vaginal examination!** 2. Stabilize patient with a premature fetus and treat accordingly. Serial ultrasound is used to evaluate fetal growth. 3. Give MgSO4 and betamethasone (to promote fetal lung maturity). 4. C-section if with signs of labor, fetal stress, fetal lung maturity, or 36-week GA.	1. For mild abruption and premature fetus: stabilize patient and treat with IV fluid, fetal monitoring, blood typing, and bed rest in hospital. 2. For moderate to severe abruption: immediate delivery. C-section if mother or fetus is in distress; vaginal delivery with life-threatening bleeding; amniotomy if mother and fetus are stable.
Complications	Increased risk of placenta accrete, vasa previa (fetal vessels crossing the internal Os), PROM, and congenital anomalies.	Hemorrhagic shock, fetal hypoxia, DIC, preterm delivery, IUGR, and recurrence.

Intrauterine Growth Retardation (IUGR)

It's defined as expected fetal weight (EFW) < 10th percentile for calculated GA; divided into 2 types:

1. **Symmetric**: About **20%**, in which all the growth variables (abdomen and head circumference, length, Wt) are equally reduced. Common causes include **congenital infections or abnormalities**, chromosomal abnormalities, and maternal drug abuse (alcohol, smoking, cocaine). Mostly occurs in early pregnancy.

2. **Asymmetric**: About **80%**, in which there is relative sparing of the head circumference (HC) and other variables are reduced more. It's usually later onset and with a better prognosis. Common causes are **chronic maternal disease** (hypertension, diabetes, etc), placental deficiency, multiple gestations, etc.

Essentials of diagnosis

1. Serial fundal height measurements: Discrepancy between fundal height (cm) and GA (week) > 4.

2. Ultrasound: It confirms the diagnosis by revealing head/abdomen circumference ratio (**HC/AC) in asymmetric IUGR** (also in oligohydramnios), and the **ratio is normal in symmetric IUGR**.

Treatment

1. Serial exams and ultrasound follow-ups every 3-4 weeks.

2. Fetal monitoring: Nonstress test, contraction stress test, or biophysical profile.

3. Steroids: Accelerate fetal lung maturity and early delivery, especially with asymmetric IUGR.

4. Continue fetal heart rate monitoring during labor and prepare for C-section if nonreassuring decelerations persist.

Differential diagnosis

Preterm newborns: Proportionately small in size, and the weight falls in the normal GA range.

Complication

Hypoglycemia, polycythemia (hypoxia), asphyxia, and fetal death.

Uterine Rupture   _- Pain, bleeding. The site of rupture can be palpated on manual exploration of the uterus._

It refers to complete separation of the wall of the pregnant uterus before or after the fetal birth, which threatens the maternal/fetal life. The rupture may be incomplete (not including the peritoneum) or complete (including the visceral peritoneum). Common **risk factors** include history of **classic uterine incision (No.1)**, myomectomy, excessive oxytocin stimulation, and grand multiparity.

Essentials of diagnosis

1. Typical findings are nonreassuring fetal monitor tracing associated with vaginal bleeding, abdominal pain, and changes in uterine contractility. Rupture may occur before or during the labor.

2. Diagnosis is confirmed by surgical exploration of the uterus.

Treatment

1. Immediate cesarean delivery of the fetus is demanded.

2. Uterine repair if the patient is stable and young, and desires further fertility.

Uterine Rupture

3. Hysterectomy if the patient is unstable or desires no more childbearing.

Hydatidiform Mole—Gestational Trophoblastic Disease (GTD)

GTD includes a group of proliferative trophoblastic abnormalities with benign or malignant nature.
Risk factors: Extreme age (< 20 or > 40), poor nutrition, or diet deficiency in folate or beta-carotene.

Classification

1. **Complete moles**: 46, XX, paternal derived; mostly due to sperm fertilization of an empty ovum.

2. **Incomplete (partial) moles**: 69, XXY; usually from an ovum fertilized by two sperms and contain fetal tissue.

3. **Invasive moles**: malignant, 10-15% of GTD.

4. **Choriocarcinoma**: 2-5% of GTD.

Essentials of diagnosis

1. **The most common symptom is 1st trimester uterine bleeding**, hyperemesis, preeclampsia or eclampsia at < 24 weeks, **uterine size > gestational dates**.

2. P/E reveals no fetal heartbeat; pelvic exam may show enlarged ovaries (bilateral theca-lutein cysts), or expelled grapelike molar clusters in the vagina.

3. **Lab tests**: **Markedly elevated serum beta-hCG** (can be > 100, 000 mIU/mL). Pelvic ultrasound shows "**snowstorm**" image. **Biopsy** confirms the disease nature.

Treatment

1. **Benign moles: D&C** along with beta-hCG monitoring is usually adequate.

2. **Invasive moles and choriocarcinoma: Hysterectomy** plus chemotherapy (methotrexate mainly) and beta-hCG monitoring are the most effective therapies. Chemotherapy is always indicated if metastasis occurs (most commonly to the lungs). Emboli can be a common complication.

Spontaneous Termination of Pregnancy (Abortion)

1st-trimester bleeding (occurring before 12 weeks of gestation) is the most common symptom associated with spontaneous abortions (miscarriage).

Genetics of pregnancy loss
Miscarriage: > 50% cases of first-trimester abortuses have abnormal chromosomes; among these, 50% are autosomal trisomies; 20% are Type "45, X" (Turner syndrome).

Indications for genetic counseling
1. Advanced maternal age (> 35): with higher risk of trisomies 21 and 18.
2. History of multiple fetal losses, neonatal death, child's mental retardation, or aneuploidy.
3. Family history of genetic disease, birth defects, intellectual disability, or aneuploidy.
4. Abnormal prenatal tests: triple marker screening or ultrasound examination.

PEARLS—Table 12-10: Comparison of Spontaneous Abortions

Type	Clinical features & diagnosis	Treatment
Threatened abortion	1. Uterine bleeding, abdominal pain may be ($\pm$); no products of conception (POC) expelled; membranes remained intact; and the fetus is still viable. 2. Os is closed and ultrasound (U/S) is normal.	1. Avoid heavy activity, coitus, and douching. 2. Bed rest for two days then gradual activities.
Inevitable abortion	1. Uterine bleeding and cramps, POC not expelled yet but tends to be inevitable. 2. Os is open and ROM may be ($\pm$).	1. D&C, PG suppository or expectant Tx. 2. Surgical evacuation if bleeding is heavy.
Incomplete abortion	1. Mild uterine cramps and bleeding; some POC is expelled and visible in the vagina. 2. Os is open and ultrasound shows retained fetal tissue.	D&C to remove retained tissue for pathology and to control bleeding. 2. If bleeding is heavy, IV fluid or blood is ingested.
Complete abortion	1. All POC is expelled; uterine cramps stop, but spotting may persist. 2. Os is closed; ultrasound reveals an empty uterus. POC sent for pathologic confirmation.	D&C if incomplete abortion is suspected.
Septic abortion	Infection with abortion. Endometritis can develop to septicemia, with > 10% maternal mortality. 1. History of using contaminated tools, purulent discharge at Os, uterine tenderness, and minimal bleeding. 2. Signs of infectious shock ($\pm$): Hypothermia, hypo-tension, oliguria, respiratory distress, increased WBCs.	1. Hospitalize patient. 2. Take sample for culture/sensitivity (C/S). 3. IV antibiotics (gentamicin + clindamycin). 4. Complete uterine evacuation; careful D&C to avoid perforation.
Missed abortion	Fetal demise but still retained in the uterus, usually for weeks, **mostly < 8-10 weeks' GA.** 1. Pregnancy symptoms disappear; no uterine growing, cramps or bleeding; no POC expelled but brownish vaginal discharge. 2. Os is closed; ultrasound reveals a fetus without cardiac activity. **Differentiation: Intrauterine fetal demise** Fetal demise, usually **> 20-week**'s gestation. Ultrasound reveals a fetus > 20 weeks GA but no cardiac activity, with > 15 mm crown-rump length.	D&C or prostaglandins to evacuate the uterus fully. **Complication**: Increased risk of DIC with increased GA. **Fetal demise Tx**: D&C to evacuate the uterus fully to avoid DIC.
Recurrent abortion	More than consecutive spontaneous abortions or totally 3 times in a year. 1. Early abortion is usually caused by chromosomal abnormalities; both parents should be examined for karyotyping. 2. With history of painless cervix dilation and normal fetus delivery between 18-32 weeks, the uterus should be examined for possible abnormalities and incompetent cervix, and cervical cultures for Gonococcus, Chlamydia, and Group-B Strep are done.	1. Activity restriction. 2. Surgical cerclage to suture the cervix until labor or ROM, followed by removal prior to delivery. **Prevention of Rh hemolysis**: Give RhoGAM to all Rh (-) mothers with history of abortion.

POSTNATAL (PUERPERIUM)

Another term is postpartum period. It's the period beginning immediately after the birth of a child and extending for about six weeks. It is the time after birth, a time in which the mother's body, including hormone levels and uterus size, returns to a non-pregnant state.

Postpartum Hemorrhage

Definition: Blood loss > 500 mL for vaginal delivery or > 1000 mL for C-section occurring before, during, or after delivery of the placenta. Common causes are summarized in the table below.

Complication: Hemorrhagic shock, Sheehan syndrome, and anemia (due to chronic blood loss).

[handwritten margin note: one hand massaging uterine fundus abd, another massaging uterus vaginally.]

PEARLS — Table 12-11: Summary of Postpartum Hemorrhage

Cause	Risk factors	Diagnosis	Treatment
Uterine atony	It's the **#1 common cause** (90%). **Risk factors:** Uterine overdistention (macrosomia or multiple gestations), exhausted myometrium (rapid/prolonged labor, or over-use of oxytocin, anesthesia, or MgSO$_4$), and uterine infection. *[forceps-assist. vag delivery]*	Palpation of an enlarged, soft, "boggy" uterus. *[above umbilicus]* *[oxytocin receptor saturation]*	1. Initially bimanual uterine massage (usually effective). *[-2 large bore IV lines, O2]* 2. If still bleeding, give oxytocin or methergine (if there is no hypertension), or PGF$_2\alpha$ (if there is no asthma).
Genital trauma	Precipitous labor, large baby, forceps/vacuum injury, or loose episiotomy cut.	Manually and visually inspect the lower genital tract for any laceration > 2cm long.	Surgical repair.
Retained placental tissue	Placenta accrete/increta/percreta/previa, preterm delivery, uterine leiomyoma, and history of C-section/curettage. *[- cord avulsion during placental delivery]*	Manually and visually inspect the placenta and uterine cavity for missing or retained tissue. Uterine ultrasound may also help.	Manually remove retained placental tissue, followed by curettage with suction (be careful not to cause uterine perforation).

[handwritten right margin notes: Hemostasis after placental delivery is achieved by clotting & by compression of placental site blood vessels by myometrial contraction. → uterine inversion. Retained placenta prevents the uterus from contracting.]

Sheehan Syndrome

Also called "**Postpartum pituitary necrosis**", it's the No.1 cause of anterior pituitary deficits in women, mostly secondary to massive obstetric hemorrhagic shock. **The most common symptom is lactation failure**; others include lethargy, weakness, cold insensitivity, genital atrophy, and menstrual disorders. **Treatment is lifelong hormone replacement therapy: prednisone, levothyroxine, estrogen, and growth hormone.**

Postpartum Infection

It's the postpartum genital tract infection with T≥38°C for >2d (beyond the 1st 24h), with endometritis most common. **Risk factors:** PROM, urgent C-Section, prolonged delivery, and multiple vaginal exams.

Treatment

For endometritis: Hospitalize patient and give IV broad-spectrum antibiotics (No.1 is **clindamycin + gentamycin**), until the patient is afebrile for 48 hours. If the case is complicated, add ampicillin.

Common causes of postpartum fever are summarized below.

PEARLS──Table 12-12: Common Causes of Postpartum Fever

Postpartum Day / Commonest cause
0: Atelectasis
1-2: Urinary tract infection (UTI)
2-3: Endometritis
4-5: Wound infection
5-6: Septic thrombophlebitis
7-21: Infectious mastitis

Lochia

Lochia is post-partum vaginal discharge, containing blood, mucus, and placental tissue. It is due to the shedding of the superficial layers of the endometrial deciduas through the vagina during the first three postpartum weeks. The initial color is red (lochia rubra), changing to pinkish (lochia serosa), ending with a whitish color (lochia alba).

Lactation and Breast-feeding

After the placental delivery, estrogen and progesterone levels decrease markedly and prolactin is released, stimulating milk production. Baby suckling also help further release of prolactin and oxytocin, leading to milk ejection ("let-down reflex").

Colostrum is the "early breast milk" containing protein, fat, secretory IgA and minerals, good for infant's nutrition and protection from infection.

Contraindications to breast-feeding: Active HBV and HCV status, HIV infection, and ingestion of certain medicines (chloramphenicol, tetracycline, warfarin, etc). **Mastitis is not a contraindication**, and both breasts should be empty by breast-feeding.

Cessation of breast milk: Use tight bra and ice pack.

TERATOLOGY

Teratology is the study of abnormalities of physiological development. It is often thought of as the study of human birth defects (Def), but it is much broader than that. A teratogen is any agent that disturbs normal fetal development and affects subsequent function. The nature of the agent and its timing and duration after conception are all critical factors to affect the fetus.

PEARLS—Table 12-13: Maternal Drug Use or Disease and Associated Fetal Effects

Maternal drug or disease / Fetal effects
Alcohol: Fetal alcohol syndrome.
Anesthetics; barbiturates: Respiratory, CNS depression; Vit-K deficiency (Def).
Androgens and derivatives: Female virilization; over-development of male genitals.
ACE-Inh: Fetal renal tubular dysplasia, neonatal renal failure, oligohydramnios, IUGR, and cranial ossification Def.
Carbamazepine: Neural tube Def, fingernail hypoplasia, microcephaly, and IUGR.
Cocaine: Bowel atresia, Def of the heart, face, limbs, and GU tract, microcephaly, IUGR, and cerebral infarctions.
Coumadin derivatives: Nasal hypoplasia, stippled bone epiphyses, IUGR, and eye Def.
Cyanotic heart disease: IUGR.
DES (Diethylstilboestrol): Clear cell adenocarcinoma of the vagina or cervix; genital Def (for both male & female).
Folate antagonists (methotrexate): Increased rate of spontaneous abortion.
Lead: Increased rate of SAB or stillbirths.
Lithium: Heart Def (Ebstein anomaly).
MgSO$_4$: Respiratory depression.
Organic mercury: Cerebral atrophy, microcephaly, intellectual disability, seizures, and blindness.
Sulfonamides: Displaces bilirubin from albumin.
Isotretinoin: Facial or ear Def, and congenital heart disease.
Phenytoin: Dysmorphic facies, IUGR, intellectual disability, heart Def, and nail Def.
Streptomycin and kanamycin: CN-8 (facial nerve) damage and hearing loss.
Tetracycline: Enamel hypoplasia or permanent tooth discoloration.
Thalidomide: Bilateral limb Def, cardiac and GI Def, anotia, and microtia.
Trimethadione and paramethadione: Cleft lip or palate, cardiac Def, microcephaly, and intellectual disability.
Valproic acid: Neural tube Def or craniofacial Def.
Vit-A and derivatives: Increasing SAB rate, thymic agenesis, cardiovascular Def, craniofacial Def, cleft lip or palate, and intellectual disability.
Graves disease: Transient thyrotoxicosis.
Hyperparathyroidism: Hypocalcemia.
Myasthenia gravis: Transient neonatal myasthenia.
ITP: Thrombocytopenia.
SLE: Congenital heart block.

Chapter 12: High-yield Questions (HYQ)

1. A 34 y/o female at 28-week's gestational age (GA) comes to the clinic for low back pain for the past week. She generally feels well except for mild polyuria without dysuria. She denies history of fever, diabetes, hypertension (HTN), and other chronic diseases. Physical examination (P/E) and urine analysis (U/A) results are mostly normal (Nl). 1-hr 50g glucose tolerance test (GTT) returns normal. What's the most appropriate next step?

A. 3-hr 100g GTT   B. 12-hr fasting glucose test   C. Urine culture

D. Empiric cephalosporins for E coli   E. Reassurance

2. The same patient as in Q1 comes for the exams again at 35 weeks of gestation. She has no special symptoms but vaginal swab test for Strep-B is (+). What's the most appropriate next step?

A. Ampicillin for 10 days   B. Ampicillin 30 min before labor

C. Gentamicin 30 min before the labor starts

D. Ampicillin 30 min before and after labor   E. Reassurance

3. A 36 y/o woman at 16 weeks of GA comes for the prenatal exams. A triple screen is done and shows high serum hCG, and low AFP and estriol. The most likely defect is

A. trisomy 21   B. trisomy 18   C. trisomy 13

D. neural tube defect   E. fragile X syndrome

4. A 30 y/o woman at 32 weeks of GA is sent to the ER with headache, nausea, blurred vision, and abdominal pain for 30 min. P/E finds BP is 170/120 mmHg with hyperactive reflexes, and cervical Os is closed. Lab tests show proteinuria of 4.5 g/24hrs, serum creatinine = 2.5 mg/dL, and elevated hepatic enzymes. What's the best next step?

A. IV MgSO4   B. IV MgSO4 + labor induction

C. IV Nitroprusside-Na   D. IV MgSO4 + betamethasone

E. IV Nitroprusside-Na + C-section

5-10: Match the following clinical scenarios with the most like condition.

A. Cord prolapse   B. Head compression   C. Uteroplacental deficit

D. Contraction stress test (CST) (+)   E. CST (-)

F. Oligohydramnios   G. Biophysical profile (BPP) score is 0-2

H. Maternal fever or anemia

5. Prenatal fetal heart rate (FHR) monitoring finds an apparent, gradual decrease in FHR with return to baseline, onset to nadir > 30 sec.

6. In a pregnant female, prenatal monitoring finds baseline FHR = 105 beats per min (bpm), BPP score = 4.

7. In a pregnant female, prenatal monitoring finds baseline FHR = 165 bpm, BPP score = 6.

8. Prenatal monitoring finds a gradual decrease in FHR with return to baseline (onset to nadir > 30 sec), whose onset, nadir, and recovery occur after the start, peak, and end of uterine contraction, respectively.

9. In a pregnant female, prenatal monitoring finds an abrupt decrease in FHR below baseline (onset to nadir < 30 sec), lasting 15 sec to 2 min.

10. In a pregnant female, prenatal monitoring finds baseline FHR = 140 bpm, no late decelerations or significant variable decelerations in 10 min and for > 3 contractions.

11. A 30 y/o female at 32-week's GA comes to the physician and complains of decreased fetal movement. She denies other symptoms. P/E results are normal. What's the most appropriate next step?

A. Vibroacoustic stimulation   B. Nonstress test (NST)   C. CST

D. BPP   E. Labor induction

12. The same patient has no response after both NST and vibroacoustic stimulation, and BPP (by real-time ultrasonography) is done with a score of 5. What's the best next step now?

A. Labor induction   B. IV steroid   C. CST

D. C-section   E. Reassurance

13. A patient at 34-week's GA comes to the physician due to moderate vaginal bleeding without pain. Her bleeding is stopped after proper treatment, and vital signs are stable. Baseline FHR = 140 bpm. She lives very close to the hospital. What's the most appropriate next step?

A. Test of fetal lung maturity   B. IV steroid   C. Forceps-aided delivery

D. C-section   E. Observation at home

14. A patient at 29 weeks of GA comes to the physician for strong uterine contraction for 2 hours. She has a history of heart disease. Pelvic exams show that Os = 5 cm, 80% effaced. BPP scores = 6. What's the best next step?

A. Acceleration of labor with oxytocin   B. Bed rest + steroid

C. MgSO4 + steroid   D. Steroid + ritodrine   E. MgSO4 + cervical culture + steroid

15. A patient at 29-week's GA comes to the physician for severe vaginal bleeding and painful uterine contraction for 30 min. P/E finds her HR = 120 bpm, BP = 88/58 mmHg; FHR is 165 bpm and with repeated late deceleration. Pelvic exams show that Os = 5 cm, 80% effaced. What's the best next step?

A. Acceleration of labor with oxytocin   B. IV fluid + steroid

C. IV fluid + MgSO4 + steroid   D. IV fluid + C-section

E. Blood transfusion + cervical culture + steroid

16. A patient at 34-week's GA comes to the physician and presents regular painful contraction every 2 min with the Os 5 cm. Two hours later, the Os is still 5 cm, and she feels less abdominal pain but tired. Her vital signs are stable and FHR is 125 bpm. What's the best next step?

A. Acceleration of labor with oxytocin   B. IV fluid + steroid

C. Test of fetal lung maturity   D. Vacuum induction   E. C-section

17-23: Match the following clinical scenarios with the most likely diagnosis.

A. Antepartum hemorrhage   B. Inevitable abortion   C. Threatened abortion
D. Uterine rupture   E. Hydatidiform mole   F. Fetal macrosomia
G. Oligohydramnios   H. Polyhydramnios   I. Ectopic pregnancy
J. Multiple gestations   K. Rh isoimmunisation   L. Prolapsed umbilical cord

M. Placenta accrete   N. Symmetric IUGR   O. Asymmetric IUGR
P. Middle pelvic contraction

17. A 35 y/o woman at 30-week's GA comes for a routine exam. Random serum glucose is 150 mg/dl. Ultrasonography reveals duodenal atresia and marginally normal fetal size. She denies a history of diabetes before pregnancy.

18. A 35 y/o woman at 32-week's GA comes to the physician for irregular fetal movements. She denies chronic diseases but admits history of abortion before this pregnancy. FHR monitoring reveals frequent late deceleration. Fetal blood sampling shows "erythroblastosis fetalis".

19. A 35 y/o woman at 30 weeks of GA comes to the physician for regular painful uterine contraction for 3 hours. P/E finds stable maternal vital signs. FHR = 110 bpm. Cervical Os is 4 cm. Ultrasonography reveals bilateral renal agenesis. The physician advises to allow spontaneous vaginal delivery.

20. A 30 y/o female at 26-week's GA comes to the physician for a regular exam. P/E finds her fundal height is lower than expected. She claims she takes methyldopa for hypertension control. Ultrasound is done and reveals that the ratio of head and abdominal circumference (HC/AC) is increased.

21. A 35 y/o woman at 34-week's GA of the 2nd pregnancy is brought to the ER. She has severe vaginal bleeding for 30 min following 4 hours of painful uterine contraction aided with oxytocin use. She has gestational diabetes and is controlled by insulin injection. P/E finds maternal HR = 110 bpm, BP = 90/58 mmHg, and irregular abdomen on palpation. Fetal monitoring is nonreassuring.

22. A 28 y/o woman has moderate vaginal bleeding 40 min after delivery of a normal sized baby. P/E finds a firm uterus without vaginal tears. Her HR = 100 bpm and BP = 90/60 mmHg.

23. A 30 y/o woman at 37-week's GA has regular, progressive uterine contraction for 5 hours with the Os of 5 cm. At 6-hour checkup, the Os is still 5 cm. Maternal and fetal vital signs are stable. Internal pelvic assess reveals prominent ischial spines.

24. A 20 y/o woman is brought to the ER because she fainted at home following abdominal pain. P/E finds HR = 118 bpm, BP = 90/58 mmHg, T = 37°C. Her abdominal is distended with diffusive tenderness, and with mild vaginal bleeding. What's the best next step for Dx?

A. Vaginal ultrasonography   B. Urine beta-hCG test   C. Dilation and curettage (D&C)

D. Laparoscopy   E. Culdocentesis

25. Culdocentesis is performed to the above patient and 100 mL of bright blood is recovered. IV fluid is given to the patient. What's your best next step now?

A. Vaginal ultrasonography   B. Laparotomy   C. D&C

D. Methotrexate   E. Laparoscopy

26. A 30 y/o woman at 38-week's GA comes to the ER for fever, regular painful uterine contraction for 2 hours. She has a history of "STD" before pregnancy. P/E finds HR = 100 bpm, T = 39°C, and BP is normal. There's diffuse tenderness over the uterus. The Os is 5 cm and still in progress. FHR = 160 bpm. What's your best next step?

A. Ampicillin + gentamicin   B. Ampicillin + gentamicin + oxytocin

C. Clindamycin + gentamicin   D. Clindamycin + gentamicin + oxytocin

E. Clindamycin + gentamicin + C-section

Answers and Explanations

1. (E). Explain to the patient that 3rd-trimester low back pain is common and it's due to increased lumbar lordosis and loose ligaments that support pelvic girdle joints, although it's a risk factor for gestational diabetes. Reassurance is proper after the necessary 50g GTT returns normal. "D" is indicated for typical UTI symptoms. Mild polyuria without dysuria is common after 2nd-trimester and does not mean UTI.

2. (D). Asymptomatic vaginal Strep-Group-B (+) during pregnancy is not easy to cure because the Strep-Group-B has resided there long; best treated by I.V. ampicillin 30 min before and after labor to prevent the newborn infection.

3. (A). Only beta-hCG is high in "A". All the 3 tests (AFP, hCG, estriol) are low in "B". AFP is high in "D".

4. (D). Patient is at < 34 weeks of gestation with HELLP syndrome, best treated with IV MgSO4 to decrease BP and prevent seizure, plus steroid to accelerate fetal lung maturity and preparing for labor in 24-48 hours. "B" is the best if the GA is > 34-weeks (with mature fetal lungs). Induction is tried first, and then C-section is chosen if it fails.

5. (B). It's typical early deceleration, common and normal.

6. (A). Fetal bradycardia due to severe hypoxia, or congenital heart defects.

7. (H). Fetal tachycardia due to relative hypoxia.

8. (C). Late deceleration due to uteroplacental insufficiency and fetal hypoxia/stress. If it repeats, delivery!

9. (F). Variable deceleration due to umbilical cord compression (oligohydramnios is #1 cause).

10. (E). CST (-), predictive of good fetal well-being. CST (+): late decelerations associated with > 50% contractions in 10 min; worrisome fetus requiring speedy delivery. BPP score of 0-2: Highly worrisome because of severe fetal hypoxia; prompt delivery regardless of GA.

11. (B). NST should be done first. If it's (-) (no response), it's mostly due to fetal sleep; "A" is followed.

12. (B). The fetus is in worrisome conditions and mother's GA is < 34 weeks, thus you should speed up delivery first by IV steroid, followed by labor induction or C-section in 24-48 hours.

13. (A). This patient is in borderline GA (34 weeks) for a risky C-section delivery (placenta previa), no forceps or vaginal exams is allowed. "A" should be done first. If the lung is mature, hospitalize the patient and prepare for C-section; if immature, give IV steroid, then prepare for C-section. If GA is before 32 weeks, the patient can stay home nearby and wait for the fetal lung maturity (with IM steroid).

14. (E). This fetus is facing premature birth with risk of RDS, neonatal infection, etc. Thus labor should be delayed best by IV MgSO4, steroid, cervical culture, antibiotics, and bed rest. Ritodrine is 2nd-line drug for uterine relaxation, and contraindicated with history of heart disease and diabetes.

15. (D). This patient is in ischemic shock most likely due to placental abruption or placenta previa, and the fetus in severe hypoxia. You can't wait for the Os to open fully or the fetal lung to be mature but an emergent C-section. Other choices are all improper without C-section.

16. (E). It's an active phase rest (#1 cause is cephalopelvic disproportion), and requires a prompt C-section since 34 weeks GA makes the fetus viable (with enough lung maturity). Oxytocin, vacuum, and forceps deliveries are forbidden in this condition.

17. (H). Dx is AFI > 20 cm on ultrasound. Causes include normal pregnancy, fetal chromosomal abnormity, maternal diabetes, multiple gestation, isoimmunisation, cystic lung defects, fetal defects (fistula or atresia). Fetal macrosomia: birth weight > 90th percentile, commonly secondary to gestational diabetes. Treatment: C-section is preferred.

18. (K). It's indicated by the history of abortion, "erythroblastosis fetalis" and late deceleration (due to fetal hypoxia or stress). Diagnosis: Test mother's Rh antibody titers. Treatment: if severe, give intrauterine blood transfusion, IV steroid, and induce preterm labor.

19. (G). Dx: AFI < 5cm on ultrasound. Cause: fetal defects (renal agenesis or pulmonary hypoplasia, making fetus not viable), PROM, uteroplacental defects, etc.

20. (O). 80% of IUGR is asymmetric, associated with chronic maternal diseases (hypertension, diabetes, etc), placental deficiency, etc. Symmetric IUGR accounts for 20% +/-, associated with congenital infections/defects and maternal drug abuse.

21. (D). Uterine rupture is commonly associated with history of classic uterine incision (#1), excessive oxytocin stimulation, grand multiparity, and myomectomy. Surgical exploration of the uterus is both diagnostic and therapeutic (C-section or hysterectomy if no more children are desired).

22. (M). Placenta accreta; Tx is hypogastric artery ligation, then manually removing the placenta.

23. (P). It's an active-phase arrest due to cephalopelvic disproportion. Tx: Low-position C-section delivery.

24. (E). This patient is in ischemic shock most likely due to ruptured tubal pregnancy and hemoperitoneum, which requires immediate Dx and surgery. "E" can supply the fastest method to confirm the internal bleeding from a ruptured tubal pregnancy, but negative result cannot rule it out. hCG can be (-) in 50% cases. Ultrasound and laparoscopy can make more accurate Dx but are slower in this case.

25. (B). Tubal rupture and hemoperitoneum is an obstetric emergency that is best treated with salpingectomy through laparotomy. Laparoscopic surgery is applied if with stable vital signs. Methotrexate is for small, unruptured ectopic pregnancy. Ultrasound is the best means of Dx for unruptured pregnancy. D&C has limited effects.

26. (C). This patient most likely has chorioamnionitis with a mildly stressful fetus in labor. Since she is in normal labor progress and has a history of STD, "clindamycin + gentamycin" is the best Tx here. C-section will be needed if the labor is arrested or conditions of the mother or the fetus are worsened.

Chapter 13

PEDIATRICS

NEWBORN DISEASES

APGAR Scoring

It's defined as 0-2 scores for each of the following 5 indexes:

1. Appearance (color): 2 scores—normal (pink) all over; 0 score—blue all over.

2. Pulse (Heart rate—HR): 2 scores—120-160/min or beats per min (BPM); 0 score—<60 BPM or asystole.

3. Grimace (reflex irritability): 2 scores—sneeze or cough; 0 score—no response.

4. Activity (muscle tone): 2 scores—active movement; 0 score—none.

5. Respiration: 2 scores—RR=40-60 breaths per min and strong; 0 score—absent.

A rapid APGAR scoring helps determine the need for neonatal resuscitation.

1. A score of **8-10 means good** cardiopulmonary adaptation.

2. A score of **4-7 reflects the possible need for resuscitation**. Monitor and stimulate the newborn, with possible ventilation support.

3. A score of **0-3 indicates the need for immediate resuscitation**.

PEARLS—**Important Screening Tests for Newborns**

All infants must be screened for these diseases prior to discharge:

1. **PKU (phenylketonuria)**: Deficiency in the enzyme phenylalanine hydroxylase (PAH) that leads to intellectual disability. Treatment is a special diet low in phenylalanine for at least the first 16 years of life.

2. **Congenital adrenal hyperplasia (CAH)**: It may result in errors in steroidogenesis and sexual development. Treatment is replacement of mineralocorticoids and glucocorticoids and possible genital reconstruction.

3. **Galactosemia**: Enzyme (GALT) deficiencies that can cause feeding problems, failure to thrive, cataracts, and sepsis. Treatment is to cut out all galactose-containing products.

4. **Congenital hypothyroidism**: It can lead to cretinism.

5. Other recommended screening tests: Homocystinuria (mainly causing thromboembolic complications); biotinidase deficiencies (causing developmental delays); beta thalassemia (serious form of anemia).

Birth Injuries

It refers to all avoidable and unavoidable injuries that occur during labor and delivery. Common birth injuries are summarized in Table 13-1 below.

Table 13-1: Summary of Common Birth Injuries

Cephalhematoma - vacuum

A subperiosteal bleed usually limited to the bone and **not crossing suture lines**. A rim can be felt around the edge. It can be associated with an overlying non-depressed skull fracture; may not present at birth with slow bleeding but increase in size over the first few days; mostly resolves spontaneously over months.

Caput succedaneum

A swelling of the scalp involving the presenting part, mostly caused by the pressure exerted on that part during labor and delivery. It usually **crosses suture lines** and resolves over several days without treatment (Tx). Caput is a common cause of jaundice.

Subcutaneous fat necrosis

Usually with a history of a difficult labor and delivery, particularly with forceps or vacuum extraction. Palpable rubbery, firm nodules are on the cheeks, buttocks, back, or extremities. Most of the lesions resolve spontaneously, though occasional Ca-deposits may be left.

Facial palsy

Usually a peripheral, flaccid paralysis secondary to difficult delivery. The affected side does not move when the baby cries.

Clavicular fracture

#1 common bone fracture during delivery, associated with babies large for gestational age and with shoulder dystocia. Physical examination (P/E) shows a fussy baby with an asymmetric Moro reflex and crepitus over the fractured area. A palpable healing callus is usually formed < 1 week without treatment.

Subconjunctival haemorrhage

Temporary lesion resulting from increased pressure during passage through the birth canal; self-limited.

Brachial palsy

It usually occurs in large infants and is secondary to traction on the head during delivery. Prognosis depends on the extent of damage to the nerves. There are two common presentations: (1) **Erb-Duchenne palsy:** Involves C_5-C_6. The arm is adducted and pronated, with wrist flexion and finger flexion ("waiter's tip"). Occasionally C_4 is affected, causing an ipsilateral diaphragmatic paralysis. (2) **Klumpke paralysis:** Involves C_7-T_1. It produces flexion and supination of the elbow, with wrist extension, finger flexion ("claw hand"), and numbness along ulnar nerve distribution. If the T_1 root sympathetic fibers are injured, an ipsilateral Horner syndrome is seen.

Neonatal Skin Diseases

Common newborn skin diseases and lesions are summarized below.

Table 13-2: Common Neonatal Skin Disorders

Erythema Toxicum (Urticaria Neonatorum, Image 96)

An autoimmune rash in newborns, with typical small, red, white or yellow, papules or pustules on an erythematous base; usually appear after the 1st day of life and resolve within 2 weeks. The pustules are benign lesions full of eosinophils if scraped for examination. The infant generally looks well otherwise. **Differentiation: SSSS** (Staph-scalded skin syndrome, **Image 98**) —The infant looks very ill; lesions are full of neutrophils; skin culture reveals Staph-aureus. Others: Pyoderma, candidiasis, etc.

Sebaceous Hyperplasia

Small yellow-white, oily, shiny papules or bumps on the face that can occur in infants and adults. Acne can be one of the symptoms but more often in teenagers.

Milia (Milk Spots)

Small, pearly white, keratin-filled inclusion cysts on the skin or mucous membrane; in the mouth, they are called "**Epstein Pearls.**" They often disappear within 2-4 weeks but need **to be differentiated from STD and whiteheads (in adults)**.

Cutis Marmorata

It's a vasomotor response to cold stress, with the skin appearing a lacy pattern similar to cobblestones. A persistent form is seen in trisomy 21, trisomy 18, and cutis marmorata telangiectasia congenita.

Neonatal Acne

It can be open and closed comedones, possibly caused by an increased level of androgen. Self-limited and no treatment is needed.

Table 13-3: Common Birthmarks

Congenital Dermal Melanocytosis (Image 118)

Also known as "Mongolian blue spot", it is a benign, flat, gray-blue, **congenital birthmark** with wavy borders and irregular shape, more common in dark-skinned races; usually over the presacral area or near the buttocks at birth and **disappearing in the first few years of life**. It is secondary to melanocytes in the dermal layer. It can be confused with a child abuse bruise, which usually fades into the surrounding skin with different colors and carries other evidence.

Salmon Patch *aka nevus simplex, macular stain, stork bite, angel kiss*

present @ birth

A vascular, *blanching*, salmon-colored, flat lesion commonly seen over the eyelids, glabella, and the nuchal area. It usually **disappears with time**, except for those in the nuchal area (may persist). **Differential diagnosis: Port wine stains**—usually unilateral and permanent.

nevus flammeus - sturge weber (encephalo trigeminal angiomatosis)
- capillary malformation that appears as blanchable erythematous patch. present from birth & don't regress

Common birthmarks

> ### Capillary (strawberry) hemangiomas (Image 119)
> *Benign capillary tumor formed from aban proliferating endothelial cells*
> It starts as bright red, strawberry-like, macular lesion(s) in the first few months and quickly grows in the first *nodule, or plaque* year of life, then **regressing spontaneously** without treatment. *Rapid growth first year of life, spontaneous regression.*
> *Tx: propranolol*
>
> ### Nevus sebaceous (Image 120)
>
> Yellow-orange, hairless plaques located on the scalp resembling flat warts. Because of the **malignant potential**, they are usually removed by adolescence.
>
> ### Cafe-au-lait spots (Image 57)
>
> Superficial, light-brown, flat birthmarks with sharply demarcated borders and various shapes. It can occur on any part of the skin **in normal persons, or with neurofibromatosis type 1**, etc.

Conj bilirubin
- *H2O soluble*
- *urine excr*
- *urine dark*
- *Ø cross BBB*
- *Ø kernicterus*

Neonatal Jaundice — *FA52 p.400*

see one notes & FA52 400

RF: prematurity, ↓birth wt, FM Hx, fetal-maternal blood group incompatibility, birth trauma

It occurs when indirect (unconjugated) bilirubin is increased and deposited in the skin. Indirect bilirubin can also deposit in CNS and cause neurotoxic symptoms. Newborn jaundice is divided into physiologic or pathologic. **Physiologic jaundice is usually seen after the first 24 hours of life and < 13 mg/dL, and is unconjugated and resolves by 1 week of age. Beyond these conditions are mostly pathologic.** *Pathologic = during 1st day of life*

uncon bilirubin
- *fat soluble*
- *Ø excreted urine*
- *Ø urine dark*
- *crosses BBB*
- *kernicterus*

Etiology

↑ hemolysis of fetal Hb + immature hepatic bilirubin metab = physiologic jaundice. day 3-8   ↑ uncons.

Hemoglobin (Hb) is the major source of bilirubin, thus increased hemolysis and RBC mass, decreased RBC survival, and defective Hb metabolism can all cause hyperbilirubinemia.

Essentials of diagnosis

1. Pathologic jaundice usually appears in the first day of life, from the face down over the body as the level rises above 13 mg/dL. *Cons or uncons.*

2. Breast milk jaundice usually presents at one week of age and resolves faster with a pause of the breast milk.

3. Infants with increased direct (conjugated) bilirubin and clay-colored, acholic stools should be suspected of having biliary atresia, although direct bilirubin is not neurotoxic. Increased indirect bilirubin can cause neurotoxicity and kernicterus. *→ p. 510, Pathoma 116*

4. Hb level, blood typing (mother-newborn ABO or Rh type), and Coombs test help diagnosis of hemolysis, polycythemia, etc. WBC count helps diagnosis of sepsis.

Treatment
Must tx uncons hyperbilirubinemia → cons (when bilirubin is high) Exchange (r/y high)

1. Phototherapy is usually started when bilirubin > 20 mg/dL. It causes isomerization of indirect bilirubin to a form that is more easily excreted.

2. Exchange blood transfusion can effectively remove bilirubin and circulating auto-antibodies, and restore Hb.

uncons: hemolysis, hemorrhage

mixed: crigler najjar, Gilbert, Dubin Johnson, Rotors, Hepatitis

cons: atresia, sepsis

Neonatal Sepsis

It's is a severe bacterial infection in the blood and serious systemic response to it. In newborns, it can be "early sepsis" occurring in the 1st week of life, or "late sepsis" occurring between 10-28 days.

Etiology

The most common causes are **pneumonia and meningitis. The most common pathogens are Group-B Strep, E. coli, Staph-aureus, and Listeria.** HSV and enteroviruses can also cause it. **Risk factors** include maternal infection during pregnancy (UTI or chorioamnionitis), prematurity, and prolonged rupture of membranes.

Essentials of diagnosis

1. Nonspecific manifestations of tachypnea, apnea, cyanosis, bradycardia, poor feeding, irritability, tremors, or seizures. Newborns usually have hypothermia rather than fever.

2. In severe cases, **DIC and purpura fulminans (Image 34)** may occur. With neonatal meningitis, full fontanelle is common but not nuchal stiffness.

3. **Lab tests**: The best tests are complete blood count (CBC), **pathogen cultures of the blood, CSF, urine, and drainage, along with CXR (to rule out pneumonia).**

Differential diagnosis

Neonatal respiratory distress syndrome and pneumonia (very similar); congenital heart disease or infection, metabolic disease, and neurologic disease.

Treatment

1. Supportive care is important: Fluids, electrolyte, and hemodynamic stability.

2. The best initial therapies while waiting for cultures are **empirical antibiotics—ampicillin plus gentamicin or a third-generation cephalosporin or vancomycin.** Treatment is adjusted according to results from culture and sensitivity testing.

Complications

Seizures, hearing loss, developmental delay, cerebral palsy, and hydrocephalus.

Neonatal Seizures

Neonatal seizures present with different features from those in adults and children due to the immaturity of the nervous system (NS).

Etiology

1. **Hypoxic-ischemic** encephalopathy is the #1 cause; usually present < 12-24 hours after birth.

2. Intraventricular hemorrhage is more common in preterm infants, usually at 1-3 days of life, presenting with a bulging fontanelle or bloody CSF on LP (lumbar puncture).

3. Other causes: Infections, fever, or metabolic disorders (hypoglycemia and hypo-Ca).

Neonatal Seizures

Essentials of diagnosis

1. **Focal seizures:** Rhythmic twitching, especially of the face and extremities; associated with structural lesions, infections, and subarachnoid hemorrhage (SAH).

2. **Multifocal clonic:** Tonic-rigid posturing or myoclonic jerks of the extremities, fixed deviation of the eyes, tongue thrusting, apnea, staring, blinking, etc.

3. **Lab tests:** EEG, CBC, and serum electrolytes should be done and may be normal. LP helps if meningitis, encephalitis, or bleeding is suspected. If it's complicated, newborn screening for metabolism, blood culture, and CT scan may be considered. Generally, diagnosis of neonatal seizures is difficult.

Treatment

Treat underlying cause together with initial antiseizure drug phenobarbital.

Neonatal Hypoglycemia   See peds P.6

It refers to normal low neonatal blood glucose levels—normally occur in the first hours after birth and may persist for several days. It can fluctuate from 40 mg/dL to 80 mg/dL (4.4 mmol/L).

Causes of pathologic hypoglycaemia include inadequate glucose supply or glycogen stores, impaired glucose production, increased glucose utilization, excessive insulin secretion, etc.

Essentials of diagnosis

1. Plasma glucose levels should be measured in infants at risk for hypoglycemia (E.g., preterm infants, infants who are large or small for gestational age, infants with perinatal stress or of mothers with diabetes or related medications) and in infants with signs or symptoms consistent with hypoglycaemia.

2. **Diagnosis**: Hypoglycemic infants are frequently asymptomatic and are usually detected by screening of at-risk infants. In symptomatic neonates (plasma glucose levels < 50-60 mg/dL), the findings are nonspecific and include tremors, hypotonia, changes in level of consciousness, apnea, bradycardia, cyanosis, tachypnea, poor suck or feeding, hypothermia, and/or seizures. Diagnosis is confirmed by **plasma glucose testing.**

Treatment

1. For at-risk neonates, the goal is to maintain plasma glucose levels > 50 mg/dL in the first 48 hours of life, and > 60 mg/dL after 48 hours of life.

2. In neonates with a suspected or confirmed genetic hypoglycemia disorder, the goal is to maintain glucose concentrations > 70 mg/dL (3.9 mmol/L).

Method: Symptomatic—IV glucose; asymptomatic—oral glucose.

Newborns of Diabetic Mothers

Diabetes in pregnancy is associated with an increased risk of fetal, neonatal, and long-term complications in the offspring. The outcome is generally related to the onset and duration of glucose intolerance during pregnancy and severity of the mother's diabetes.

Maternal Hypoglycemia [handwritten]

Essentials of diagnosis

1. Maternal hyperglycemia causes **fetal hyperglycemia** (leading to **fetal hyperinsulinemia**), a **large fetus/newborn**, birth trauma, and **post-birth hypoglycemia** (tremors, jitters, excitability).

2. Other associated presentations: Hypo-Ca, hypo-Mg, hypertrophic cardiomyopathy, hyperbilirubinemia, polycythemia, respiratory distress syndrome (due to surfactant inhibition by insulin), and **congenital anomalies** (cardiac defects, lumbosacral agenesis, and small left colon).

Treatment

1. Start treatment in utero by controlling the mother's blood glucose in normal ranges and close follow-up.

2. After birth, monitor infant's blood glucose closely and treat the hypoglycemia aggressively.

Complications

Infants have higher risks of developing subsequent obesity and diabetes (DM).

Acute Respiratory Distress Syndrome (ARDS) *FA51 p 607* [handwritten]

Neonatal ARDS is mostly caused by **surfactant deficiency** in preterm babies. The surfactant deficiency leads to increased surface tension and collapse in the alveoli, resulting in atelectasis and ventilation-perfusion ratio mismatch.

Essentials of diagnosis

1. Soon after birth, the preterm baby shows signs of respiratory distress: tachypnea, dyspnea, cyanosis, or apnea. The baby's conditions are worst on the 2nd or 3rd day, improved with a spontaneous diuresis.

2. **Diagnosis** is clinical and supported by **CXR** showing a reticular pattern and hazy, **ground-glass** appearance.

Differential diagnosis

Sepsis (especially from Group-B Strep).

Treatment

1. **Prevention is the most importance treatment: Glucocorticoteroids** adminstered to the mother 48 hours before delivery is helpful with decreased incidence.

2. Exogenous surfactant supply greatly reduces mortality from ARDS. Mechanical ventilation and good supportive care are all important treatment.

Complications [handwritten: And NEC]

Pneumothorax, mucous plugging, sepsis, intraventricular hemorrhage, pulmonary interstitial emphysema, chronic lung disease, and patent ductus arteriosus.

[Handwritten marginalia:]

IVH - FA51 P. 470, 581
pt: premie, as x screen, L>shunts, death
- ↑ICP. Bulging fontanelle, siezure, coma, lethargy
- Dx: Cranial doppler
- Tx: ↓ICP

Broncho pulm dysplasia: chronic lung dz in premature infants exposed to prolonged mech vent & O₂ tx, (causing barotrauma, O₂-tox, & inflammm) for NRDS.
- ↓ surfactant, Alveoli derecruitment.
- scarring → fibrosis
pt: ↑ O₂ demand ⇒ ↑ FiO₂, Lung protective strategy
Dx: CXR ⇒ ground glass opacities
F/u: lung dz
Tx: surfactant, antenatal steroids post-natal

Retinopathy of Prematurity: Neonatal Resp distress Sx ⇒ conc O₂ tx ⇒ Retinal neovascularization ⇒ blindness (ROS) pt: worsened by ↑ FiO₂ reqs.
Dx: eye exam, visualize blood vessels. Asx screen,
Tx: photo ablation. F/u early glaucoma.

diffuse parench → 28 weeks

Meconium Aspiration Syndrome

Meconium aspiration syndrome (MAS) is defined as respiratory distress in newborn infants born through meconium-stained amniotic fluid whose symptoms cannot be otherwise explained. MAS can present with varieties of severity from mild respiratory distress to life-threatening respiratory failure.

Clinical features and diagnosis *most common in post premature neonates.*

It occurs when meconium is aspirated after delivery. The baby mostly presents with respiratory distress—tachypnea and hypoxia. CXR shows patchy infiltrates. *Meconium plugging of airways traps distal gas, promoting alveolar overdistension & rupture = pneumo thorax*

Complications

Pneumothorax, pneumomediastinum, and primary pulmonary hypertension of the newborn.

Treatment

Mechanical ventilation, inhaled nitric oxide (alleviating meconium injury), and supplemental oxygen or extracorporeal membrane oxygenation (ECMO).

Persistent Fetal Circulation

(PFC; Primary Pulmonary Hypertension of the Newborn—PPHN)

It is a condition caused by a failure in the systemic circulation and pulmonary circulation to convert from the antenatal circulation pattern (high pulmonary vascular resistance) to the "normal" pattern.

Clinical features and diagnosis

It occurs when severe hypoxemia causes pulmonary vasoconstriction, leading to right-to-left shunting through a patent ductus arteriosus or a patent foramen ovale. Echocardiogram usually shows increased pulmonary artery pressures and shunting.

Treatment

1. Hyperventilation to avoid acidosis.

2. Treat pulmonary hypertension: Maintaining optimal oxygenation to decrease pulmonary vasoconstriction. Pulmonary vasodilators (nitric oxide, etc.) and ECMO can be helpful.

Necrotizing Enterocolitis

Path: dead gut
pt: premie, has either RDR, NRDS, or IVH, & then bloody bowel movement
Dx: Air in intestine wall = pneumatosis intestinalis

NEC is a devastating disease that affects mostly the intestine of premature infants. The wall of the intestine is **invaded by bacteria**, which cause local infection and inflammation that can ultimately destroy the wall of the intestine. *due to impaired bowel perfusion & defective immunity*

Essentials of diagnosis

1. It's the most common surgical GI emergency in the newborn, mostly in the preterm. GI-related symptoms usually occur in the first 2 weeks of life: bloody stools, dyspnea, lethargy, and abdominal distension.

Necrotizing Enterocolitis *air in bowel wall, portal venas air.*

2. **Pneumatises intestinalis** found on plain abdominal X-ray films is the pathologic mark.

Treatment

NPO   *IV Abx*   *TPN*
1. Feed cessation, gut decompression, systemic antibiotics, and supportive care.

2. Surgical resection of necrotic bowel may be necessary if severe.

Sudden Infant Death Syndrome (SIDS)

Definition and Etiology

It's an unexplained death of an infant < 1 y/a. It's the #1 cause of death in infants < 1 y/a. The peak incidence occurs at 2-3 mo of age, between midnight and dawn, and in the winter. There is no clear etiology found for SIDS, because many factors in respiratory-cardiovascular systems may lead to SIDS. **Risk factors** include **prone sleep positions**, air bed, preterm birth, inadequate prenatal care, maternal smoking or drug abuse during pregnancy, lower socioeconomic status, life stress, SIDS history among siblings, etc.

Essentials of diagnosis

1. All cases are < 1 y/a, and the death is unexplainable either by history or by post-mortem examination. Presently there is no diagnostic means to determine the risk for SIDS.

2. On autopsy, mild pulmonary edema, diffuse intrathoracic petechiae and tissue markers of chronic asphyxia may be found.

Treatment

→ flatten occiput, turn head to one side, ant to the other side the next night
back to sleep w2 it can't roll.

Prevention and adjust sleep position are important. Latest data suggest that using air mattresses or air beds for infant sleep increases the risk of SIDS and thus should be avoided.

– don't share a bed.   *Don't: EKG SpO2,*
– smoking cessation.   *EEG,*

DEVELOPMENT AND RELATED PROBLEMS

Definition: Development reflects changes in and acquisition of new functions. It includes neuromotor, cognition, and psychosocial development.

Important Developmental Milestones in Children

Apparent Life-Threat Event (ALTE):
– change in color, tone, breathing – parent or caregiver
– answer in hx most of the time, 50% = nothing
– GERD, LRI, seizure – MC → abn eye movements / limb jerks
– sepsis, CV disease, abuse – next up injuries
– FTT, difficult eating, nv nm

Brief Resolved Unexplained Event (BRUE):
1st time ≤ 1yo + <1 min duration
DC PR
∅ Hx – Δ in color, tone, breathing, responsiveness
∅ PE ® Low risk   High risk
*   – monitor + investigate*
497 term – don't tx
*   60 days*
Age premie – reassurance
*   ≥32 weeks*
*   GA,*
*   ≥35 days PC*

Table 13-4: Important Developmental Milestones

Age, motor, language, cognitive/social
2 m: Lifts head/chest while prone, tracks past midline; attends to sound, coos; social smile; recognizes parents.
4-5 m: Moves head, rolls; grasp objects and brings to mouth, sits with aid; orients to voice, making consonant sounds; laughs out, looks around.
6-7 m: Sits without aid, rolls over; babbles, repeats vowels, transfer objects; stranger anxiety. _6 = babbles_
9-10 m: Crawls, pulls to stand; says non-specific "mama/dada"; waves bye-bye. _respond to name_
12 m: Stands and walks alone, uses mature pincer grasp; says specific "mama/dada", understands 1-2 word; imitates actions, plays ball. _Separation anxiety_
15 m: Walks backward, uses a bowl/cup; uses > 4 words; temper tantrums.
2 y: Runs well, jumps, walks up/down steps with help, makes 4-cube tower, takes off clothes; uses 2-word phrases; follows 2-step orders. _stranger/ Sep. anxiety resolves._
3 y: Rides tricycle, copies a circle; uses > 3-word sentences; washes hands with help.
4 y: Hops, throws a ball, copies a square; tells a story, knows numbers; group playing, toileting alone.
5 y: Skips, copies a triangle, uses > 5-word sentences; role and dress-up playing. _Skip_

6m–12m, object permanence

Top Three Reasons for Infant Deaths

1. Birth defects;
2. Sudden infant death syndrome (SIDS);
3. Low birth weight (<1,500g) and ARDS.

The Black population has the highest rates of infant mortality, mostly from low birth weight and infections.

Sociologic Risk Factors for Children

Maternal immaturity (< 19 y/a) and poverty are major risk factors for premature birth and other unfavorable outcomes. The single-parent family is also associated with higher rates of child abuse, truancy, delinquency, and suicide.

Failure to Thrive

It's also known as **weight faltering**, defined as failure or deceleration of gaining weight in a child.
Etiology

FTT

It can result from malnutrition (starvation, deprivation, abuse), malabsorption (infection, celiac disease, cystic fibrosis, enzyme deficiency), allergy, immunodeficiency, and chronic diseases.

Essentials of diagnosis

1. **Growth charts** are the best standard: In infants, birth weight is doubled by 4-5 months and tripled by 1 year.

2. Patients show little subcutaneous fat, muscle wasting, poor tone, rashes, and weak cry, and may need to be hospitalized for records of caloric intake and weight, and need tests of CBC, urinalysis, liver function, serum protein, and sweat chloride.

Treatment: Target underlying cause.

Beckwith-Wiedemann Syndrome

It is a **sporadic pediatric overgrowth disorder** usually present at birth, characterized by variable **omphalocele (exomphalos), macroglossia, and macrosomia (gigantism)**, and an increased risk of childhood cancer, certain congenital features, and mortality.

Treatment

1. Assessment for airway and feeding sufficiency in the presence of macroglossia.

2. Assessment of neonates for hypoglycemia and alpha fetoprotein (AFP) for hepatoblastoma.

3. Abdominal ultrasound examination to assess for organomegaly, structural abnormality, and tumors.

4. Comprehensive cardiac evaluation including electrocardiogram (ECG) and echocardiogram prior to any surgical procedures or for a suspected cardiac abnormality.

Child Abuse

① SXS, intentional active harm. doing bad

① SXS, passive, not doing good

Child abuse is defined as any physical, sexual, or emotional abuse, including **battery or neglect (most common), tissue damage, sexual exploitation, and/or mental cruelty**. It should be suspected when the history is inconsistent with P/E results or the needed medical care is delayed.

Essentials of diagnosis

1. An abused infant may present with feeding intolerance, apnea, seizures, excessive irritability or somnolence, or failure to thrive. *absence of crying in presence of caretaker. Running from caretaker. Comfort from healthcare provider.* *injury*

2. An abused child may present with poor hygiene or abnormal behavior (social withdrawal, etc.).

3. **Typical P/E results (Image 121):** *bruises in diff stages of healing, location on body & development level* *strange*

(1) Genital bleeding, swelling, or discharge. *Anal, vaginal, penis trauma*

(2) Injuries in atypical places (the face, thighs), or unusual types (cigarette burn, belt marks).

(3) Posterior rib fractures; spiral fractures of long bones (humerus or femur); usually < age 3. *also skull*

(4) Epiphyseal/metaphyseal injuries in infants (resulted from limb pulling or twisting).

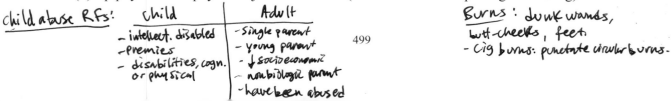

child abuse RFs:

child	Adult
- intellect. disabled	- single parent
- premies	- young parent
- disabilities, cogn. or physical	- ↓ socioeconomic
	- nonbiologic parent
	- have been abused

Burns: dunk wands, butt-cheeks, feet
- cig burns: punctate circular burns.

Child Abuse

any STD

4. Lab tests for suspected sexual abuse: Testing for Gonorrhea, Chlamydia, syphilis, or HIV.

Differential diagnosis

First rule out mimic conditions: Mongolian spots, osteogenesis imperfecta with fractures, bleeding disease, "coining treatment", etc.

Shaken baby syndrome (SBS): It's multiple traumatic injuries including the brain, eyes, neck, spinal cord, and bones caused by violent shaking. **It's a serious form of child abuse ("abusive head trauma").** Bone fractures (ribs), retinal bleeding (by an ophthalmologic examination), or/and subdural hematomas (by a CT scan) may be found.

Treatment

and to abusive family.
explain why you're doing what you're doing. express that it's for pt safety.

1. Document injuries and report to child protective services or authorities immediately for evaluation and child protection. **It's a mandatory reportable offense up to age 18.** Failure to do so is a criminal offense.

2. Hospitalize the child if necessary to treat and protect the child. *or child treatment unit*
last resort, if no safe alternative.
cope: help parent cope, id stressor. Abuse may be alleviated.
from common abuser.

Adolescence

It is the transitional stage of physical and psychological development generally occurring during the period from puberty to legal adulthood (approximately from **11 to 21 y/a**). During this period the adolescent experiences many changes—completing puberty and somatic growth; developing socially, emotionally, and cognitively; moving from concrete to abstract thinking; establishing an independent identity; preparing for an occupation. **Adolescence includes puberty**, but does not correspond with it.

Risk factors

The adolescent is at more risk for mortality and morbidity of **accidents** (#1 is from motor vehicles), **suicide** (girls have more attempts and boys have more success), **homicide**, and **cancers** ("BBC" cancers **for the adolescent—blood, bone, CNS**).

Adolescent Sexual Behavior and Pregnancy

In the US, adolescents reach puberty and sexual maturity at earlier ages than ever. Approximately 50% of high schoolers report having had sexual intercourse, and one-third report being currently sexually active. Prevalence of sexual activity increases with age, 80% of boys and 70% of girls have sexual activities by the end of the twelfth grade.

Adolescent pregnancy: Approximately one million adolescent girls each year and 20% of teenage girls with sexual intercourse become pregnant in the US. Most of these pregnancies are unwanted or unintended. About 50% of the pregnant girls had the child; for the other 50%, 1/3 had man-made abortions and 2/3 had spontaneous abortions. More than 50% of adolescents did not use birth controls during the first sexual intercourse and 31% of them believed they could not get pregnant at the time of intercourse. Adolescents with mental health symptoms or major mental illness (e.g., major depression, bipolar disorder, psychotic disorders) appear to be at increased risk of pregnancy.

Consequences

1. Increased **risk of STD** (sexually transmitted disease) and marriage problems: About 20% teenagers with sex will catch an STD.

2. **For the teenage mother**: Usually with school dropout; many never work and then become welfare dependent.

3. **For the child**: Commonly with neonatal deaths and prematurity; lower level of education and intelligence; increased risk of delinquency and suicide in future.

Table 13-5: Puberty and Tanner Stages

Tanner Stage	Male	Female
1 (Prepuberty)	Basal growth in height; no genital enlargement or pubic hair.	Basal growth in height; no genital enlargement or pubic hair.
2	Basal growth in height; minimal pubic	Accelerated growth; minimal pubic hair on labia;
3	Accelerated growth; moderate pubic hair; enlarged testes and penis; gynecomastia.	Peak growing period; breast and areola enlarge; pubic hair crosses mons pubis; axillary hair appears.
4	Peak growing period; pubic hair widens; penis and testis enlarge further; axillary hair appears; voice changes.	Slower growth rate; areola form 2nd mound; pubic hair coarsens and widens.
5	No further growth in height; mature genital size; adult pubic hair distribution; with facial hair.	No further growth in height; adult breast contour with recession of 2nd areola mound; adult pubic hair quality and distribution.

NUTRITION AND RELATED DISEASES

At birth: All newborns should receive **Vit-K** to prevent hemorrhagic disease because Vit-K is inadequate in breast milk.

At 6 months: Solids, iron, and fluoride are added to breast-feeding for most infants. Vit-D is needed if the infant has limited sun exposure or mother has limited intake.

Table 13-6: Nutritional Comparison of Different Types of Feedings

Breast feeding
1. Preferred food for full-term babies. Advantages: right temperature, concentration and mother-baby bonding; 2. With protective IgA, lactoglobulin, and macrophages against infections and allergic disease. 3. Feeding mothers return to pre-pregnancy weight and uterine status faster. **Contraindications:** 1. Active/untreated TB, syphilis, HIV, galactosemia, varicella, and breast herpes. 2. Taking drugs: anti-cancer and radioactive drugs, ergot alkaloids, iodides, lithium, chloramphenicol, smoking, and alcohol. 3. Relative contraindications: atropine, neuroleptics, sedatives, metronidazole, tetracycline, sulfonamides, and steroids. 4. **Mastitis is not** a contraindication to nursing, and frequent nursing on the affected side helps prevent engorgement.

Formula feeding
Most commercial formulas are cow's milk-based and modified to approximate breast milk, containing 20 calories per ounce.
Whole Cow's Milk
1. Good for baby cows and > 1 y/o human baby. 2. It has a higher protein level but also higher renal solute load and harm. 3. Also with potentials for protein intolerance and iron deficiency anemia.
Adjusted Cow's Milk
Same water:solids ratio, 20 calories/ounce, 3.3% (whey/casein), 4.5% lactose, 3-4% fat, low in iron, copper, Vit-C, and Vit-D; contains harmless bacteria, same digestibility as mother's milk after 45 days.

Protein Malnutrition (Kwashiorkor)

It's the result of a severe protein deficiency and inadequate caloric intake.

Essentials of diagnosis

1. Early symptoms: Lethargy, apathy, or irritability. Late: Lost muscle mass and tone, edema, dermatitis, sparse hair, and secondary infections.

2. **Lab tests**: Decreased albumin, glucose, Hb, vitamins (Vit), and minerals in the blood.

Treatment

Gradually increase feeding of dilute milk or protein added with Vit and minerals.

Complications

Permanent mental and physical retardation may occur. Mortality can be up to 30-40% even with appropriately treatment.

Vitamin Deficiencies

See "Chapter 5: Endocrine, Nutritional and Metabolic Diseases."

Pediatric Diarrhea

(Details in "Chapter 1: INFECTIOUS DISEASES").

Pediatric diarrhea is an important cause of malnutrition.

Common causes

1. **Acute:** Gastroenteritis, food poisoning, systemic infection, or antibiotic use.

2. **Chronic:** Lactase deficiency, indigestion, celiac disease, cystic fibrosis; older children: irritable bowel syndrome (IBS), IBD (inflammatory bowel disease), Giardiasis, or laxative abuse.

3. **In infectious diarrhea: Viruses**: the most common—**#1** is **rotavirus** (especially in winter), then adenovirus, Norwalk virus; **bacteria:** E. coli, Campylobacter, Salmonella, Shigella, Yersinia, and Clostridium; **parasites** (usually with immunodeficiency): Entamoeba, Giardia, and Cryptosporidium.

Treatment

Treat underlying cause.

PEDIATRIC IMMUNIZATIONS

Definitions and immunization rules

See "Chapter 17: Preventive Medicine" for details.

PEARLS—**Table 13-7: Important Immunization Schedules for All (USA)**

Vaccine \ Schedule
HAV: 2-dose series between 12-23 months (mo).
HBV: At birth, 1-2 mo, 6-18 mo; total 3 doses.
DTaP: 2 mo, 4 mo, 6 mo, 15-18 mo, 4-6 y/a; total 5 doses; Td per 10 yrs.
IPV: 2 mo, 4 mo, 6-18 mo, 4-6 y/a; total 4 doses.
Rotavirus: 2 mo, 4 mo; total 2 doses.
Hib: 2 mo, 4 mo, (6 mo), 12-15 mo; total 3-4 doses.
MMR: 12-15 mo, 4-6 y/a; total 2 doses.
Varicella: 12-15 mo, 4-6 y/a; add shingles vaccine at 60 y/a.
HPV: 2 doses with 6 mo gap under 15 y/a; 3 doses over 24 weeks above 15 y/a.
Influenza (IIV): Starting at 6 mo, annually.
PCV: 2 mo, 4 mo, 6 mo, 12-15 mo; add PPSV at 65 y/a or older.
MCV: 1st at 11-12 yrs; booster at 16 y/a.

PEDIATRIC INFECTIONS

CONGENITAL INFECTIONS

TORCH Infections

It refers to **T**oxoplasmosis, **O**ther (Syphilis), **R**ubella, **C**MV, and **H**SV (Herpes simplex v) infections.

Table 13-8: Summary of Congenital Infections

Infection / Clinical features, diagnosis, and treatment
CMV
1. **#1 common,** transmitted in #1-2 trimesters. 2. Intrauterine growth retardation, prematurity, petechiae, jaundice, hepatosplenomegaly, hearing loss, chorioretinitis, microcephaly, and periventricular calcification. **Dx:** Confirmed by virus culture or PCR. **Tx: Ganciclovir. Prognosis** is poor.
Varicella
1. Congenital varicella is associated with infection in #1-2 trimesters: Limb hypoplasia, cataracts, microcephaly, chorioretinitis, cutaneous scars, and cortical atrophy. 2. Neonatal or perinatal: < 1 week after birth; all neonatal varicella is **treated with valacyclovir or acyclovir plus VZIG** (Varicella-Zoster IG).
Rubella (German measles)   *Cephalo caudal spread of maculopapulo rash. Posterior auricular LAD*
1. It occurs in 80% of babies if the mother is infected in the 1st trimester. 2. **Intrauterine growth retardation (#1)**, mental retardation, cataracts, microcephaly, heart defects (patent ductus arteriosus, pulmonary artery stenosis, etc.), hepatosplenomegaly, deafness, and "blueberry muffin." **Dx:** Confirmed by virus culture or IgM titers. **Tx:** Symptomatic. **Prevention is the most important** management--immunization is effective. *ages 1 & 4*
Herpes simplex (Image 29-30)
Usually acquired from passage through an infected birth canal. Primary infection in the mother has a high rate of transmission to baby due to lack of maternal Ab in the baby, whereas recurrent maternal or 3rd-party infection has a low incidence. Features: 1. Local lesions (5-15 days)--**red, painful vesicles with ulcers (Type 1 in the mouth/facial area; Type 2 in the anogenital area)**; 2. Disseminated diseases--pneumonia, shock, and hepatitis at 5-7 days, with high risk of mortality; 3. CNS--lethargy, seizures at 3-4 weeks. 4. **Dx:** Clinical features, virus culture, PCR in CSF, and antibody titters. **Tx: Acyclovir or valacyclovir. Prevention:** Delivery by C-section greatly lowers infections if mother has active genital HSV infection.
Syphilis (Images 24-26)
1. Transmittable to the fetus at any stage of pregnancy, with 40% fetal or perinatal death. 2. Early stage (usually < 2 y/a): fever, anemia, snuffles, failure to thrive, a maculopapular rash, hepatosplenomegaly, periostitis of the long bones, and thrombocytopenia. 3. Late-stage: skeletal abnormalities including saber shin, Hutchinson teeth, rhagades, saddle nose, and Clutton's joints (knee synovitis). 3. **Lab:** VDRL and RPR are sensitive but non-specific screening tests. FTA-ABS is the specific, confirmatory test. **Tx:** Large-dose penicillin.
Toxoplasmosis
Presentations: Chorioretinitis, hydrocephalus, and multiple ring-enhancing lesions [*intracranial calcifications*] on CT caused by Toxoplasma gondii. **Dx:** The best initial test is IgM to Toxoplasma (increased); most accurate test is PCR for toxoplasmosis. **Tx:** Pyrimethamine plus sulfadiazine and folinic acid (leucovorin).

Forchheimer spots

VIRAL INFECTIONS IN CHILDREN

PEARLS—Table 13-9: Important Viral Infections in Children

Infection / Clinical features, diagnosis, and treatment
Erythema Infectiosum ("The 5th Disease", Image 122)
1. **Cause: Parvovirus B₁₉.** 2. Usually no prodrome or fever. 3. **Rash: "Slapped face"**, erythematous, pruritic, maculopapular; spreads from the arms to the trunk and legs. It worsens with fever and sun exposure. _aplastic crises_ **Tx:** Supportive, IVIG, +/- blood transfusion for anemia. **Complication:** Arthritis, hemolytic anemia, or encephalopathy. Congenital B₁₉ infection can cause fetal hydrops and death. _Dx clx_ _isolated mom_
Measles (Image 123) _simultaneous fever + rash.   Shouldn't get bc MMRV_
1. **Cause:** Paramyxovirus. 2. Prodrome: Low fever with **"3Cs"** _4 c's_—cough, coryza, and conjunctivitis. **Koplik's spots** (small, irregular red/grey spots) on the buccal mucosa after 1-2 days. 3. **Rash:** Erythematous, maculopapular spots spreading from the head/neck down to the feet. **Tx:** Supportive care for symptoms and complications. **Complication:** Pneumonia, otitis media, or laryngotracheitis. **Prevention:** Immunization is effective.
Mumps _parotitis, orchitis.   MMRV._
1. **Cause:** Mumps virus (a Paramyxovirus); incubation period 14-24 days, transmitted by airborne droplets, direct contact, and saliva-fomites. Outbreaks are related to lack of immunization. 2. Prodrome: Fever, headache, muscle pain, and malaise, followed by pain and swelling in the **parotid**, unilateral or bilateral. 3. **Lab: Elevated serum amylase, Anti-mumps IgM and IgG (+)**; virus can be isolated in the saliva, urine, CSF, blood, etc. **Tx:** Supportive and NSAIDs. It's preventable by immunization. **Complication:** Orchitis is #1 (postpuberty); meningoencephalomyelitis, arthritis, and mild pancreatitis are also common.
Rubella (Image 124) _simultaneous fever + rash.   MMRV   Adults get same + arthralgias/arthritis_
1. **Cause:** Rubella virus. 2. Also known as **"3-day measles"** _"german"_; prodrome: asymptomatic or low fever with generalized tender lymphadenopathy. 3. **Rash:** Erythematous, maculopapular, tender spots starting on the face and spreading distally. **Tx:** Supportive care. **Complication:** Polyarthritis, encephalitis, or thrombocytopenia. Congenital rubella is associated with congenital anomalies. **Prevention:** Immunization is effective.
Roseola Infantum (Exanthema Subitum) _HHV6 & 7   Fever THEN Rash_
1. **Cause:** HHV-6, age 5 months to 5 years. 2. Incubation: 5-15 days with upper respiratory symptoms, acute onset of high fever (> 40°C); when **fever fades in 3-4 days, a maculopapular rosy rash** appears, spreading from the trunk to the face and extremities and lasting < 24 hours. **Tx:** Supportive care. **Complication:** Seizure (with high fever). Prognosis is good. _f/u febrile seizures, cuba4 v benzo if > 5 min._
Varicella (Chickenpox, Image 80) _Rash, NO Fever_
1. **Cause: Primary infection by VZV.** 2. Prodrome: Mild fever, anorexia, and malaise for 24 hours. 3. **Rash:** generalized, pruritic, **teardrop-like** vesicles often at different stages of healing; infectious from 24 hours before eruption until lesions crust over. **Tx: Supportive care for children < age 12.** Systemic valacyclovir or acyclovir is only for adults and immunodeficient children. **Prevention:** Immunization is effective. **Complication:**

SSPE, PAST P.154

Prodrome: q fever > 104°F. Fever THEN Rash

useAPAP.

vesicles on an erythematous base, diff stages of healing

don't do Tzanck, don't do PCR.
dx: clx
~~pox parties~~
PPX: MMRV

[handwritten: varicella VZV]

[handwritten left margin: shingles vx!]

[handwritten left margin: post-herpetic neuralgia: TCAs or gabapentin]

[handwritten left margin: VDVx]

Meningoencephalitis and hepatitis in the immunodepressed. Congenital varicella is associated with congenital anomalies.

Varicella Zoster (Image 81) *[handwritten: Shingles]*

1. **Cause:** The reactivation of varicella by VZV, usually **in immunodepressed patients**. 2. Pain in the affected area. **Rash:** Pruritic "teardrop" vesicles in a dermatomal distribution. **Tx:** Systemic **valacyclovir** or acyclovir. **Complication:** Meningoencephalitis, pneumonitis, TTP, etc. *[handwritten: never crosses midline]*

Hand-foot-mouth Disease (Syndrome) *[handwritten: looks exactly like varicella, except only → hand, foot, mouth]*

1. **Cause: Coxsachie A.** 2. Prodrome: fever, anorexia, and painful oral ulcerations. 3. **Rash:** maculopapular vesicles on the hands and feet. **Tx:** Symptomatic. Complication: Rare.

Arboviral Encephalitis

1. **Cause:** Different arthropod-borne viruses: (1) St. Louis encephalitis (spread by birds); (2) California encephalitis (by mosquitoes); (3) Western equine encephalitis (by mosquitoes and birds); (4) Eastern equine encephalitis (by mosquitoes and birds); (5) Colorado tick fever (by wood tick). 2. **Features:** Similar to those of aseptic meningitis, but with more mental dysfunctions (confusion, delirium, etc.). 3. **Dx:** History, clinical features, along with specific ELISA for the pathogen. **Tx:** Supportive. **Prognosis:** Good except for E. equine (1/3 deaths).

RESPIRATORY TRACT INFECTIONS IN CHILDREN

PEARLS — Table 13-10: Important Respiratory Tract Infections in Children

Infection / Clinical Features, diagnosis, and treatment

Pharyngitis (Image 22)

1. **Cause:** Virus (most) or bacterium (**Strep-A #1, Staph-aureus #2**), often difficult to differentiate types of pathogens clinically. 2. **P/E:** Erythema, exudates, petechiae, enlarged tonsils, and cervical adenopathy are common to both. 3. Viral cause usually has a gradual onset; vesicles and ulcers are more common with herpes simplex and coxsackievirus; conjunctivitis is more with adenovirus. 4. Bacterial cause is more rapid and associated with tonsil exudates with a blanching, erythematous, sandpaper rash often prominent in inguinal and antecubital areas. 5. **Lab tests: Rapid Strep-Ag** test is both sensitive and specific; suspected (-) results is confirmed by **throat culture**.

Tx: (1) Viral pharyngitis: Symptomatic-supportive. (2) **Strep pharyngitis: Penicillin (V, G)** is the #1 choice; if allergic, erythromycin, azithromycin, clindamycin, or first-generation cephalosporins (cephalexin) is used. **Complication (Strep-A):** (1) **Peritonsillar abscess:** mostly > 10 y/a; high fever, severe sore throat, trismus, muffled "hot potato" voice, and drooling; the tonsil bulges medially, and the uvula deviates to the normal side. Treat with IV antibiotics, drainage, and possible tonsillectomy. (2) **Retro-pharyngeal abscess:** more common in **6 months to 6 years**, with risk of airway obstruction; lying with the neck extended, trismus, muffled "hot potato" voice, drooling, and cervical lymph node (LN) enlarging; lateral neck X-film reveals a soft tissue mass. Treat with IV antibiotics and drainage of abscess. (3) **Rheumatic fever** (later). (4) **Glomerulonephritis** (later).

[handwritten left margin: - anterior unilateral lymphadenopathy - tender mass that is the abscess]

[handwritten bottom: dx: CT Tx: drain aspirate IV abx]

[handwritten top right margin: Peritonsillar absc / path: oral cav / pt. 10 yrs + dvool / hot potato voice / + dysphagia, / dysphagia. / -(+) Uvula devi- / tion! / +c/o / tx dvain / Abx]

Scarlet Fever

1. **Cause: Strep-A**; usually associated with pharyngitis; may also follow wound/burn skin infections; rare in infancy. 2. Typically with abrupt fever, chills, headache, sore throat, and nausea/vomiting, followed by a maculopapular rash starting in the axilla, groin, and neck and spreading all over in 24 hours. 3. P/E usually shows a "strawberry" tongue, circumoral pallor, sandpaper rash, and small vesicular lesions over the limbs and abdomen; inflamed tonsils with exudates; desquamation from the face to the trunk/limbs. 4. **Lab tests**: Rapid Strep-Ag first for suspected pharyngitis; if (-), throat culture. **Differential Dx:** Roseola, rubella, measles, Kawasaki disease, etc.

Tx: The same as for Strep-A pharyngitis. Complication: (1) Early: Peritonsillar abscess, sinusitis, otitis media, and bacteremia. (2) Late: Rheumatic fever and glomerulonephritis.

Croup (Laryngotracheobronchitis) — [handwritten: edema & erythema, narrowing of proximal trachea (subglottis) Prevention: hand washing / ventilation / surface decontamination]

1. **Cause**: #1 is **parainfluenza** virus; then adenovirus, RSV and influenza. 2. Age group: **5 months—5 years**. [handwritten: rhinorrhea, congestion] Prodromal URI symptoms for 1-7 days, then low fever, barking cough, hoarseness, dyspnea, and inspiratory stridor worsened by agitation; [handwritten: dx:] improved by racemic epinephrine (EP). 3. **CXR**-AP: "**Steeple sign**" [handwritten: => Subglottic narrowing] [handwritten: or dexamethasone]

Tx: (1) Mild: nebulized cold steam at home. (2) Severe (with respiratory distress): PO/IV corticosteroids and nebulized racemic epinephrine (EP) plus supportive care in a hospital. **Complication**: Middle ear or lung infections.

[handwritten right margin: -stridor w / agitation/crying / => + dose / dexamethason / stridor@rest / => corticosteroids / & nebulized / epinephrine]

Epiglottitis [handwritten: - sick as fuck]

1. **Cause: Mostly Hib; then Strep-spp**, virus. 2. Age group: **3-7 years**. Rapid onset (4-12 hours) of high fever, [handwritten: Hot potato] dysphagia, drooling, muffled voice, and respiratory [handwritten: stridor] distress with a seated & neck extended position; not improved by epinephrine. 3. **Do not examine the throat** unless the anesthesia or tracheostomy is ready in case of laryngospasm. 4. **Lateral X-film**: Swollen epiglottis as "**thumbprint sign**".

Tx: Treat as a true **emergency**! (1) Keep patient calm, prepare for anesthesia, and then perform endotracheal intubation or tracheostomy. (2) IV a **3rd-generation cephalosporin** (ceftriaxone or cefotaxime) +/- vancomycin.

(Bacterial) Tracheitis — [handwritten: croup that doesn't improve]   [handwritten: more toxic]

1. **Cause**: An uncommon infection mostly initiated by respiratory **viruses followed by aggressive** bacteria (**Staph-A#1**, Strep-A, pneumococcus, Hib). 2. Age group: **3 months-6 years**. Prodrome for a few days, then moderate fever, dry cough, **stridor, hoarseness**, and varied respiratory distress. [handwritten: dx] Symptoms are not improved by epinephrine (adrenaline) use. 3. CXR may find narrowing of the subglottic trachea. Laboratory tests are not helpful with diagnosis, but microbiologic testing is necessary to guide antimicrobial therapy. Endoscopy can be used to confirm the diagnosis and often is necessary to remove adherent or copious pseudomembranous exudates.

[handwritten right margin: -do tracheal / culture / Tx: IV Abx]

Tx: 1. Maintenance of the airway is the mainstay of treatment. Many patients with bacterial tracheitis require endotracheal intubation. 2. Empiric antibiotics includes coverage for Staph-A, Strep-A, pneumococcus, and Hib. Antiviral therapy may be warranted when influenza is the predisposing viral etiology. Glucocorticoids in the initial Tx is not suggested.

Bronchiolitis
[handwritten: Lower resp tract]   [handwritten: winter months,]

1. An acute inflammation of the small airways mostly **caused by RSV** and affecting infants **< 2 y/a**. 2. Initial [handwritten: fever] URI symptoms followed by apnea, [handwritten: SOB,] tachypnea, wheezing, crackles, prolonged expiration, and hyperresonance (to percussion). 3. **Lab:** CXR shows lung hyperinflation, interstitial infiltrates, and atelectasis. **ELISA** of nasal

[handwritten bottom: r/o PNA, no need tx]

Bronchiolitis

---

washings for RSV is both very sensitive and specific.   *Sx peak @ day 3-9*

Acute hypox resp fail (AHRF)   or ARDS

Tx: (1) Hospitalize patient with respiratory distress, hypoxia, dehydration, risk factors of prematurity, immuno-deficiency, history of cardiorespiratory disease, and < 6 months of age, because it may potentially progress to fatal respiratory failure. (2) Treat them with O2, hydration, and aerosolized albuterol and glucocorticoids with contact isolation. **Prevention: Cloned RSV-Ab or palivizumab** is recommended for patients with above risk factors.

Pertussis

1. **Cause: Gram⁻ bacillus Bordetella pertussis**; also called "**whooping cough**". Usually in **5months-5years'** children; immunized by a vaccine or disease history. 2. Incubation period of 3-12 days for infants; presenting with long cough, post-tussive emesis, apnea, and cyanosis. 3. Older children usually experience **three stages** of the disease: (1) The catarrhal stage: mild URI symptoms, lasting 1-2 weeks and most contagious. (2) The paroxysmal stage: a paroxysmal cough followed by a forceful inspiratory gasp (whoop), emesis, and conjunctival/facial petechiae; lasting 2-4 weeks. (3) The convalescent stage: Decreased symptoms, lasting 1-2 weeks. 4. **Lab: Elevated WBC and LC ratio** (>70%). **Culture (+)** is the best Dx standard.

Tx: (1) Supportive care in hospital. (2) **Azithromycin or clarithromycin** (better than erythromycin) for 14 days to patient and close contacts. (3) Patient is allowed to return to school after 5-day antibiotics or 3-week break without Tx. **Complication:** Pneumonia, pneumothorax, encephalopathy, or death (mostly in patient < 6 months).

Occult Bacteremia

Definition: A condition with bacteria in the blood without an obvious focus of infection. It's commonly due to **S. pneumonia, N. meningitis, Hib, and Salmonella in 3month-3year's children; Listeria and E. coli are mostly in infants < 1 month of age. Risk factors:** < 24 months of age, T > 39°C, history of chronic diseases, immunodeficiency, day-care center, etc.

Essentials of diagnosis

1. Most infants have fever (> 38°C) but appear relatively well. Some can be ill appearing, lethargic, irritable, or with petechiae.

2. **Lab tests**: WBCs > 15 x 10³/uL with predominant neutrophils and bands. Cultures of blood, urine, and CSF should be performed for suspected cases, particularly for an ill-appearing child.

Treatment

For most patients with T < 39 °C: Obtain CBC and blood culture, and administer empirical **ceftriaxone** (or ampicillin for Listeria, or clindamycin as an alternative). Adjust therapies according to the culture results. Without treatment, it may resolve spontaneously, persist, or lead to localized infections (abscess, meningitis, or septic arthritis).

[handwritten, top right]: Laryngeal vascularring: congenital malformation. Aberrant vessel encircles the airway ⟹ chronic stridor from airway narrowing

CONGENITAL ABNORMALITIES

Eye, Neck, and Chest Abnormalities

Table 13-11: Congenital Abnormalities of the Eye, Neck, and Chest

Disease / Clinical features, diagnosis, and treatment
Aniridia: Absence of the iris. If there is hemihypertrophy, always suspect Wilm tumor.
Coloboma: An iris/retina/eyelid defect, ranging from a small notch to a large cleft.
Branchial cleft cysts: It can be formed from incomplete closure of the branchial clefts; usually unilateral. **Tx:** Antibiotic therapy is used for infected cases.
Congenital torticollis ("wry neck"): It usually results from injury to the sternocleidomastoid during delivery; cause from congenital cervical anomaly is less common. **Tx:** Stretching exercises are helpful with muscular torticollis.
Breast hypertrophy: A temporary condition in the neonate secondary to increased circulating estrogen.
Pectus excavatum (funnel), pectus carinatum (pigeon): Usually benign, isolated deformities of the chest, requiring surgical correction for cosmetic purpose.
Tracheoesophageal fistula: Commonest type: Atretic esophagus and a fistula between the trachea and the distal esophagus, leading to the air into the stomach and small intestine. **Cause:** Malformation of the foregut. **Dx:** 1. Coughing or choking with swallowing or feeding. It may also be associated with polyhydramnios, cyanosis, etc. 2. Lab: Inability to pass a catheter into the stomach (CXR shows an NG tube coiled in the esophagus) or bronchoscopy to confirm Dx. **Tx:** Surgical repair. **Complication:** Increased risk of congenital heart disease ("CHD", such as patent ductus artery, coarctation of the aorta) and multiple other defects (spinal cord, rectum, kidney, limbs). *gastric reflux into lungs ⟹ Aspiration PNA ⟹ crackles, pulm infiltrates* *[fetus can't swallow amniotic fluid]*
hole in diaphragm= bowel in chest =   Polyhydramnios from esophageal compression **Diaphragmatic hernia:** Failure of the diaphragm development causes abdominal contents to enter the chest, resulting in pulmonary hypoplasia on the affected side. Patients are born with respiratory distress and a scaphoid abdomen. P/E reveals bowel sounds in the chest, and CXR shows bowel in the chest. **Tx:** Surgical correction, *surfactant* *give corticosteroids to help develop the lung*

L>R, Posterior > lateral. Dx xray

CHARGE Syndrome

--**It's a set of congenital defects occurring in** connective tissues.
C: Coloboma of the eye, central nervous system anomalies. *missing eye tissue*
H: Heart defects.
A: Atresia of the choanae.
R: Retardation of growth and/or development.
G: Genital and/or urinary defects (hypogonadism).
E: Ear abnormalities and/or deafness.

[handwritten right]: -FA5 1 p.453 Neural Tube Defect path: genetic disorders, folate def caudal spine fails to form. Pt: prenatal care, Quad screen: ↑AFP. U/S= dz. ↑Achase no prenatal care: -tuft hair -meningomyelocele Dx: prenatal screen, clx Tx surg, s/o-arnold chiari malf, -hydrocephalus, -SND ↑level of lesion

[handwritten bottom left]: cleft lip or palate: failure to grow or fuse. -soft, hard palate. Lip. -superficial—D deletions. -BL, UL, midline. -cosmetic, failure to thrive.   Dx clx. recurrent infxn Tx: surg correct Lip 11-12weeks 11-12 months palate

Gastrointestinal Tract (GIT) Abnormalities

Table 13-12:　Congenital GIT Malformations

Disease / Clinical features, diagnosis, and treatment
Umbilical hernias
Arise from incomplete closure of the fascia of the umbilical ring; associated with diastasis recti and usually close spontaneously by 5 y/a.
Omphalocele
A herniation of peritoneum and abdominal contents into the base of the umbilical cord, forming a sac covered by peritoneum and amniotic membranes. **Clinical features:** Polyhydramnios in utero, often premature and associated with other GIT and cardiac defects. **Tx:** (1) Initially covering and wrapping the exposed bowel sterilely to minimize heat and fluid loss. (2) Surgical repair ASAP. _Silo_
Gastroschisis
A herniation without a sac, through an abdominal wall defect to the right of the umbilicus. **Clinical features:** Polyhydramnios in utero, often premature and associated with GIT stenosis or atresia. **Tx:** (1) Initially covering and wrapping the exposed bowel sterilely. (2) Urgent surgical repair. _Silo_
Hypertrophic Pyloric Stenosis
A gastric outlet obstruction; M:F = 4:1. **Clinical features: 1. Nonbilious projectile vomiting is the hallmark.** Vomiting usually begins 2-3 weeks after birth. 2. Jaundice, weight loss, and signs of dehydration may appear. 3. **P/E will find a palpable olive-size mass** in the abdomen, occasionally with a peristaltic wave. 4. **Dx tests:** Abdominal ultrasound reveals a thickened, elongated pylorus. **Ba** study shows a dilated stomach with elongated pylorus (**string sign**). **Lab tests** show **hypo-K, hypo-Cl metabolic alkalosis**. **Tx:** First correct fluid deficit and electrolyte imbalance; then fix the stenosis by surgery.
Meckel Diverticulum
#1 common congenital GIT anomaly, a vestigial remnant of the omphalomesenteric duct. **Clinical features:** 1. Known as **"the disease of 2s"**: Present in about 2% of infants, the peak age is 2, with 2 types of tissue (ectopic gastric and pancreatic-duodenal mucosa), about 2 cm long, and located about 2 feet from the ileocecal valve. 2. **Painless rectal bleeding is #1 symptom ("currant jelly" stool).** Occasionally, it causes obstruction or intussusception, becomes inflamed (mimic appendicitis), or may perforate and cause peritonitis. 3. **Dx:** The **Tech**[99] **scan** is the most sensitive means. **Tx:** Endoscopic therapy or surgical removal.
Duodenal Atresia (Image 126)
Partial or complete failure of the duodenal lumen to recanalize during gestational week 8-10. **Clinical features:** 1. Polyhydramnios in uterus; bilious vomiting within hours with every feed. 2. It's associated with Down syndrome and other cardiac or GIT anomalies (pancreas, anus). 3. Abdominal X-ray: shows typical **"double bubble"** sign. **Tx:** Surgical correction.

Handwritten annotations:

(beside Omphalocele, top) midline, sac around bowel

(left margin, beside Omphalocele) Silo: sterile bowel, overtime you twist bowel back into baby

(beside Gastroschisis) Right of midline, no covering

(left margin, bottom) pathoma 116 Biliary Atresia:
- Failure to form or early destruction of extrahepatic biliary tree ⇒ biliary obstruct. < 2 months of life, about 2 weeks
- progressing jaundice ⇒ cirrhosis. direct hyperbilirubinemia. acholic stools.
Dx: U/S = no ducts. HIDA scan after 5-7 days of phenobarbital ⇒ stim biliary tree to secrete bile.
Tx: resect atretic segment & reconnect.

[handwritten top margin: - 60% pts - chronic diarrhea w overflow incontinence - Dx: Anal rectal manometry]

[handwritten: Dx Best Bx]

[handwritten right margin: 90% pts - palpable colon from distension - explosive diarrhea on DRE finger liberates contracted colon stool shoots out.]

Hirschsprung Disease (Aganglionic Megacolon)

[handwritten: - fails to innv. distal colon.]

Results from absence of the ganglion cells in the distal colon, causing obstruction and dilation. **Clinical features:** 1. Newborn fails to pass meconium in the first 48 hours of life; the rectal exam typically shows an empty vault. 2. Ba-enema reveals a dilated megacolon, best confirmed by a biopsy showing absence of the ganglion cell. **Tx:** Surgical resection. *[handwritten: Dx: Xray. good colon = dilates, bad colon = looks normal ① Contrast enema → ① Best initial: Xray]*

Differentiation: Intussusception

Clinical features: 1. Results from a bowel portion slipping into the distal portion; mostly ileocolic, in 6-24 months of age. 2. Causes are unknown; may be associated with viral enteritis, lymphoid hyperplasia, Meckel diverticulum, polyps, cystic fibrosis, and Henoch-Schonlein purpura. 3. **Typically with acute colicky abdominal pain**, vomiting, fever, and lethargy, and later **with bloody stool** and shock. **P/E: A sausage-shaped mass** in the upper abdomen. 4. **Lab: Barium/air enema** is both diagnostic and therapeutic. A **coil-spring sign** is seen as the Ba fills the obstruction. Ultrasound helps. **Tx:** It's fatal without immediate Tx. Hydrostatic reduction is effective if < 48 hours; urgent surgery if > 48 hours and with peritonitis or perforation.

Differentiation: Colic

[handwritten: ≥3 hr/day, usually evening, healthy infant age <3 months]

Clinical features: 1. A paroxysmal, functional abdominal pain in an infant without clear reasons, mostly < 3y; may be associated with air swallowing by overfeeding or hunger. 2. Attacks often occur at the same time of day, causing baby crying and abdomen distended and rigid; relieved after hrs or passing gas/stool. Lab tests are mostly normal. **Tx**: Abdominal warming and massage. **Differentiation:** Intussusception, hernia, intestinal obstruction.

[handwritten: Review soothing techniques]

Genitourinary Tract (GUT) Abnormalities

Table 13-13: Summary of Congenital GUT Malformations

Disease / Clinical features, diagnosis, and treatment

Polycystic kidney disease (Also see Chapter 7)

It can be autosomal dominant (most, with 10% renal failure) or recessive (30% renal failure). It's the most commonly palpated abdominal mass in the newborn. Another common mass is a distended bladder from posterior urethral valves.

Epispadias

The urethral opening is located on the dorsum of the shaft of the penis (and in female urethra less frequently). **Tx**: Surgical repair by 6-12 months.

Hypospadias

A urethral opening located on the ventral side of the shaft of the penis (and in female urethra less frequently), usually with a ventral hood. Circumcision should be avoided because the foreskin is needed in the treatment of surgical repair.

Undescended testes: Usually in the inguinal canal; if not descended by 1 year, surgery should be done to avoid sterility or malignant degeneration. **Necessary differentiation**: Retractile testes—This is the result from an active cremasteric reflex that needs no Tx.

[handwritten bottom: Bladder exstrophy: midline defect, wet w urine, shiny, red. No bowel! Dx clx, tx surg]

[handwritten bottom: Vesico ureteral Reflux: hydroureter, hydronephrosis. Recurrent UTIs, dx w voiding cysto urethrogram. Renal U/s - screen for hydronephrosis.]

Hydrocele

A collection of fluid in the scrotum, particularly the tunica vaginalis; may also be associated with maternal high levels of lead in the blood. Most cases resolve by 1 y/a; if not, surgical correction is indicated. **Diagnosis** is made on transillumination. **Differentiation**: Hernia.

Hernia

Usually inguinal, indirect hernias in children, presents as a bulge in the inguinal area or reducible scrotal swelling. If a hydrocele is reduced by compression, it's probably a hernia. **Tx**: Surgery. Also refers to Chapter 15.

GENETIC SYNDROMES

Table 13-14: Summary of Genetic Syndromes

Disease or syndrome / Clinical features, diagnosis and treatment
Down syndrome (Image 125)   1. Genetic defect: Trisomy 21; rate: 1:700; translocation: recurrent. **#1 common chromosomal disease and cause of congenital intellectual disability**; with advanced maternal age as #1 etiology. 2. Presenting with typical **intellectual disability, a flat facial profile** (a flat nasal bridge, thin upper lip), small chin, large tongue, slanted eyes with brushfield spots in the irises, **prominent epicanthal folds, simian crease, wider space between the eyes and the first and second toe,** poor muscle tone, etc. 3. **Associated with duodenal atresia, Hirschsprung disease, congenital heart disease (#1 as ASD, VSD with valve defects), and increased risk of acute lymphoblastic leukemia (ALL) and Alzheimer disease.**
Edwards syndrome   1. **Trisomy 18, 1:8000.** 2. Severe intellectual disability, rocker-bottom feet, micrognathia, prominent occiput, low-set ears, and clenched hands. 3. Associated with congenital heart/kidney disease, and early death < 1 y/a.
Patau syndrome   1. **Trisomy 13, 1:6000.** 2. Severe intellectual disability, small head and eyes, "punched-out" scalp lesions, polydactyly, etc. 3. Associated with congenital heart disease and early death < 1 y/a.
Klinefelter syndrome   1. **45, XXY,** inactivated X̲ chromosome (**Barr body**) present, **male only, 1:850.** 2. **#1 cause of congenital hypogonadism in males.** 3. Testis atrophy, tall body and long limbs, gynecomastia, female hair distribution, etc.
Turner syndrome   1. **45, XO, no Barr body, female only, 1:3000; #1 cause of primary amenorrhea.** 2. Short stature, neck webbing, ovary dysgenesis, aorta coarctation, etc. 3. May be associated with horseshoe kidney and limb lymphedema.
Double Y male   1. **47, XYY, 1:1000;** seen more in penal institutions. 2. It carries a normal phenotype, but showing **very tall stature with severe acne and antisocial behavior.**

[handwritten margin notes: "FAp 7α", "FAp 585", "extra" (above X chromosome in Klinefelter), "↑estrogen or ↓androgen = 2° hypogonadism" (right margin of Klinefelter), "Normal intelligence" (next to Turner syndrome)]

FA73 **Fragile X syndrome**　　*methylation silences the fragile x mental retard protein*

　　hyper　　　　　　　　　　　　　　　　　　　　　　trinucleotide repeat

　　1. **X-linked deficiency** in the methylation and expression of **FMR1 gene**; a triplet repeat disease with genetic anticipation. 2. **#2 cause of genetic intellectual disability.** 3. Macroorchidism, long face, large jaw/ears, autism. +DHD

Uworld: MCC inherited intellect disability. Begin

GENETIC METABOLIC ABNORMALITIES

PEARLS—Table 13-15: Important Congenital Metabolic Abnormalities

FA95 **Phenylketonuria (PKU)**

　　It's caused by **a deficiency (Def) in hydroxylation of phenylalanine to tyrosine,** with an autosomal recessive trait (1/10,000). **Clinical features:** Affected infants are normal at birth until sufficient toxic metabolites are accumulated, showing **fair hair and skin, blue eyes, a musty odor, and severe intellectual disability**. Vomiting can be projectile as in pyloric stenosis. **Lab tests:** Routine newborn screening for PKU now establishes the Dx before most symptoms, best performed after 48-72 hours of life. With a (+) screening result, blood levels of phenylalanine (high) and tyrosine (low to normal) should be tested.

　　Tx: Early phenylalanine restriction in diet for life time. **Complication:** Unless PKU is diagnosed and treated in time, infants can easily develop intellectual disability, microcephaly, heart disease, and spontaneous abortions.

FA 92

　　Galactosemia

　　It results from a **deficiency of galactose-1-phosphate uridyl transferase (GALT),** causing galactose-1-P accumulation, and brain, liver and kidney damage. It is inherited in an autosomal recessive trait (1/60,000). **Clinical features:** Multi-organ symptoms including jaundice, vomiting, seizures, cataracts, hypoglycemia, hepatosplenomegaly, and lower body weight (growth delay). It's with higher risk of **sepsis by E coli**. **Lab tests:** Newborn blood screening and reducing substances for galactosemia in the urine (+) help with initial Dx, confirmed by specific **RBC GALT activity**. Prenatal and carrier testing also help with Dx.

　　Tx: Eliminating galactose from the diet. **Complication:** Developmental delay, speech/learning disabilities may still occur despite early Dx and Tx.

FA 366, Pathoma /23

　　Special disorder: Reye syndrome　　*Acute liver failure, encephalopathy, ↑ICP*

　　It's a rare **encephalopathy associated with fatty degeneration and dysfunction of the liver** of unknown etiology, which may be associated with **aspirin use in children**, a viral infection (influenza A/B, EBV, varicella), medium-chain acyl-coenzyme A dehydrogenase (MCAD) deficiency, or urea cycle disorders. It mostly occurs around 6 y/a. **Clinical features and Dx:** 1. Following recent aspirin use or viral infection, patient presents with abrupt onset of protracted vomiting, combative behavior, delirium, and confusion, and rapid progress to seizures, coma, and death. No focal neurologic signs. 2. Clinical Dx is supported by elevated levels of **LFTs** and **blood ammonia**, and **by exclusion**. Definite Dx is by **liver biopsy**.

- ↑ aminotransferases
- ↑ ammonemia
- ↑ Prolonged PT
- hypoglycemia from depletion of glucose stores & ↑ use

　　Tx: 1. **Urgent supportive care!** ICP is monitored; if it's increased, reduction by IV mannitol and corticosteroids is essential to treat lethal cerebral edema. 2. Supply glucose for hypoglycemia, Vit-K, and fresh frozen plasma to reverse the coagulopathy. Use oral lactulose and neomycin to decrease ammonia levels. 3. **Prevention**: Aspirin is contraindicated in most infections in children.

LYSOSOMAL STORAGE DISEASES

Lysosomal storage diseases (LSDs) are a group of rare inherited disorders that result from defects in lysosomal function and metabolisms of lipids, glycoproteins or mucopolysaccharides. Most of these disorders are autosomal recessively inherited. LSDs affect mostly children and they often die at a young and unpredictable age, many within a few months or years of birth and with various symptoms of their particular disorder. LSDs are summarized in the table below.

Table 13-16: Lysosomal Storage Diseases ﹛AS2-100

Disease / Clinical features and diagnosis
Fabry disease: 1. X-linked recessive; deficiency (Def) of alpha-galactosidase A causing build-up of ceramide trihexoside in the brain, heart and kidneys. 2. Renal failure and increased risk of stroke and myocardial infarction.
Krabbe disease: 1. Autosomal recessive trait; deficiency of galactosylceramidase causing accumulation of galactocerebroside in the brain. 2. Optic atrophy, spasticity, and early death.
Gaucher disease : 1. Autosomal recessive trait; deficiency of glucocerebrosidase causing build-up of glucocerebroside in the brain, liver, spleen, and bone marrow (showing "crinkled paper"). 2. Usually with anemia, hepatosplenomegaly, and thrombocytopenia. 3. Classified into 3 subtypes. Type 1 is the most common one, which does not affect the brain and patient may live a normal life.
Niemann-Pick disease: 1. Autosomal recessive trait; sphingomyelinase deficiency causing accumulation of sphingomyelin cholesterol in cells. 2. Type A patient die by 3 y/a.
Metachromatic Leukodystrophy (MLD): Also known as "sulfatide lipidoses", a rare autosomal recessive disease that causes progressive demyelination of the central and peripheral nervous system; deficiency of arylsulfatase A causing sulfatide build-up in the brain, kidney, liver, and peripheral nerves.
Tay-Sachs disease: 1. Deficiency of hexosaminase causing GM2 ganglioside build-up. 2. A typical cherry-red spot on the macula. 3. Weakness and slowed development; die by 3 y/a; more among Jews.
Hurler syndrome: 1. Autosomal recessive trait; deficiency of a-L-iduronidase. 2. Corneal clouding, visual and hearing loss, and intellectual disability.
Hunter syndrome: 1. X-linked recessive trait; iduronate sulfatase deficiency. 2. A milder form of Hurler syndrome; no corneal clouding.

GLYCOGEN STORAGE DISEASES (GSD)

Glycogen storage disease, also called glycogenosis and dextrinosis, is a group of rare metabolic diseases caused by inborn error of defective enzymes involved in the processing of glycogen synthesis or breakdown in the muscle, liver, and other organs. There are 11 distinct GSDs briefly summarized below.

FAS7-98

Table 13-17: Glycogen Storage Disease (GSD)

Type	Enzyme deficiency	Eponym	Hypo-glycemia	Hepato-megaly	Hyper-lipidemia	Muscular symptoms	Development / prognosis	Other symptoms
I	Glucose-6-phosphatase	von Gierke disease	Yes	Yes	Yes	None	Growth failure	Lactic acidosis, hyperuricemia
II	Acid maltase	Pompe disease	No	Yes	No	Muscle weakness	Death by age 2 (infantile variant)	heart failure
III	Glycogen debrancher	Cori or Forbes disease	Yes	Yes	Yes	Myopathy		
IV	glycogen branching enzyme	Andersen disease	No	Yes, also cirrhosis	No	None	Growth failure, death by age 5	
V	Muscle glycogen phosphorylase	McArdle disease	No	No	No	Exercise-induced cramps, rhabdomyolysis		Renal failure by myoglobinuria
VI	Liver glycogen phosphorylase	Hers disease	Yes	Yes	No	None		
VII	Muscle phospho-fructokinase	Tarui disease	No	No	No	Exercise-induced muscle cramps and weakness	Growth retardation	Hemolytic anemia
IX	Phosphorylase kinase, PHKA2	-	Yes	No	Yes	None	Delayed motor development and growth	
XI	Glucose transporter, GLUT2	Fanconi-Bickel syndrome	Yes	Yes	No	None		

Chapter 13: High-yield Questions (HYQ)

1-4: Match the following clinical scenarios with the most likely diagnosis (Dx).

A. Cephalhematoma   B. Caput succedaneum   C. Subcutaneous fat necrosis

D. Facial palsy   E. Clavicular fracture   F. Erb-Duchenne palsy

G. Klumpke paralysis   H. Newborn jaundice   I. Subconjunctival hemorrhage

J. Capillary hemangiomas

1. 24 hours after a vacuum-aided delivery, a newborn presents with a swelling of the scalp crossing the suture lines. Mild fever and conjunctival yellowing are also found. There are no other abnormal findings.

2. Five days after a difficult, vacuum-aided delivery, a newborn presents with palpable, rubbery, firm nodules on the cheeks and forehead. There are no other abnormal findings.

3. 24 hours after a forceps-aided delivery with shoulder dystocia, a newborn is found fussy with regular feeding, but no vomiting. Physical examination (P/E) finds an asymmetric Moro reflex and crepitus over the left shoulder. There are no other abnormal findings.

4. 24 hours after a forceps-aided delivery with shoulder dystocia, a newborn is found fussy with regular feeding, but no vomiting. P/E finds ptosis and miosis on the right side, flexion and supination of the right elbow, and a "claw right hand." There are no other abnormal findings.

5-9: Match the following clinical scenarios with the most likely diagnosis (Dx).

A. Congenital dermal Melanocytosis   B. Erythema toxicum

C. Cutis marmorata   D. Milia   E. Neonatal acne

F. Sebaceous hyperplasia   G. Nevus sebaceous   H. Capillary hemangiomas

I. Cafe-au-lait spots   J. Salmon patch   K. Child abuse

L. Staph scalded skin syndrome (SSSS)

5. A 6-month infant is brought to the clinic for feeding intolerance and irritability. P/E finds a large flat blue lesion on the buttock, with relatively clear margins that fade into the surrounding skin with dark-red discoloration. There are no other abnormal findings.

6. A 1-year infant is brought to the clinic for feeding intolerance and irritability. P/E finds multiple flat dark-brown lesions over the body, with clear margins and of various sizes. CBC reveals anemia. There is a family history of neurofibromatosis and no other abnormal findings.

7. 24 hours after a forceps-aided delivery, a newborn is found fussy with regular feeding, but no fever or vomiting. P/E finds multiple small papules on an erythematous base. Dominant eosinophils are identified in the scraped papules. The infant looks well and quiets down after a while.

8. A 1-year infant is brought to the clinic and found with two 3-mm yellow-orange, hairless, wart-like plaques on the scalp. There are no other abnormal findings.

9. A 1-year old infant is brought to the clinic. The mother says that there were only two "strawberry-like warts" on the trunk 6 months ago but now there are many of them. P/E reveals ten bright red, strawberry-like macules of 3 mm in diameter on the trunk. The color fades after pressing. There are no other abnormal findings. The physician tells the mother to observe them and bring the infant back if they do not disappear in 6 months.

10. 24 hours after a preterm delivery, a newborn has yellowish skin and begins to vomit milk and greenish fluid. The mother says that the infant is breast-feeding and has sparse, clay-colored stool. P/E finds a weak but alert newborn with generalized jaundice without fever. Lab tests reveal that serum bilirubin is 20 mg/dL, with predominant direct bilirubin. What's the best treatment (Tx) for this condition?
A. Stop breast-feeding   B. Observation   C. Surgery
D. Phototherapy   E. Exchange blood transfusion

11. 24 hours after a preterm and forceps-aided delivery, a newborn presents with conjunctival yellowing, blue lips, coughing, and tachypnea. P/E finds a weak but alert newborn with mild jaundice, cyanosis, tachycardia, and tachypnea, but no fever. Lab tests reveal moderate hypoxia and bilirubin of 5 mg/dL (mostly indirect bilirubin). CXR shows patchy infiltrates. Blood is taken for culture and mechanical ventilation with oxygen is supplied. What's the best next treatment?
A. Upper chest tubing   B. Phototherapy   C. Nitric oxide
D. Exogenous surfactant + steroid   E. Ampicillin + 3rd-generation cephalosporins

12. A toddler is brought for a regular developmental check-up. He can run, jump, and walks up and down the stairs. He can also undress himself, make a 4-cube tower, say "I want," and follow instructions of "Put the toy down and come here." What's his most likely age?
A. 1 year   B. 2 years   C. 3 years
D. 4 years   E. 5 years

13. A 12 y/o boy is given a 6-month medical Tx for a chronic disease. He runs out of the drug and comes to refill his prescription. P/E finds generally pale and dry skin with scratching tracks, and decreased pain sensation. CBC reveals a microcytic, normochromic anemia. What's the most likely vitamin deficiency?
A. B1   B. B2   C. B3
D. B5   E. B6

14. A 2 y/o girl is brought to the clinic for a regular check-up and immunization. Her mother says the girl's required immune shots were completed for the 6-month schedule, and her last immune shots were done a year ago for DTaP and MMR only. P/E finds a thin girl with normal lab results. The most appropriate vaccination needed at this time is
A. Hib   B. PPV   C. Varicella
D. HAV   E. Meningococcus

15. When the girl in Q14 is between the ages of 4-6 years and in the fall season, she should receive all of the following immunizations EXCEPT
A. DTaP   B. PPV   C. IVP
D. influenza   E. MMR

<u>16-21</u>: Match the following clinical scenarios with the most likely diagnosis.

A. Measles	B. Mumps	C. Rubella
D. Varicella	E. Erythema infectiosum	F. Pertussis
G. Viral pharyngitis	H. Croup	I. Epiglottitis
J. Hand-foot-mouth syndrome	K. Bronchiolitis	L. Tracheitis
M. Scarlet fever	N. Exanthem subitum	

16. A 5 y/o boy is brought to the physician for a "spreading itchy rash" starting yesterday. P/E finds an alert boy without fever. There are generalized erythematous macules and papules on the face, trunk, and legs, and several older rashes on his arms. Lab tests reveal decreased Hb and increased indirect bilirubin.

17. A 4 y/o boy is brought to the physician for a painful rash spreading from his face to body since yesterday. P/E finds an alert boy with mild fever. There are generalized erythematous macules and papules on his face (old), trunk, and limbs (fresh) with tenderness, and several swollen lymph nodes. CBC reveals mildly decreased platelets.

18. A 3 y/o girl is brought to the physician for fever and a painful rash. The mother says that she had high fever 3 days ago and the rash appears today spreading from the trunk to the face and limbs. P/E results: alert, no fever; with generalized rosy macules and papules on the face, trunk, and limbs. CBC shows increased lymphocytes (LC).

19. A 3 y/o boy is brought to the physician for fever and a spreading itchy rash over his body for the past 2 days. P/E finds an alert boy with mild fever. There are generalized pruritic, "teardrop"-like vesicles over the body in different stages of crusting and healing. CBC reveals increased LC.

20. A 4 y/o boy is brought to the physician for fever, barking cough, hoarseness, and dyspnea for the past 3 days. P/E finds T = 38°C, RR = 25/m, and rough respiratory sounds on auscultation. CXR-AP shows "Steeple sign."

21. A 2 y/o toddler is brought to the physician for fever, tachypnea, dyspnea, and wheezing today. P/E finds T = 38°C, cyanosis, crackles, prolonged expiration and hyperresonance to percussion. CXR shows lung hyperinflation and interstitial infiltrates.

<u>22-26</u>: Match the following clinical scenarios with the most likely diagnosis.

A. Diaphragmatic hernia	B. Tracheoesophageal fistula	C. Umbilical hernias
D. Omphalocele	E. Gastroschisis	F. Duodenal atresia
G. Hypertrophic pyloric stenosis	H. Meckel diverticulum	I. Hirschsprung disease
J. Intussusception	K. Colic	

22. A newborn presents with coughs and chokes with cyanosis whenever he is fed. CXR shows an NG tube coiled in the esophagus with evidence of aspiration.

23. A newborn presents with a mass without a sac extending through the abdominal wall to the side of the umbilicus. The mother has a history of polyhydramnios in uterus and premature delivery.

24. A 2-week old male newborn presents with frequent vomiting and yellowish skin. The mother describes the vomiting as projectile and with milk only. P/E finds an alert infant with mild jaundice and a small mass in the abdomen. Lab tests show hypo-K and hypo-Cl. Abdominal ultrasound (U/S) and Ba-study are scheduled.

25. A 1 y/o infant presents with periodic crying due to abdominal pain shortly after feeding, which is relieved after a few hours. He has no fever, vomiting, or diarrhea. P/E finds an alert infant without jaundice or rash; the abdomen is distended and rigid with mild tenderness. Blood and stool tests are normal.

26. A 2 y/o girl presents with recurrent fever, cough with sputum, dyspnea, cyanosis, greasy stool, and flatulence for the past 3 months. P/E finds T = 39°C, tachypnea, tachycardia, cyanosis, and pulmonary rales. Abdomen is soft. CXR shows bilateral pulmonary infiltrates. CBC reveals increased WBC with bands. What's the best next step?

A. Supply antibiotics, digestive enzymes and vitamins

B. Start diet modification   C. Test sweat Cl

D. Take sputum for culture (C/S)   E. Screen for genetic deficiencies

27. A 3 y/o boy had fever, headache, polyuria, and dysuria for the past 3 days. His mother gave him amoxicillin and aspirin for the past 2 days. Now he has started to vomit and has become combative and confused. P/E finds T = 40°C, delirium, tachycardia, hypotension, jaundice, hepatosplenomegaly, and renal tenderness. Urine analysis (U/A) shows WBC and protein. Blood tests show increased WBC with bands, hypoglycemia, and normal LFTs. What's the most appropriate test to determine the original pathologic condition?

A. Blood culture (C/S)   B. Blood ammonia levels   C. Liver biopsy

D. Urine culture   E. RBC GALT activity   F. Urinary reducing substances

Answers and Explanations

1. (B). It's usually associated with delivery injury and jaundice, and resolves over several days without treatment (Tx). A cephalhematoma is mostly limited to the bone with a palpable rim and does not cross suture lines.

2. (C). Most of the lesions resolve spontaneously without Tx.

3. (E). It's the #1 bone fracture during delivery; associated with a large baby with dystocia. A palpable healing callus usually forms within a week without Tx.

4. (G). It's one of the brachial nerve injuries (C7-T1), with an ipsilateral Horner's syndrome. The other type is Erb-Duchenne palsy—involves C5-C6 and shows "waiter's tips."

5. (K). Most likely it's an abusive lesion on the buttock. Parents usually hide the true history. If abuse is prolonged, evidence of delayed development may be found. A similar lesion on the differential Dx is congenital dermal melanocytosis, which are flat blue or grey lesions with well-defined margins commonly present over the presacral area. They usually disappear in the first few years of life.

6. (I). It's associated with rare genetic disease like neurofibromatosis, tuberous sclerosis, Fanconi anemia, etc.

7. (B). Differential Dx: Staph-scaded skin syndrome (SSSS) —older infant, looks very ill, +/- fever and hypotension; diffuse erythema with crusting full of neutrophils; skin culture reveals S. aureus.

8. (G). Because of malignancy potential, they are usually removed by adolescence. Sebaceous hyperplasias are very small, benign, yellow-white papules commonly found on the nose and cheeks.

9. (H). They start in the first few months and quickly grow in the first year of life, then regress spontaneously without Tx.

10. (C). Patient most likely has duodenal or biliary atresia causing obstructive jaundice, diagnosed by ultrasound or X-ray, followed by surgical correction. Phototherapy is best Tx for most indirect bilirubin > 20 mg/dL, and 'E' is performed if the hyperbilirubinemia persists, especially with autoimmune antibodies.

11. (C). Most likely meconium aspiration, best treated with mechanical ventilation, inhaled nitric oxide, etc. 'A' is for complicated pneumothorax. 'B' is for indirect bilirubin > 20 mg/dL. 'D' is for respiratory distress syndrome (RDS), which will show severe respiratory distress; CXR shows a hazy, ground-glass appearance. 'E' is best for neonatal sepsis, which is commonly caused by Strep-B, E. coli, or Listeria.

12. (B). Review and remember the important developmental milestones.

13. (E). "DNA"—dermatitis, neuritis, and anemia, mostly due to prolonged INH use for TB. B_1 deficiency (Def): "HEN"—heart failure, encephalopathy, and neuritis. B_2 deficiency: "ACC"—angular stomatitis, cheilosis, and corneal vascularization. B_3 deficiency: "DDD"—dermatitis, diarrhea, and dementia. B_5 deficiency: Rare.

14. (D). Please review the vaccination table. By 6 months of age, the girl has received most of the required three vaccinations but missed the Hib (the 4th), PPV (the 4th), and Varicella (the 1st) for the 12-15 month schedules. She should skip these missed ones and receive the required HAV for the 2-year's schedule. 'E' is done by 11-12 y/a.

15. (B). The patient's vaccination for PPV was completed by 12-15 months of age. By 4-6 y/a, she should have the 5th DTaP, 4th IPV, and the 2nd MMR completed. Influenza shot is recommended for this thin girl in the fall season with more risk of catching the flu.

16. (E). This is a case of "the 5th disease" ("Slapped face") complicated by hemolytic anemia. It's caused by parvovirus B19.

17. (C). It's a typical case of rubella caused by rubella virus.

18. (N). Roseola infantum is caused by HHV-6 in 5 months—5 years' children, with 3 days of high fever plus rosy papules.

19. (D). Varicella is caused by VZV, and infectious from 24 hours before eruption until the lesions crust over. Acyclovir is only needed for adults and immuno-Def children.

20. (H). Laryngothacheobronchitis: The #1 cause is "para influenza virus", age 5 months—5 years. Severe cases require IV steroids and nebulized EP. Epiglottitis is mostly caused by HIB and Strep-spp in older children, with high fever, dysphagia, drooling, muffled voice, and respiratory distress not improved by EP. CXR-LP shows "thumbprint sign."

21. (K). It's mostly caused by RSV and affects infants < 2 y/a. ELISA is the best Dx test. Tracheitis is mostly caused by S. aureus in children aged 3 months—2 years. Middle-grade fever, dry cough, hoarseness, and varied respiratory distress; not improved by administration of epinephrine.

22. (B). T-E fistula is caused by mal-formation of the foregut. Tx is surgery. Diaphragmatic hernia usually presents with respiratory distress and a scaphoid abdomen, with bowel in the chest (CXR, P/E). Tx is surgery.

23. (E). Tx: Urgent surgical repair. Differential Dx: Omphalocele—A sac covered by peritoneum and amniotic membranes in the base of the umbilical cord; associated with polyhydramnios and premature birth. Tx is surgical repair ASAP.

24. (G). Pyloric Stenosis occurs primarily in male infants with symptom presenting 2-3 weeks after birth. Ultrasound or Ba-X-ray confirms Dx and surgery corrects the stenosis. Duodenal atresia presents within hrs of birth with bilious vomiting upon feeding. Abdominal X-ray shows "double bubble" sign.

25. (K). Colic is paroxysmal, functional abdominal pain in an infant with unclear reasons, mostly < 3 y/a. Intussusception shows acute colicky abdominal pain, vomiting, fever and lethargy, and later with bloody stool and shock. P/E finds a sausage-shaped mass in the upper abdomen. Ba-study is both diagnostic and therapeutic.

26. (C). It's most likely cystic fibrosis (CF), an autosomal recessive disease due to the CFTR gene mutation on chromosome 7, causing Cl-channel deficiency, recurrent respiratory infections, and exocrine dysfunction. Dx is confirmed by sweat Cl test. 'A' is needed after Dx by 'C'. 'B' is for sprue disease. 'D' is better before 'A'. 'E' can be used initially for PKU, CF, galactosemia, etc.

27. (E). This is most likely a case of galactosemia complicated by E. coli pyelonephritis and sepsis. The original condition can be screened by testing reducing substances for galactosemia in the urine and confirmed by specific RBC GALT activity. Blood culture/sensitivity (C/S) is important to guide Tx of the infection. Reye syndrome is associated with recent aspirin use or viral infection in children, with similar symptom but mostly with elevated LFTs and blood ammonia levels; definitive Dx is by liver biopsy.

Chapter 14

EMERGENCY MEDICINE

Emergency Medicine is the specialty that focuses on the stabilization, diagnosis, and management of individuals with acute illness and injury. It also includes the management of trauma resuscitation, advanced cardiac life support, advanced airway management, poisonings, pre-hospital care and disaster preparedness.

SHOCK AND CARDIOPULMONARY RESUSCITATION

Shock, Cardiopulmonary Arrest, and Resuscitation—Important!

Etiology

Many conditions can cause cardiopulmonary shock and arrest, including:

(1) Cardiac—coronary or ischemic heart disease (major cause), cardiomyopathy, arrhythmia, hypertensive heart disease, and congestive heart failure.

(2) Non-cardiac—trauma, intoxication, infection, anaphylaxis, pulmonary embolism, suffocation, and drowning, etc. They are fatal and require emergent resuscitation.

Essentials of diagnosis

1. **Severe hypoxia and impending respiratory arrest**: Tachycardia, respiratory distress with cyanosis, stridor, agitation, confusion, exhaustion, and poor chest movement.

2. **Cardiogenic shock**: Pale, cold extremities, hypotension, pulmonary edema, jugular vein distention (JVD), heart murmurs (+/-); decreased cardiac output (CO); increased central venous pressure (CVP), systemic vascular resistance (SVR), and pulmonary capillary wedge pressure (PCWP). These signs mostly indicate more than 40% left ventricular myocardial infarction (LVMI, the No.1 cause) and over 80% in-hospital mortality.

3. **Hypovolemic shock**: Pale, cold extremities, an orthostatic BP drop > 20 mmHg; decreased cardiac output, CVP, and PCWP; increased SVR. Supine hypotension with systolic BP < 90 mmHg is a late sign of shock. Massive hemorrhage is the most common cause.

4. **Neurologic shock**: Warm extremities; decreased cardiac output, CVP, SVR, and PCWP. Spinal cord injury in the cervical or thoracic region is the most common cause.

5. **Septic shock**: Warm and faint; increased cardiac output; decreased CVP and SVR. E. coli and Staph-aureus are the most common pathogens.

6. **Lab tests**: Increased BUN/creatinine ratio, AST, and ALT.

Emergent management

1. **Follow the order of "ABC"** — "Airway, Breathing, and Circulation."

(A) Airway: Assessment of airway. Endotracheal intubation is immediately indicated for severe stridor, cyanosis, hypoxia, hypoventilation, chest wall exhaustion, apnea, or unconsciousness with vomiting.

Foreign-body airway obstruction: Back blows-chest thrusts (if < 1 y/a); Heimlich maneuver (if > 1 y/a).

(B) Breathing: Mechanical ventilation, along with high-flow oxygen. For cardiopulmonary arrest, compression-ventilation ratio is 5 to 1.

(C) Circulation: IV access and fluid, along with cardiac monitoring (by ECG). Large volumes of fluids are needed for hypovolemic shock.

2. **Cardiac arrest** (unresponsive, pulseless):

(1) **Ventricular (Ventr) fibrillation or Ventr-tachycardia** (V-tach): Immediate defibrillation with 200, 300 and 360j as needed. If the ventricular fibrillation (Ventr-fib) or Ventr-tachycardia persists, cardiopulmonary resuscitation (CPR), tracheal intubation, oxygen and IV lines are started. IV **amiodarone** (most effective) or lidocaine is the drug of choice for Ventr-fibrillation or Ventr-tachycardia. Other options are bretylium, $MgSO_4$, etc.

(2) **Asystole** (or pulseless electrical activity, PEA):

The treatment of choice is epinephrine (EP) or adrenaline (Ad) 1 mg IV push every 3 min; electrical therapy is not effective.

(3) **Reversible asystole:**

Hypoxia: Treat with oxygen and ventilation.

Hyper-K: Treat with IV 10% $CaCl_2$ and $NaHCO_3$.

Hypothermia (rectal T < 30°C): Supply warmed IV fluid, oxygen, etc.

ALTERED MENTAL STATUS

It refers to changes in consciousness from confusional states to coma, indicating a continuing status of the disease.

Etiology

Multiple: Trauma, stroke, heart failure, infections, intoxication, drug overdose, or metabolic disorders (hypoglycemia, hyper/hypo-Na, hyper/hypo-Ca, low Mg or P); through dysfunction of either the reticular activating system or bilateral cerebral cortices.

Clinical features, diagnosis, and treatment

1. History is usually not reliable from patients. Better sources include clinical manifestations and history provided by family members or friends.

2. **Physical examination (P/E) and treatment always begin with "ABC"** ("**A**irway, **B**reathing, and **C**irculation"). Vital signs should be recorded. Special attention should be paid to possible hypoventilation, pinpoint pupils, track marks, skull fracture, fruity breath, or paralysis. A complete neurologic exam should be done.

3. **Lab tests**: First test arterial blood gas (ABG) and glucose; then electrolytes, toxicology, and complete blood count (CBC).

4. **Diagnosis** is by clinical impression. In many cases, immediate **"IV thiamine (100 mg) + glucose (50%, 50 mL) + naloxone (2 mg) + oxygen" can be both diagnostic and therapeutic** without much adverse effects. Glucose with Vit-B1 is very effective in preventing permanent brain damage from hypoglycemia. Definitive treatment is targeting the specific cause.

Coma

Definition: It's a **status of unconsciousness** marked by a profound suppression of responses to external and internal stimuli.

Etiology

Usually catastrophic structural CNS injury or diffuse metabolic dysfunction caused by brain **infarction, hemorrhage, infection**, **inflammation**, herniation, abscesses, tumors, exogenous **toxins** (medicines, ethanol), electrolyte or metabolic disturbances, major seizures, etc.

Essentials of diagnosis

1. Obtain a complete history on the above etiology.

2. Perform thorough P/E and especially neurologic exams: mental status, breathing patterns, eye movements, pupil and motor response, response to noxious stimuli, etc.

3. Necessary lab tests: blood glucose, electrolytes (especially Ca), ABG, renal and liver function tests (LFTs), toxin screen, and blood or CSF culture if indicated.

4. Imaging: Should be performed before LP if it's risky of herniation. CT is best for suspected hemorrhage and MRI for non-hemorrhagic lesions.

5. **Diagnosis is made by history, P/E, important lab results,** and excluding other causes.

Treatment

1. Stabilize the patient: Following **"ABC"** ("Airway, breathing and circulation").

2. Treat the **reversible factors**: Empiric IV "**D**extrose + **N**aloxone + **T**hiamine (B1)", plus O_2 supply.

3. Treat **underlying causes** and prevent further damage.

Differential diagnosis

Delirium, syncope, "locked-in" syndrome, persistent vegetative state, etc.

Syncope:

It's defined as a sudden temporary loss of consciousness and postural tone due to cerebral hypoperfusion. Causes include cardiac (arrhythmias, valvular disease, cardiac tamponade, aortic dissection, and pulmonary embolism), and noncardiac (orthostatic hypotension, transient ischemic attack—TIA, vasovagal syndrome, metabolic abnormalities). Diagnosis is based on history, suspected causes, (+) signs, along with related lab tests (including ECG, echocardiogram, etc.) and "ruling-out".

"Locked-in" syndrome:

It's mostly caused by basilar artery thrombosis. Patients are alert and awake but cannot have verbal communication except moving the eyes. Usually it's associated with brain stem stroke, central pontine myelinolysis, advanced amyotrophic lateral sclerosis (ALS), etc.

Persistent vegetative state:

Patients have normal wake-sleep cycles but poor awareness of self or the environment--disorientation. It's mostly associated with hypoxic ischemic injury or diffuse cortical injury.

Delirium

Definition: It's a short and fluctuating conscious status with prominent confusion and disturbances in alertness.

Etiology

It's usually caused by an acute metabolic disorder or substance intoxication. Commonly associated medical conditions include systemic infections, metabolic diseases, hepatic/renal disease, head trauma or seizure, and rapidly changing levels of drugs in elderly and severely ill patients.

Essentials of diagnosis

1. Agitation, stupor, hallucinations, delusions, fear, emotional lability, and disturbed psychomotor activity.

2. **P/E:** Commonly shows motor abnormalities (incoordination, tremor, asterixis, and nystagmus) and incontinence, and signs of general medical conditions or drug effects.

3. **EEG** often reveals either generalized slowing of activity, fast-wave activity, or focal abnormalities.

Treatment

1. Correction of underlying disease is essential.

2. Frequent orientation, reassurance, emotional support, and protective physical restraints and treatment of dangerous agitation.

ANAPHYLAXIS

It's a life-threatening, IgE-mediated, abnormal, hypersensitive immune reaction that occurs upon re-exposure to a stimulus in a person with previous sensitization. Common causative agents include drugs (Penicillin is the No.1 cause), protein (foods, insect venoms), and plants.

Essentials of diagnosis

1. History of exposure to allergic agents and early manifestations of pruritic rash, a lump in the throat, hoarseness, abdominal cramps, or nausea and vomiting.

2. **P/E** may find signs of anaphylactic shock (tachycardia, hypotension, wheezing, stridor), dyspnea, wheezing, angioedema (facial swelling), and urticarial rashes. Lab tests have little value.

3. **Diagnosis is clinical**. Two common lethal complications are laryngeal edema and refractory hypotension.

Treatment

1. **Follow "ABC"** — "**A**irway, **B**reathing, and **C**irculation." Immediate injection of epinephrine (EP) 0.3 mL SC will relieve both the airway with angioedema and the hypotension. Perform intubation or cricothyroidotomy if necessary; supply oxygen and treat hypotension with IV EP and bolus N.S. (1-2 L in adults and 20 mL/kg in children).

2. Remove the offending substance if possible, and administer an antihistamine (diphenhydramine) routinely. Glucocorticoids can help alleviate late reactions.

TRAUMA AND INJURY

See "Chapter Surgery".

TOXICOLOGY

Toxicology is the study of the nature, effects, mechanisms, and detection of poisons and the treatment of poisoning. **Poisoning** is injury or death due to swallowing, inhaling, touching, or injecting various drugs, chemicals, venoms, or gases. Many substances (such as drugs and carbon monoxide) are poisonous only in high concentrations or dosages. Some others (such as cleaners) are dangerous only if ingested.

<u>Guidelines for Evaluation and Management of Poisoning</u>

Early recognition is the key to successful management. First, try to find out the nature of the toxin and the time ingested based on patient's history and manifestations, and then manage accordingly. If patient's vital signs are compromised, follow the above emergent principles of "ABC".

Induced vomiting

Ipecac can be used within 1-2 hours after ingestion; it is most useful at home but often too late and unnecessary in the hospital (emergency room). It only decreases absorption by < 30% after 1 hour of ingestion. Furthermore, it takes 15-20 min for the ipecac to work and delays the antidote administration.

Gastric lavage

It is best used within 1 hour of ingestion in patients with normal consciousness. It removes 50% of the pills at 1 hr of ingestion with good efficiency, and only 15% at 2 hours of ingestion, which is useless.

Both ipecac and lavage are contraindicated with (1) altered mental status (may cause aspiration); (2) ingestion of caustic substances (acids or alkalis, may cause injury of the esophagus and oropharynx).

Charcoal

It is harmless and the mainstay of therapy for most patients with 1-2 hours after toxic ingestion or after gastric emptying of the toxin. It works to accelerate the removal of already absorbed toxins. Charcoal administration is not dangerous but is ineffective for hydrocarbon ingestions (such as methanol or ethylene glycol). **Cathartics** (sorbitol, etc.) are only useful when used in combination with charcoal administration.

Whole bowel irrigation

It's the flushing-out of the GI contents with polyethylene glycol-electrolyte solution by a gastric tube. It has limited indications in large-volume pill ingestions such as iron, lithium, and drug-filled packets seen on an imaging exam.

Dialysis

This is only used when there are very serious symptoms such as hypotension, coma, or apnea, especially with renal or hepatic failure that compromise removal of toxins from the body.

Diuresis

It refers to administration of fluids and diuretics to accelerate urinary excretion may cause more harm such as pulmonary edema than benefits.

INTOXICATIONS OF SPECIAL TOXIC SUBSTANCES

Legal drugs usually cause more poisoning and deaths than illegal drugs because they are more available and less expensive. Common drugs causing acute overdose and poisoning are **acetaminophen, salicylates, iron, and TCAs** (antidepressants). Salicylates are a major source of chronic poisoning. Carbon monoxide (CO) poisoning kills more people among common toxins.

Carbon Monoxide (CO)

CO poisoning occurs with exposure to burning materials such as natural gas, gasoline (automobile exhaust), and wood, and with entrapment in fires causing smoke inhalation. It's the No.1 cause of death in fires. Low levels of CO poisoning are always present in tobacco smokers.

Pathogenesis

CO binding to hemoglobin (Hb) is more than 200 times stronger than that of oxygen, which acts like acute anemia. Carboxyhemoglobin (CO-Hb) decreases release of oxygen to tissues and inhibits mitochondria, which results in tissue hypoxia and eventual death.

Essentials of diagnosis

1. History of exposure to burning materials or environment, followed by "**cherry-red skin**" and dysfunctional manifestations of the lungs (dyspnea and tachypnea), the heart (chest pain, arrhythmia, and hypotension), and the CNS (headache, confusion, and syncope).

2. Lab tests: CO-Hb levels determine the severity and outcome. It may be fatal if it's higher than 50%. The PO_2 is usually normal. CPK may be elevated.

Treatment

1. **Urgently remove patient from intoxicating source and supply 100% oxygen to compete with CO-Hb**.

2. **Hyperbaric oxygen is indicated in**: (1) Significant CO poisoning; (2) Severe decompression sickness or arterial gas embolism; (2) Severe anemia, actinomycotic brain abscesses, acute crush injuries, prior radiation therapy, aggressive soft tissue infections, nonhealing ulcers, or compromised skin grafts and flaps.

Methemoglobinemia

It is the condition that methemoglobin is oxidized hemoglobin locked into the ferric state (brown color), which does not carry oxygen and causes similar effects and symptoms of CO-Hb. Methemoglobinemia is resulted from an idiosyncratic reaction of Hb with certain medicines (local anesthetics, nitrites, nitroglycerin, dapsone).

Essentials of diagnosis

1. History of taking certain drugs as mentioned above, followed by headache, tachypnea, dyspnea, cyanosis, confusion, and seizures.

2. Lab tests may show normal PO_2 and evidence of metabolic acidosis. The most accurate test is **obtaining a methemoglobin level**.

Treatment

1. In asymptomatic patients, usually methemoglobin levels are < 20%, discontinuation of the offending agent(s) and observation.

Methemoglobinemia

2. For symptomatic cases: (Commonly **dapsone, local anesthetic agents, aniline dyes, and high nitrate** levels in water supplies are administered). If severe, **100% oxygen** may help decrease tissue damage and save life, along with adjunctive blood transfusion or exchange transfusion.

3. **Methylene blue** (MB) may reduce the level of methemoglobin but should **not be used in patients with symptomatic methemoglobinemia and known G6PD deficiency**, since the reduction of methemoglobin by MB is dependent upon NADPH generated by G6PD.

Organophosphate (Insecticide)

It has **the same effects as nerve gas** (faster and more severe). It inhibits acetylcholinesterase (AChE) and ACh metabolism, and causes a marked increase in ACh level and cholinergic effects in the body. **Organophosphate poisoning from insecticides and suicides is one of the most common causes of poisoning worldwide.**

Essentials of diagnosis

1. History of exposure to toxic insecticides or nerve agents. Symptoms can be acute or chronic depending on the specific exposure.

2. Effects on muscarinic receptors (M-R) are memorized by the mnemonic **SLUDGEM** (Salivation, Lacrimation, Urination, Diarrhea, GI motility, Emesis, Miosis). Additional presentations include diaphoresis, bradycardia, hypoglycemia, excitation, bronchospasm, and even respiratory arrest.

3. Chronic effects include neuropsychiatric disorder, infertility, and growth retardation.

Treatment

1. **First administer anti-cholinergic atropine** to block the toxic cholinergic (M-receptor) effects immediately, **followed by specific antidote pralidoxime (or trimedoxime, obidoxime)** early to reactivate acetylcholinesterase.

2. Stop and remove sources of absorption if possible. Supportive care is also important.

Caustics or Corrosives (Acids and Alkali)

Oral ingestion, inhalation, or cutaneous/ocular contact with a wide range of corrosive substances (acids or alkali) causes mechanical damage to the oropharynx, esophagus, and stomach including perforation. The most common serious injury is from the oral ingestion of liquid drain cleaner.

Essentials of diagnosis

1. History of ingestion of caustics, followed by typical symptoms of oral pain, drooling, odynophagia, and abdominal pain. Esophageal injury with subsequent stricture formation may occur from either acid or alkali ingestion, and gastric perforation may occur. Usually, alkali injuries last longer and are more serious than acid injuries.

2. Upper endoscopy is the major diagnostic tool to access the extent of the injury.

Treatment

Caustics, Chemical Burns

1. Immediately wash out the mouth (or skin) **with large volumes of cold water. Do not ingest either acids or alkaline to neutralize the base or acid because this can cause further lesions!**

2. For ocular exposures, flush the eyes with large volumes of saline or water, followed by fluorescent staining to determine possible corneal injury. Charcoal, steroids, and antibiotics are not helpful.

Lead

Millions of children per year only in the US may have lead poisoning, which results from ingestion of lead in paint, soil, dust, drinking water, and/or old gasoline. GI absorption is increased by deficiencies of zinc, iron, and Ca. More than 80% of the body's lead is found in bone and excreted through stool.

Essentials of diagnosis

1. **Chronic**—Abdominal pain, anemia, renal disease, lethargy, headache, memory loss; "lead lines" at the metaphyseal plate of the long bone in children.

2. **Acute**—seizure and coma; ATN (acute tubule necrosis); mostly in children.

3. **Lab tests**: Blood lead levels > 10 mg/dL is most accurate for the diagnosis. An increased level of free erythrocyte protoporphyrin can be the best initial test. Sideroblastic anemia co-exists.

Treatment

1. Removal of exposure source.

2. Early use of chelating agents to remove lead from the body: **Succimer** is the preferred oral lead chelator and main therapy for lead poisoning, especially for children. IV **CaNa2EDTA, dimercaprol** (BAL) or **penicillamine** may be administered if it's severe.

Mercury

It is a heavy metal poisoning with toxic effects in high doses. The consumption of fish is the most common source of ingestion-related mercury poisoning.

Clinical features

Oral: neurologic toxicity—sensory impairment (vision, hearing, speech), disturbed sensation, lack of coordination, nervous, jittery, twitchy, or/and hallucinatory.

Inhaled: lung toxicity—irreversible interstitial fibrosis.

Treatment

1. Patients with **inorganic mercury ingestion** mostly require aggressive fluid resuscitation, given the high risk of severe gastrointestinal symptoms leading to shock and renal failure. All patients should be followed closely for electrolyte abnormalities or kidney injury from fluid and electrolyte losses.

2. A chelator is indicated when the urine or blood concentrations of mercury is > 100 ug/L. **Both dimercaprol and succimer** are effective.

Methanol (Methyl Alcohol)

The poisoning of methanol is a toxic effect of ingestion, inhalation, or absorption of methanol (through the skin), which may impair the CNS and cause characteristic visual deficiency or blindness, anion gap metabolic acidosis, shock, and even death. Methanol is found in antifreeze, varnish, and de-icing agents.

Diagnosis

It's confirmed by blood test of methanol levels.

Differentiation

Methanal (formaldehyde): It's a flammable, poisonous, colorless gas with a suffocating odor, used in the preparation of dyes, production of plastics, and synthetic resins. Ingestion of certain amount of its solution can cause severe corrosive GI injury, CNS damage, and even death.

Treatment

Alcohol dehydrogenase (ADH) inhibition therapy with fomepizole should be initiated in any suspicious poisoning with either methanol or ethylene glycol. Sodium bicarbonate is added with academia. If fomepizole is not available, **ethanol** infusion can be used to stop production of toxic metabolites. Vit B1 and B6 are helpful. Hemodialysis is indicated if it's severe.

Ethylene Glycol

Ethylene glycol is the primary ingredient in antifreeze and hydraulic brake fluid. It's a toxic, colorless, odourless liquid with a sweet taste, which may be accidentally consumed by children and dogs. Symptoms of poisoning (mainly by its metabolites) follow a three step progression: (1) vomiting and metabolic acidosis; (2) cardiovascular dysfunction; (3) finally acute kidney injury or failure.

Diagnosis

It's based on a history of ingestion and characteristic oxalate crystals and stones in the urine, hypocalcemia, anion gap metabolic acidosis, increased BUN:creatinine ratio, and renal failure, confirmed by urinary fluorescence test with an ultraviolet Wood's lamp, or blood test of the substance (most accurate).

Treatment

Treatment is the **same as for methanol poisoning—fomepizole or ethanol**, sodium bicarbonate, Vit B1, and Vit B6 are administered. Hemodialysis is indicated if it's severe.

Isopropyl Alcohol

It is a colorless, flammable chemical compound with a strong odor. It is the simplest example of a secondary alcohol. Isopropyl alcohol and its metabolite, acetone, act as CNS depressants. Symptoms of poisoning include flushing, headache, dizziness, CNS depression, nausea/vomiting, anesthesia, and coma.

Diagnosis

Poisoning is implied by a history of "alcohol ingestion" with ketosis but no anion gap acidosis, and confirmed by blood test of the chemical.

Treatment

Supportive care and **fomepizole** plus Vit B1 and B6 are effective. Hemodialysis is indicated if severe.

PEARLS — **Table 14-1: Special Toxins and Specific Antidotes**

Toxin:	Antidote
CO	100% O_2 and hyperbaric O_2
Methanol, ethylene glycol (antifreeze):	Fomepizole, ethanol + B_1, B_6; hemodialysis
Lead	Succimer, CaNa2EDTA, dimercaprol
Arsenic, gold, mercury	Succimer, Dimercaprol
Copper, arsenic, lead, gold	Penicillamine
Cyanide	Nitrite or thiosulfate-Na
Methemoglobinemia	Dapsone, aniline dye, methylene blue

INTERACTION, INTOXICATION AND DETOXIFICATION OF DRUGS

PEARLS — **Drug Interactions**

1. Drugs metabolised by p450:

Amide anesthetics, barbiturates, diazepam (BZ), nifedipine, propranolol (-olol), phenytoin, quinidine, theophylline, and warfarin

2. Drugs that induce p450:

Barbiturates, phenytoin, carbamazepine, and rifampin

3. Drugs that inhibit (Inh) p450:

Cimetidine, flutamide, and ketoconazole

4. Drugs that compete for albumin binding sites (increasing free T4, Ca, etc):

Aspirin, warfarin, and phenytoin

5. Drugs that cause hemolysis in G6PD deficient persons:

Aspirin, ibuprofen, sulfonamides, INH, and primaquine

6. Drugs that increase digoxin levels and toxicity:

Ca-blockers, amiodarone, and quinidine.

Acetaminophen (Tylenol)

Also known as **paracetamol,** its intoxication mainly causes liver injury, and is one of the most common causes of drug poisoning and acute liver failure.

Essentials of diagnosis

Patient has a history of ingestion (overdose) of the above drug, usually no symptoms in the first 24 hours, followed by GI symptoms (abdominal pain, nausea/vomiting, etc), CNS symptoms (headache, altered mental status), etc. Fulminant hepatitis (low blood sugar, low blood pH, easy bleeding, and hepatic encephalopathy) may occur but rare.

Treatment

Evaluate symptoms and blood level first before gastric lavage is determined. **Antidote is N-acetylcysteine**, usually administered if several grams of acetaminophen are ingested, and not administered if the overdose is over 24 hours or ALT is normal.

Salicylates (ASA, Aspirin)

Salicylate (aspirin) poisoning remains a common clinical problem and can be acute or chronic. The use of aspirin in children has declined since it was associated with Reye syndrome. A single overdose may cause acute poisoning. Chronic overdose is more commonly lethal in children and the elderly, with a mortality rate as high as 25%. No specific antidotes are currently available for aspirin poisoning.

Essentials of diagnosis

History of ingestion (overdose) of the above drug, followed by tinnitus, altered mental status, hyperventilation, respiratory alkalosis, metabolic acidosis, hyperpyrexia, cerebral edema, renal toxicity, and increased anion gap and PT (prothrombin time).

Treatment

NaHCO3 is usually administered to alkalinize the urine and increase excretion of aspirin. Watch out for aspirin-coexistent hypoglycemia and add glucose if needed. Dialysis is performed if it's serious.

Digoxin

Digoxin poisoning can occur acutely or over an extended period of use. Initial presentations may be nonspecific.

Essentials of diagnosis

1. History of ingestion (overdose) of digoxin, followed by GI upset (nausea/vomiting, diarrhea, abdominal pain), headache, dizziness, confusion, blurred vision, typical change in color vision ("yellow vision"), hyper-K, and characteristic cardiac arrhythmias (A-V block, ventricular inhibition). Toxicity is increased by hypo-K/hypo-Mg or hyper-Ca.

2. **Diagnosis**: The best initial tests are a serum K-level and an ECG (will show a depressed ST segment in all leads).

Treatment

1. Gastric lavage plus **active charcoal or cholestyramine** for GI decontamination.

2. Arrhythmia: **Atropine** for bradycardia; lidocaine or electrical cardioversion for severe arrhythmia.

3. **Correction of hypo-K, hypo-Mg, or hyper-Ca**, which can increase toxicity of digoxin.

4. For resistant cases or high levels of digoxin: **Anti-digoxin Fab** to remove digoxin rapidly.

Toxicity and Specific Treatment of Common Drugs

PEARLS—Table 14-2: Toxicity and Specific Treatment of Common Drugs

Drug / Toxicity and Specific Treatment/Antidotes
Acyclovir: Renal tube crystal and obstruction, may lead to renal failure. **Tx**: Large fluid intake.
ACE inhibitors (Captopril, etc.): **Cough** (#1 common), rash, proteinuria, angioedema, taste changes, hypo-Na, and hyper-K.
Aminoglycosides: Ototoxicity, nephrotoxicity, etc.
Amiodarone: Pulmonary fibrosis (also with bleomycin), arrhythmia (prolonged Q-T as with quinidine), peripheral deposit (skin discolor, photosensitivity), hypo/hyper-thyroidism
Amphotericin: Fever, chills, and nephrotoxicity; (Mnemonic: "Ampho-terror").
Amantadine: Ataxia and livedo reticularis.
Antimuscarinic, anticholinergic agents: Urinary retention, constipation, sedation, orthostatic hypotension, and paralysis. **Antidote: Physostigmine**.
Antipsychotics: **Extrapyramidal symptoms** (dystonia, akathisia, and convulsion) —**Treat with propranolol** or diazepam; neuroleptic malignant syndrome (**NMS**) —**Treat with dantrolene** +/- bromocriptine or amantadine; anticholinergic effects—Treat with physostigmine.
Azathioprine: Dose-related diarrhea, liver toxicity, and WBC decrease.
AZT: Thrombocytopenia and megaloblastic anemia.
Benzodiazepines (BZ): Psychological and physical dependence; addictive effects with other CNS depressants. Antidote: **Flumazenil**. Caution: Flumazenil can cause seizures in chronic BZ-dependent patients.
Beta-R-blockers (-olol): Asthma exacerbation, A-V block, CHF, masking of hypoglycemia, and impotence. **Antidote: Glucagon,** IVF, *bradycardia, HoTN, hypoglycemia, altered mental status, seizures* 3, atropine
Bile acid resins: GI upset and malabsorption of lipid-soluble vitamins and medicines.

Clonidine: α₂ agonist that tx HTN. OD: ↓ sympathetic activity mimicing opioid OD.

Ca-blockers: Cardiac depression, peripheral edema, and constipation. *Not N, hyperglycemia*
Carbamazepine: Agranulocytosis, aplastic anemia, and induction of p450.
Chloramphenicol: Aplastic anemia and grey baby syndrome.
Clonidine: Severe rebound headache and hypertension.
Clozapine: Agranulocytosis.
Corticosteroids: Mania (acute toxicity), immunosuppression, bone mineral loss, thin skin, and easy bruising, and myopathy (chronic use).
Cisplatin: Nephrotoxicity and acoustic nerve damage.
Colchicine, meclocycline, and lithium: Renal desensitivity to ADH (causing renal DI).
Cyclophosphamide: Myelosuppression and hemorrhagic cystitis.
Cyclosporine: Nephrotoxicity, hyper-K, hypertension, gingival hyperplasia, hirsutism, and tremor.
Doxorubicin: Cardiotoxicity.
Fluoroquinolones (quinolones): Cartilage damage in children.
Fluconazole (-azoles): Inhibits liver p450 enzymes and increases toxicity of other drugs metabolized by p450.
Furosemide: Hypo-K, Hypo-NaCl, ototoxicity, and nephritis.
Gemfibrozil, -statins: Myositis and reversible hepatic enzyme increase.
Halothane: Hepatotoxicity.
Heparin: Bleeding trends, thrombocytopenia, and drug-drug interactions. **Antidote: Protamine**.
Hydralazine: Orthostatic hypotension and lupus syndrome (also for procainamide).
Isoniazid (INH): B6-deficient neuritis, hepatoxicity (rare), and seizure (overdose). **Tx**: Stop INH and use B6.
Iron salts: GI upset and bleeding, hyperglycemia, and **"3 Cs"** (cardiotoxicity, convulsion, and coma). **Antidote: Deferoxamine**.
MAOIs: Hypertension crisis with tyramine (in cheese, wine, etc.).
Methyldopa: Hemolysis, lupus syndrome, and sexual dysfunction.
Metronidazole: Disulfiram reaction (with alcohol) and CN8 toxicity.
Opiates: Respiratory inhibition, miosis ("pinpoint pupils"), and coma. Antidote: **Naloxone**.
Penicillin: Anaphylaxis. **Tx:** "ABC", epinephrine (**EP**), and antihistamine.
Phenytoin: Diplopia, nystagmus, ataxia, gingival hyperplasia, and hirsutism.

Prazosin: 1st-dose hypotension and priapism.
Quinidine: Arrhythmia, cinchonism (headache and tinnitus), and thrombocytopenia. **Tx: NaHCO₃**.
SSRIs: **More sexual dysfunction, GI** stimulation (N/V) and **CNS toxicity** (headache, insomnia and tremor) than TCAs. Toxicity increases with MAOIs or TCAs. **Treatment of overdose**: Use BZs (**lorazepam**) for agitation, tremor, or seizures; NaHCO₃ for arrhythmia; avoidance of serotonergic medications.
tachycardia, AMS, sedation **TCAs**: **More serious adverse effects than SSRIs**— "**3 Cs**": Cardiotoxicity (typical QRS widening in ECG), Convulsion, and Coma; anticholinergic effects (dry mouth, constipation, and urinary retention). **Tx: NaHCO₃** is effective in treating arrhythmia (but not increasing excretion of TCAs); use **lorazepam** for seizures.
Theophylline: Ventr-arrhythmia, GI upset, hyper-ventilation, convulsion, hypo-K, hypo-Mg, hypo-P, hyper-Ca, and hyperglycemia. **Tx:** 1. **Active charcoal**; 2. hemodialysis; lorazepam for convulsion; amiodarone for ventricular arrhythmia; avoid lidocaine.
Thiazides: Mnemonics— "**3 lows 3 highs**": Hypo-K, -Na, and -Cl; Hyper-glycemia, -lipidemia, and -uricemia.
TPA, streptokinase: Bleeding tendency. **Antidote: Aminocaproic acid**.
Valproic acid: Neural tube defects (congenital) and hepatotoxicity (rare).
Vancomycin: CN8 toxicity, nephrotoxicity, and "red man syndrome" (due to histamine release, not allergy).
Warfarin: Bleeding tendency, teratogen, and drug-drug interactions. **Antidote: Vit-K** or FFP (fresh frozen plasma), recovering in 1-2 days.

THERMAL INJURIES

Burns

Burn injuries can be divided into several types. Fire injury is the most dangerous one because respiratory injury and infection are usually involved. The most common cause of death from fire injury is smoke inhalation and CO poisoning in a closed environment.

Degrees of skin burns

1st-degree: The skin may be discoloured but is fully intact (no blister); with mild pain.

2nd-degree: Blister formation with severe pain.

3rd-degree: Deeper burns, with destroyed skin appendages (such as sweat glands, hair follicles, even pain receptors) and painlessness.

Body surface area (BSA) of skin burns

BSA% affected by skin injury is used to guide fluid resuscitation efforts after burns and is estimated using the "**Rule of 9s**." The head and arms are 9% each; the chest, back, and legs are 18% each; the genitalia or perineum is 1%; one hand's width is about 1% (to estimate patchy burns). Hand's width is used to estimate the BSA% of patchy burns.

Burns

Essentials of diagnosis

1. Altered mental status, headache, dyspnea, and chest pain suggest severe CO poisoning. Stridor, hoarseness, and dyspnea imply laryngeal edema and airway compromise.

2. Severe burns are defined as combined 2nd- and 3rd-degree burns > 20% or 3rd-degree burns > 5% of BSA.

3. **Lab tests**: (1) Tests of levels of carboxyhemoglobin (CO-Hb) and amylase (from secondary pancreatitis) to determine if 100% oxygen should be given.

(2) With suspension, CXR and especially bronchoscopy can help determine the exact extent of respiratory injury (in a closed building).

(3) Foley catheter helps determine the adequacy of fluid resuscitation.

Treatment

1. **Follow "ABC"** (Airway, Breathing, and Circulation): If patient has severe respiratory injury (laryngeal edema), intubate the patient before the airway is blocked.

2. If the **CO-Hb level** is significantly elevated (**> 5-10%**), **100% oxygen** must be given.

3. **Fluid resuscitation:**

Day 1 (first 24 hours)—based on the **Parkland** Memorial Hospital formula: **4 ml/kg x BSA% burned**. Ringer's lactate is the preferred fluid. Give half the fluid in the first 8 hours, 1/4 in the next 8 hours, and 1/4 in the final 8 hours.

Day 2: Administration of ½ **of the total amount, with colloids**.

Day 3: A brief diuresis, no further fluid; urine > 4 mL/kg/hour.

It's important for adequate IV fluid to maintain a urine output > 0.5-1 mL/kg/hr. Higher amounts are needed in patients with respiratory tract burns, electrical burns, or recent escharotomies.

4. **Administer preventive H2 blockers** (for stress ulcer) and **topical antibiotics** (silver sulfadiazine), but **do not use steroids**.

5. **Escharotomy** is useful in circumferential burns to avoid limb circulation decrease. Do not break blisters. Skin grafting may be needed for severe 3rd-degree burns (< 40% BSA).

Heat Disorders

They are divided into two main groups: exertional and nonexertional. Exertional disorders include heat cramps, heat exhaustion, and heat stroke. Nonexertional disorders are malignant hyperthermia and neuroleptic malignant syndrome (See "NEUROLOGY" chapter).

I. Heat Cramps

I. Heat cramps

This is a mild heat disorder that can happen to any healthy person with fluid and electrolyte depletion. The patient has painful muscular contractions lasting a few minutes. Sweating and neurologic functions as well as body temperature (T) are all normal.

Treatment: Rest along with oral fluid with salts.

II. Heat Exhaustion   *prolonged exercise*
Hyperthermia w normal mental status, sweat, N/V, HA, dizziness, tachy ♥, HoTN

It's a more severe heat disorder, with more systemic symptom (headache and anxiety) and slightly elevated body temperature. Sweating and neurologic functions are still normal. It can progress to heat stroke if not treated.
cool pt (Air conditioning, cool water shower) Salt-containing beverages

Treatment: Oral fluid with electrolyte supplements, plus IV hydration if the patient is too weak.

III. Heat Stroke   *CNS dysfxn*

It's a very severe and potentially lethal heat disorder. Most patients have lost the ability to sweat and remove heat from the body, resulting in a high body temperature, and symptoms of nausea, disorientation, blurred vision, confusion, and seizures. Anuria, DIC, and lactic acidosis may also occur.

Lab tests: Rhabdomyolysis, and increased CBC, WBC, and BUN:creatinine ratio.

Treatment: (1) Bolus IV fluid replacement and rapid cooling of the body. The body should be placed in a cool environment with a fan and sprayed with water. Ice water immersion should not be used as it can result in hypothermia.

(2) Convulsions or shivering can be treated effectively with chlorpromazine and diazepam.

Hypothermia

It's defined as a reduction of core body T < 35^{0}C (normal T = 37^{0}C, rectal); T < 30^{0}C is severe hypothermia. The most common cause is **alcohol intoxication in the elderly**. Patients usually have lethargy, confusion, and weakness. Very severe hypothermia can cause death from arrhythmia. Typical ECG results are J-point elevation, ventricular tachycardia, and even ventricular fibrillation.

Treatment

Patient can be effectively treated with a warm bed, bath, or heating blanket. Warmed IV fluids or humidified oxygen can be administered in severe cases. Be watchful to avoid fast and excessive re-warming, which can lead to arrhythmias.

DROWNING

It's often associated with alcohol and drug abuse. The presentations depend on the severity of the injury, varying from cyanosis, coughing, and signs of pulmonary edema, to coma or death.

Treatment

1. Time is crucial to save patient's life. Remove patient from water and follow resuscitation "ABC".

[handwritten: drownings — Sx. Maintain oxygenation & ventilation. continuous pulse ox. suppl. O2, bronchodilators]

2. Endotracheal intubation and O2 can be used as needed. *[handwritten: CXR, EKG, ABG, CBC, e⁻, drug screen]*

3. Continuous positive pressure mechanical ventilation (**CPPMV**): It's the most effective treatment for hypoxia. *[handwritten: asx: observe ≥ 8 hr, continuous pulse ox, D CXR @ end, serial exam.]*

[handwritten right margin: Aspiration of water — direct tissue damage → inflam — washout of alveolar surfactant → alveolar collapse — disruption of osmotic gradient at alveolar-capillary membrane → ↑ fluid permeability]

VENOMOUS BITES

Snake Bites

Most snakes are non-poisonous, and deaths from venomous snakebites are < 20% and mostly caused by rattlesnakes. Lethal toxins include hemolytic toxin (causing hemolysis and DIC), cardiotoxin (causing heart failure), and neurotoxin (causing muscular and respiratory paralysis). Proteases and lipase in the venom result in local tissue damage (local wound).

Treatment

1. **Transport** the patient immediately to the nearest medical unit, and **immobilize** the patient to decrease the spread of venom through the blood-lymphatics, which increases with muscular contraction. Place a compression bandage to decrease lymphatic flow, but avoid making it so tight as to decrease venous flow.

2. **Antivenin**: It binds and removes toxins. Be aware of potential anaphylactic reactions with horse serum.

3. **Supportive treatment**: Supportive ventilation and IV fluid for hypotension may be needed. Avoid ineffective or risky treatment such as suction of the bites, incision, tourniquets, or ice immersion.

Spider Bites

It is an unusual type of injury and the effects of most confirmed spider bites are trivial, even though nearly all species of spider are venomous.

Clinical features and diagnosis

1. Patient usually feels a sudden, **sharp pain as if "Stepping on a nail or a piece of glass."**
2. **Black widow bite**: Causing a neurotoxic condition known as **Latrodectism**—abdominal pain, muscle pain, and hypo-Ca.
3. **Brown recluse bite**: Causing a condition called **Loxoscelism— "necrotic arachnidism"** —local skin necrosis, bulla, and blebs.

Treatment
Black widow bite: Administration of Ca and antivenin.
Brown recluse bite: Debridement, corticosteroids, and dapsone.

Cat, Dog, and Human Bites

Pathogens in cat and dog bites—**Pasteurella** multocida is the most common one. Rabies (virus) is rare but fatal. Rabies vaccination is required if patient is bit by a raccoon, a stray dog that cannot be observed or diagnosed, or a dog with bizarre behavior or altered mental status.

Pathogens in human bites: S. aureus and Eikennella (Bacteroides) corrodens are common.

Treatment

1. **Empirical therapy with amoxicillin plus clavulanate.**
2. Give a booster tetanus vaccination if the last immune shot was more than 5 years ago.

Chapter 14 High-yield Questions (Combined into the next chapter)

Chapter 15

SURGERY

TRAUMA AND INJURY

Advanced Trauma Life Support

Advanced Trauma Life Support (ATLS) is a training program for medical doctors in the management of acute trauma cases, developed by the American College of Surgeons. **The most common causes of death in trauma patients in the hospital are subdural and epidural hematomas, major blood loss, pneumothorax, hemothorax, spleen or liver rupture, and pelvic fractures.**

Management— "ABC":

1. **Airway:** The airway is normal if the patient is conscious and speaking in a normal tone of voice. The airway will soon be compromised if there is a **relaxed tongue** (the most common cause), an expanding hematoma or emphysema in the neck. The airway needs to be secured if the patient is unconscious or the breathing is noisy.

(1) For a relaxed tongue: Perform chin lift or jaw thrust.

(2) For an unconscious, apneic patient: Perform cricothyroidotomy if the patient is in the field or in the emergency room with an orotracheal intubation to prevent aspiration, with monitoring of pulse oximetry.

(3) For a patient with head injury: Keep the neck immobilized at all times until cervical spine injury is ruled out.

2. **Breathing:** It's normal (Nl) if breath sounds are heard on bilateral (B/L) chest and pulse oximetry is satisfactory. Oxygen is usually supplied for a severe trauma case. Absent breath sounds may indicate a hemothorax or pneumothorax, which requires immediate chest tube insertion.

3. **Circulation:** A rapid, flimsy pulse with low BP indicates severe bleeding (or **hemorrhagic shock**) and the need of immediate fluid infusion.

(1) For external bleeding, first use direct pressure to stop it; for suspected internal bleeding, take the patient to the operation room (OR) for immediate exploration. Meanwhile, place two large-bore peripheral IV lines. If it's too difficult, use a percutaneous femoral vein catheter or saphenous vein cut down. If this fails in children, use intraosseous lines.

(2) Fluid: IV infusion of 2-3 liters of Ringer's lactate or normal saline (N.S.), and type-matched (or type "O") blood (packed RBC) if available, until urinary output reaches 0.5-2 mL/kg/hr. Maintain central venous pressure (CVP) < 15 mmHg, and avoid vasopressors or $NaHCO_3$ in the treatment of hypovolemic shock.

CHEST TRAUMA

Pericardial Tamponade

Also known as **cardiac tamponade**, it is an acute type of pericardial effusion in which blood, fluid or clot accumulates in the pericardium, resulting in slow or rapid compression of the heart. It's mostly caused by penetrating wounds medial to the left nipple. The classical **Beck's triad**—three signs are **hypotension**, jugular-venous distension (**JVD**) on inspiration, and **distant (muffled) heart sounds**. Other clinical signs include tachycardia, pulsus paradoxus or absent pulse, and shock. It can rapidly progress to death without emergent treatment. Diagnosis is usually clinical. If time allows, echocardiography is the diagnostic test of choice.

Treatment

Supply oxygen and monitoring, and perform an emergent evacuation of the pericardial sac by pericardiocentesis, tube, pericardial window, or open thoracotomy. Anti-shock/heart failure therapies with fluids and blood products following the evacuation are also important.

Rib Fracture

Fractures of the first and second ribs may be more associated with head and facial injuries than other rib fractures. The middle ribs are the ones most commonly fractured. Fractures usually occur from direct blows or from indirect crushing injuries. The most commonly fractured ribs are the 7th and 10th. A lower rib fracture has the complication of potentially injuring the diaphragm, which could result in a diaphragmatic hernia. Rib fractures are usually very painful with breathing, and the continuous pain can be deadly in the elderly, causing hypoventilation, atelectasis, and pneumonia.

Essentials of diagnosis

1. History of a major injury followed by pain with breathing or movement.

2. Physical examination (P/E) finds flail chest, a grating sound with breathing or movement.

3. CXR or CT scan confirms the fracture.

Treatment

1. Symptomatic and effective analgesic therapy by local nerve block is the mainstay of treatment.

2. Large-area chest trauma can cause multiple rib fractures, resulting in flail chest and paradoxical breathing. It may be necessary to use a respirator and bilateral chest tubes with occlusive dressing to prevent tension pneumothorax.

Complication

Pulmonary contusion, penetration, aortic injury, flail chest, atelectasis, and pneumonia.

Pulmonary Contusion

It is usually caused directly by **blunt chest trauma** but can also result from explosion injuries or a shock wave associated with penetrating trauma. The use of seat belts and airbags reduces the risk to vehicle occupants.

Essentials of diagnosis

Pulmonary contusion can appear immediately after chest trauma or delay for 1-2 days, with typical manifestations of **chest pain, hemoptysis, and cyanosis**. Lab findings include deteriorating blood gases and "**white-out lungs**" on CXR.

Treatment

The contused lung is very sensitive to fluid overload, and thus the treatment includes supportive care, fluid restriction, use of colloids (plasma or albumin, not saline) and diuretics. Arterial blood gases (ABG) must be monitored.

Myocardial Contusion

- blunt chest trauma can induce myocardial edema, hemorrhage, & necrosis.
- can cause structural, ischemic, & electrical complications
- 24-48 hr continuous cardiac monitoring
- significant findings, ie. arrhythmias, HoTN, HF) = echo

It is an uncommon consequence of **blunt trauma** to the anterior chest wall and injuries may include rupture of the ventricular or atrial wall, septum, or a valve; cardiac dysfunction; arrhythmia. The right heart is more frequently affected due to its anatomic location as the most anterior surface of the heart. Myocardial contusion should be suspected in **sternal fractures**, although it's rare. **ECG monitoring** is the best way of diagnosis and 4-6 hours of observation is usually sufficient in a hemodynamically stable patient. Cardiac enzyme tests may be less reliable.

Treatment

Give supportive care and treat arrhythmias and other complications. Immediate surgical consultation is required for severe injury, such as a valve tear, or septal or ventricular wall rupture.

Pneumothorax

A primary spontaneous pneumothorax (PSP) is one that occurs without a precipitating event in a person who does not have known lung disease. Most patients with PSP actually have unrecognized lung disease, with the pneumothorax resulting from rupture of a subpleural bleb. The incidence is increased in men, smokers, and patients with a family history of PSP.

A secondary spontaneous pneumothorax (SSP) is one that occurs as a complication of underlying lung disease, most commonly COPD.

Spontaneous pneumothorax mostly shows acute moderate dyspnea and pleuritic chest pain at rest.

Traumatic pneumothorax is usually caused by penetrating trauma by a broken rib or a penetrating weapon. Typical manifestations include moderate painful dyspnea and absent breath sounds on one side of the thorax, which is hyperresonant to percussion.

Pneumothorax   ↑ tightness over affected hemi thorax on chest transillumination

Diagnosis of plain pneumothorax is established by detection of a visceral pleural line on the chest X-ray of a patient with underlying lung disease or injury. If the diagnosis is unclear, a chest CT scan may confirm diagnosis.

→ ↑ intrapleural pressure ⇒ ↓ venous return & ↓ CO.

pPnx risk by ↑ transpulm pressure

Tension pneumothorax is a life-threatening injury with increased air pressure inside the pleural space. The potential risk of an expanding pneumothorax is greater in patients receiving positive pressure ventilation during surgery or for long-term pulmonary support. The patient typically has **dyspnea, JVD, hyperresonance of the chest on the lesion side** (mediastinal shift to opposite side), **hypotension, and hypoxia/cyanosis** or shock. **Diagnosis of tension pneumothorax is clinical and this emergency requires immediate decompression** without wasting time for CXR or ABG results. In the absence of hemodynamic compromise, the suspicion for tension pneumothorax should ideally be confirmed on CXR prior to thoracostomy. Accumulation of intrapleural air can cause ♡ displacement, mediastinal deviation

Treatment of plain pneumothorax

1. Clinically unstable patients with SSP require an upper-anterior chest tube connected to underwater seal. emergency needle thoracostomy

2. For clinically stable, asymptomatic patients with a very small pneumothorax, close observation (+/-oxygen) in hospital may be sufficient. Onset of symptoms or an enlarging pneumothorax would be indications for pleural drainage.

Treatment of tension pneumothorax

Immediately insert a **large-bore needle or IV catheter (24 or 28 Fr) into the upper pleural space for decompression** followed by a chest tube connected to underwater seal.

Hemothorax and Traumatic Aortic Injury

Hemothorax is mostly caused by penetrating trauma similar to pneumothorax, resulting in blood in the pleural space. The major different sign from pneumothorax is that **the affected side is dull to percussion**. Diagnosis is made by **CXR showing a liquid level** after trauma. Bedside this, ultrasonography is a critical tool for diagnosing traumatic pericardial tamponade. Ultrasonography is more sensitive for diagnosing pneumothorax than CXR and is also useful for diagnosing hemothorax.

Blunt aortic injury (BAI): Patients involved in high-energy, rapid-deceleration blunt chest trauma are at significant risk for it. It's often a "hidden injury" occurring at the junction of the arch and the descending aorta. Almost 80 percent of BAIs cause immediate death. No clinical signs, P/E findings or CXR results possess adequate sensitivity or specificity for BAI. The following CXR findings increase the likelihood of BAI and the need for further investigation, usually a chest CT scan:

(1) Wide mediastinum; (2) Obscured aortic knob or abnormal aortic contour; (3) Left hemothorax; (4) Deviation of trachea or nasogastric tube rightward; (5) Wide left paravertebral stripe.

Traumatic rupture of the aorta: It should be suspected after high-energy, rapid-deceleration chest trauma, particularly with "firm chest bone fractures" (first rib, scapula, or sternum) and the above CXR findings. It's usually asymptomatic until the hematoma contained by the adventitia bursts and results in sudden death. **Spiral CT** will confirm a widened mediastinum.

Hemothorax ; traumatic Aortic injury

Treatment

1. Hemothorax: Place a large-bore tube (> 28Fr) into the lower chest to evacuate blood and prevent empyema. The pulmonary hemorrhage will mostly stop by itself as a low-pressure system. Surgery (thoracotomy) is rarely needed, unless >1,500 ml of total blood or > 600 mL/6hrs is drained out.

2. Traumatic rupture of the aorta: Emergent surgical repair in time is lifesaving! Morbidity (cardiovascular, pulmonary, and renal complications) and mortality rates following open thoracic aortic aneurysm repair remain high.

3. Malignant effusion: The management depends on the patient's symptoms and rate of re-accumulation. A small-bore catheter (8 to 18 Fr) placed under ultrasound or CT guidance is usually adequate to drain a malignant pleural effusion or perform pleurodesis.

4. Empyema: The initial treatment is antibiotics covering anaerobics plus surgical decortication versus chest tube. A chest tube is usually effective within clinical stage 1-2 of the empyema whereas surgery is needed beyond stage 2.

Pneumohemothorax

It is the combination of pneumothorax and hemothorax, also caused by penetrating trauma to the chest. **CXR (Image 127) usually shows increased lucency of the injured hemi-thorax with a liquid level, and mediastinal shift to opposite side.**

Treatment

Treatment for this condition is the same as for hemothorax and pneumothorax independently. Usually surgery is required to close off whatever injuries caused the blood and air to enter the cavity (e.g., stabbing, broken ribs).

Diaphragmatic Injury

Diaphragmatic injury or rupture is uncommon. There is usually a history of the left chest or abdominal trauma followed by persistent pain and respiratory distress. P/E usually reveals reduced or absent breath sounds on the left chest. Both P/E and CXR will demonstrate **bowel in the left chest**. CXR may also display the inserted **NG tube curling up** into the left chest. **Early diagnosis is important** because delayed diagnosis and management may cause herniation and strangulation of abdominal organs, which can be life-threatening. Penetrating injury usually leads to smaller rents which are more likely to be missed compared with blunt rupture which typically causes large radial tears.

Treatment

Immediate surgical repair is required and usually performed from the abdomen in conjunction with abdominal exploration to identify and repair other associated injuries. Hemodynamically stable patients with diaphragmatic injury with negative physical exam and imaging results can be observed.

- esophageal rupture : dyw esophago graphy w
  H2O- soluble contrast
  - spillage of GI contents can cause systemic
    inflamm. response (tachy cardia, fever)   from esophageal rupture

Tracheobronchial Injury

Tracheobronchial injury is damage to the tracheobronchial tree (the airway structure involving the trachea and major bronchi). It can result from blunt or penetrating trauma to the neck or chest, inhalation of harmful fumes or smoke, or aspiration of liquids or objects. Though rare, it may cause obstruction of the airway with resulting life-threatening respiratory insufficiency. About 50% of cases are associated with other injuries in the chest. Early diagnosis is important to prevent complications, which include stenosis of the airway, respiratory tract infection, and damage to the lung tissue. Signs and symptoms vary based on the location and severity of the injury, commonly including dyspnea, dysphonia, coughing, and abnormal breath sounds.

Tracheobronchial rupture is characterized by a history of major trauma followed by subcutaneous emphysema in the upper chest and lower neck, or by a large "**air leak**" from a chest tube. **CXR reveals air in the tissues**, and fiberoptic bronchoscopy confirms the lesion and allows intubation to secure an airway beyond the lesion.

Treatment

It is usually difficult to diagnose and treat. Follow "ABC". Emergent surgical repair is required.

Air Embolism

Small amounts of air often get into the blood circulation accidentally during surgery and other procedures (e.g., from an IV fluid line), but most of these air emboli enter the veins and are stopped at the lungs, and thus a venous air embolism showing symptoms is rare. A large amount of arterial air embolism in the coronary artery or cerebral circulation can be fatal. Surgery, trauma, vascular interventions, and barotrauma from mechanical ventilation and diving are the most common causes of air embolism.

Essentials of diagnosis

1. An injured or intubated patient suddenly shows respiratory distress (venous air embolism) and/or neurologic deficits—loss of coordination, control of bodily functions, vertigo, convulsions, or consciousness (arterial embolism). If severe enough, cessation of breathing and death may occur.

2. A large bubble of air in the heart will present with a constant "machinery" murmur, usually in an intubated patient. Air embolism is typically a retrospective clinical diagnosis, based upon a high index of suspicion and the exclusion of other life-threatening processes.

Treatment and prevention

1. Patients should be rapidly assessed for ABC, and appropriate supportive therapies should be administered (e.g., high flow oxygen, mechanical ventilation, volume resuscitation, vasopressors, advanced cardiac life support).

2. Administration of **high percentage oxygen** is recommended. **Trendelenburg position** with left side down and cardiac massage are effective prevention and treatment.

ABDOMINAL TRAUMA

It can be blunt or penetrating trauma. Initial clinical assessment in an unstable patient is to confirm or exclude the abdomen as a source of concealed bleeding that requires immediate surgery, for example by using Focused Assessment with Sonography for Trauma (FAST). Secondary survey preferably by the same surgeon may be necessary. Exploratory laparotomy is generally necessary for most penetrating trauma to the abdomen, regardless of the hemodynamic status.

PEARLS—**Indications for trauma laparotomy:**

(1) Intra-abdominal bleeding;

(2) Gunshot wound;

(3) Hemodynamically unstable from stab wounds and blunt abdominal trauma;

(4) Hollow viscus injury on CT or signs of peritonism;

(5) Penetrating truncal injuries with potential peritoneal injury.

Gunshot Wound to the Abdomen

Intra-abdominal injuries from gunshot wounds are generally defined as below the level of the nipple line, and they tend to cause significant damage to major intra-abdominal structures—the small bowel (50%), colon (40%), liver (30%) and abdominal vascular structures (25%). Important historical information includes the number of shots heard, the type of gun used, the position of the patient when shot, and the distance of the patient from the gun.

Diagnosis and treatment

X-ray film and CT scan with IV contrast are usually performed in patients with abdominal gunshot wounds to visualize the bullet path and solid organ injuries. Exploratory laparotomy is generally required for accurate diagnosis and repair of the intra-abdominal injury (instead of "bullet removal"), particularly with evidence of hemodynamic instability, peritonitis, or evisceration.

Stab Wound to the Abdomen

Stab wound is situational and the treatment is individualized based on the specific injury. Visceral bleeding or protrusion may be present.

Diagnosis and treatment

1. Exploratory laparotomy is required for accurate diagnosis and repair of the intra-abdominal injury.

2. In the absence of the above, finger exploration of the wound in the ER and observation may be sufficient.

Blunt Trauma to the Abdomen

It's commonly seen in motor vehicle accidents and working situations, etc.

Blunt Abd Trauma

Diagnosis and treatment

1. Indications of abdominal trauma include nausea, vomiting, fever, hematuria (kidney contusion), abdominal pain, tenderness, distension, or rigidity to the touch, and bowel sounds may be diminished or absent. Abdominal guarding or pneumoperitoneum may be an indication of rupture of a hollow organ. Associated trauma may include rib fractures, vertebral fractures, pelvic fractures, and injuries to the abdominal wall. The initial clinical examination of the abdomen can often be misleading for the unwary. Initially blood may cause little peritoneal irritation, and drugs, alcohol, head injury and other distracting injuries may act to mask abdominal signs.

2. **CT scan** is the most accurate means of diagnosis for abdominal bleeding in a stable patient.

3. It requires **exploratory laparotomy with signs of peritoneal irritation** (an acute abdominal condition) or signs of internal bleeding (hemorrhagic shock without obvious external blood loss).

4. **Liver rupture** is the most common cause of intra-abdomen bleeding in blunt abdominal trauma, but **spleen rupture** causes the most significant and fatal bleeding. Best efforts should be made to repair the spleen rather than remove it (especially in children) to reserve its immunologic functions. If the spleen is smashed into pieces, it has to be removed to save life.

5. Other conditions are treated accordingly. Surgery is not necessary if the patient has minor internal injuries and prompt recovery from fluid resuscitation.

PELVIC AND UROGENITAL TRAUMA

Pelvic Fracture and Hematoma

Pelvic fracture is a disruption of the bony structure of the pelvis, including the hip bone, sacrum and coccyx. The most common cause in elderly is a fall, but the most significant fractures involve high-energy forces such as a motor vehicle accident, cycling accidents, or a fall from significant height. **It may produce significant invisible internal bleeding.**

Pelvic hematoma is usually caused by gynecologic surgical injury, trauma, ruptured ectopic pregnancy, ruptured abdominopelvic aneurysm, anticoagulant overdose, or a coagulation disease.

Essentials of diagnosis

1. Rectal exam and proctoscopy for rectal injury.
2. Pelvic exam for vaginal injury in women.
3. Retrograde urethrogram for urethral or bladder injury.
4. Diagnosis of pelvic fracture and bleeding is based on clinical features and evidence of hypovolemic shock with a pelvic injury in the absence of other bleeding sources; X-ray and CT scan may be necessary aids. Ultrasonography is helpful for hematoma.

Treatment

1. Emergent treatment consists of advanced trauma life support management. However, treatment of pelvic fractures with significant bleeding is very difficult, usually with **external fixation** as the first choice. After stabilisation, the pelvis may be surgically reconstructed. Patients with severe pelvic fractures have multiple risk factors for deep vein thrombosis and should receive thromboprophylaxis.

2. **Pelvic hematoma**: If it's not expanding, hematoma should be left alone for natural resolution and follow-ups. Otherwise, surgery may be indicated.

Urologic Injuries

Both blunt and penetrating injuries may involve the kidney, the bladder, or urethra. The typical sign of urologic injury is blood in the urine after abdominal or pelvic trauma. Further examinations are necessary for gross hematuria after trauma, but not for microscopic hematuria without symptoms. Congenital defects may be discovered during the investigation.

Essentials of diagnosis

1. **Hematuria** occurs after abdominal or pelvic trauma. Gross hematuria requires further urogenital examinations.

2. Anterior urethral injury: Occurs typically in men with a pelvic fracture, presenting with blood at the meatus, a scrotal hematoma, or a "high-riding" prostate on rectal exam.

3. Posterior urethral injury: The patient feels the need to void but cannot do so. It's necessary to do a retrograde urethrogram for the diagnosis of urethral injury, but do not insert a Foley catheter as this may cause further injury.

4. **Bladder injury**: It's usually caused by pelvic fracture, and diagnosed by **retrograde cystogram**. It's necessary to have pelvic X-ray to include postvoid films to see extraperitoneal leaks at the base of the bladder.

Treatment

1. **Penetrating injury**: Always requires surgical exploration and repair.

2. **Anterior injury**: Perform surgical repair right away.

3. **Posterior injury**: Perform suprapubic drainage and delayed repair.

4. **Bladder injury**: Perform surgical repair protected with a suprapubic cystostomy.

Kidney Trauma

It is usually secondary to abdominal blunt trauma (accounting for 10% of all kidney injuries and mostly **renal contusion**). The major causes include motor vehicle accident and falls. Patient typically presents with abdominal pain, **renal (angle) tenderness, and hematuria**; lower rib fractures may be present. **Diagnosis** is confirmed by a **CT scan (Image 128)**.

Treatment

Treatment is mostly conservative without surgery--analgesia, IV fluids, and close monitoring. If renal artery stenosis develops after trauma, it can lead to renovascular hypertension. Most patients with significant GU injuries require urgent urologic consultation.

Scrotal and Testicular Trauma

Scrotal and testicular injuries are rare and include **blunt trauma (#1)**, penetrating trauma, and degloving trauma. A thorough history and detailed physical examination are essential for an accurate diagnosis. Significant scrotal trauma includes marked testicular pain, scrotal swelling, laceration into or through the dartos layer, or a large scrotal hematoma. Blood at the meatus or ecchymosis of the penis, perineum or scrotum suggest urethral injury. Scrotal **ultrasonography with Doppler** flow evaluation is particularly helpful in determining the nature and extent of injury.

Treatment

1. **Penetrating trauma** usually requires scrotal exploration to determine the severity of testicular injury, to assess the structural integrity of the testis, and to control intrascrotal hemorrhage. Conservative management can be an option when ultrasonography demonstrates an intratesticular hematoma without obvious fracture planes or disruption of the tunica albuginea.

2. **Blunt trauma** is mostly minor (even with a scrotal hematoma) and only conservative therapy is required. Operative indications for blunt trauma include suspicion of rupture, expanding hematomas, dislocation refractory to manual reduction, avulsion, and scrotal degloving.

Testicular Torsion

It is the twisting of the spermatic cord leading to arterial occlusion and venous outflow obstruction. Ischemia can lead to testicular infarction. It's uncommon and mostly seen in young male adolescents.

Clinical features and diagnosis

Patient typically presents with **sudden, severe testicular pain**, but no history of recent infection (such as mumps), fever, or pyuria. P/E reveals a swollen testicle and scrotum with intense tenderness, "high riding", and with a "horizontal lie". The cord is not tender and the cremasteric reflex is typically absent. **Ultrasound** of the scrotum is a useful adjunct in equivocal cases but should not delay surgical exploration.

Differential diagnosis

<u>Acute epididymitis:</u> This occurs mostly in a sexually active young man, starting with sudden, severe testicular pain, fever, and pyuria. The swollen and very tender testis and cord are in their normal positions. Treat it with antibiotics. If testicular torsion is suspected, ultrasound is indicated.

Treatment

It's a urologic **emergency requiring immediate untwisting and surgical orchiopexy** to scrotum bilaterally (to protect the normal testicle from torsion in future) to maintain viability of the testis. It's recommended also to evaluate and fix the other side. Manual detorsion is not recommended. If surgery is delayed beyond 6 hours, infarction may occur, and the testicle may have to be resected.

Penis Fracture

It's the fracture of the corpora cavernosa or tunica albuginea, typically occurring to the erect penis during aggressive sexual intercourse with the woman on top position. Patient usually presents with an abrupt popping or cracking sound, significant pain, immediate flaccidity, and a large penile shaft hematoma. The glans appears normal. **The patient usually hides the history and makes up a story!**

Treatment
Immediate surgical repair is needed. Delayed treatment increases the complication rate.

EXTREMITY TRAUMA

Penetrating Trauma to the Extremities

It is a common complex injury that **foremost requires the evaluation for vascular injury**.

Treatment

1. If no major vascular injury is found, treatment is wound cleaning plus tetanus prophylaxis.

2. If the penetration is near major vessels and the patient is asymptomatic, detailed peripheral nerve and vascular assessment, extremity radiography, and antibiotics are considered.

3. If there is an obvious **vascular injury** (hemorrhage, absent distal pulses, expanding hematoma), control of hemorrhage **and surgical exploration and repair** are required.

4. If it's a **combined injury** (vessels, nerves, and bone), <u>**first fix the bone, then the vessels (artery and vein), and finally the nerve.**</u> A fasciotomy may be needed to avoid a compartment syndrome by prolonged ischemia.

5. High-velocity gunshot wounds can cause a large cone of tissue destruction and thus requires extensive debridements and potential amputations.

Crushing Extremity Injury

This form of injury is common following a natural disaster or after some form of trauma from a deliberate attack. There are high concerns and risks of myoglobinemia, myoglobinuria, acute kidney injury or tubular necrosis (increased BUN:creatinine ratio), crush syndrome, and compartment syndrome.

Therapeutic and preventive guidelines
Advanced trauma life support, large-volume IV fluid, osmotic diuretics, urine alkalinisation, and fasciotomy.

Fat Embolism (Syndrome)

Usually it's a complication of multiple long bone fractures, which allow fat globules to enter the bloodstream through tissue (bone marrow or adipose tissue). It can lead to sudden respiratory distress and even death.

Essentials of diagnosis

The syndrome typically manifests 24 to 72 hours after major trauma, presenting as the classic triad of abrupt hypoxemia (dyspnea, tachycardia), neurologic abnormalities, and a petechial rash over the body. Fever and low platelet count may be found. CXR shows bilateral patchy infiltrates. Diagnosis is clinical.

Treatment

Respiratory support is the mainstay of treatment. For patients at high risk for fat embolism syndrome, low-dose systemic corticosteroids are suggested for prophylaxis.

ORTHOPEDIC TRAUMA AND INJURIES

Fractures

Fractures are common orthopedic injuries characterized by local pain, swelling, and deformity. Fractures are always diagnosed with x-ray films. Fractures can be classified into the following **five types**:

I. Comminuted fracture: a fracture in which the bone is broken into several pieces; mostly caused by crush injuries.

II. Stress fractures: a fracture from repeated stress or insults to the vulnerable bone.

Metatarsal fracture is the No.1 common type, usually in an athlete or similar profession. X-ray results are usually (-), and thus a CT or MRI must be performed for diagnosis.

Treatment: Rehabilitation, reduced physical activity, and casting. Surgery is indicated if it's persistent.

III. Compression fractures: a specific fracture of the vertebra associated with osteoporosis. In origin, about 1/3 are lumbar, 1/3 are thoracolumbar, and 1/3 are thoracic.

IV. Pathologic fractures: a brittle fracture that occurs from minimal trauma to bone that weakened by certain diseases, such as bone tumors, metastatic carcinoma, multiple myeloma, Paget disease, etc.

Treatment: Surgical realignment of the bone; treating the underlying disease.

V. Open fractures: a fracture when injury causes a broken bone to pierce the skin.

Treatment: Open reduction and internal fixation (ORIF) along with antibiotics to prevent high-risk bacterial infections.

PEARLS——**General therapeutic guidelines for fractures**

1. **Closed reduction**: For mild fractures without displacement.

2. **Open reduction and internal fixation (ORIF):** For open/segmented fractures, multiple trauma, pathologic fracture, vessel-associated fracture, and inadequate closed reduction. For open fractures, the bone must be set in the operation room with debridement, and the skin must be closed.

Common orthopedic injuries are summarized in Table 15-1, 15-2, 15-3, and 15-4 below.

Upper Extremity Injuries

Common upper extremity injuries are summarized in Table 15-1 below.

Table 15-1: Summary of Common Upper Extremity Injuries

Injury / Clinical features, diagnosis (Dx), and treatment (Tx)
Shoulder dislocation (Image 129)   1. **Anterior dislocation:** #1 common, caused by strain on the glenohumoral ligament (Lig.). Patient has painful arm turned outward on anterior chest, in a shape of "**shaking hands.**" X-ray confirms Dx. There's risk of injuries of the axillary artery and nerve. **Tx:** Closed reduction and immobilization. Physical therapy may help.   2. **Posterior dislocation:** Usually seen in seizure or electric shock; arm is medially rotated and rested on the side; X-ray must be on lateral view. **Tx:** Closed reduction under general anesthesia or sedation followed by sling and swathe. Traction or surgery is done if pulses are diminished.   3. **Inferior dislocation:** Patients hold the involved arm above their head and are unable to adduct the arm. Most patients have some neurologic dysfunction (#1 axillary nerve compression; resolves after reduction) and rotator cuff tears or greater tuberosity fractures. **Tx:** Closed reduction with or without local lidocaine.
Scaphoid fracture—Carpal navicular fracture   **#1 common carpal bone fracture**, usually due to falling on an outstretched hand or a focal trauma; tenderness in the anatomical snuff box. X-ray may not show the fracture until 1-2 weeks later. Avascular necrosis (**AVN**) may occur with the 3rd scaphoid fracture. **Tx: Mostly short-arm thumb spica cast** for 6-10 weeks. Open or displaced fracture requires surgery.
Metacarpal neck fracture (Boxer's fracture)   It usually results from a direct blow to the hand or from **striking an object with a clenched fist**. The 5th metacarpal neck fracture is the most common one. **Tx:** Closed reduction and ulnar gutter splint. If skin is broken, amoxicillin and clavulanate IV is given, plus surgical irrigation and debridement. If fracture is angulated, perform pinning.
Distal radius fracture (Colle's fracture, Image 131)   **It's the most common wrist fracture.** It involves the distal radius usually from a **fall onto an outstretched hand**, resulting in a dorsally angulated and displaced fracture. It is mostly seen in children with high-energy trauma and the elderly with **osteoporosis. Tx: Closed reduction** followed by long arm cast.
Humerus fracture   Caused by direct trauma. 1. **Middle shaft fracture** often causes **radial nerve palsy** (wrist drop and thumb abduction deficits); 2. **Proximal** fracture may cause **axillary artery** injury; 3. **Distal (supracondylar) fracture** **(Image 132)** mostly in children and causes **brachial artery injury** (decreased radial pulse, Volkmann contracture). **Tx:** Closed reduction and fixation by hanging arm cast; coaptation splint and sling, and bracing. If it's not getting well, perform **ORIF**.
Monteggia fracture

(Handwritten margin notes: "abducted & ext. rotated arm"; "D to sensation lateral shoulder"; "Axillary n: t. minor, deltoid, weakened short er abd. muscles")

Dislocation of the radial head along with diaphyseal fracture of the ulna; also known as "**nightstick fracture**" ("self-defense injury"). **Mnemonic: "Radius mounting ulna"**. **Tx:** All Monteggia fractures are unstable and require surgical Tx—mostly by ORIF.

Galeazzi fracture

Distal radius dislocation and fracture. **Mnemonic: "2-radius Gallery"**. **Tx: ORIF** of the radius and casting of the forearm in supination.

Knee Injuries

Common knee injuries are summarized in Table 15-2 below.

Table 15-2: Summary of Common Knee Injuries

Injury / Clinical features, diagnosis, and treatment

Vulgar knee injuries
Commonly include: 1. Medial meniscus tear; 2. Medial collateral ligament (MCL) injury; 3. Anterior cruciate ligament (ACL) injury. Patient usually gets injured with a half-flexed position and presents with knee instability, edema, and hematoma.
   I. Medial meniscus tears: Caused by acute twisting injury or a degenerative tear in the elderly; showing knee clicking/locking, joint line tenderness, McMurray's test (+). **Tx:** Conservative (rest, ice pack, bracing, etc).
   II. MCL: Leg bent outward more than normal ranges. **Tx:** Conservative.
   III. Lateral Col ligament: Leg bent inward more than normal. **Tx:** Conservative.
   IV. ACL: Caused by twisting, forced hyperextension, or strike to an extended knee; showing anterior drawer and Lachman tests (+). **Tx:** Surgical grafting from the patellar or hamstring tendons.
   V. Posterior Col ligament (PCL): By forced hyperextension; shows a (+) posterior drawer test. **Tx:** It depends on the severity. Surgical repair is reserved for competitive athletes.

Chondromalacia patella A common "**overuse syndrome**" of the knee in **teenagers**, characterized by anterior knee pain worsened by movement or exercise, grating or crepitating sensation, and tenderness on medial patella.   **Tx:** 1. Rest with acute pain; active resistance exercise to strengthen quadriceps. 2. NSAIDs are helpful.
Osteochondritis dissecans Subchondrial bone necrosis and separated joint fragments due to repeated trauma to vessel tenuous segments of bone. It most commonly occurs in the knees of active teenagers. Patient has gradual knee pain, stiffness, clicking, joint swelling, and locking, worsened by exercise and relieved by rest; may be associated with muscular atrophy. X-ray may show "**notch view**".   **Tx:** 1. Early diagnosis and conservative treatment are important--exercise reduction, joint immobilization, physical therapy, and NSAIDs. 2. If symptoms persist > 3 months, an arthroscopy plus surgery are suggested.
Osgood-Schlatter disease (Tibial tuberosity avulsion) Apophysitis of the tibial tubercle usually due to **overuse in active adolescent boys**, causing localized **tibial pain**, worsened with activities or quadriceps contraction and relieved with rest. It's benign and self-limited.

Tx: Conservative measures are the mainstay of therapy. An icepack, NSAID, neoprene brace or/and physical therapy helps alleviate the pain. Reduced activities for a few months help further.

Hip and Other Lower Extremity Injuries

These are summarized in Table 15-3 below.

Table 15-3: Summary of Hip and Other Lower Extremity Injuries

Injury / Clinical features, diagnosis, and treatment
Hip dislocation (Image 130)   **Posterior** dislocation most often, by the same direction force on internally rotated, flexed and adducted hip ("**dashboard injury**").   **Tx:** 1. For infants <6 months, the Pavlik harness is the #1 used abduction splint. 2. For older ages, Tx is closed or open reduction under anesthesia followed by abduction pillow/bracing and regular X-ray follow-up.
Hip fracture (Image 133)   **1. Intertrochanteric hip fracture**: It's commonly caused by falls in **osteoporotic females**, presenting with the affected leg shortened and externally rotated. It's risky of subsequent **DVT**. **Tx:** ORIF, femoral neck pinning or sliding screw, anticoagulation, and early exercise.   **2. Displaced femoral neck fracture**: Caused by direct trauma. Patient may have history of long steroid or alcohol use; often associated with **avascular femoral head necrosis** (diagnosed by MRI) **and fracture nonunion.** **Tx:** The best is surgical arthroplasty in elderly patients. **Preventive antibiotics and anticoagulation** are suggested for potential, severe **complications—infection and thromboembolism.**   **3. Isolated trochanteric fractures**: Usually result from forceful muscular contraction of a fixed limb in young, active adults. **Tx:** Non-weightbearing for 3-4 weeks; self-limited.
Femur (shaft) fracture   Caused by direct, powerful trauma; risk of **major hemorrhage and fat emboli syndrome** (showing fever, scleral petechiae, dyspnea, hypoxia, confusion, and shock).   **Tx:** 1. Closed fracture with intact skin: intramedullary nailing of the femur. 2. Open fracture: early, thorough irrigation and debridement (to prevent fat embolism), along with fixation plus antibiotics and tetanus prophylaxis.
Tibial fracture   Closed tibial shaft fracture is the **#1 common long-bone fracture**, occurring in both high/low energy traumas.   **Tx:** Conservative therapies, casting and intramedullary nailing, or ORIF depending on specific fracture. **Watch for compartment syndrome** (signs: pain on passive toe extension, with sensory or motor deficits).
Ankle fracture (Image 134)   Commonly due to external rotation or supination, causing fractures of medial and lateral malleoli. **Tx:** Initially **splinting, ice, elevation** above the level of the heart, and analgesics. Unstable fractures require surgery or ORIF.
Achilles tendon rupture   Typical "**sudden pop with pain**" during an intense activity followed by decreased ankle movement. **P/E:** Limited plantar flexion and Thompson's test (+) (no foot plantar flexion after pressure on the gastrocnemius).   **Tx:** Mostly it requires **surgical repair and long leg cast for > 6 weeks.**

Common Orthopedic Injuries in Children

Table 15-4: Summary of Common Orthopedic Injuries in Children

Injury / Clinical features, diagnosis, and treatment
Clavicular fracture It's the #1 common long bone fracture in newborns and children. Usually it occurs in the middle third of the clavicle, with the proximal fractured end displaced superiorly (deformity and tenderness), and may cause brachial nerve palsy (**Erb's palsy**). In newborns, a large baby and asymmetric Moro reflex are often seen.
Tx: Conservative treatment with **arm support and immobilization** in a sling is adequate in most children. In adults, a figure-of-8 sling vs arm sling is used (but it's not enough arm support for type 2 fracture and not used for this, in which the proximal fragment loses its ligamentous attachment and is displaced superiorly). Note: If "bruit" is heard under it, an angiography should be done for suspected artery injury.
Radial head subluxation (Nursemaid elbow) It's radial head subluxation due to sudden pulling or lifting by the hand. Patient presents with pain and will not bend the elbow; often associated with Erb's palsy. **Tx**: Manual reduction by gentle **hyperpronation maneuver** or supination of the elbow at 90 degree of flexion. No immobilization is needed. If the reduction fails, patient is referred to an orthopedic surgeon.
Greenstick fracture Also known as cortex breach—incomplete fracture involving the bone cortex of one side only. **Tx**: Reduction with **casting** followed by X-ray films at 7-10 days.
Torus fracture It's buckling of the bone cortex after trauma; the cortex continuing without breaking. Mostly it occurs in the distal radius and ulna. **Tx**: **Cas**t immobilization for 3-5 weeks.
Supracondylar humerus fracture (Image 132) Usually it occurs at 6-8 y/a; risk of the **brachial artery injury**, **compartment syndrome** of the forearm and **Volkmann contracture**. Radial nerve injury can cause wrist drop. **Tx**: **Cast** immobilization; open reduction for vascular injury; closed reduction with percutaneous pinning for displaced fracture.
Salter-Harris fracture Physeal (growth plate) fracture of the bone in children. It's divided into five Salter-Harris types. Type I and II can be treated conservatively. Other types are unstable and must be treated by surgery to prevent complications (e.g., growth arrest, leg length inequality). The timing of physeal closure in the extremities varies by age, sex, etc.
Developmental dysplasia of the hip (Previously as "Congenital hip dislocation", Image 130) Varying displacement of the proximal femur from the acetabulum. The hip may be subluxed or dislocated; more common in **first-born female and breech presentation** (with excessive uterine packing). **P/E**: 1. **Barlow's** maneuver to check if it's dislocated posteriorly; 2. **Ortolani's** maneuver as a reduction test (hearing a soft click); 3. Allis' (Galeazzi) sign: The knees are at unequal heights. 4. Other signs: Waddling gait, asymmetric skin folds, and limited hip abduction. **Dx**: Made by P/E + ultrasound (>10weeks).

 DDH

Tx: 1. < 6 months: Splint with a Pavlik harness to maintain the hip flexed and abducted. 2. 6-18 months: Reduction under anesthesia (closed or open) with spica cast. 3. > 18 months: Reduction plus concomitant procedures (e.g., adductor tenotomy, iliopsoas release, capsulorrhaphy, femoral shortening) may be necessary. Early correction is important to prevent progressive deformity and AVN (avascular necrosis) of the femoral head.

Legg-Calve-Perthes disease

Osteochondrosis due to idiopathic **avascular necrosis of the femoral head**; mostly unilateral, in **2-10 years' boys** and self-limited. It may be **associated with high-dose use of glucocorticoids**. Patient presents with one **shorter leg and painless limp**. P/E: Limited hip abduction and internal rotation. X-ray (2 views): showing increased joint space and collapsed femoral head.

Tx: Controversial but targeting joint reservation. Options depend on the symptoms, stage of the lesion, and the comorbidities: (1) nonoperative management (age < 5 years; hip abduction, bracing); (2) joint-preserving procedures; (3) joint replacement.

Slipped capital femoral epiphysis (SCFE, Image 135)

Separation of the proximal femoral epiphysis through the growth plate leading to displaced femoral head medially and posteriorly to the femoral neck. Mostly it's in **obese adolescent boys**; maybe associated with hypothyroidism; 30% bilateral. Patient presents with **thigh or knee pain and a limp**. P/E: Tenderness and limited internal rotation and abduction of the hip, and external rotation at the hip flexion. X-ray: Displaced femoral head posteriorly and medially.

Tx: 1. Mild (< 30%): Conservative treatment or gentle closed reduction, no weight-bearing. 2. Moderate to severe: Mostly requires immediate surgical correction and fixing. **Complications** include osteonecrosis of the femoral head and femoroacetabular impingement.

PREOPERATIVE EVALUATION

Surgical patients must be optimized prior to surgery so that perioperative and postoperative complications can be reduced.

Risk Assessment of Cardiovascular Diseases (CVD)

Cardiovascular risk factors with implications for anesthetic management include myocardial ischemia, congestive heart failure, and cerebrovascular or proximal aortic atherosclerosis. Potentially modifiable noncardiac risk factors include preexisting renal insufficiency and anemia. Detailed cardiovascular risk factors and the assessment include:

1. **A history of CVD (including diabetes): It's the No.1 limiting factor prior to surgery. A recent myocardial infarction (MI) must defer the surgery 6 months.** Stress the patient during the interval. An ECG, stress testing and echocardiogram for organic disease must be done.

2. **Ejection fraction < 35%:** It increases the risk for non-cardiovascular surgery.

3. **Congestive heart failure** (CHF, with JVD, pulmonary or lower limb edema): It requires medical treatment with ACE-I (inhibitors), beta-blockers, and potassium-saving diuretics (spironolactone, etc.) to decrease mortality.

Risk assessment of CVD

4. Most patients with valve repair or replacement, as well as for the majority of patients scheduled to undergo coronary artery bypass grafting (CABG) need echocardiography and diagnostic cardiac catheterization. Patients without history of CVD and under age 35 only need an ECG test.

Risk Assessment of Pulmonary Diseases

Patient-related risk factors include: age > 50 years, chronic obstructive pulmonary disease, congestive heart failure, poor general health status, obstructive sleep apnea, cigarette smoking, pulmonary hypertension, low oxygen saturation, and serum albumin < 3.5 g/dL. Patients with a history of lung disease or smoking require **CXR and pulmonary function tests** for the vital capacity evaluations, and smoking must be stopped for 6-8 weeks prior to surgery.

Risk Assessment of Renal Diseases

Patient with a history or presence of renal disease: **Adequate hydration before and during surgery** must be maintained in order to decrease renal hypoperfusion, adverse activation of rennin-angiotensin system, and postoperative mortality. **Patients on dialysis have an increased perioperative mortality** and should be well dialyzed 24 hours prior to surgery. ACE inhibitors, angiotensin receptor blockers and diuretics should be discontinued in most dialysis patients two days prior to surgery to reduce the hemodynamic instability.

COMPLICATIONS OF SURGERY

It refers to any postoperative condition that adversely affects the patient's morbidity or mortality. Complications may be specifically associated with the surgery performed or with the general conditions that can follow any operation. The incidence and severity are directly related to the patient's general health. Early prevention and treatment can reduce risk of serious consequences. Thus it is important to collect the following information in the preoperative history:

1. Smoking or alcohol consumption;
2. Medications and allergies;
3. Chronic diseases (COPD, CAD, diabetes, etc.);
4. History of past surgery and complications.

PEARLS—Common Postoperative Complications

I. Fever

(1) **Postoperative fever** is usually in 38-39°C and caused by **atelectasis (#1, < 24 hours), pneumonia (1-2 days), UTI (3-4 days), wound infection (5-7 days), deep venous thrombophlebitis (DVT, 5-7 days), or deep abscesses (> 7 days).**

1) Post of fever

(2) **Malignant hyperthermia** develops shortly after the start of the anesthetic (halothane or succinylcholine), with high fever (> 39.5°C), metabolic acidosis, hyper-Ca, and psychological symptoms. Family history may be positive. **Treatment**: IV dantrolene, 100% oxygen, acidosis correction, and cooling blankets. Watch for evidence of myoglobinuria and renal failure.

II. Respiratory Complication

It's the most common one, especially with a history of chronic lung disease or smoking.

(1) **Atelectasis** is the most common postoperative complication within 24 hours of most surgeries. Typical presentations include fever, tachycardia, and decreased breath sound and rales; CXR reveals platelike opacities. Prevention is by encouraging patient to cough, taking frequent deep breaths, and incentive spirometry.

(2) **Aspiration pneumonia**: Mostly caused by inhalation of oropharyngeal or gastric contents.

III. Infection

The most common sites of postoperative infection are "**4 Ws**": **Wind** (pneumonia), **Walk** (phlebitis), **Water** (UTI), and **Wound** (wound infection).

Risk factors: Presence of foreign bodies, necrotic tissue, hematomas, chronic diseases, malnutrition, and steroid use. Bacterial infections typically present with chills and T > 39.5°C within an hour of invasive procedures. afebrile, confusion, HoTN, tachycardia, leukocytosis.

Treatment: Three blood cultures followed by empiric antibiotics. Incision and drainage first if abscess forms.

IV. DVT

Virchow's triad (Risk factors): (1) Trauma or surgery; (2) venous stasis; (3) hypercoagulability. Other factors include obesity, aging, steroid use, malignancy, etc.

DVT: Typical signs are fever, swollen and tender calf, and Homan sign (calf pain with dorsiflexion of the foot). Confirmative diagnosis is by ultrasound (first), plethysmography, or venography.

Treatment: Heparin for 5 days followed by coumadin for 3-6 months.

V. Pulmonary embolism (PE)

See Chapter 3: "Pulmonary Embolism".

ANALGESIA AND ANESTHESIA IN SURGERY AND OBSTETRICS

Patient request is usually clinical indication for analgesia during labor and other painful conditions. Anesthesia is divided into general and regional anesthesia. Regional anesthetic techniques can be divided into central and peripheral techniques. The central techniques include so called neuroaxial blocks (epidural anesthesia, spinal anesthesia). The peripheral techniques can be further divided into plexus blocks such as brachial plexus blocks, and single nerve blocks.

The goal of anesthesia is to provide the desired combination of analgesia, amnesia, and optimal operating conditions (including muscular relaxation) while ensuring physiologic homeostasis. Careful assessment of the patient's preoperative conditions and consideration of anesthetic choices will improve the operative outcome. The types of anesthesia include general anesthesia, neuraxial anesthesia (spinal and epidural), peripheral nerve blocks, monitored anesthetic care (including deep sedation), and light or moderate sedation. Multimodal analgesia may be used to decrease opioid side effects. This may include utilizing a combined technique (E.g., general anesthesia plus epidural or peripheral nerve block analgesia) or the addition of non-opioid analgesics into the perioperative analgesic plan. Absolute **contraindications for regional anesthesia include** refractory hypertension, coagulopathy, daily use of low-molecular-weight heparin, elevated ICP, and serious infection.

Features of commonly used anesthetic methods

1. **Local anesthesia (lidocaine**, etc.): It is usually used for small local operations, before episiotomy, during laceration repair, or for pudendal block. Topical anesthesia is commonly used to anesthetize the upper airway, nasal passages, and trachea, for awake laryngoscopy and intubation, etc.

2. **Epidural anesthesia**: It's a type of neuraxial anesthesia in the epidural space that is used for thoracic, abdominal, pelvic, and lower extremity procedures. It provides the **most effective** pain relief for normal delivery as well as elective C-section, tubal ligation, and other abdominal operations.

3. **Spinal anesthesia**: It's a type of neuraxial anesthesia in the subarachnoid space at the lumbar level that is used for a variety of lower extremity, lower abdominal, pelvic, and perineal procedures. It provides rapid-onset analgesia but with more adverse effects (bradycardia, hypotension, dyspnea, secondary headache, etc.). Thus, the patient must be monitored as for general anesthesia.

4. **General anesthesia**: It causes hypnosis/unconsciousness, amnesia, analgesia, muscle relaxation as appropriate for the procedure, and autonomic and sensory blockade of responses to noxious surgical stimulation. It is usually indicated in a major surgery, emergency C-section, serious FHR abnormalities, and cases with absolute contraindications for regional anesthesia. It's associated with most adverse effects and risks (patient's aspiration, death, neonatal respiratory depression, etc.).

VOLUME DISORDERS

Normal body fluid distribution

1. Men: Total body water (TBW) = 60% of body weight.
2. Women: TBW = 50% of body weight.
3. Percentage of TBW decreases with age and obesity (because fat contains little water).
4. 2/3 of TBW (or 40% of body weight) is intracellular fluid (ICF, mostly in skeletal muscle mass), and 1/3 of TBW (or 20% of body weight) is extracellular fluid (ECF).

Assessing volume status

1. This is a difficult task. Monitoring urine output is very important in the assessment of volume status. **Normal urine output in adults is more than 1.0 mL/kg/hour**. Lower urine output could be a sign of volume depletion.
2. Daily weight may give a more accurate assessment of volume trends.
3. Patient's conditions can influence the volume status:

(1) Generally patients with fever, sepsis, burns, or open wounds have higher metabolic demands and insensible losses.

(2) Patients with liver failure, nephrotic syndrome, renal failure, and other conditions causing hypoalbuminemia tend to have increased third-space fluid and total body fluid, but they are intravascularly depleted.

(3) Patients with CHF may have pulmonary edema (left-ventricle failure) or anasarca (right-ventricle failure).

Fluid replacement therapy

1. Normal saline (N.S.): Usually used to increased intravascular volume in dehydrated patients; not the best option with CHF unless urgent resuscitation is needed.

2. 5% Dextrose (D5) 1/2NS: Usually used as the standard maintenance fluid, often given with 20 mEq/L KCl fluid.

3. Lactate Ringer's solution (contains potassium): It's good for replacement of intravascular volume (especially for trauma resuscitation), but not good for maintenance fluid or patients with hyperkalemia.

4. 5% Dextrose water (D5W): This can be used in correcting hypernatremia or diluting powdered medicines, but not as an efficient maintenance fluid.

5. Blood loss: This can be replaced with crystalloid at a 3:1 ratio.

6. Total fluid replacing volume = Deficit + Maintenance + Ongoing losses. Frequent monitoring of HR, BP, urine output and weigh is necessary. Urine output should be maintained at 0.5-1 mL/kg/hr.

Hypovolemia and Dehydration

Hypovolemia represents the loss of sodium and water.

Etiology

1. Inadequate intake plus insensible losses—evaporation through skin and the respiratory tract.
2. GI losses due to vomiting, nasogastric suction, diarrhea, fistula drainage, etc.
3. Third-spacing: Effusions, ascites, bowel obstruction, burns, crush injuries, etc.
4. Trauma, open wound, sequestration of fluid into soft tissues.
5. Others: Polyuria, sepsis, inflammation, etc.

Classification, clinical features, and treatment

Summarized in the table below.

PEARLS—**Table 15-5: Classification, Clinical Features, and Treatment of Dehydration**

I. By Degree / Clinical features and treatment (Tx)
Mild (5%): Thirsty, alert, and restless; otherwise normal.
Moderate (10%): Thirsty, restless, irritable, tachypnea, tachycardia, weak pulses, dry mucous membranes, slightly depressed skin turgor and fontanelle, oliguria, and orthostatic hypotension.

> **Severe (15%):** Lethargic, limp, cold, sweaty, cyanotic, hypotensive, deep-rapid respiration, very dry and mottled skin, sunken fontanelle, tachycardia with decreased pulses, anuria or severe oliguria, and comatose.

II. By Serum Sodium (Na) Level

Isotonic: Serum Na is 130-150 mEq/L, with proportional losses of fluid and electrolytes from the extracellular space. **Tx:** The deficit should be replaced over 8-24 hours normal saline (**N.S.**).

Hypotonic: Serum Na < 130 mEq/L, with more Na loss than water, or with excess water. **Tx:** The deficit should be replaced over 8-24 hours with **Ringer lactate or NS plus 3% NaCl** 100 mL IV if severe (Na < 120 mEq/L). **Colloid** (with 5% albumin) IV may be used to replace blood loss.

Hypertonic: Serum Na > 150 mEq/L, with more water loss than Na, or with Na excess. **Tx:** The deficit should be replaced over 48 hours with 5% dextrose water (D5W), or D5 1/2NS.

Hypervolemia

Also known as fluid overload, hypervolemia is an abnormal increase in the body's blood volume, particularly in the sense of blood plasma.

Etiology
1. Fluid-retaining status: CHF, cirrhosis, nephritic syndrome, renal failure, etc.
2. Iatrogenic: Parenteral overhydration, etc.

Clinical features and diagnosis
1. **P/E**: Weight gain, JVD (jugular venous distention), peripheral edema, pulmonary edema (rales), ascites, etc.
2. **Lab**: Low hematocrit and albumin concentration.

Treatment
1. Fluid restriction; judicious use of diuretics; correction of underlying causes.
2. Monitoring urine output and daily weight, and treating patient accordingly.

ABDOMINAL SURGERY

Differentiation of Abdominal Pain

Abdominal pain is a common symptom. Most patients have a benign and/or self-limited etiology, and the initial goal and challenge is to identify those patients with a serious etiology that may require urgent intervention. A detailed history and focused physical examination are important for differential diagnosis, which may require further evaluation with laboratory testing and/or imaging.

Important differentiations of abdominal pain by clinical features are summarized in the table below.

PEARLS—Table 15-6: **Important Differentiations of Abdominal Pain**

I. Left upper quadrant (LUQ)
Gastritis: LUQ or epigastric pain or discomfort, heartburn, nausea, vomiting, and hematemesis.   **Gastric ulcer**: LUQ or epigastric pain or discomfort associated with food.   Others: splenic rupture, IBS (splenic flexure syndrome); splenomegaly, splenic infarct, splenic abscess, splenic rupture.
II. (Middle) epigastrium
Acute pancreatitis: Acute, persistent upper abdominal pain radiating to the back; usually after meal/alcohol.   **Chronic pancreatitis**: Chronic epigastric pain radiating to the back; associated with pancreatic insufficiency.   **Peptic ulcer disease**: Epigastric pain or discomfort; occasionally localized to one side.   **GERD**: Epigastric pain associated with heartburn, regurgitation, and dysphagia.   **Gastritis/gastropathy**: Abdominal discomfort/pain, heartburn, nausea, vomiting, and hematemesis; may have history of ingestion of alcohol or NSAIDs.   **Functional dyspepsia**: The presence of one or more of the following: postprandial fullness, early satiation, epigastric pain, or burning; no evidence of structural disease.   **Gastroparesis**: Nausea, vomiting, abdominal pain, early satiety, postprandial fullness, and bloating. Most causes are idiopathic, diabetic, or postsurgical.
III. Right upper quadrant (RUQ)
Biliary colic: Intense, dull pain located in the RUQ or epigastrium; associated with nausea, vomiting, and diaphoresis; usually lasting > 30 min and alleviated within 1 hour; generally benign P/E results.   **Acute cholecystitis**: Prolonged (> 4 hours) RUQ or epigastric pain, fever. Patients will have abdominal guarding and Murphy's sign.   **Acute cholangitis**: Triad of fever, jaundice, RUQ pain; may have atypical presentation in older or immuno-suppressed patients.
Sphincter of Oddi dysfunction: RUQ pain similar to other biliary type pain without other apparent causes.   **Acute hepatitis**: Dull RUQ pain with fatigue, malaise, nausea, vomiting, and anorexia; +/- jaundice, dark urine, and light-colored stools. Causes include hepatitis A, alcohol, and drug-induction.   **Perihepatitis (Fitz-Hugh-Curtis syndrome)**: RUQ pain with a pleuritic condition; pain may radiate to the right shoulder; aminotransferases are usually normal or only slightly elevated.
Budd-Chiari syndrome: Fever, abdominal pain and distention (from ascites), lower extremity edema, jaundice, gastrointestinal bleeding, and/or hepatic encephalopathy.   **Portal vein thrombosis**: RUQ pain, dyspepsia, or gastrointestinal bleeding; most commonly associated with cirrhosis.   Others: duodenal ulcer (perforation), hepatic abscess.
IV. Right lower quadrant (RLQ)
Appendicitis: Periumbilical pain initially that radiates to the right lower quadrant; associated with anorexia, nausea, and vomiting.   **Cecal diverticulitis**: Constant RLQ pain and low fever for several days; may have nausea and vomiting but no lower GI bleeding. Others: ectopic pregnancy, ovarian torsion.
V. Left lower quadrant (LLQ)

(Sigmoid) diverticulitis: Constant LLQ pain and low fever for several days; may have palpable sigmoid mass but no lower GI bleeding.

(Sigmoid) diverticulosis: LLQ colicky pain and relieved by defecation; may also have typical painless rectal bleeding or hematochezia (melena).

Others: sigmoid volvulus, ectopic pregnancy, ovarian torsion.

VI. Lower abdomen (left or right)

Infectious colitis: Diarrhea and associated abdominal pain +/- fever. Clostridium difficile infection can show acute abdomen and peritoneal signs in the setting of perforation and fulminant colitis.

Nephrolithiasis: Usually mild to severe flank pain (left or right); may have back or abdominal pain.

Ectopic pregnancy: Triad of amenorrhea, unilateral lower abdominal pain, and spotting vaginal bleeding (1-2 weeks after LMP).

Others: twisted/ruptured ovary cyst, endometriosis, intestinal obstruction, abdominal abscess.

Bowel Obstruction

It is a mechanical or functional obstruction of the intestines due to varieties of causes. After the lumen's occlusion, gas and fluid build up proximally and cause increased pressure within the lumen that leads to decreased blood perfusion of the bowel and necrosis. Bowel obstruction can be classified as small bowel and large bowel obstruction; partial and complete obstruction.

PEARLS—Table 15-7: Comparison of Small and Large Bowel Obstruction

	Small Bowel Obstruction (SBO)	**Large Bowel Obstruction (LBO)**
Causes	**#1** is postsurgery **adhesion**; hernias, tumors, volvulus, intussusception, gallstone ileus, Crohn disease, hematoma; younger patient.	**Fecal impaction, volvulus, or colon cancer** is common; diverticulitis, benign tumors; older patients: suspect cancer until proven otherwise
Diagnosis	1. Cramping abdominal pain, copious emesis, fever, and dehydration. 2. **Abdominal distention** (distal SBO), **high-pitched bowel sound** (±), scars, or hernias. 3. AXR may show "ladder-like" pattern; Ba-study can determine partial or full SBO; CT scan if complicated.	1. Deep **cramping abdominal pain and distention**, vomiting with **feculent emesis**, and constipation. 2. Abdominal tenderness, **high-pitched bowel sound** perforation, peritonitis, fever, or shock; ± mass. 3. AXR is helpful, Ba or water contrast enema for perforation; if stable, sigmoid/colonoscopy can be performed as both diagnosis and treatment.
Treatment	1. Hospitalize; treat partial SBO with nasogastric decompression and observation. 2. Full SBO: NPO, NG tube, IV fluid, and surgical exploration.	1. Hospitalize and treat underlying causes. 2. **Perform surgery in most cases**: gangrene, tumor, etc. Rectal tube or colonoscopy may solve some cases.

FAST P. 560

Appendicitis

It's inflammation of the appendix, mostly due to lymphoid hyperplasia or fecalith obstruction of the appendiceal lumen. It may lead to infection, abscess, and/or perforation if diagnosis and treatment are delayed. It's the most common abdominal emergency in young patients < 35 y/a.

Essentials of diagnosis

1. Initial dull periumbilical **pain migrating to RLQ then becoming sharp, intensified, and fixed**; anorexia, nausea, vomiting, and fever may exist.

2. **P/E:** Localized tenderness at **McBurney point (#1 diagnostic mark), positive psoas** or **obturator** or **Rovsing sign** (RLQ pain on palpation of the LLQ). A **rectal exam** is mandatory and a positive tenderness suggests posterior appendicitis. A **pelvic exam** is required in a young female to exclude PID.

3. **Lab diagnosis:** WBC is typically > 12,000/ul with predominant neutrophils. Ultrasound is helpful in diagnosis. CT is only needed for complicated cases.

Differential diagnosis

Ectopic pregnancy (ruptured):

For sexually active females, obtaining beta-hCG test and history of last menstrual period (LMP) is always necessary. Pelvic exam and ultrasonography confirm most of the diagnosis. Surgery may be both diagnostic and therapeutic.

Pelvic inflammatory disease (PID):

It mostly occurs in sexually active females. Pelvic exam and secretion tests confirm diagnosis.

Acute ileitis:

It's caused by Yersinia E., typically with RLQ pain, fever, and diarrhea without a mass. Appendicitis is usually associated with RLQ pain and constipation, not diarrhea.

Others: Ovary torsion, gastroenteritis, volvulus, diverticulitis, Crohn disease, pyelonephritis, mesenteric ischemia, Meckel diverticulum, colon cancer with perforation.

Complications

Abdominal abscess, appendiceal perforation (with a stiff abdomen and X-ray shows free air under the diaphragm), hepatic abscess, septic pylephlebitis, etc.

Treatment

1. Appendectomy is the best treatment. Emergent surgery is necessary if it is perforated.
2. With stable abscess, CT-guided drainage is performed followed by elective appendectomy.
3. If the appendix is normal after the abdomen is opened, appendectomy is recommended.
4. Antibiotics can be used prior to surgery and continued for 2-3 days after an uncomplicated operation.

Anal Fissure

It refers to a tear or ulcer in the anal canal that mostly results from trauma due to passage of large and hard stool. Other causes include STD, IBD, and anatomical abnormalities. If the fissure is on the internal sphincter, it may cause sphincter spasm and secondary avoidance of defecation and hard, constipated stools.

Essentials of diagnosis

1. Pain during and after defecation, and bleeding upon wiping. A skin tag may be seen outside the anus.

2. Diagnosis is based on clinical manifestations.

Treatment

1. High-fiber diet, stool softeners, glycerine suppositories, local anesthetic or botulism, laxatives, frequent sitz baths, etc.

2. If it's refractory to 3-4 week's conservative treatment, associated diseases (Crohn disease, cancer, syphilis, etc.) should be suspected and excluded. Afterwards, sphincterotomy can be chosen.

Hemorrhoids

It refers to varicose veins of the anus and rectum. The basic cause is increased pressure in the anorectal vessel network, which is usually secondary to excessive straining with defecation/constipation, portal hypertension, CHF, obesity, pregnancy, prolonged sitting or standing, or anal intercourse.

Classification

I. External hemorrhoids—dilated veins arising from inferior hemorrhoidal plexus; distal to dentate line (sensate area).

II. Internal hemorrhoids—dilated submucosal veins of superior rectal plexus.

Essentials of diagnosis

1. Bright rectal bleeding on stool or toilet paper. Internal hemorrhoids are usually painless, whereas external hemorrhoids can be itchy, prolapsed, and painful when they are thrombosed. The pain lasts for several days and then subsides gradually.

2. P/E of the rectum may reveal a tender bluish swelling +/- reducibility. Anoscopy is used to diagnose an internal hemorrhoid.

3. Occult rectal hemorrhage should never be attributed to hemorrhoids until other more serious causes (such as cancer) are ruled out.

Treatment

1. Asymptomatic hemorrhoids do not require treatment. Initial therapies for symptomatic cases are stool softeners (psyllium), sitz baths, ice packs, increased fiber-fluids in diet, avoidance of prolonged sitting, and topical pain creams or topical steroids.

2. Rubber band ligation is effective by causing necrosis and sloughing of the protruding hemorrhoid.

3. If there is no effect after 1-2 weeks of conservative treatment or the conditions get worse, surgery is indicated and can be performed in an ambulatory setting.

(1) Injection sclerotherapy: Injecting sclerosing agent into the protruding vein.

(2) Hemorrhoidectomy: Most effective but rarely done.

Hernia

It is a protrusion of a viscous or intra-abdominal tissue through a weakness or defect in the abdominal wall. **Inguinal hernias are the most common type**, affecting male more than female and classified as direct or indirect (the differentiation is of limited clinical significance). Other types include femoral and ventral (umbilical or incisional) hernias. A hernia is usually apparent when intra-abdominal pressure increases, which is mostly caused by excessive straining, chronic cough, obesity, pregnancy, or ascites.

Essentials of diagnosis

1. **Inguinal hernia**: Mostly asymptomatic and found on routine P/E, which reveals a palpable mass in the groin (inguinal canal)—finger at the superior border of the sacrum in men, noticeable with coughing and with aching.

2. **Femoral hernia**: Just below the inguinal ligament, viscous in the femoral canal; more risk of incarceration.

3. **Severe hernias**: Occasionally **incarcerated** in which hernia contents become strangulated and may even infarct. Patient presents with a non-reducible, tender mass on palpation.

Treatment

Most hernias require **laparoscopic surgical repair** to avoid a worsening defect and bowel incarceration. Attempts of gentle reduction can be tried before surgery. If it fails, emergent surgery is required to avoid incarceration.

Intra-abdominal Abscess

It is a collection of pus or infected fluid that is surrounded by inflamed tissue inside the abdomen. It can be caused by surgery, spontaneous bacterial peritonitis, pelvic infection/abscess, pancreatitis, perforation of the GI tract, inflammatory bowel disease, parasite infection, or osteomyelitis. Most cases are polymicrobial in origin. Risk factors include a history of appendicitis, diverticulitis, perforated ulcer disease, or any surgery that may have infected the abdominal cavity.

Essentials of diagnosis

1. History of the above causes or risk factors, followed by lack of appetite, nausea/vomiting, fever, abdominal pain, change in bowel movements, and focal mass with tenderness.

2. CT scan or ultrasonography usually confirms the diagnosis.

Treatment

It is best treated with drainage of the abscess plus broad-spectrum antibiotics against Gram-negative rods (particularly P. aeruginosa and Enterobacteriaceae), enterococci, and anaerobes.

Miscellaneous: Decubitus Ulcer

It is defined as necrosis of tissue and subsequent ulceration mostly in areas with bony prominences; also known as a "bed sore or pressure sore." It is usually the complication of localized pressure after prolonged immobilization in debilitated, bedridden patients. These patients usually have decreased or absent sensation of pain caused by the chronic ischemia, which eventually leads to the ulceration.

Risk factors: Poor nutrition, anemia, infection, contact with perspiration, urine, or feces.

Essentials of diagnosis

1. Based on history and clinical impression.

2. Ulcers are graded by **3 degrees or phases**: (1) persistent redness; (2) ulceration; (3) destruction of structures beneath the skin (muscle, fat, etc.). The depth of the ulcer determines the severity of disease and symptoms.

Treatment

1. The best treatment is prevention—relieving the local pressure on bony prominences by frequent position changes (every 2 hours).

2. In early stages, it's essential to give good care and to help keep patients clean, dry, and with optimal nutrition. Underlying diseases (anemia, infection, etc.) should be treated adequately.

3. In late stages, surgery is required for any ulcer > 2cm thickness to debride necrotic tissue, close a large defect, or remove affected bone. Protective dressings (wet to dry) should be used to cover the wound.

Chapter 14-15: High-Yield Questions (HYQ)

1. A 5 y/o boy has a headache and fever and ingests several pills from a drawer at home. Four hours later he is brought to the ER for worsening headache, dizziness, nausea, and vomiting. P/E shows T = 38°C, HR = 120/min (bpm), RR = 28/min, BP = 90/60 mmHg, and normal (Nl) other results. The most appropriate next step is

A. ipecac-induced vomiting   B. gastric lavage
C. drug screening and concentration test   D. acetylcysteine administration
E. charcoal administration

2. A farmer spraying a chemical at his ranch is brought to the ER. He's dizzy and disoriented, with tachypnea, abdominal pain, sweating, and incontinence of stool and urine. P/E shows T = 37.5°C, HR = 60/min, RR = 27/min, BP = 90/60 mmHg, and muscle shivering. His clothes are removed. The best initial treatment (Tx) is
A. IV fluid   B. atropine   C. pralidoxime (PAM)
D. diuretics   E. mannitol

3. A 19 y/o girl is brought to the emergency room from bed after breaking up with her boy-friend and taking "half a bottle of sleeping pills" about 40 min ago for a suicide. She is mostly conscious but refuses to answer any question. P/E results: HR = 68/min, RR = 15/min, BP = 110/75 mmHg, and respiration is normal. The most appropriate next step is
A. consultation for the truth   B. flumazenil   C. gastric lavage
D. ipecac   E. a laxative   F. drug screening

4. A 50 y/o man has been unemployed for the past 3 months. He feels fatigue, sleepless, irritable, and hopeless. He takes two prescribed medicines including a TCA for his symptoms for the second day. He has seizures after ingesting flumazenil for altered mental status today. His vital signs are normal except for tachycardia. The best initial test is
A. Drug screening   B. ECG (EKG)   C. Electrolytes
D. Head CT   E. Head MRI

5. A 17 y/o boy was burned when playing fire with gasoline in the countryside yesterday and is brought to the ER. The burned areas include the head, one arm, and two hand-width patchy areas on the chest, with blister formation and severe pain. His vital signs are stable with tachycardia, and his body weight is 50 kg. IV fluid is ready for ingestion. According to the Parkland's Formula, the immediate fluid need for the first 8 hours is
A. 2000 mL of Ringer's lactate   B. 3000 mL of Ringer's lactate
C. 4000 mL of Ringer's lactate   D. 2000 mL of Ringer's lactate with colloids
E. 3000 mL of Ringer's lactate with colloids   F. 4000 mL of Ringer's lactate with colloids

6. A 15 y/o boy is accidentally electrocuted by a high-tension electrical power line. He has both entrance and exit burn wounds in the thigh. What's the most appropriate next step?

A. Extensive surgical debridement   B. Arteriogram   C. Exploratory surgery
D. Large volume of IV fluid, osmotic diuretics, and alkalinisation of the urine
E. Support and observation

7. A 50 y/o female is rescued from a burning building. She has burns around her entire face with a dark, "smoked" throat. She is alert and her vital signs are stable. What's the most appropriate next step?

A. Tests of blood carboxyhemoglobin and arterial blood gas

B. 100% oxygen therapy

C. Bronchoscopy

D. Respiratory support (including tracheotomy and PPMV)

E. A large volume of IV fluid

8. A student was performing a laboratory test with a chemical when his sleeves suddenly caught on fire, and both of his arms were burned severely. Five days later now, both his arms appear dry, white, leathery, and painless. The burns are circumferential all around the arms and forearms. His vital signs are stable. What's the best next step?

A. Monitoring of peripheral pulses and capillary filling   B. Escharotomy

C. Fasciotomy   D. Eschar removal   E. Respiratory support

9. A 50 y/o man who weighs 70 kg has third-degree burns over all the legs and genitalia/perineum areas. During the first 8 hours in the hospital, he needs all the following therapies EXCEPT

A. oxygen   B. 2300 mL of Ringer's lactate   C. a H2-R blocker

D. antibiotics without steroid   E. colloids or diuretics

10. During a fight, a 20 y/o man was stabbed twice on the abdomen. In the emergency room (ER) he is pale and shivering but alert, with weak breathing at 28/min (RR). Other findings: a weak pulse of 130/min, BP = 65/50 mmHg, and a firm abdomen with extensive tenderness. What's the most appropriate next step?

A. High pressure oxygen   B. Fast IV fluid infusion   C. Foley catheter

D. Exploratory laparotomy   E. Preventive antibiotics

11. A 25 y/o man is stabbed in the chest with a long knife. The wound entry is just to the left of the sternal border, at the fourth intercostal space. He is pale, shivering, and perspiring heavily. P/E results: BP = 60/50 mmHg, HR = 120/min; jugular vein distention (JVD); heart sounds and bilateral breath sounds are weak. What's the immediate next step?

A. Large-bore IV lines for fluid infusion   B. Upper chest needle

C. Lower chest tube   D. Median sternotomy   E. Exploratory surgery

12. A 70 y/o tall man fell off the curb while walking and is brought to the ER for severe chest pain. He is short of breath, pale, and perspiring heavily. P/E results: BP = 80/60 mmHg; HR = 120/min; JVD; heart sounds are weak; bilateral breath sounds seem normal. He has a history of hypertension for the past 10 years. What's the most likely diagnosis?

A. Tension pneumothorax   B. Ruptured aorta aneurism   C. Myocardial infarction (MI)

D. Pericardial tamponade   E. Hemothorax

13. A 30 y/o man is stabbed in the right chest. He presents with moderate dyspnea, with BP = 90/60 mmHg, HR = 80/min. No breath sounds are heard on the right side and there is hyperresonance to percussion. What's the best next step?

A. Big-bore IV lines for fluid   B. Upper chest tube   C. Lower chest tube

D. CXR for plain pneumothorax   E. Chest CT

14. A 70 y/o man falls down the stairs and hurt his chest wall. He has persistent pain and tenderness over the 6th rib below the right nipple. CXR confirms a right 6th rib fracture. No other abnormal signs are found. What's the most appropriate next step?

A. CT scan for other injuries   B. Strapping or binding of the fractured rib

C. Local pain relief   D. NSAIDs   E. External fixation

15. An 18 y/o man is stabbed in the right chest and brought to a distant clinic. He is moderately short of breath. P/E results: BP = 90/60 mmHg, HR = 100/min, distant breath sounds at the apex, and no breath sounds over the lower half of the right chest. What's the most appropriate next step?

A. Big-bore IV lines for blood supply   B. Upper chest needle

C. Lower chest tube   D. Chest CT   E. Antibiotics

16. A 17 y/o girl is involved in a high-speed car collision. She presents with severe dyspnea, cyanosis, JVD, and multiple tender points on the right chest. Her BP is 70/50 mmHg and HR is 140/min. No breath sounds are heard on the right hemithorax and it is hyperresonant to percussion. The best next step is

A. big-bore IV lines for fluid and blood supply   B. upper chest needle

C. lower chest tube   D. CXR   E. surgery

17. A 70 y/o man receiving total parenteral nutrition (TPN) through a central venous line falls off the bed and has his central line disconnected from the IV tubing. When the nurse hears the alarm and comes to the bed, the patient is dead. What's the most likely diagnosis?

A. Pulmonary embolism (PE)   B. Air embolism   C. Tension pneumothorax

D. Apnea   E. ICH

18. A 20 y/o man is stabbed in the left chest. He has a large, flap-like, painful wound in the chest wall, and he sucks air through it with every inspiration. His vital signs are stable. What's the best next step?

A. Local pain relief   B. Cover the flap with Vaseline gauze

C. On-site upper chest needle insertion   D. Transfer to a nearby hospital for a chest tube

E. Mechanical ventilation

19. A 20 y/o man crashes his car against a tree at high speed and is brought to the ER. He has multiple bruises and tender points over the lower left chest. P/E reveals that a segment of the left chest wall caves in when he inhales and bulges out when he exhales. CXR has confirmed multiple rib fractures on the left without signs of pneumothorax. His vital signs are stable. What's the most appropriate next step?

A. Spiral CT scan of the chest and abdomen

B. Aortogram

C. Abdominal ultrasound

D. Fluid restriction, diuretics, and respiratory support

E. IV fluid and respiratory support

20. A 20 y/o man crashes his car against a tree at high speed and is brought to the ER. He has moderate respiratory distress and multiple bruises and tender points over the lower left chest. His vital signs are stable. P/E reveals no breath sounds over the entire left chest. Percussion is uncertain. A nasogastric (NG) tube is inserted, and CXR shows the NG tube curling up into the left chest with multiple air fluid levels. What's the best next step?

A. Spiral CT scans of the chest and abdomen   B. Aortogram

C. Abdominal sonogram   D. Respiratory support and surgery

E. IV fluid and respiratory support

21. A 30 y/o man with multiple severe fractures of the left leg has developed abrupt tachypnea, tachycardia, petechial rashes around the neck, and disorientation. CXR shows bilateral patchy infiltrates, and CBC reveals low platelet count. What's the most appropriate next step of treatment?

A. Heparin   B. Steroid   C. Thrombolytics

D. Respiratory support   E. Fluid and diuretics

22. A 17 y/o boy was shot with a bullet, which entered in the left middle clavicular line, 2 inches below the nipple without an exit wound. His HR is 100/min and BP is 90/60 mmHg. He's conscious but irritable. CXR is done with uncertainty. What's the most appropriate next step?

A. Exploratory chest surgery   B. Exploratory laparotomy   C. IV fluid and close observation

D. Chest tube insertion   E. Chest CT

23. A 20 y/o man wrecks his car and presents with multiple fractures of the extremities and abdominal pain. CXR is unremarkable. His HR is 140/min and BP is 70/50 mmHg. He has low hematocrit and central venous pressure (CVP). IV fluid is started. What's the best next step?

A. Abdominal CT   B. Abdominal sonogram   C. Diagnostic peritoneal lavage

D. Exploratory laparotomy   E. Blood transfusion

24. A 40 y/o female has a major surgery for multiple abdominal wounds. She's been given a large volume of IV fluid. One day after the surgery, she develops respiratory distress and a very tense, distended abdomen. The surgical retention sutures are cutting through the abdominal wall. What's the most appropriate next step?

A. Stop IV fluid and observe

B. Stop IV fluid and place an absorbable mesh over the incision

C. Open the incision and place an absorbable mesh over it

D. Stop IV fluid and place a non-absorbable plastic to cover the incision

E. Exploratory surgery again

25. A 40 y/o female suffers severe pelvic injuries in a car crash. She is found to have a pelvic fracture and hypotension. Large volume of IV fluid is given but her hypotension does not improve. Sonogram shows no intra-abdominal fluid but a pelvic hematoma. What's the most appropriate next step?

A. Pelvic surgical exploration   B. Exploratory laparotomy   C. Foley catheter

D. External pelvic fixation of and arteriographic embolization

E. Support and close observation

26. A 20 y/o man is involved in a motorcycle accident with a severe pelvic fracture. His vital signs are stable. He feels the urge to urinate but is unable to do so. P/E reveals blood at the meatus, a scrotal hematoma, and a high-riding prostate. What's the most appropriate next step?

A. Retrograde urethrogram   B. Foley catheter   C. Repair of the anterior urethral injuries

D. Repair of the posterior urethral injuries   E. Observation

27. In a car accident, a 20 y/o man has multiple rib fractures and abdominal contusions. His vital signs are stable. Retrograde urethro-cystogram shows normal results. A Foley catheter reveals gross hematuria. The most appropriate next step is

A. abdominal CT　　　　　　　　B. abdominal sonogram　　　　　　C. exploratory laparotomy

D. support and close observation　　　　　　　　　　　　　E. retrograde urethrogram

28. A 40 y/o man suffers from a blunt abdominal trauma in a car collision. His vital signs are stable and P/E results are unremarkable. Urine analysis finds microscopic hematuria. What's the most appropriate next step?

A. Abdominal CT　　　　　　　　B. Abdominal sonogram　　　　　　C. Exploratory laparotomy

D. Supportive treatment and close observation　　　　　　　　E. Retrograde urethrogram

29. A 10 y/o boy has his arms crushed in a traffic accident, and arrives to the ER looking bruised, battered, and swollen. X-rays show normal bones. His vital signs are stable. What's the most appropriate next step?

A. Fasciotomy　　　　　　　　　B. Arteriogram　　　　　　　　　C. Exploratory surgery

D. IV fluid with NaHCO3 and diuretics　　　　　　　　　　　E. NSAIDs

30. A 20 y/o man suffers a gunshot, with the entrance wound in the anteromedial aspect of his upper thigh and the exit in the posteromedial aspect of the thigh. He has normal pulses in the leg and normal X-rays of the femur. What's the most appropriate next step to do?

A. CT scan　　　　　　　　　　B. Arteriogram　　　　　　　　　C. Exploratory surgery

D. Support and close observation　　　　　　　　　　　　　E. Analgesics and antibiotics

31. After a 7-hour abdominal surgery, a 50 y/o female has developed lethargy, confusion, and coma. Her medical charts show that her serum Na is 154 mEq/L and urinary output is 450-550 mL/hr since the surgery, despite IV fluids being given at 150 mL/hr. What's the best next treatment?

A. IV 1.5 L of 5% dextrose　　　　　　　　B. IV 1.5 L of 5% dextrose in normal saline

C. IV 3 L of 5% dextrose in normal saline　　　　D. IV 3 L of 5% dextrose in half normal saline

E. IV 3 L of normal saline

32. A 20 y/o female has acute lower abdominal pain and a vaginal discharge for the past 5 hours, with mild fever and nausea. Her vital signs are stable and her last menstrual period (LMP) was 4 weeks ago. P/E shows diffuse lower abdominal and adnexal tenderness. What's the most appropriate next step?

A. Pelvic ultrasound　　　　　　　　B. Gram stain and culture of the cervical discharge

C. Blood beta-hCG test　　　　　　　　D. Oral ceftriaxone and doxycycline for 4 weeks

E. Surgical exploration

33. A 20 y/o female has acute lower abdominal pain for the past 5 hours, with mild fever, nausea, and distress. Her HR is 130/min and BP is 80/60 mmHg. Her LMP was 4 weeks ago. P/E shows RLQ abdominal and adnexal tenderness. What's the most appropriate next step?

A. Pelvic exam　　　　　　　　　B. Abdominal CT　　　　　　　　C. Blood beta-hCG test

D. Culdocentesis　　　　　　　　E. Surgical exploration

34. A 20 y/o female has acute lower abdominal pain for the past 5 hours, with mild fever and nausea. Her vital signs are stable and her LMP was 2 weeks ago. P/E shows RLQ abdominal tenderness. What's the most appropriate next step?

A. Abdominal and pelvic ultrasound   B. Abdominal CT
C. Blood beta-hCG test   D. Culdocentesis   E. Surgical exploration

35. A 70 y/o man has acute abdominal pain, tachypnea, and tachycardia for the past few hours. P/E shows a silent abdomen with diffuse tenderness and mild rebound, and threads of blood in the rectal exam. Careful history taking reveals that he has previously been diagnosed with atrial fibrillation (AF) and has intermittently received medical treatment. His vital signs are stable. What's the most appropriate next step?
A. CXR   B. Angiogram   C. Surgical exploration
D. Abdominal X-rays   E. Abdominal CT

36. A 70 y/o man is brought to the ER after having two bowel movements with dark red blood over the past two days. He is pale and weak but has stable vital signs. His past history is unremarkable. What's the most appropriate next step?
A. Angiography   B. Upper endoscopy   C. Lower endoscopy
D. Both upper and lower endoscopy   E. NG tube aspiration

37. A 70 y/o man is diagnosed with a 0.5 cm ureteral stone, which is expected to pass spontaneously with large volumes of water intake. Two days later, he develops chills, fever, and flank pain on the side with the stone. What's the most appropriate next step?
A. Massive IV antibiotic therapy   B. Stone extraction
C. Abdominal X-rays   D. Ureteral stent or percutaneous nephrostomy
E. Abdominal CT

38. On the 6th postoperative day after a big obstetric surgery, a 40 y/o female suddenly develops severe pleuritic chest pain and short of breath (SOB). P/E shows that she is anxious and diaphoretic with tachycardia and JVD; BP = 90/70 mmHg. What's the most appropriate next step?
A. ECG   B. Pulmonary angiography   C. Ventilation-perfusion (V/Q) scans
D. CXR   E. ABG test

39. A 70 y/o woman just had a big hip surgery. On the 6th postoperative day she develops a tense, distended abdomen with occasional bowel sounds and no tenderness. X-rays show a distended colon, with a few distended loops of small bowel. What's the most appropriate next step?
A. Nothing by mouth (NPO)   B. GI-dynamic drug   C. Colonoscopy
D. Colostomy   E. Cecostomy

40. A 65 y/o woman is very weak with acute cholecystitis not responding to medical treatment. She had a history of myocardial infarction (MI) about 5 months ago and currently has an irregular pulse and JVD. Her BP is normal. What's the most appropriate next step?
A. Fast cholecystectomy   B. Percutaneous radiologic tube cholecystectomy
C. Supportive treatment and observation   D. CVS support and delaying cholecystectomy
E. Add new antibiotics

41. A 60 y/o man had a difficult abdominal surgery 10 days ago. Now he begins to leak 1-1.5 L of green fluid per day through the subcostal abdominal wound. He has stable vital signs. What's the most important next management?
A. Total parenteral nutrition (TPN)   B. Surgical exploration
C. Adequate normal fluid and nutrition supply   D. Antibiotics

E. Abdominal ultrasound

42. A 70y/o man presents with confusion and short of breath on the 5th day after a colon resection. P/E results: T = 38.5°C, HR = 90/min, RR = 28/min, BP = 100/70 mmHg; orientation to time and space is unclear; chest and abdominal signs are unremarkable. All the following steps of management are necessary EXCEPT

A. ABG test   B. ECG   C. blood cultures
D. CXR   E. urine culture   F. abdominal CT

43-45: Match the following clinical scenarios with the most likely diagnosis.

A. Medial meniscus tear   B. Anterior cruciate ligament (Lig) injury
C. Posterior cruciate Lig injury   D. Chondromalacia patella
E. Osteochondritis dissecans   F. Osgood-Schlatter disease
G. Medial collateral Lig injury   H. Lateral collateral Lig injury

43. A soccer athlete had an acute twisting injury on the right knee 4 hours ago. P/E shows instability, edema, hematoma, tenderness, and locking of the right knee.

44. A 13 y/o boy complains of localized right tibial pain for a month, worsened with activities and relieved with rest. He is a soccer lover and almost plays it every day. P/E finds a normal right knee but mildly swollen frontal tibial area with tenderness. X-ray shows a normal image.

45. A 16 y/o boy has progressive anterior knee pain for the past 2 months, which is worsened by activities and relieved moderately with rest. P/E finds swelling and tenderness on the medial patella with crepitating sensation.

46. An 8 y/o girl falls in a fast running with her right arm touching the ground. She feels great pain and difficulties in moving her right arm, and is brought to the ER 4 hours later. P/E shows no open cut or bleeding, but marked swelling and tenderness around the right elbow, decreased radial pulse, and difficulties in moving the forearm and wrist. X-ray confirms the fracture. The most likely specific injury is

A. radial nerve   B. ulnar nerve   C. axillary artery
D. brachial artery   E. medial nerve

47--53: Match the most likely orthopedic injury with the following clinical scenarios.

A. Posterior shoulder dislocation   B. Anterior shoulder dislocation
C. Posterior hip dislocation   D. Scaphoid fracture
E. Boxer's fracture   F. Colles fracture
G. Middle-shaft humerus fracture   H. Proximal humerus fracture
I. Supracondylar fracture   J. Monteggia fracture
K. Galeazzi fracture   L. Intertrochanteric hip fracture
M. Ankle fracture   N. Achilles tendon rupture
O. Femoral neck fracture

47. A 17 y/o boy is brought to the ER with a painful right arm after a serious fight with a gang of teenagers involving repeated pushing and dragging of the right arm. P/E finds stable vital signs, tenderness on the right shoulder, and the right arm turned outward on anterior chest. X-ray confirms the diagnosis.

48. A 17 y/o boy is brought to the ER with a painful right hand after a serious fight with a gang of teenagers involving repeated hand-hits. P/E finds stable vital signs and tenderness in the anatomical snuff box of the right hand. Local X-ray result is normal.

49. A 70 y/o female is brought to the ER with a painful right hand after a fall on an outstretched hand. P/E finds stable vital signs, a deformed right wrist, and dorsally angulated right hand with tenderness. Local X-ray confirms a displaced fracture.

50. A 17 y/o boy is brought to the ER with a painful right arm after a serious car accident involving the right arm trauma. P/E finds stable vital signs, deformation and tenderness on the right arm, and wrist drop and decreased thumb abduction. X-ray confirms the fracture.

51. A 17 y/o boy is brought to the ER with a painful swollen right forearm and hand after a hit by a heavy blunt object. P/E finds stable vital signs, swelling and tenderness on the right forearm and wrist. X-ray confirms dislocation of the radial head along with diaphyseal fracture of the ulna.

52. A 70 y/o female is brought to the ER with tachypnea, tachycardia, and chest pain. 10 days ago she fell at home with the right hip touching the ground first. She has stayed home by herself since the fall. P/E finds tachypnea, dyspnea, tachycardia, and a shortened and externally rotated right leg. ABG reveals decreased P_{O2} and P_{CO2}. CXR is normal and bone X-ray confirms a dislocation and fracture in the hip.

53. An athlete is in a strenuous jump when he feels a severe pain on the right ankle. He cannot move his right ankle or stand with his right foot. P/E finds limited plantar flexion and positive Thompson's test (no foot plantar flexion after pressure on the gastrocnemius). X-ray is scheduled immediately.

<u>54—57</u>: Match the following orthopedic injuries and disorders in children with the most likely diagnosis.

A. Radial head subluxation   B. Clavicular fracture
C. Greenstick fracture   D. Torus fracture
E. Salter-Harris fracture   F. Supracondylar humerus fracture
G. Developmental hip dislocation/dysplasia   H. Legg-Calve-Perthes disease
I. Slipped capital femoral epiphysis

54. A 10 y/o boy is brought to the ER 2 hours after a fight with another boy involving repeated hits on the right neck, chest, arm, and elbow. He feels severe pain when moving his neck and right shoulder. P/E finds obvious swelling and tenderness between the neck and the right shoulder but no deformity. X-ray film confirms diagnosis.

55. A 10 y/o boy is brought to the ER 2 hours after a car accident involving a severe right forearm hit. He feels severe pain in the right forearm and wrist at rest and moving. P/E finds obvious swelling, tenderness and deformity on the distal right forearm and wrist. X-ray reveals buckling of the distal radius and ulna with continuous cortex.

56. A 2 y/o boy presents with a shorter left leg and painless limp. P/E finds limited left hip abduction and internal rotation. X-ray (two views) reveals increased joint space and collapsed femoral head on the left side.

57. A 16 y/o obese boy presents with pain in the left thigh and knee with limping after a running competition 3 days ago. P/E finds tenderness and limited internal rotation and abduction of the left hip, and decreased external rotation at the hip flexion. X-ray reveals displaced femoral head posteriorly and medially.

58. A 17 y/o boy receives a hard blow on his right knee when playing football. He feels severe progressive pain in the right knee and has difficulty standing or walking. The physician advised daily use of an icepack as the initial treatment. 5-6 days later, the pain and swelling remain the same. Then the doctor orders an MRI scan of the knee, which shows a torn anterior cruciate ligament (ACL). The best next step is

A. NSAIDs   B. arthroscopic repair   C. rehabilitation

D. surgery to replace the knee   E. joint fluid analysis

59. A 40y/o man takes a nap with his head on his arms. When he wakes up, he feels a severe pain in the index finger and finds it flexed while other fingers are extended. When he pulls the index finger free, he hears a "pop" sound with a sharp pain. What's the best next step of management?

A. Reassurance   B. Rehabilitation   C. NSAIDs

D. Steroid injection   E. Surgical repair

60. A 15 y/o boy ingests an unknown substance for suicide and survives after emergent treatment. 2-days later, his lab results show that Ca = 7.5 mg/dL; BUN and creatinine are increased; BUN:creatinine ratio = 15: 1; urinalysis is abnormal. The most likely substance taken by the boy is

A. acetaminophen   B. aspirin   C. opiates

D. insecticides   E. ethylene glycol

Answers and Explanations

1. (C). It's most likely a case of acetaminophen intoxication, mostly with GI and CNS symptoms. Treatment (Tx) is to first check symptoms and blood levels of the drug before other choices. Ipecac and gastric lavage can be used within 1-2 hours of ingestion. Charcoal is the safe therapy 1-2 hours after ingestion, but after "C" is performed. Antidote N-acetylcysteine is used only when symptoms are serious.

2. (B). This patient most likely has organophosphate intoxication with severe symptoms. Therefore, Tx with atropine is first needed for symptomatic relief, followed by administration of the specific antidote PAM (to reactivate anticholinesterases) and other Tx to ensure patient stability.

3. (C). It's most likely that the patient has taken benzodiazepine but the specific antidote flumazenil is not necessary yet because the ingestion is as recent as 40 min ago and the vital signs are normal (Nl). Ipecac-induced emesis and gastric lavage can be used within 1-2 hours of ingestion but emesis has very limited value because the time for the pills to pass the pyloric sphincter (not removable) is not long enough. Thus gastric lavage is the best initial management here to remove the pills. A laxative is unnecessary since most of the pills are not in the intestine yet. Other steps may be helpful but are not as immediate as "C".

4. (B). This patient has probably ingested overdosed antidepressive (TCA) and BZ (diazepam) for his symptoms. When the patient is dependent on diazepam, ingestion of flumazenil may induce seizures, but it may not be the mechanism here because diazepam is taken only for the 2nd day. It's more likely in this case that blocking the seizure-inhibitive effect of diazepam released the toxicity of TCA and resulted in seizures. ECG is thus the best initial test because typical widened QRS waves will be present with TCA intoxication. Others may be done later.

5. (A). This is a case of second-degree, 20%-area burn (head and one arm for 9%/each, plus 2x1% hand-sized burn). The first day's (first 24 hours) fluid: 4mL/kg x 50 x 20 = 4000 mL; 1/2 of 4000 mL is given during the initial 8 hr; ¼ for each of the following 8 hr. The 2nd-day's fluid: ½ of the total, mixed with colloids. The 3rd day's fluid: mild diuresis, no more IV fluids; maintaining urine > 4 mL/kg/hr.

6. (D). Electrical burns are usually much larger and more severe than they appear, often with deep tissue destruction. The patient will first need "D" to prevent renal failure, and then "A".

7. (A). She has CO poisoning and respiratory burns from a fire inside a closed building. All treatment steps are needed in the order of (A, B, C, D, and E). If the blood level of CO-Hb is > 5%, put the patient on 100% oxygen. After the diagnosis of respiratory tract lesion with bronchoscopy, "D" may be chosen.

8. (A). This is a 3rd-degree, circumferential burn: the leathery eschar will not expand, but the area under the burn will develop massive edema that can decrease circulation (as circumferential burns of the chest can compromise breathing). First monitor the peripheral circulation, and then perform escharotomy with signs of decreased circulation. 'C' may be needed for deeper burns. An open space burn is rarely associated with respiratory burn.

9. (E). This has a burn injury of about 20% total BSA (9% for each leg and 1% for genitalia/perineum). Fluid resuscitation for Day 1 (first 8 hrs): 4 mL/kg x BSA% = 4 x 70 x 20 x ½ = 2300 mL, giving Ringer's lactate and avoiding colloids or diuretics. Oxygen, antibiotics (to prevent infection), and a H2-R blocker (to prevent stress ulcer) are all needed. From the 3rd day on, no further fluid is needed and a brief diuresis may be helpful. Steroids may be harmful and should be avoided.

10. (B). "B, C, D, and E" are all therapies needed to save this patient under hemorrhagic shock. After assuring a stable airway and breathing and supplying oxygen, treat following the order of "B, C, D, and E." "A" may be harmful and unnecessary.

11. (D). It will open the pericardial sac, relieve the tamponade, and save the patient's life.

12. (C). A severe MI should be suspected immediately in an old man with hypertension, history of fall, chest pain, and cardiogenic shock. "A" would not have normal bilateral breath sounds. "B" is the most likely 2nd Dx. Either "B" or "D" usually follows trauma.

13. (D). This is a case of plain pneumothorax, not a tension pneumothorax. Patient has stable vital signs and thus CXR should be done to confirm the Dx before Tx.

14. (C). This is the #1 common chest injury--a plain rib fracture. The most effective Tx is local pain relief (best by nerve block) to avoid hypoventilation and pneumonia, especially in the elderly.

15. (C). This is a case of hemopneumothorax. Contaminated blood has to be evacuated to avoid empyema. Upper chest tube connected to a vacuum bottle can be used for this case of plain pneumothorax (not tension pneumothorax).

16. (B). Typical tension pneumothorax: insert an upper chest needle followed by a chest tube to get the air out. Later, CXR is done to rule out widened mediastinum (aortic rupture) or hemothorax.

17. (B). Most sudden deaths occurring during IV procedures are due to air embolism.

18. (B). This is a sucking chest wound, best to be covered with Vaseline gauze to prevent further air intake, and to be taped on three sides to create a one-way flap (to allow air to move out). Once hospitalized, the patient will need an upper chest tube for plain pneumothorax.

19. (A). The patient has labored paradoxical breathing and flail chest, with high risk for other hidden injuries (aortic rupture and Abd injuries) that need to be ruled out. Follow the order of "A, B, C, and D" for this case: if "A" is (+), avoid "B or C"; continue "B, C, and D" only if the previous evaluation result is (-). "D" is for underlying pulmonary contusion.

20. (D). It's traumatic diaphragmatic rupture--always on the left and requires immediate surgical repair.

21. (D). This is a case of multiple traumatic injuries with fat embolism symptoms, respiratory distress, hypoxia, etc. The major problem is respiratory distress and the crucial Tx is respiratory support (oxygen and positive pressure mechanical ventilation—PPMV). "A" or "C" may be helpful with a serious pulmonary embolism.

22. (B). A penetrating wound on the abdominal always requires exploratory laparotomy, but not on the chest. This is a penetrating chest-abdominal wound, and thus a laparotomy is required to search for additional injuries in the abdomen. An upper or lower chest tube may be needed later.

23. (D). Most likely it's a ruptured spleen, requiring emergent laparotomy because the patient has developed on-going hemorrhagic shock. If he's stable, serial CT scans will be the best choice to diagnose the abdominal hemorrhage. "B" and "C" are older, noninvasive diagnostic ways for abdominal bleeding.

24. (C). This is a post-surgery abdominal compartment syndrome. The abdomen needs to be decompressed by opening the incision and using a temporary cover, while delaying reclosing procedures until a later date. "B and D" are used for a surgical cut with high tension that cannot be closed normally.

25. (D). This is a tough case with continuous pelvic bleeding, which is very difficult to stop and may lead to death. Surgical exploration may not always work. "D" is thus the best choice here. "C" is needed after "D". Pelvic hematoma with stable vital signs can be left for observation.

26. (A). This is a case of combined anterior and posterior urethral injuries. Tx steps: (1) first perform retrograde urethrogram for Dx; (2) insert a suprapubic catheter and repair anterior urethral injuries; (3) delay repairing posterior urethral injuries for 6 months.

27. (A). The blood is most likely from the kidneys since lower UT injuries have been ruled out. CT scan is the best Dx for renal injuries. Generally, traumatic hematuria from blunt trauma does not require surgery even if the kidney is smashed. "D" is after "A".

28. (D). Most traumatic microhematuria in adults requires no further investigation, but gross traumatic hematuria always requires work-up. Non-traumatic hematuria of any type must be investigated to rule out cancer of the kidney, bladder, or ureter. Most traumatic microhematuria in children needs to be investigated because it often indicates congenital anomalies, and ultrasound or IVP is usually the first means of Dx.

29. (D). Crush injuries can lead to two complications: (1) myoglobinemia-myoglobinuria acute renal failure; (2) swelling-compartment syndrome. "D" (large volume of IV fluid, osmotic diuretics, and alkalinisation of the urine) is done first to help protect the kidney. "A" is for the compartment syndrome later.

30. (B). Gunshot or stab wounds of the extremities may cause injury to major vessels. "B" is preferred over "C". "D" is required later. If there's a hematoma or vascular injury at the wound site, surgery is done first.

31. (D). This is hypotonic dehydration with more water loss than salt. Every 3 mEq/L of Na rise above the normal 145 mEq/L represents 1 L of water loss. This patient has 9 mEq/L of Na rise and 3 L of fluid loss from the urine. She needs "D" or 3 L of 5% dextrose (D5W) over 48 hours.

32. (C). Though it's most likely pelvic inflammatory disease (PID), pregnancy must be excluded before the appropriate choices for PID ("B and D").

33. (D). This is most likely a ruptured ectopic pregnancy (or less likely, an ovarian cyst). Because her vital signs are unstable, culdocentesis is the fastest way to Dx the bleeding. If it's (-), ectopic pregnancy cannot be excluded. Perform a quick ultrasound to confirm Dx, then surgery ("E") to cure. "B" and "C" are both too late for the necessary surgery. If the patient is stable, both ultrasound and beta-hCG should be done first.

34. (A). This is most likely a simple appendicitis. The most cost-effective Dx and Tx steps are "A" followed by "E"—appendix removal even if it's not appendicitis. CT is indicated for complicated cases. "C" is needed if LMP is > 4 weeks.

35. (D). Mesenteric embolism is the most likely Dx for this elderly patient with a history of AF. Abdominal X-rays usually show distended small bowel and ascending-transverse colon. As it's early in the case implying that the bowel can be saved, the next step is an angiogram followed by an urgent embolectomy. If it's too late and the bowel is dead, resection is the only choice.

36. (D). It's either upper or lower GI bleeding. For an elderly patient, cancer, diverticulosis, polyps, and angiodysplasias have to be considered. For a young patient, an upper site is more likely. Angiography is not much effective in detection of slow bleeding. For this case, "D" is the best choice. "E" is helpful if the patient has recent onset of upper GI bleeding.

37. (A). It's a difficult, urgent condition of both UTI and obstruction. First do "A" to control the infection, then "D" to decompress, and finally "B" to cure the cause when the patient is stabilized. In a septic patient, stone extraction would be very risky.

38. (E). This is a late postoperative pulmonary embolus (PE). ABG is usually done first to show decreased O_2 and CO_2. If ABG is normal, it's not PE. V/Q scan is then performed to confirm the Dx, but can be spared if the patient is unstable—respiratory support and heparin can be given after ABG Dx. Pulmonary angiography is the most specific Dx test for PE but is too invasive and thus rarely used. CXR is not very helpful.

39. (C). An elderly patient with a recent major surgery and immobilization can easily develop massive colonic dilatation. Colonoscopy will suck out the gas, rule out mechanical obstruction (cancer), and allow long rectal tube placement.

40. (B). She has several predictors of operative cardiac risk, and thus should not undergo any major surgery such as "A". The best option to treat the cholecystitis here would be "B", plus "C" or "D".

41. (C). It's best to help the wound heal by itself without further operation. "A"--total parenteral nutrition and "D" are 2nd choices. If he is febrile, unstable, or with an acute abdominal condition, he needs "B".

42. (F). This elderly patient has postoperative confusion, low fever, and hypoxia—tachypnea and tachycardia. An initial ECG followed by an ABG should be tested for suspected pulmonary embolism. An ECG may also exclude an atypical myocardial infarction in an elderly. A CXR is for atelectasis or pneumonia. CBC, blood and urine cultures are for suspected sepsis, pneumonia, or UTI in this patient. An abdominal CT scan may be necessary when evidence of the abdominal complication (abscess, bleeding, etc) is present or suspected.

43. (A). It's one of the vulgar knee injuries, usually with a positive McMurray's test. MCL: Leg bent outward more than normal range. Lateral Col Lig: Leg bent inward more than normal range. ACL: By twisting or forced hyperextension; positive anterior drawer and Lachman tests. PCL: By forced hyperextension; positive posterior drawer test.

44. (F). It's a common "overuse disorder" of the tibia in active adolescent children.

45. (D). It's a common "overuse syndrome" of the knee in teenagers. "E" is subchondral bone necrosis and separated joint fragments due to repeated trauma; commonly occurs in the knee in active teenagers with swelling, tenderness and clicking; X-ray shows "notch view".

46. (D). It's most likely a supracondylar fracture causing the Volkmann's contracture, treated with closed reduction and fixation by hanging arm cast. Middle shaft humerus fracture often causes radial nerve palsy (wrist drop and thumb abduction deficiency). Proximal fracture often causes axillary artery injury affecting the whole arm.

47. (B). Anterior dislocation is the No.1 common type of shoulder dislocation, caused by strain on the glenohumoral Lig. Painful arm turned outward on anterior chest, in a shape of "shaking hands". It's risky of injuries of auxiliary artery and nerve. Posterior dislocation: Seen in seizure or electric shock. Arm is medially rotated and rested on the side. Posterior hip dislocation is caused by the same direction force on internally rotated, flexed and adducted hip.

48. (D). A typical case of scaphoid fracture—carpal navicular fracture, the most common carpal bone fracture. X-ray may not show the fracture until 1-2 weeks later. Avascular necrosis (A-V-N) may occur with the 3rd scaphoid fracture. Boxer's fracture: The 5th metacarpal neck fracture, often from punching a hard object with a closed fist.

49. (F). Colle fracture is the most common wrist fracture. It involves the distal radius usually from a fall onto an outstretched hand, resulting in a dorsally angulated and displaced fracture. The disorder is mostly seen in children and the elderly with osteoporosis.

50. (G). Middle shaft humerus fracture often causes radial nerve palsy (wrist drop and thumb abduction deficiency). Proximal humerus fracture may cause auxiliary artery injury. Distal (supracondylar) fracture mostly in children and causes brachial artery injury (decreased radial pulse, Volkmann contracture, etc).

51. (J). Monteggia fracture is also known as "nightstick fracture" ("self-defense injury"); X-ray confirms dislocation of the radial head along with diaphyseal fracture of the ulna. Galeazzi fracture: distal radius dislocation and fracture.

52. (L). It's most likely a case of intertrochanteric hip fracture complicated by a pulmonary embolism. This fracture is commonly caused by falls in osteoporotic females, presenting with the affected leg shortened and externally rotated and with increased risk of subsequent DVT. Displaced femoral neck fracture is caused by direct trauma; associated with avascular femoral head necrosis and fracture nonunion. Femur fracture is also caused by direct trauma, risky of major bleeding and fat emboli syndrome.

53. (N). A typical case of Achilles tendon rupture: sudden "pop" with pain during an intense activity followed by decreased ankle movement. Ankle fracture: injured by external rotation/supination, causing fractures of medial and lateral malleoli; Tx is ORIF.

54. (B). Clavicular fracture is the most common long bone fracture in newborns and children. Usually in the middle third of the clavicle, with the proximal fractured end displaced superiorly (deformity and tenderness), and may cause brachial nerve palsy (Erb's palsy. Nursemaid's elbow is the radial head subluxation due to sudden pulling or lifting by the hand. X-ray confirms both Dx.

55. (D). A typical case of torus fracture; the cortex continuing without breaking. Greenstick fracture--also known as cortex breach-- incomplete fracture involving the bone cortex of one side only.

56. (H). A typical case of Legg-Calve-Perthes disease, osteochondrosis due to idiopathic avascular necrosis of the femoral head; mostly unilateral, in 2-10 year boys, and self-limited. Developmental hip dislocation/dysplasia: varying displacement of the proximal femur from the acetabulum. The hip may be subluxed or dislocated. More common in first-born female and breach presentation.

57. (I). A typical case of slipped capital femoral epiphysis (SCFE), separation of the proximal femoral epiphysis through the growth plate; mostly seen in obese children. Salter-Harris fracture is the fracture of the growth plate in children, which is divided into five types.

58. (B). Arthroscopic repair is the most definitive therapy for this young patient with ACL injury, followed by rehabilitation. Knee replacement is only for total knee joint destruction such as in elderly osteoarthritis. Joint fluid analysis may be helpful if joint inflammation or sepsis is suspected.

59. (D). Steroid injection is very effective in decreasing pain and recurrence of "trigger finger", which is an acutely flexed and painful finger caused by a stenosis of the tendon sheath. Surgical repair should be considered only after steroid injection is ineffective. NSAIDs may have limited effects. Other choices are inappropriate.

60. (E). This patient has acute kidney injury (AKI) due to acute tubular necrosis (ATN), supported by increased BUN and BUN:creatinine ratio < 20:1 after ingestion of a harmful substance. Ethylene glycol can cause ATN by oxalate crystal precipitating in the kidney tubules. The crystal precipitates as Ca-oxalate so that the serum Ca is low. Acetaminophen is hepatotoxic. Aspirin is kidney toxic but not associated with hypo-Ca and abnormal urinalysis. Opiates are associated with respiration suppression and focal-segmental glomerulonephritis. Organophosphate poisoning from insecticides causes cholinergic effects ("SLUDGEM"), not AKI.

Chapter 16

MENTAL AND BEHAVIORAL DISORDERS

(Mainly by DSM-5: Diagnostic and Statistical Manual of Mental Disorders, 5th Ed, 2014)

BASICS

Psychiatry is the medical specialty devoted to the study and treatment of mental disorders, which include various affective, behavioral, cognitive, and perceptual disorders.

Mental Status Examination (MSE)

MSE is used to describe the physician's observation and impression of the patient during the interview. Combined with the patient's history (Hx), it is the best way to make an accurate diagnosis (Dx) for most psychiatric diseases and disorders.

MSE includes appearance, attitude, behavior, mood (emotions perceived), affect (emotional responses), thought (form and content), speech, sensorium (alertness, level of consciousness, and orientation), cognition (memory, concentration, capacity to read, write and learn, abstract thinking, judgment, and insight), reliability, and self-control ability.

Neuropsychological tests used to detect organicity from any psychiatric disorder include Bender-Gestalt, Luria-Nebraska, and Halted-Reitan tests.

Interviewing Techniques

Open-Ended Questions: Allow patient to speak in his own words as much as possible. E.g., "Can you tell me more about this?"

Closed-Ended Questions: Ask for specific information without much choice in answering. E.g., "Are you feeling the pain now?"

Facilitation: The physician helps the patient continue by providing verbal or nonverbal clues. E.g., "Yes, continue, please."

Confrontation: The doctor points something out to the patient directly. E.g., "You look angry today. I'd like to know why."

Reassurance: If it's truthful it can lead to increased compliance, but if it's false it can lead to decreased compliance. E.g., "His conditions are serious, but we'll do our best to treat it." (True) "Don't worry. Everything will be fine." (False)

Leading: The answer is suggested in the question. E.g., "Is the voice telling you to kill yourself?"

Defense Mechanisms

The way and means that the ego reduces anxiety and controls instinctive urges and unpleasant affects (emotions). Most defense mechanisms are unconscious (except suppression), discrete, and dynamic, and can be adaptive or maladaptive.

Types of Defense Mechanisms

Acting out: The outburst display of previously inhibited emotions or behavior (often in actions rather than words); usually considered to be healthy and therapeutic. E.g., harshly criticized by his father, the boy had a temper tantrum.

Blocking: Temporary block in thinking. E.g., "What were we talking about?"

Denial: A defense used to avoid becoming aware of some painful aspect of reality. E.g., "I know they gave me a wrong diagnosis as cancer."

Displacement: An emotion or drive is shifted to another object with similar but with more tolerable nature. E.g., someone kicked the dog after having a fight with his supervisor.

Humor: A mature defense; permitting the expression of feelings and thoughts with comfort or release to self and others. E.g., a patient said to the doctor, "It's good that I have all these conditions to keep you busy."

Introjection: Features of the external world are taken into part of the self. E.g., a secretary dresses like her supervisor.

Intellectualization: Excessive use of intellectual processes to avoid affective expression or experience. E.g., "It's interesting to see there are more people getting the same cancer as mine."

Isolation: Separation of an idea from the affect that accompanies it. E.g., when he saw the dead body of a friend, he appeared to show no emotion.

Projection: Attributing one's own wishes, thoughts, or feelings onto someone else. E.g., (1) "I'm sure he did it intentionally!" (2) A nurse has been ignoring a patient with late-stage cancer, and replied when asked why, "He wants to be left alone." (It is actually the nurse who wants to be alone. If she made excuses for ignoring the patient, it's "rationalization").

Regression: Returning to an earlier stage of immature behaviour. E.g., a 66 y/o physician begins to help his colleague occupy a seat at a routine meeting.

Repression: An idea or feeling is withheld from consciousness; unconscious forgetting. E.g., someone said he did not remember the car accident he had 2 years ago.

Reaction formation: An unacceptable impulse is transformed into its opposite, resulting in the formation of character traits. E.g., a frustrated man smiled at his supervisor after an immediate fight with a co-worker.

Rationalization: Using rational explanations to justify unacceptable attitudes, beliefs, or behaviors. E.g., "It's good I lost the job so that I have more time to do exercise."

Defense Mechs

Somatization: Psychic distress is converted into bodily symptoms. E.g., after hearing the bad news, she suddenly became blind.

Splitting: Dividing external objects into all good or all bad categories. E.g., "All car dealers are cheaters!"

Sublimation: Most mature defense. Instincts are led to change the aim or object from unacceptable to acceptable, to achieve impulse gratification. E.g., a boy who enjoyed ripping things becomes a surgeon.

Suppression: Conscious forgetting; the only conscious defense mechanism. E.g., "After becoming a Christian, Peter forgave his colleague's insult and made a good friend with him."

Undoing: It's an "after behavior" —trying to "undo" an unhealthy, destructive, or unacceptable thought or action by acting out or engaging in the contrary behavior that is more acceptable. E.g., (1) A man quit smoking and alcohol drinking and advocated his friends to do so; (2) A man insulted someone but immediately gave praising words.

NEURODEVELOPMENTAL DISORDERS

Intellectual Disability *Disorder*

↓ cognitive skill
↓ adaptive fxn

Definition: Previously known as "**Mental retardation**", also as "**Intellectual developmental disorder**", it is defined as intelligence quotient **(IQ) < 70**, significantly decreased intellectual function (such as cognitive abilities), and must be accompanied by concurrent impairment in adapting to demands in school, work, social, and other environments. The onset is before 18 y/a, accounts for about 1% of the population, and is more common in school-age boys.

Etiology

Down syndrome, velocariofacial syndrome, and fetal alcohol syndrome are the three most common inborn causes. Other causes include genetic and chromosomal abnormalities (lipidoses, aminoacidurias, glycogen storage diseases, cri du chat syndrome, and fragile X syndrome); intrauterine or postnatal exposure to infections (rubella or CMV), toxins, alcohol, hypoxia, malnutrition (iodine deficiency, etc), heavy metals, physical trauma, and social deprivation.　*Lead poisoning*

Essentials of diagnosis　*dt: clx ~~IQ~~*
How severe ∝ loss of adaptive fxn

1. **Mild intellectual disability (IQ 50–69)**: Patient attains academic skills to elementary 6th-grade level; can live independently or with minimal supervision; may have problems with impulse control and self-esteem; associated with conduct disorders, drug abuse, and ADHD.

2. **Moderate intellectual disability (IQ 35-49):** Academic skills to a *3rd* 2nd-grade level; may be able to manage activities of daily living and working with serious supervision, and have significant problems conforming to social norms. Patient with Down syndrome has higher risk of early development of Alzheimer disease.

Intellectual disability disorder   *20 = infants total care*

3. **Severe (IQ 20-34) and profound intellectual disability (IQ ≤ 20):** Little or no speech, very limited abilities to manage self-care; requires more intensive support and a continuously, highly supervised environment. *Pre-school Age, below everything.*

4. **P/E** may show evidence of underlying disorder or injury. **Amniocentesis** may reveal chromosomal abnormalities associated with intellectual disability in high-risk pregnancies (mother >35 y/a).

1) Genetic screen, must be willing to terminate

Differential diagnosis

Borderline intellectual functioning (IQ 70-100), learning disorders, autistic disorder, sensory impairment, and environmental deprivation.

Treatment

1. Primary prevention such as genetic counselling, good prenatal care, and safe environments for expectant mothers.

2. Treating and monitoring associated disease may improve level of cognitive and adaptive function. Special education techniques and behavioral therapy may improve ultimate level of function. All children with disabilities are mandated to receive a comprehensive education in the least restrictive environment, using an Individualized Education Plan. *Social Skills*

Global Developmental Delay (GDD)

Definition: GDD is a generalized intellectual disability that is usually characterized by lower than average intellectual functioning along with significant limitations in at least two other areas of development. Most children with this disorder are < 5 years. Common signs include delayed acquisition of milestones (e.g., sitting up, crawling, walking), limited reasoning or conceptual abilities, poor social skills and judgement, aggressive behavior as a coping skill, and communication difficulties.

Etiology and risk factors

These include genetic (Fragile X syndrome), metabolic (PKU, etc.), prenatal (rubella or birth trauma), perinatal (prematurity, injury, or infection). Sometimes the cause is unknown.

Treatment

Treat underlying cause.

Specific Learning Disorder and Language Disorder

Definition: Learning achievements in specific areas are substantially below expectations, considering the patient's age, intelligence, sensory abilities, and educational experience. Types include reading disorder (No.1 common), math disorder, and written expression disorder.

Etiology and risk factors

There is more association with males, genetic factors, low socioeconomic status (**SES**), and coexisting conditions (cerebral palsy, lead poisoning and fetal alcohol syndrome). Many cases have no obvious causes found. Prevalence is 5% among school-age children.

Speech Learning/Language Disorder

Essentials of diagnosis

1. Onset is usually during elementary school, presenting with reading, math, or written expression disorder; poor self-esteem and social-maturity, school failure, and behavioral disturbances may occur. It may persist into adulthood.

2. Perceptual-motor problems, conduct disorder, oppositional defiant disorder (ODD), and ADHD may be present.

3. IQ and academic achievement tests are the major diagnostic tools.

Differential diagnosis

It's necessary to rule out hearing or vision impairment, environmental deprivation, and intellectual disability.

Treatment

The main treatment is special education (remedial or individual classes; quality instructions) to improve general learning and skills in the deficient areas. Counselling of patients and families to improve self-esteem, social behavior, and family functioning is helpful.

Communication Disorders

Phonological disorder and stuttering are now called communication disorders—which include **language disorder, speech sound disorder, childhood-onset fluency disorder**, and a new condition characterized by impaired social verbal and nonverbal communication called **social (pragmatic) communication disorder**. They should be treated by speech therapists according to individual's needs.

Attention-Deficit Hyperactivity Disorder

It is a disorder characterized by inattention, short attention span, hyperactivity, and impulsivity that interfere with daily social or academic functioning in school and at home. Prevalence is 3-5% in school-age children; male:female = 9:1. The onset is mostly before 7 y/a, and symptoms persist throughout childhood (about 30% into adulthood).

Etiology

Unknown. It may be associated with family history, trauma, and other disorders—mood and anxiety disorder, drug abuse, antisocial personality disorder, conduct disorder, and learning disorder.

Essentials of diagnosis

1. A child with ADHD usually presents with symptoms **both in school and at home**, and causes marked **social and academic impairment for over 6 months**.

2. Multiple symptoms of attention deficits: Short attention span for schoolwork, play or eating, difficulty following instructions or staying quiet, easily distracted and forgetting, and poor school performance and relationships with siblings.

ADHD

3. Multiple symptoms of hyperactivity and impulsivity: Fidgety and over-active, unexpectedly leaving and running around, excessive talk, interrupting others, disobedient, and fighting.

4. IQ tests and structured symptom-rating scales: Useful for teachers and parents.

Differential diagnosis

Major rule-outs: Normal active behavior, adverse effects (S/E) of drugs, brain trauma, conduct disorder, autistic disorder, and mood disorders.

Treatment

1. Initial treatment should be non-medical—psychobehavioral. Behavior therapy and environmental changes that can be used by parents or teachers to shape the behavior of children with ADHD include:

Maintaining a daily schedule; reducing distractions; setting small, reachable goals; providing places for the child to keep his personal things; rewarding positive behavior; using charts/checklists and calm discipline; limiting choices; encouraging healthy activities (sports, hobbies).

2. Medical treatment: Psychostimulants (**methylphenidate #1,** amphetamine, or pemoline) can effectively alleviate ADHD, given only on school days. S/E: Headache, tics, decreased appetite, sleep, and growth rate. If there is no response to psychostimulants or no tolerance to the adverse effects, an antidepressant, **atomoxetine** (a norepinephrine reuptake inhibitor) or desipramine (a TCA) may be effective.

3. Combined psychobehavioral and medical treatment is better than a single therapy.

f/u absence seizures => Tx w ethosuximide

Autism Spectrum Disorder (ASD)

Previously it was in **Pervasive Developmental Disorders (PDDs)** and known as **autism or autistic disorder. ASD is a neurodevelopmental disorder characterized by (1) persistent deficits in social communication and interaction and (2) restricted, repetitive patterns of behavior, interests, or activities in early childhood** (mostly < age 3). ASD is four times **more common in boys** than in girls.

Etiology

Unclear; may be associated with genetics, environmental causes (heavy metals, pesticides, or childhood vaccines), CNS damage, and other diseases (encephalitis, maternal rubella, perinatal anoxia, phenylketonuria, tuberous sclerosis, fragile X syndrome). All these can affect brain development and information processing in the brain. No obvious causes are found in many cases.

Essentials of diagnosis

1. ASD-specific screening tests should be used in children with (1) delayed language/communication *+ eye contact* milestones; (2) regression in social or language skills; (3) a sibling diagnosed with ASD; (4) ages of 18-24 months; (5) concerns by parents or care providers regarding ASD.

2. **Diagnostic criteria**—requiring all of the following three aspects:

(1) Persistent deficits in social communication (verbal and non-verbal) and social interaction in multiple settings; demonstrated by deficits in all three of the following:

Autism Spectrum Disorder
Dx criteria

A. Social-emotional reciprocity (eg, absent or bizarre use of speech); B. Nonverbal communicative behaviors used for social interaction (eg, abnormal eye contact or body language); C. Developing, maintaining, and understanding relationships (eg, difficulty adjusting behavior to social setting; difficulty making friends with peers).

(2) Restricted, repetitive patterns of behavior, interests, or activities; demonstrated by ≥ 2 of the following:

A. Stereotyped or repetitive movements, use of objects, or speech; B. Insistence on sameness, unwavering adherence to routines, or ritualized patterns of behaviour; C. Highly restricted, fixated interests that are abnormal in strength or focus (eg, bizarre manners, swinging and bumping, attracted by inanimate objects); D. Bizarre response to the environment (sounds, smells, temperature, etc.).

(3) The symptoms must impair social or academic functions, exist in the early developmental period, and not better explained by intellectual disability or global developmental delay, although intellectual disability may be present in about 75% of cases.

3. P/E: May show evidence of self-injuries by head banging or biting, or by seizures.

4. Lab tests: May reveal abnormal EEG and brain morphology.

5. Course: About 30% of patients become semi-independent in adulthood, but almost all have severe residual disabilities. Poor outcome is associated with intellectual disability and speech failure.

Differential diagnosis

Major rule-outs: intellectual disability, hearing impairment, environmental deprivation, and selective mutism.

Treatment *early intervention*

Helpful therapies include family counseling, special education, and behavior training all together. Antipsychotics can be used to control episodes of severe hyperactivity, aggression, anxiety, agitation, compulsive or self-destructive behavior, or depression. No single therapy is very effective.

Asperger Disorder (Syndrome)

It is considered a milder form of autism spectrum disorder, more common in school age boys. Clinical features include extreme behavioral rigidity, perseverative/obsessive interests in a single object/topic and rules; with deficits in social interactions and behaviors, but not in language or intelligence.

Treatment

It mainly involves improvement of relationship with others. It requires a multidisciplinary approach that makes use of the child's strengths (verbal cognitive ability, formal language skills, etc.) to address the child's weaknesses (e.g., nonverbal and social problem-solving skills, pragmatic language). Atomoxetine may be tried if non-medical therapies fail.

Rett Syndrome

In DSM-4, it is a neurodevelopmental disorder of the grey matter of the brain that almost exclusively affects girls. Clinical features include a period of initially normal development followed by loss of normal speech and purposeful hand use, stereotypic hand movements, gait abnormalities (ataxia), and psychomotor disabilities. Additional features include deceleration of head growth, seizures, autistic features, and breathing abnormalities. Most cases result from mutations in the MECP2 gene.

Treatment

Symptomatic therapy; behavioral therapy for self-injurious behavior; physical therapy for muscular dysfunction. No specific therapy is available for Rett syndrome.

MOTOR DISORDERS

A new sub-category, motor disorders, encompasses **developmental coordination disorder, stereotypic movement disorder, and the tic disorders including Tourette disorder** (syndrome).

Tourette Disorder

It is characterized by the onset of multiple motor and vocal tics in childhood (mostly before the age 18), lasting more than one year. Prevalence for male to female is 3 to 1. The average onset age is 7. The course can be fluctuated for many years.

Etiology

Mixed genetics may be associated, and may include abnormity in the dopaminergic (DA) and adrenergic system, ADHD and obsessive-compulsive disorder (OCD).

Essentials of diagnosis

1. Motor tics: Usually involve the muscles of the face and neck, presenting with head shaking, blinking, or twitching of the face, trunk, or extremities. It may also involve complex behaviors such as grimacing, swearing at people, pacing, touching, etc.

2. Vocal tics: Commonly include grunting, coprolalia, counting, throat clearing, etc.

3. Chronic multiple motor and vocal tics: Over one year and before 18 y/a, with remissions and exacerbations.

Treatment

Education and counselling are initiated for mild cases. **Tetrabenazine** (Monoamine-Depleting Agent) is preferred over high-potency dopamine-R blockers (risperidone, pimozide or haloperidol). Clonidine and clonazepam may useful for suppressing tics. Severe focal motor and vocal tics may be treated with injections of botulinum toxin into the affected muscles.

ELIMINATION DISORDERS

Handwritten left margin: begin potty training ① age 2-4 w aquisition of - walking - imitating others actions (eg, sit on toilet) - follow 2-step commands - remove pants - communicate need to urinate & stool - voluntary sphincter ctrl

Enuresis

Handwritten: - assoc w constipation, fecal retention => ↓ bladder capacity? age instability of detrusor - bed wetting is normal ≤5

Handwritten right margin: - Voluntary (acting out) - Anatomic (ectopic ureter) - meds - dz (DM 1 - regression (abuse, new sibling)

It is a disorder characterized by repeated urine voiding into the patient's clothes or bed usually at night in a child > 6 y/a. **Diagnosis is by excluding** a medical condition, and considering possible etiology of psychological stress, UTI or UT-defects, and Family history of enuresis. Prevalence is 3%.

Treatment   *Handwritten:* dx: urinalysis first.!.

1. **Enuresis alarms** (alarm with pad) for 3-4 months are the most effective long-term therapy and have few adverse effects. It's important to reduce the patient's emotional stress and reward the child for "a dry bed/clothes day," to practice appropriate toilet training and to avoid large amounts of fluids before bed.

Handwritten right margin: for noct-urnal incontinence, age ≤5

2. Medications: Oral **desmopressin (DDAVP, No.1)** is good for short-term effect, but with a high relapse rate.

Handwritten: ① Urinalysis, screen for UTI, DM, DI. when incontinence persists beyond age 4 ② 2° enuresis, return of incontinence after ≥6 months dryness, often due to social stressors (divorce, new school). Address those in therapy.

Encopresis

Encopresis, also called stool holding/soiling, or paradoxical diarrhea, is voluntary or involuntary fecal soiling in children who have usually already been toilet trained. It usually occurs when a child after age 4 resists having bowel movements, as a symptom of chronic constipation.

Diagnosis: When encopresis occurs (1) in a child > 4 y/a at least once a month for > 3 months; (2) in inappropriate places (e.g., clothing or floor); (3) without a general medical condition, it may be diagnosed as a developmental or emotional disorder (elimination disorder).

Treatment: It can usually be treated successfully with patient positive reinforcement. Chronic constipation (with or without fecal incontinence) of children is treated with a combination of daily laxatives and behavior modification after disimpaction.

DISRUPTIVE, IMPULSE-CONTROL, AND CONDUCT DISORDERS

(ICD-10: Habit and Impulse Disorders)

This group of disorders involves problems in the self-control of emotions and behaviors, in which individuals are unable to resist an impulse. Different from other emotional and/or behavioral disorders, this group is unique in that these problems are manifested in behaviors that violate the rights of others (e.g., aggression, destruction) and/or that bring the individual into significant conflict with societal norms or authority figures. The underlying causes are various and mechanisms are poorly understood but mostly associated with the serotonin system and anxiety state.

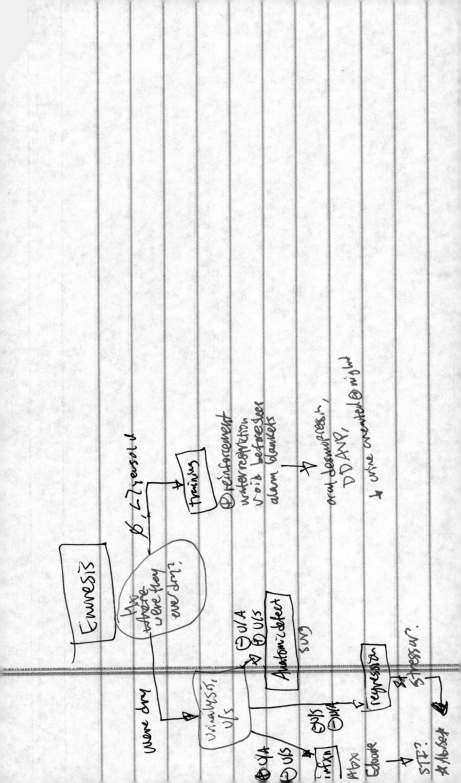

, Arya Stark, teen acting out
- coops w peers

Oppositional Defiant Disorder (ODD)

Definition and features: Persistent pattern of negativistic, defiant, and hostile behaviors toward adults and authorities, including arguments, temper outbursts, deliberate annoyance, and vindictiveness. It's considered an **initial, milder form of conduct disorder.** Prevalence is **10%** in school-age children, more common in boys before puberty and about equal after puberty. **ODD coexists with ADHD in approximately 50-80% of cases.**

Etiology

Associated causes may include family conflict, poor parenting, learning disorder, school failure, low self-esteem, mood lability, ADHD, drug abuse, and over-activity.

Treatment

Tx: parenting

Cognitive-behavioral modification is the effective therapy. It's important to advise parents to **spend time interacting with a child,** to care and reward desired behavior and not simply punish undesired behavior, and to be **consistent in parents' words and deeds.** Without special care in time, it will develop into conduct disorder. Co-therapy for ADHD may be needed in many cases.

Conduct Disorder

, Joffrey Baratheon
Pretty much Antisocial PD
- Bullying, cruelty to animals

Definition and features: Conduct disorder refers to a repetitive and **persistent violation in four areas (aggression, property destruction, deceitfulness/theft, and rules) lasting over 6 months in a child younger than 18 y/a.** These behaviors are often referred to as "antisocial behaviors" and often seen as the precursor to antisocial personality disorder. It is the **No.1 reason for a child or adolescent to be sent to a psychiatrist.** It affects **10%** of school children; **male:female = 9:1.** Symptoms usually gradually remit.

Etiology

It may include genetic factors, family stress, school environment, ADHD, mood disorder, and substance abuse (especially alcohol).

Essentials of diagnosis

1. The main manifestations are repetitive aggression, fighting, cruelty, property destruction, cheating, theft, robbery, and school truancy lasting over 6 months in a patient younger than 18 y/a.

2. **The major outcome or progress is "antisocial personality disorder" diagnosed when the individual with conduct disorder is over 18 y/a.**

3. The major differential diagnosis is oppositional defiant disorder.

Treatment

1. **Cognitive-behavioral modification is the relatively effective therapy.** It's very important to build up healthy group identity and role models. Punishment/incarceration is often ineffective.

Conduct Disorder

2. **Medications:** Risperidone or quetiapine can be the initial option but usually not used until the phase of antisocial personality disorder. Lithium can be used for aggressive behavior, carbamazepine for aggression with emotional lability, and haloperidol for rage and impulsion.

| PEARLS | Order of Progression of Associated Disorders |

ADHD → Oppositional disorder → Conduct disorder → Antisocial personality disorder → Alcoholism

Intermittent Explosive Disorder

It's a disorder characterized by discrete episodes of failure to resist aggressive impulses that result in serious consequence. The aggression degree is usually out of proportion to the stressor, and tends to resolve spontaneously. Prevalence: young male > female. Associated risk factors include CNS trauma or diseases, genetics, hyper-androgen levels, bad occupational and lawful records, poor marital status, etc.

Treatment

Helpful therapies include psychotherapy combined with medications (**fluoxetine#1**, or phenytoin, *SSRI* *Anti-epileptic* or oxcarbazepine) plus cognitive-behavioral therapy (CBT). *Antiepileptic*

Kleptomania

It's a rare disorder characterized by the recurrent failure to resist impulses to steal objects with trivial values or not needed. Patient feels less anxious after the stealing but guilty or ashamed of the actions. Prevalence is female > male. Associated disorders include stress in life, mood disorder, OCD, and mild mental retardation.

Treatment

Insight-oriented therapy, behavioral therapy (aversive conditioning and systematic desensitization), or/and SSRIs may be helpful.

Pyromania

It's a disorder characterized by deliberate fire-setting on more than one occasion. It is seen more frequently in men associated with intellectual disability, alcohol abuse, and history of truancy and cruelty to animals. Patient usually lacks remorse for the consequences. Prevalence: male > female.

Differential diagnosis

Necessary rule-outs: arson, conduct disorder, and antisocial personality disorder.

Treatment

There is no effective treatment. SSRIs, antiepileptic agents, atypical antipsychotics, lithium, or anti-androgens have been proposed. Cognitive behavioral therapy has shown some promise. Incarceration may be necessary.

DEPRESSIVE DISORDERS

Disruptive Mood Dysregulation Disorder (DMDD)

DMDD is a condition in which a child is chronically irritable and experiences frequent, severe temper **outbursts** that are grossly **out of proportion** to the situation at hand. These occur, on average, $\geq$ 3 times each week for $\geq$ 1 year up to age 18 years. DMDD (previously as a bipolar disorder) is at increased risk for depression and anxiety as adults, but not adult bipolar disorder. It occurs more often in boys than girls.

Essentials of diagnosis

1. Symptoms go far beyond temper tantrums in children to temper outbursts that are grossly out of proportion in intensity to the situation, which is severe enough for clinical attention.

2. Between outbursts, children display a persistently irritable or angry mood, most of the day and nearly every day.

3. A DMDD diagnosis requires the above symptoms to be present in at least two settings (at home, at school, or with peers) for 12 or more months, and symptoms must be severe in at least one of these settings. During this period, the child must not have gone 3 or more consecutive months without symptoms. The onset of symptoms must be before age 10, and a DMDD diagnosis should not be made for the first time before age 6 or after age 18.

Treatment

Individualized medications (atypical antipsychotics), psychotherapy and a combination of the two are helpful therapies.

Major Depressive Disorder (MDD)

It is also called **Major Depression** or **Unipolar Depression**, including **single and recurrent episodes**, defined as depressed mood or anhedonia (loss of pleasure or interest) more than 2 week's course that changes from the patient's previous level of functioning. The course is mostly **between 2 weeks and 2 years**. Prevalence is 15-25%; **female:male = 2:1**. Onset is usually 20-40 y/a. **Suicide mortality is 10-15%**. Subclasses are Single Episode and Recurrent MDD. The prognosis is better than other mood disorders if treated properly, and is worse if psychotic symptoms are present.

Etiology

Studies have shown that depression is influenced by both biological and environmental factors – associated with genetics (first degree relatives of patients with higher risk), low levels of serotonin (5-HT)

MDD

and norepinephrine (NE), abnormal dopamine (DA), sex hormone imbalances, chronic diseases, stress (divorce, job loss), and loneliness.

Essentials of diagnosis

1. DSM-5 criteria: $\geq$ five of the following symptoms must have been present **for 2 weeks**: (1) **Depressed mood** (feeling sadness or emptiness) **most of the day** and nearly every day; (2) **Loss of energy, anhedonia, or fatigue most of the day**; (3) **Reduced interest** in activities that used to be enjoyed, sleep disturbances (insomnia or hypersomnia); (4) **Difficulty concentrating, memorizing**, or making decisions; (5) **Feelings of worthlessness** or guilt and recurrent **suicide thoughts** or intentions; (6) Others: psychomotor **agitation** or retardation; significant **weight loss or gain**. (7) Absence of a manic or hypomanic episode. r/o Suicidal ideation

2. The symptoms cause clinically significant distress or impairment in social, occupational, or other important areas of functioning.

3. The episode is not attributable to the physiological effects of a substance/drug or to another medical condition (hypothyroidism, chronic fatigue syndrome, etc), and is not better explained by other psychotic disorders.

4. P/E is usually normal but **dexamethasone suppression test** or thyrotropin-releasing hormone test is abnormal.

Differential diagnosis

Dysthymia (with milder symptoms lasting more than 2 years); normal grief; drug abuse; drug effects; hypothyroidism; Parkinson disease; dementia; postpartum depression/Blues/psychosis, etc.

Postpartum Blues ("Baby Blues"):   usually 1st baby

Mild depression sometimes occurs immediately after birth and lasts **up to 2 weeks**. Mother may have sadness, mood lability, and tearfulness, but cares about the baby. It's self-limited and **no treatment** is necessary.

Postpartum depression: usually After 1st baby   onset <1 month duration ongoing unless Tx

Typical depressed symptoms usually occur within **1-3 months after birth** (mostly the 2nd baby) and symptoms may continue more than 1 month. Patient usually has depressed mood, excessive anxiety, sleep disturbances, and weight changes. The mother may have negative **thoughts of hurting the baby. Treat the patient with antidepressants.** SSRIs   Mom doesn't care about baby

Postpartum psychosis: effectively brief psychotic disorder. usually not 1st baby. Mom fears baby, will kill.

Severe depression and psychosis may occur **2-3 weeks after the first birth** and may continue. Patient usually has depression and delusion, and may have thoughts of hurting the baby. **Treat with antidepressants and mood stabilizers or antipsychotics.** onset <1 month, duration ongoing if untreated.

Normal grief:

- Anhedonia,
  focused on 4
  deceased.

Also known as **Bereavement**, it usually begins **after the death of a loved one**, presenting with feelings of sadness, tearfulness, worrying about the deceased, irritability, disturbed sleep, and poor concentration. It typically lasts < 6 months and only needs **supportive care (psychotherapy).** <12 months?.

- Can be harm in future
- Suicide ideation normal in grief if focus is on the deceased

Treatment

- If ⊕ Suicidal Ideation & ⊕ Plan → Hospitalization
⊕ SI   ∅ Plan → contract safety

In principle, combined pharmacotherapy and psychotherapy are the most effective therapies.

1. **Cognitive psychotherapy** is the **initial treatment**, which will help change the patient's distorted thoughts about self, future, and the world, and help the patient deal with conflicts, stress, sense of loss, etc. **Combined with an SSRI**, it will be the **most effective** treatment. Patient must first be protected from suicide.

Uworld: 4-6 weeks, @ therapeutic dosage

2. **Pharmacotherapy—requires 3-4 weeks** for initial effects and 6 months for maintenance.

- ≥6 weeks to see @ dose
Tx
- ≥6 months @ effective dose
- ≥6 weeks of washout

(1) **SSRIs** (Selective serotonin reuptake inhibitor, increasing 5-HT): *or SNRI, trial & error*

They are the 1ˢᵗ line medications for both depression and anxiety disorder. With low toxicity but more **sexual S/E**, CNS and GI toxicity; avoid use with MAOIs (**Serotonin syndrome:** fever, CVS collapse), avoid TCAs. **Fluoxetine—most commonly used; sertraline—safe with CVD; paroxetine— good with compulsive and panic disorder; newer and stronger: citalopram and escitalopram. Escitalopram and sertraline provide the best combination of efficacy and acceptability.**

(3)
- max the dose
- combo of therapy + pharm >> than therapy or pharm alone

(2) **TCAs** (Tricyclic antidepressants, increasing 5-HT and NE):

They are the 2ⁿᵈ line drugs for depression, anxiety, chronic pain (amitriptyline), and enuresis (imipramine). Among them, nortriptyline has sedation while desipramine has not. This group of drugs has low cost but **significant adverse effects**—Cardiac arrhythmias, anticholinergic effects, orthostatic hypotension, sexual dysfunction, and seizures.

(3) **MAOIs** (Monoamine oxidase inhibitor, increasing NE):

Phenelzine and tranylcypromine are used mostly. **It's the best treatment for atypical depression with brief psychosis, phobia,** hypersomnolence, or hyperphagia. It requires dietary restrictions (avoid cheese, red wine, and anti-cough agents) to avoid serious "**hypertensive crisis**". Other S/E: Sexual dysfunction, orthostatic hypotension, weight gain, and sleep disorder.

(4) **Heterocyclics:** 2ⁿᵈ and 3ʳᵈ-generation antidepressants with varied actions, better for **atypical depression**.

Bupropion—increasing both DA and NE; best for depression with ADHD, alcohol/smoking cessation, or confusion; with risk of seizure but least S/E on sexual function.

Trazodone—inhibiting 5-HT reuptake, good choice for depression with sleep disorder; S/E: It may cause priapism.

3. **ECT** (Electroconvulsive therapy): ** Best, used for severe, refractory, catatonia, or psychosis MDD.*

Indicated in patients with serious **suicidal ideas** or adverse effects of medication. It's also safe in the 1st trimester pregnancy. Adverse effects include headaches, transient memory loss, and posterior shoulder dislocation (rare).

Persistent Complex Bereavement Disorder
- 6months after event, can last ≥ 12 months
- focus on deceased w/ dysphoria, guilt, anhedonia
- persistent ↓ mood, can't imagine being happy
- hallucinations, psychotic
- suicidal ideation based on deceased
- Tx: SSRI, SNRI

Persistent Depressive Disorder—Dysthymia

Definition and diagnosis: A chronic disorder characterized by a depressed mood lasting most of the time during the day and most of the days in a week but milder than major depression for **more than 2 years** (In DSM-4, it's "Chronic major depression"). *< 2 months at a time*
r/o Hypothyroid w TSH

Risk factors: More common in females with low social-economic status (SES). Most patients have other psychiatric disorders such as anxiety, substance abuse or borderline personality disorder.

Treatment

1. Long-term individual insight-oriented psychotherapy: Effective in helping patient overcome long-term despair sense and childhood conflicts.

2. Antidepressant therapy: If the above therapy fails, a small dose of SSRIs can be started.

Differential diagnosis: Same as for major depression. *Hypothyroid*

Atypical Depression

Atypical MDD: mood reactivity (positive response to pleasant events)

It is characterized by reverse vegetative changes such as increased sleep, appetite, and weight. Depressed mood tends to be worse in the evening. Patient complains of "feeling heavy." Atypical depression is more common in females and in individuals with bipolar I, bipolar II disorder, major depressive disorder, and "seasonal affective disorder". Depressive episodes in bipolar disorder tend to have atypical features, as does depression with seasonal patterns.

Treatment

Lifestyle modification plus medications are helpful. A SSRI (with less S/E) can be initially used. If it's not effective, a MAOI is chosen.

Premenstrual Dysphoric Disorder (PMDD)

PMDD is a condition in which a woman has severe depression symptoms, irritability, and tension before menstruation. The symptoms of PMDD are more severe than those seen with premenstrual syndrome (PMS, emotional symptoms +/- physical symptoms), occurring in 3-8% of women with menstruations.

Etiology

The causes of PMS and PMDD are unclear. They may be associated with the lack of serotonin and mediated by the fluctuations of the levels of sex hormones in the luteal phase of the menstrual cycle.

Essentials of diagnosis

1. Anxiety (feelings of tension or anxiety, panic attacks), severe depression (feelings of sadness or despair, mood swings, lasting irritability, lack of interest in daily activities, difficulty focusing, thoughts of suicide), seasonal affective disorder (SAD), and eating/sleeping disorder.

2. Physical symptoms, such as bloating, breast tenderness, headaches, and joint or muscle pain.

3. The presentations occur during the week before menstruation, and go away once it starts. A diagnosis of PMDD requires the presence of at least five of the above symptoms.

Treatment

1. The goal is to reduce the patient's suffering and the disruption to their social relationships. **SSRIs** are used as the first-line therapy. L-**tryptophan**, a serotonin precursor, is also helpful with symptoms.

2. Hormonal birth control containing drospirenone and low levels of estrogen helps relieve severe PMDD symptoms.

3. Lifestyle changes such as regular exercise and a well-balanced diet may be helpful.

Seasonal Pattern Specifier for Mood Disorders

Formerly known as **Seasonal Affective Disorder (SAD)** or seasonal depression, it is characterized by seasonal, recurrent major depressive disorder that occurs at a specific time of the year (mostly during autumn and winter) and fully remits otherwise. Lethargy and increased weight and sleep may be present. In DSM-5, it is no longer classified as a unique mood disorder, but a "Seasonal Pattern Specifier".

Treatment

Phototherapy and antidepressive (bupropion) are helpful.

Mix: Serotonin Syndrome

This is a potentially **life-threatening** condition occurring during therapeutic use of SSRIs, usually with inadvertent interactions between medications or abused substances with serotonic nature.

Common manifestations

1. Cognitive effects: agitation, confusion, hallucinations, and hypomania.
2. Automatic effects: sweating, hyperthermia, tachycardia, shivering, nausea, and diarrhea.
3. Somatic effects: tremors, myoclonus, etc.

Treatment

1. Stop the SSRI.
2. Symptomatic treatment of fever, tachycardia, hypertension, diarrhea, etc.
3. Use serotonin antagonist—**cyproheptadine** if it's severe.

BIPOLAR AND RELATED DISORDERS

Definition: Bipolar disorder is a mood disorder that is characterized by episodes of mania, hypomania, and major depression causing significant functional impairment. The onset age is about 30. Prevalence is 1-4% for both males and females. The subtypes include bipolar I and bipolar II.

Subtypes

1. **Bipolar I:** More than **one manic episode or mixed depressive-manic** episode.

2. **Bipolar II:** More than one **major depressive** *at some point* and one **hypomanic episode**. This type does not meet the criteria for full manic or mixed depressive-manic episodes.

BP1: Et 35x

3. Other subtypes may include (1) Rapid cycling type: more than four episodes (major depressive, manic, mixed, or hypomanic episode) in 1 year; (2) Cyclothymic type: chronic and less severe, with alternating periods of hypomania and moderate depression for more than 2 years.

Etiology

Unknown. It's more prevalent among high-income and low-education population and **has a strong genetic component**. It may coexist with anxiety, alcohol dependence, and substance abuse. Suicide mortality is up to 10%.

BP1:
r/o stimulants, BP2, cyclothymia

BP2:
r/o catatonia, psychosis, if either → BP1

Essentials of diagnosis

Manic Sx:

Distractability
Irresponsibility
Grandiosity

1. Patient usually has persistently elevated, expansive mood lasting longer than 1 week—increased self-esteem or grandiosity, sexual activity, and distractibility; excessive goal-directed activities and talkativeness (pressured speech); decreased need for sleep; flight of ideas; psychomotor agitation.

2. P/E results are mostly normal. Diagnosis is made based on the above symptoms and by excluding other relevant disorders and drug effects (e.g., using an antidepressant may trigger manic episode).

Flight of ideas
Agitation
Sleep, ↓ need
Talkativeness

Differential diagnosis

Schizophrenia; personality disorders; hyperthyroidism; drug effects.

Treatment

IM
BS2, Haloperidol 5ms
Benadryl diphenhydramine 50mg
lorazepam 2mg — not right t answer on test

Tx: Agitated
ED: Benzos

1. **Acute mania**: Hospitalize the patient who is usually a risk to self and others. Most patients are **initially treated with valproate or lithium** +/- an **antipsychotic as the first-line therapy**. Mood stabilizer **lithium is also used for maintenance. It takes 2-4 weeks** to be fully effective and is tapered off in 1 year. Carbamazepine or lamotrigine is used as the second-line drug. Antipsychotics (haloperidol) are used in severe psychic or refractory agitation due to shorter onset of action. *④ quetiapine → ↑ IM admin*

olanzapine

Acute psychosis:
~escalating agitation
give IM anti-psychotic
olanzapine

2. **Bipolar depression**: **Mood stabilizers should be used first** to avoid inducing mania; **antidepressants SSRIs may be added but not alone**. ECT is only indicated only in refractory cases.

3. Combined psychotherapy is helpful.

Lamotrigine (anticonvulsant mood stabilizer): fw Bipolar depressive episodes s/e of rash, SJS
Quetiapine, lurasidone (SGA): are effective for the depressed phase of bipolar.

PEARLS—**Table 16-1: Main Indications and Adverse Effects (S/E) of Mood Stabilizers**	
Valproic acid	**Indications: Acute mania and bipolar I disorder (first-line)**; convulsion. **S/E**: GI toxicity, tremor, sedation, alopecia, and weight gain; rarely, pancreatitis, hepatotoxicity, thrombocytopenia, agranulocytosis.
Lithium	**Indications**: **Acute mania (first-line and maintenance therapy)**; bipolar disorder (prophylaxis). **S/E**: Thirst, polyuria, diabetes insipidus, hypothyroidism, GI, teratogenicity, tremor, ataxia, delirium, seizure. Avoid use if renal function is impaired.
Carbamazepine	**Indications**: 2nd-line for bipolar disorder; convulsion; peripheral neuralgia. **S/E**: Skin rash, cardiac A-V block, leukopenia; rarely, aplastic anemia or Stevens-Johnson syndrome.
Lamotrigine	**Indications**: 2nd-line for bipolar disorder; convulsion; peripheral neuralgia. **S/E**: Blurred vision, GI, Stevens-Johnson syndrome.

Cyclothymic Disorder

Definition and diagnosis: It's a chronic disorder characterized by many periods of depressed mood and hypomanic mood for **more than 2 years**. It's considered a **milder form of bipolar II disorder**.

Risk factors: More frequent in females and in association with bipolar disorder, borderline personality disorder, substance abuse, and marriage problems.

Treatment

1. Antimanic drugs (lithium, valproic acid, or carbamazepine) are usually the drugs of choice.

2. Psychotherapy can help patient gain insight into their illness and how to cope with it.

Differential diagnosis

Substance abuse; bipolar disorder; personality disorder.

NEUROTIC, STRESS-RELATED AND SOMATOFORM DISORDERS

ANXIETY DISORDERS

It's a group of psychological and physiological disorders characterized by **excessive worries, hypervigilance, fears,** restlessness, difficulty concentrating, and sleep disturbance; may be accompanied with autonomic hyperactivity and motor tension. Anxiety disorders cover several different forms of abnormal and pathological fear and anxiety, including generalized anxiety, phobic, panic disorders, Obsessive-compulsive disorder (OCD), acute stress disorder, and post-traumatic stress disorder (PTSD). Each of them has its own characteristics and symptoms and requires different treatment.

Etiology

Anxiety Disorders

1. Psychodynamic theory: Anxiety occurs when instinctual drives are thwarted.

2. Behavioral theory: Anxiety is a conditioned response to environmental stimuli originally paired with a feared situation.

3. Biologic theory: Various neurotransmitters (especially GABA, NE, and 5-HT) and various CNS structures (especially reticular activating system and limbic system) may be involved.

Generalized Anxiety Disorder

It's defined as excessive, poorly controlled anxiety about events or activities in life that causes significant impairment or distress for > 6 months; usually with both psychological and somatic symptoms (fatigue, restlessness, irritability, insomnia, muscle tension, etc.).

Risk factors

There may be a genetic predisposition for an anxiety trait. Prevalence is male:female = 1:2. Associated disorders include depression, somatic symptoms, and substance abuse.

Treatment

1. Cognitive-behavioral therapy (CBT, such as relaxation training and biofeedback) combined with SSRI antidepressants are effective.

2. **Medications** (SSRIs—paroxetine, venlafaxine; buspirone) are commonly used with good effects. **Benzodiazepines (BZD)** are used for immediate relief of acute symptoms but long-term use should be avoided for **risk of dependence**. Other adverse effects: sedation, confusion, memory deficits, and respiratory depression.

Benzodiazepines (BZD) include: diazepam, lorazepam (IV use for emergencies), clonazepam (longer half-life, less addiction risk), alprazolam (more use in panic disorder), oxazepam and chlordiazepoxide (more use in alcohol withdrawal), temazepam, flurazepam.

Flumazenil: a benzodiazepine antagonist that is used only in acute BZD overdose and not in chronic dependence (may cause tremor or seizures similar to delirium tremens).

Panic Attack and Panic Disorder

Panic disorder is recurrent, unexpected panic attacks—intense anxiety accompanied with marked physical symptoms such as tachycardia, hyperventilation, dizziness, and sweating. Panic attacks usually last for a few min. The disorder is associated with agoraphobia, depression, generalized anxiety, and substance abuse. The prevalence of male:female is 1:2.   *avoidance behavior*

Risk factors

Possibly include genetic factors, separations during childhood and interpersonal loss in adulthood. Most patients have panic symptoms in response to "panicogens" (lactate, CO_2, yohimbine).

Treatment

Panic

1. 1st line drug: **Paroxetine, fluoxetine**, alprazolam. Clonazepam (BZD) is only used for immediate symptomatic relief.

2. **Cognitive-behavioral therapies (CBT)**: Relaxation training for panic attacks and systematic desensitization for agoraphobic symptom are both effective.

Phobic (Anxiety) Disorder

It's defined as irrational fear and avoidance of objects and situations. Subtypes include:

1. **Agoraphobia**: Fear or avoidance of places from which escape would be difficult in the event of panic conditions (public places, crowds, outside alone, etc). It occurs more in females and often leads to severe restrictions on the individual's travel and daily routine.

2. **Social phobia**: Fear of humiliation or embarrassment in either general or specific social situations (e.g., at public speaking, "stage fright"). *No panic attacks.*

3. **Specific phobia**: Fear or avoidance of objects or situations other than agoraphobia or social phobia, such as animals or insects, natural environments (e.g., storms), injury (e.g., injections, blood), and situations (e.g., heights, darkness).

Treatment

1. **CBT**: Very effective for phobia, combined with **systematic desensitization** and assertiveness training.

2. Pharmacotherapy: A **benzodiazepine** (lorazepam) or **SSRI** (sertraline) is effective on social phobias, and a **beta-R blocker is** effective on performance anxiety ("stage fright").

Separation Anxiety Disorder (SAD)   *extreme, persistent anxiety w separation.*
excess worry about losing major attachment figures.

Definition and diagnosis: It is an anxiety disorder among children in which the child experiences excessive anxiety, fear and distress regarding separation from home or from people to whom the individual has a strong emotional attachment (e.g. a parent). Major presentations include inappropriate anxiety, clinging to the parent, crying, throwing tantrums, fear of harm, and difficulties sleeping. SAD can also cause significant negative effects within a child's everyday life. Symptoms must persist for at least four weeks and must be present before a child is 18 years of age to be diagnosed. Etiology is unknown.

Treatment

Behavioral, cognitive and individual psychotherapies are helpful. When these are failed in extreme cases, SSRIs (sertraline, etc.) can be used.

Selective Mutism (SM)

Definition and diagnosis: SM is an anxiety disorder in which a person who is normally capable of speech consistently ~~fails~~ *or refuses* to speak in specific social situations or to specific people, mostly in children. Children with SM stay silent even when the consequences of their silence include shame, social ostracism, or even punishment. Symptoms must persist for at least one month to be diagnosed. SM usually co-exists with shyness or social anxiety. Etiology is unknown. *Can impair academic & social development*

- No Autism, childhood onset psychosis,
- comorbid S A D.

Treatment

family therapy

CBT, self-modelling, mystery motivators, stimulus fading, desensitization, shaping, spacing and antidepressive (SSRIs) may be helpful. SM does not necessarily improve with age. **Treat individual early to avoid chronic depression**.

Mixed Anxiety and Depressive Disorder

This category should be used when symptoms of anxiety and depression are both present, but neither is clearly predominant, and neither type of symptom is present to the extent that justifies a diagnosis if considered separately. When both anxiety and depressive symptoms are present and severe enough to justify individual diagnoses, both diagnoses should be recorded and this category should not be used.

OBSESSIVE-COMPULSIVE AND RELATED DISORDERS

Obsessive-Compulsive Disorder (OCD)

Can be violent

OCD is characterized by recurrent obsessions or/and compulsions that are recognized by the individual as unreasonable, affecting the individual's level of functioning. **Obsessions** are persistent, unwanted, intrusive, and anxiety-provoking thoughts or impulses, commonly concerning contamination, doubt, guilt, aggression, and sex. **Compulsions** are peculiar behaviors to reduce anxiety, commonly hand-washing, checking, and counting. *cause problems*
5-4-3-2-1, to "get rid of" violent/scary thoughts/images

Etiology

It may be associated with 5-HT metabolism, genetics, depression, and other psychiatric disorders. Onset is insidious during childhood or early adulthood.

Diagnosis

OCD is diagnosed by recurrent, unreasonable obsessions or/and compulsions, occurring more frequently among young people, with similar incidence in male and female. It may coexist with Tourette disorder.

Treatment *PsychoT x > meds*

<u>OCD</u>

ERP = Exposure & response prevention. exposure to obsession & prevention of compulsion.

ctrl anxiety w meds, then give stimulus/obsession

1. **CBT**: Exposure and desensitisation relaxation training, response prevention, thought-stopping techniques, and modelling. Patient education and counselling are highly important. *or redirect compulsion to something else (unocvae)*

2. **Medications**: A <u>SSRI</u> (paroxetine, fluoxetine, sertraline, or fluvoxamine) is the first-line medicine. Higher doses of SSRIs or clomipramine are more effective for OCD. ~~Benzos~~ *use for panic attack anxiety*

TCA: clomipramine.

PEARLS — **Table 16-2: Comparison of Obsession and Compulsion**

Obsession: Intrusive, senseless, and distressing thoughts that increase patient's anxiety. E.g., fear of contamination.
Compulsion: Rituals, such as recurrent counting and checking, that are done to neutralize thoughts; time-consuming and tend to lower anxiety.

Body Dysmorphic Disorder

Definition and diagnosis: A disorder characterized by the patient's **irrational belief that some body part is abnormal**, defective, or misshapen despite constant reassurance. The disorder causes the patient's functional level impaired. The patient's most common concern is for facial flaws, with constant mirror-checking, attempts to hide the claimed deformity and avoidance of social activities. It's more common in adolescent and young females, who are difficult to get married or keep the marriage. It may be Assoc/w 5-HT system abnormalities, depressive disorder, anxiety disorder, and OCD.

Muscle dysphoria: M, preocc. w ↑ muscle mass, does (compulsive) excess exer, Anabolic steroid use
can cause
- Rhabdo → ↗ Acute Renal failure
- roid rage, copper disorder,
testicle Atrophy
- Anabolic steroids ↑ ceruloplasmin ↑ Free Cu+ levels

Treatment

Individual psychotherapy to help the patient deal with stress of claimed deformity. If persistent, antidepressants (SSRIs) may help.

Hoarding Disorder (HD)

HD is a pattern of behavior that is characterized by the excessive acquisition of and inability or unwillingness to discard large quantities of <u>low-value objects</u> *trash* that cover the living areas of the <u>home</u> and cause significant distress or impairment. Compulsive hoarding behavior has been associated with health risks, impaired functioning, economic burden, and adverse effects on friends and family members.

unsafe environment

Treatment: No effective treatment is available.

Trichotillomania (Hair-Pulling Disorder)

compulsion

It's a disorder characterized by recurrent, <u>uncontrolled pulling of one's own hair</u>, resulting in significant hair loss. Prevalence is female > male. Associated disorders include OCD, depression, etc.

Alopecia: hair growing in varying lengths - no fungus.

Bezoar: eating hair which causes a small bowel obstruction

Treatment

Use behavior-modification techniques to decrease patient's anxiety, along with SSRIs.

Excoriation (Skin-Picking) Disorder

Also known as **dermatillomania, compulsive skin picking**, etc, it is an impulse control disorder characterized by the repeated urge to pick at one's own skin, often to the extent that damage is caused. Research has suggested that the urge to pick is similar to an OCD but others have argued that the condition is more akin to substance abuse disorder.

Treatment

The two main therapeutic strategies are pharmacological (SSRIs; opioid antagonists; glutamatergic agents) and behavioral intervention.

TRAUMA- AND STRESSOR-RELATED DISORDERS

Acute Stress Disorder (ASD) and Post-traumatic Stress Disorder (PTSD)

Definition and diagnosis

1. **Both hold these characteristics**:

(1) **Re-experiencing the overwhelming traumatic event or stressor** (nightmare, flashbacks of war, rape, or disaster experience) to which the individual reacts with fear and helplessness. Patients continuously relive the event and avoid anything that reminds them of the event. Symptoms adversely affect the individual's level of functioning.

(2) **Increased arousal** (anxiety, sleep disturbances, hypervigilance, or impulsivity), "survivor guilt", depression, or feelings of fear or helplessness.

(3) **Avoidance** of stimuli associated with the trauma, or numbing of responsiveness.

(4) **Etiology: Stressors** usually precipitate ASD. **Traumatic events (sexual assault, warfare, serious injury)** usually precipitate PTSD.

2. **Differentiation: When post-stressor symptoms last from 2 days to 30 days, it is defined as ASD.** When **post-traumatic symptoms last more than 4 weeks (1 mo), it is PTSD.** Symptoms usually begin immediately after trauma, but may also occur after months or years. Depression and substance abuse must be ruled out because both of them worsen the diagnosis.

Treatment

1. Cognitive-behavioral therapy (**CBT**) is the mainstay of therapies. Psychological counselling after a stressful event may prevent PTSD from developing. Supportive group psychotherapy with other survivors, relaxation techniques and hypnosis (**with short-term clonazepam**) following the stress are all helpful.

2. **Adjunctive medication** for resistant cases: **Antiadrenergic medications** (clonidine, guanfacine, or prazosin) or SSRIs may be helpful.

604

Adjustment Disorder

Definition and diagnosis

doesn't meet criteria for MDD
marked distress 3/or fxnal impairment

Maladaptive reactions to an identifiable psychosocial *non-life-threatening →* stressor that **occur within 3 months of the** *Mood Δ (usually depressed, no suicidal or homicidal ideation*

stressor and last 1-6 months. It's very common in all age groups and associated with social and occupational malperformance, erratic or withdrawn behavior.

r/o bereavement
Dx: onset <3 months
*   duration < 6 months*

Treatment

Remove the stressor and use brief psychotherapy to improve adjustment skills. If severe, an anxiolytic or antidepressant can be used to alleviate symptoms.

Differential diagnosis

ASD; PTSD; generalized anxiety disorder.

Reactive Attachment Disorder (RAD) — *Pairs too little*

RAD/DSED
. Abuse/ neglect in infancy
Dx < 5yo
*   r/o autism*
Tx: caregiver = better attn
-f/u: MDD,
Anxiety, substance
-f/u: learning
disability?

Definition and diagnosis

RAD is an uncommon disorder in children characterized by markedly disturbed and developmentally inappropriate ways of relating socially in most contexts. It can take the form of a persistent failure to initiate or respond to most social interactions in a developmentally appropriate way—known as the "inhibited form".

Clinical features—The disorder can manifest itself in two ways:

1. Indiscriminate and excessive attempts to receive comfort and affection from any available adult, even relative strangers. *DSED?*

2. Extreme reluctance to initiate or accept comfort and affection, even from familiar adults, especially when distressed.

Treatment

Management may include psychosocial support services for the family unit (including financial or domestic aid), psychotherapeutic interventions, education (basic parenting skills and child development), and monitoring of the child's safety within the family.

Disinhibited Social Engagement Disorder (DSED) — *Pairs too much*

Definition and diagnosis

DSED or Disinhibited Attachment Disorder of Childhood is an attachment disorder that consists of "a pattern of behavior in which a child actively approaches and interacts with unfamiliar adults." and which "significantly impairs young children's abilities to relate interpersonally to adults and peers." For example, sitting on the lap of a stranger or peer, or leaving with a stranger.

DSED is not diagnosed before the age of 9 months or after 5 y/a. Risk factors include inconsistent or insufficient care from a primary caregiver.

Treatment

Two effective treatment approaches are play therapy and expressive therapy, which help form attachment through multi-sensory means.

PERSONALITY DISORDERS

(ICD-10: DISORDERS OF ADULT PERSONALITY AND BEHAVIOR)

Definition: **These are disorders of personality patterns that are pervasive, inflexible, and maladaptive causing impaired social-behavioral functions.** They are a group of common psychiatric disorders that lack proper care.

PEARLS—General features of personality disorders:

(1) They can be classified into three clusters ("3 Ws": A—Weird, B—Wild, C—Worried); (2) Long history dating back to childhood; (3) Recurrent maladaptive behavior and major difficulties with interpersonal relationships or society; (4) Low self-esteem and lack of confidence; (5) Minimal introspective ability with a tendency to blame others for all problems; (6) Depression with anxiety when maladaptive behavior fails.

Etiology: Unknown. It may be associated with genetic factors, "original family", and childhood experiences.

Prevalence: More males have antisocial and narcissistic personality disorders, and more females have borderline and histrionic personality disorders.

Onset: Late adolescence or early adulthood.

Course: It's usually chronic over decades and very difficult to treat because the patient is not willing to seek treatment. Mostly symptoms of paranoid, schizoid, and narcissistic personality disorder worsen with age, whereas symptoms of antisocial and borderline personality disorder usually ameliorate.

Principles of treatment: Psychotherapy is the mainstay of therapies, mostly long-term, intensive psychodynamic and cognitive therapy.

Specific Types and Clinical Features

I. Cluster A Personality Disorders — "Weird"

The so-called odd-eccentric cluster, is composed of schizoid, schizotypal, and paranoid personality disorders. This cluster is mainly characterized by peculiar thought processes and inappropriate affect.

Schizoid personality disorder

Schizoid = distant. No odd thinking or perceptual distortions

Socially isolated "loners" with restricted and distant emotions and friendship; lack of desire for intimate human connection; disinterested in others and indifferent to joy, praise, or criticism. Patients who have more awareness of their interpersonal needs are more likely to form a therapeutic relationship.

Schizotypal personality disorder

Schizotypal = magical thinking. Perceptual distortions.

Odd thought, behavior, appearance, and perceptions; socially isolated and uncomfortable with others. It's differentiated from schizoid personality disorder by magical or weird thinking and affect, ideas of reference and persecution, and **brief psychotic episodes**. Patients may be wishing for a close, special or romantic relationship with therapists while simultaneously feeling aggressive or negative toward them. *Be clear, honest, & non threatening.* *– socially awk, ↓ friends, diff close r'ships due to social anxiety that does not diminish w familiarity.*

– suspiciousness & paranoid ideation can occur but are not of delusional proportions, as in psychotic disorders

Paranoid personality disorder

Pervasively **distrustful/mistrustful, suspicious**, taking other's motivation as malevolent, socially isolated, and emotionally cold. Individuals are irrationally alert for threats that others do not see. They also frequently defend an extremely fragile self-concept. Challenges to build up a therapeutic relationship are pronounced due to "confrontation". *Be clear honest, & non threatening.*

Clinical strategy for Cluster A

Cluster A patients are suspicious and distrustful of physicians and rarely seek treatment unless dealing with acute problems such as substance use. Even they seek treatment they usually have great difficulty establishing a therapeutic relationship. Therapists should be clear, honest, non-controlling and non-defensive. Maintain emotional distance and avoid humor.

II. Cluster B Personality Disorders — "Wild"

Mainly characterized by mood lability, dissociative symptoms, and preoccupation with rejection.

Histrionic personality disorder

Colorful, exaggerated behavior, emotions and appearance to **draw attention**; extremely self-centered; theatrical and sexually seductive. It's mostly seen in female.

Management: Psychotherapy is the main treatment. Attention-seeking attributes can be helpful in establishing a preliminary therapeutic relationship. However, the clinician must be prepared to manage dramatic acting-out.

Borderline personality disorder

Unstable affect, mood, relationships, and self-image; **chronic feelings of emptiness, impulsivity**, recurrent suicidal behaviors, and **inappropriate anger**. Psychotic symptoms may be present with stress. The main defense mechanism is splitting.

Management: ~~Psychotherapy~~ *dialectical Behavioral therapy* is the main treatment. Patients and families need education about the disorder. For patients who experience symptoms of emotional dysregulation (lability, inappropriate anger, and dysphoria), impulsivity and aggression, or cognitive-perceptual problems despite evidence-

Borderline PD

based psychotherapy, additional pharmacotherapy—an antipsychotic, mood stabilizer, or antidepressant—is suggested.

Antisocial Personality Disorder (ASPD)

Definition and diagnosis: A pervasive personality pattern of disregard for, or violation of, the rights of others; with continuous antisocial or criminal acts, inability to conform to social rules, marked impulsivity, violation of the rights of others, deceitfulness, and lack of remorse. There may be a history of crime, legal problems, and impulsive and aggressive behavior. It usually starts around 15 y/a as conduct disorder and is **diagnosed after the age 18**.

Etiology: It may include hormones and neurotransmitters (high testosterone, low 5-HT), limbic neural maldevelopment, head trauma, cultural influences, and environment.

Management: ASPD is considered to be among the most difficult personality disorders to treat. Because of their very low or absent capacity for remorse, patients usually lack sufficient motivation and fail to see the costs associated with antisocial acts. Therapeutic techniques should be focused on rational and utilitarian arguments against repeating past mistakes. (1) For children, early intervention with group parent training may help prevent antisocial personality in adolescence. (2) Cognitive-behavioral therapy is for persons with mild disorder who possess some insight and reason to improve. (3) For patients with ASPD and severe aggression who are willing to take medication, a second-generation antipsychotic (risperidone or quetiapine) is indicated. *Trying to tx antisocial = make them better @ lying*

Narcissistic personality disorder

Sense of **self-importance**, **grandiosity**, and entitlement; in need of admiration and lack of empathy; jealousy and improper rage with criticism. It occurs mostly **in low-educated patients**.

Management: Patients pose significant challenges in establishing a therapeutic relationship. The clinician may have to tolerate a lengthy period of time of vulnerability and self-protection before trust develops.

Clinical strategy for Cluster B

Cluster B patients are associated with testing and pushing the limits of the treatment relationship. They are manipulative and demanding (attention), and tends to change the rules. Clinicians should be firm (stick to the treatment plan), fair (not punitive or derogatory), and consistent in rules and boundaries in a quest to build a relationship.

III. Cluster C Personality Disorders — "Worried" *weak, shy, timid*

Mainly characterized by anxiety and preoccupation with criticism or rigidity.

Avoidant personality disorder
want friends, r'ships, & promotions but don't go for them.

Patients are socially inhibited, feeling inadequate or inferior, shy and lonely, hypersensitive to criticism, preoccupied with rejection, and unwilling to get involved with people. Some patients may be similar to vulnerable narcissists and/or social anxiety disorder. It is important to understand underlying self, interpersonal and emotional schemas to optimize treatment alliance.

- *fear of rejection, unrealistic*
- *Avoid power struggles, let make them choose*

Dependent personality disorder

Submissive and clinging, feeling inadequate and helpless; **avoiding responsibility and making decisions**; always in need of care. *unrealistic fear of rejection.*

Management: Psychotherapy is the main treatment. The clinician must be alert to the potential for the patient to withdraw emotionally and psychologically. Additional challenges may occur when the clinician attempts to encourage more independence. *Give clear advice, make sure pt doesn't sabotage own tx*

Obsessive-compulsive personality disorder (OCPD) *~ego syntonic*

Preoccupied with details, orderliness, perfectionism, and control; often consumed by the details of everything and lose the efficiency (goals); inflexible morals and values. It is different from obsessive compulsive disorder (OCD), an anxiety disorder. OCD is manifested by the patient's experience of obsessive thoughts and compulsive behaviors. There is only modest co-occurrence between OCPD and OCD. Both disorders are mainly treated with cognitive-behavioral therapy (CBT). OCD may also need SSRIs.

Passive-aggressive (negativistic) personality disorder

This diagnosis was initially included in Cluster C, but shifted to disorders in need of further study in DSM-IV, and deleted altogether in DSM-5.

Clinical strategy for Cluster C

Patients are worried but controlling, and their words may be inconsistent with actions. These may ruin the treatment. Therapists should give clear recommendations, but not force the patient into decision. Be caring, sympathetic, and patient. Building a therapeutic relationship with patients with Cluster C disorders is facilitated because these patients are willing to take responsibility for their problems and more readily engage in a dialogue with the clinician to try to solve them in comparison to patients with more severe Cluster A or B disorders.

SCHIZOPHRENIA SPECTRUM AND OTHER PSYCHOTIC DISORDERS

Schizophrenia

Definition: It is a mental *Thought disorder* disorder characterized by a disintegration of the process of thinking and of emotional responsiveness, which impairs judgment, behavior, and ability to interpret reality. It most commonly manifests as auditory hallucinations, paranoid or bizarre delusions, or disorganized speech and thinking, accompanied by significant social or occupational dysfunction. The onset of symptoms typically occurs in young adulthood, with a global lifetime prevalence of around 1.5%. Symptoms must be present for **more than 6 months** to make the diagnosis. The incidence is higher in males and the onset is earlier in males (male: 20's y/a, female: 30's y/a). Suicidal rate is about 10%.

Etiology and risk factors

→ ⊕Sx   ↑↑ S-HT ⇒ ⊖Sx

1. Unknown; associated with high levels of dopamine (DA) and abnormal 5-HT in the brain.

Schizophrenia

2. Strong genetic trend or family history: General prevalence is 1%; monozygotic twin is 47%; dizygotic twin, first-degree relative, and one schizophrenic parent are all about 12%; patient with two schizophrenic parents has 40% of prevalence.

3. Environment: More prevalent in patients with low social-economic status (SES), a conflicting environment, and a birth season in the winter and early spring (may include viral infection). If family members are critical, intrusive, and hostile to the patient, the relapse rate is high. If family members are supportive, understanding, and loving, the relapse rate is low.

Essentials of diagnosis

Pt: ≥2, one must be from 1-3.

1. **More than two of the following characteristic psychotic symptoms affecting social or occupational functions for at least 6 months:**

⊕ Sx
1) delusions, persec or grandiose
2) hallucinations
3) disorganization, speech or behavior
4) catatonia

(1) **Positive symptoms:** Delusions (mostly bizarre), hallucinations (mostly auditory), disorganized speech, and disorganized or catatonic behaviour.

⊖ Sx
⑤ flat affect, poverty speech or movement, anhedonia, cognitive delay.

(2) **Negative symptoms:** Flat affect, poverty of speech, decreased emotional reactivity, and anhedonia.

2. P/E: Usually normal, but may show saccadic eye movements, hypervigilance, etc.

3. Brain imaging: CT and MRI usually reveal **lateral and third ventricular enlargement**, reduction in cortical volume (associated with negative symptoms and neuro-psychiatric impairment).

PET: May show hypoactivity of the frontal lobes and hyperactivity of the basal ganglia relative to the cerebral cortex.

4. Psychological Tests:

(1) IQ tests—lower on all IQ tests.

(2) Neuropsychological tests: Usually are consistent with bilateral frontal and temporal lobe dysfunction (deficits in attention, retention time, and problem-solving ability).

MSx same for these

(3) Personality tests: May show bizarre ideations, etc.

Malig Catatonia — Psych Sx, 0 meds
- rigidity, lead pipe
- ↑ CK from muscle breakdown
- ↑ resistance

Neuroleptic Malig Sx — Psych Sx, Antipsychotic meds
ANS dysfxn
- ↑HR, BP, temp
- hypertonicity, hyperreflexia

S-HT Sx — Psych Sx, SSRI

Differentiation

<u>Catatonia</u>: a modifier of illnesses

Malig Hyperthermia
- Halothane gas & anesthesia
- same Sx
- No Psych
- Ask Fam Hx
- also succinyl choline

Catatonia is a state of neurogenic motor immobility and behavioral abnormality manifested by stupor. It is not a separate disorder, but is associated with psychiatric conditions such as schizophrenia (catatonic type), bipolar disorder, post-traumatic stress disorder, depression and other mental disorders, as well as drug abuse or overdose (or both). It may also be seen in many medical disorders including CNS infections, autoimmune disorders, focal neurologic lesions, metabolic disturbances, and alcohol or benzodiazepines (BZD) withdrawal. **Treatment: BZD is** the first-line option. Electro-convulsive therapy is sometimes effective. NMDA antagonists can be tried for BZD resistant catatonia.

Treatment of Schizophrenia

Psychotic break:
- Schizophrenia is active.
- occurs w meds are stopped, or can happen w meds.
- ↑ cognitive impairment w each break
- Teen - 20s: ↓ stressor, ∆ behavior, old substances, fxntion ↑/↓ mood, Tx w short acting benzos

Catatonia Sx:
stupor
catalepsy
waxy-flexibility → Retarded ↓ Sx
negativism
mutism

stereotypy
agitation/grimace
echolalia/praxia } Excited ↑Sx

Dx: clx, Lorazepam & it goes away → dx
Tx: Lorazepam, short acting IV benzos
s/w malnutrition
- track Albumin
- may need parenteral or enteral nutrition
- DVT, low nutrition

Schizophrenia
Tx:

1. Hospitalization is recommended to make patient safe and stabilized. Supportive psychotherapy mainly aims at building up a relationship of mutual trust and understanding between the patient and physician.

2. **Antipsychotic drugs: They are first-line treatment for schizophrenia.** Specific selection of medicine is based on patient's situations.

(1) **Typical antipsychotics: Blocking DA-R (D2, D4 subtypes).** Indicated for psychotic disorders, acute agitation or mania, and Tourette syndrome.

High-potency: Haloperidol, droperidol, fluphenazine, and thiothixene.   *Combative ED pt*
                                                                              Haloperidol depot

Adverse effects of typical antipsychotics:

(a) **More extrapyramidal symptoms (EPS):** acute dystonia or dyskinesias (pseudo-parkinsonism, tremor, and rigidity)—treated with **bentropine, amantadine** or diphenhydramine; akathisia—treated with propranolol or a BZD.

(b) **Tardive dyskinesia** (lip smacking, etc.)—It's treated by changing to clozapine or risperidone, no anticholinergics.

(c) **Neuroleptic malignant syndrome**: fever, rigidity, and autonomic instability (instable HR, BP and conscious status). **Treatment**: Stop neuroleptic; give **dantrolene or bromocriptine** along with IV fluid.

(d) Hyperprolactinemia: amenorrhea, gynecomastia, and galactorrhea. Treatment depends on specific cases.

Low-potency: Thioridazine (S/E: retinal pigmentation), **chlorpromazine** (with **more anticholinergic S/E**: dry mouth, orthostatic hypotension, constipation, and urine-retention).

(2) **Atypical antipsychotics**: Blocking DA2-R and 5HT2-R. Cariprazine, clozapine and   *aats,*
olanzapine are more effective on negative symptoms; **risperidone is effective on both positive and   *Normal Pt*
negative symptoms.** Similar new medicines include **quetiapine, ziprasidone, aripiprazole. Except for clozapine and olanzapine, currently these are the 1st-line medicines for schizophrenia**, with fewer EPS and anticholinergic S/E.

Note: Clozapine is best reserved for patients who have no response to adequate therapies of typical and atypical antipsychotics, and who have severe negative symptoms and tardive dyskinesia. It is never used as a first-line therapy, as with olanzapine.

Adverse effects of atypical antipsychotics:

Clozapine—the main adverse effect is agranulocytosis and thus weekly CBC testing is necessary.

Olanzapine—higher incidence of weight gain and diabetes; avoid use in obese/diabetic patients.

Risperidone—higher incidence of movement disorder; quetiapine has less.

Ziprasidone—higher incidence of prolonged QT interval; avoid in patients with **conduction** defects.

Specific sub-types of schizophrenia dropped by DSM-5

Paranoid, disorganized, catatonic, residual, and undifferentiated types.

ICD-10 defined two additional subtypes
                                            - Antipsychotics can cause
                                            Neuroleptic Malig Sx,
                                            Tx w. dantrolene.

Post-schizophrenic depression: A depressive episode arising in the aftermath of a schizophrenic illness where some low-level schizophrenic symptoms may still be present.

Simple schizophrenia: Insidious and progressive development of prominent negative symptoms with no history of psychotic episodes.

Other Psychotic Disorders

Schizophreniform Disorder

It's defined as **psychotic symptoms** (hallucinations, delusions, disorganized speech or behaviour, affective or negative symptoms, and impaired social function, etc.) for **more than one month but less than 6 months**. Most patients can return to their functional level at baseline after treatment. Be watchful that depressive suicide is a risk factor after the psychotic symptoms resolve.

Treatment

1. Physician must first evaluate if it's necessary to hospitalize the patient for safety purpose.

2. Antipsychotic medicine is indicated for a 3-6 month course. Individual psychotherapy may help the patient assimilate the psychotic experience into real life.

Schizoaffective Disorder

— mostly psychotic + a little bit of mood

It's defined as complex symptoms of **major depressive-manic episodes and schizophrenia** (delusions or hallucinations) for **more than 2 weeks**. The prognosis is better than that for schizophrenia, but worse than that for affective disorder. *— MDD or manic episodes concurrent w schizophrenia sx, ≥6 months, AND*
— delusions or hallucinations ≥2 weeks in absence of major mood episode, depress or manic.

Treatment

1. Physician must first evaluate the necessity of the patient's hospitalization for safety purpose. Multimodal, integrated care for patients may be necessary.

2. An antidepressant with or without anticonvulsant is used first to control the mood symptoms. If it's not effective, an antipsychotic agent is used to control the symptoms. *1st mood,*

(Persistent) Delusional Disorder

Fixed false belief

It's defined as **non-bizarre delusions** more than 1 month and **no impairment in level of functioning**. Specific features and types include erotomanic, jealous, grandiose, somatic, mixed, and unspecified. For example, the patient may believe the government will collapse soon and the leader will be replaced by him/her, but the patient still follows the law and goes to work.

Risk factors: More commonly in low SES, married, employed women.

Treatment

First-line treatment is antipsychotic medication rather than other clinical interventions. Because patients with this disorder often reject psychiatric treatment, it is particularly important that medication be prescribed in the context of a therapeutic relationship that includes support, education, encouragement of healthier pursuits, and discouragement of damaging, delusion-inspired actions. Individual psychotherapy should be focusing on helping the patient understand how the delusions are distressing and interfere with normal life. *Gentle confrontation?*

Brief Psychotic Disorder

>1 day, <1 mo

It's defined as sudden onset of **psychosis lasting for a few days to a month** and returning to a normal premorbid functional level in a month.

Risk factors: More common in the low SES and in those with pre-existing personality disorders or psychological stressors.

Treatment

1. Physician must first evaluate the necessity of the patient's hospitalization for safety purpose.

2. Antipsychotics (risperidone) can be used for short-term treatment of psychotic symptoms. *<1mo* *FE if persists, it's probably schizo-phrenia*

PEARLS—Differentiation of psychotic disorders by duration

Pay special attention to the **duration of psychotic symptoms**, which is key to the differentiation of **brief psychotic disorder (1 day—1 month), schizophreniform disorder (1 month—6 months), and schizophrenia (more than 6 months).**

Schizotypal (Personality) Disorder (STPD)

It's a disorder characterized by **eccentric behavior and abnormalities of thinking and affect** which resemble those seen in schizophrenia, though no definite schizophrenic anomalies occur at any stage. The symptoms may include a cold or inappropriate affect; anhedonia; odd behavior; social withdrawal tendency; paranoid or bizarre ideas not amounting to true delusions; obsessive ruminations; thought and perceptual disturbances; occasional transient psychotic episodes with intense illusions, auditory or other hallucinations, and delusion-like ideas, usually occurring without external provocation. There is no definite onset, and evolution and course are usually those of a personality disorder.

Treatment

STPD is among the most difficult psychotic and personality disorders to treat because patients usually consider themselves to be simply eccentric, creative, or nonconformist, not "patients". When patient's social maladaptation is significant, psychotherapy and antipsychotics should be used.

DISSOCIATIVE DISORDERS

Definition: Dissociation is the fragmentation or separation of aspects of consciousness, including _thoughts_ memory, identity, and perception. Some degree of conscious dissociation is normal, but if it's too fragmented, it may be a pathologic dissociative disorder that interferes with patient's normal adaptive ability. _due to severe, prolonged stressors._

dx: r/o malingering, substance abuse
Tx: deal w/ initial stressor w/ psychotherapy

Dissociative Amnesia

Archer→Bob's Burgers or lose entire autobiography

It refers to significant episodes in which the individual is unable to recall general or important events, usually during emotional or psychological stress. It's more common in young women. _Also, loss of daily occurrences or routines, i.e. forget where to order at coffee shop, DOB._

i.e. rape - can't remember rape or rapist

Treatment

1. First evaluate and exclude general medical conditions (head trauma, seizures, stroke, substance abuse, etc).

2. Psychotherapy may help resolve underlying emotional stress.

Differentiation

Fugue state (Dissociative fugue or psychogenic fugue): _Jason Bourne_

Sudden, unexpected <u>travel</u>; unable to remember one's past and confused about personal identity; usually following a stressful life event, mood disorder, or substance abuse. Most episodes are isolated and with rapid resolution, but amnesia may persist for months. **Treatment:** Same as for dissociative amnesia.

Dissociative Identity Disorder (Multiple Personality Disorder) _-most severe stressor most severe disorder, dissoc_

switching _≥2_ _identity states_

It's defined as presence of multiple, distinct personalities that recurrently control the individual's behavior, together with personal identity confusion. Childhood sexual abuse is a strong risk factor. Usually it occurs in a female with an occult onset, subtle clinical presentations, and delayed diagnosis for years. _Psyche creates an additional identity to absorb trauma so primary identity doesn't experience. After stressor is over, the 2nd identity persists_

Associated problems and differential diagnoses include chaotic interpersonal relationships, self-destructive behaviors, impulsivity, major depression, suicide attempts, sexual disorder, eating disorder, substance abuse, borderline personality disorder, PTSD, etc.

Treatment

Psychodynamic <u>psychotherapy</u> plus hypnosis is helpful in uncovering psychologically traumatic memories of patients and to resolve the associated emotional conflicts.

pt: self has
- memory gaps (blackouts)
- hx severe trauma
- other dissoc sx
other: paradoxical behaviors
- appearance change, facial muscles.

Depersonalization or Derealization Disorder _least severe stressor least severe dissoc. disorder_

From body   _from environment (unreal, or in a dream)_

It's a condition of persistent or recurrent feeling of being detached from one's mental processes or body, accompanied by intact sense of reality. It may follow a stressful event, and show jamais vu (a sense

- Ketamine.
- intact reality testing
- nonsevere trauma/stressor in an adolescent

Depersonalization or Derealization Disorder

of familiar things being strange), deja vu (a sense of unfamiliar things being familiar), and other forms of perceptual distortion.

Treatment

Psychotherapy is helpful in decreasing anxiety. Naltrexone, an opioid antagonist, is helpful with pronounced emotional numbing. Lamotrigine and transcranial magnetic stimulation have shown promising results. SSRIs, benzodiazepines and antipsychotics are not very helpful.

Dissociative Stupor

It is a condition of a profound diminution or absence of voluntary movement and normal responsiveness to external stimuli such as light, noise, and touch, but examination and investigation reveal no evidence of a physical cause. In addition, there is positive evidence of psychogenic causation in the form of recent stressful events or problems. Diagnosis is clinical.

Treatment

Treatment may include emergency "ABCs" (including 50% glucose + thiamine IV +/- phenytoin for seizures if necessary), removal of patient from the stressful environment, individual psychotherapy (including hypnosis), and atypical antipsychotics if necessary.

SOMATIC SYMPTOM AND RELATED DISORDERS

- distress about dz, no organic cause

This is a group of disorders characterized by the presentation of physical symptoms without full medical explanations, and the symptoms are severe enough to interfere with the patient's social or occupational activities.

Primary gain: Keeps internal conflicts outside patient's awareness.

Secondary gain: Benefits received from being "sick".

La belle indifference: Patient seems unconcerned about impairment. *Conversion disorder* *Dx: use H/P to decide* *r/o organic w img/blood work*

Identification: One models one's behavior on someone who is important to him/her. *r/o factitious, malingering*

Somatic Symptom Disorder

excess preoccupation ;, anxiety about sx

* multiple physicians, many tests
* Anxiety or depression
* mult surg/procedures

Formerly known as a **somatoform disorder**, it is a mental disorder characterized by multiple physical symptoms that affect multiple organs and systems without full medical explanations. They are suggestive of physical illness or injury but not attributable to another mental disorder. It more often affects low-socioeconomic, unmarried females in the 30's. *- chronic childhood illness* *- child abuse/neglect* *; sexual trauma*

- pain, fatigue
- don't wanna hurt, lots of docs
- +/- dz preocup, is disproportionate

Diagnosis

1. Many physical symptoms affecting multiple organs that cannot be explained fully by a general medical condition or drug effects. Most cases include more than four pain, two GI, one sexual, and one neurological symptoms.

- ≥1 somatic sx causing distress/fxnal impairment
- excess thoughts, anxiety, or behaviors related to sx
- ≥ 6 months

- High healthcare ;, specialist utilization
- repeated testing not reassuring

Somatic Symptom Disorder (aka somatoform disorder)

2. Patient usually has a long, complicated medical history and impaired psychosocial functions.

Treatment

limit # of visits, tests, procedures, specialists

— & setting rules & boundaries. ONE provider. New complaints that can be real.

Both psychotherapy and pharmacotherapy (antidepressants <u>SSRIs</u>) may be needed. Therapists should have sympathy for the patient. Try to keep the same physician and make regular schedules for the patient. Individual psychotherapy can help patient aware of the possible psychological nature of the symptoms and help with coping skills. *SNRI, TCA*

Conversion Disorder (Functional Neurological Symptom Disorder)

It's a disorder in which the individual experiences one or more neurologic deficits after a special event that cannot be explained by any medical or neurologic diseases. It's more common in young, low-socioeconomic and low-IQ females, and military persons. Associated disorders include passive-aggressive, dependent, antisocial, and histrionic personality disorders. *— La Belle Indifference, don't care about*

— won't hurt self.   *neuro Sx.*

— unwanted.   *— Assoc w acute stressor, Neuro defect is*

Diagnosis   *r/o MS, stroke*   *proportionate to stressor.*

Patient typically has 1-2 neurologic symptoms that affect **voluntary motor or sensory functions** (commonly mutism, blindness, paralysis, or paresthesia) following psychological factors. Patient is usually unconcerned about his/her impairment.

Treatment

Symptoms usually resolve spontaneously. Psychotherapy can help establish a caring relationship with the patient and help relieve stress and deal with illness.

Factitious Disorder *any sx, intentional w intent to deceive*

Also known as factitious disorder imposed on self (Munchausen syndrome)", it is a disorder characterized by the conscious or deliberate production of false or exaggerating symptoms and signs of both medical and mental disorders in order to **assume the sick role for attention (rather than obvious external rewards)**. Typically, patients have faked symptoms and signs and demand treatment in the hospital, and become angry when they are confronted or rejected, or accuse the physician or nurse if the test result is negative (indicating faked sample). It's more frequent in male health workers. Pediatric patients may have a history of being abused and thus seek the sick role.

If the manifestations are faked for another person (as in mother and child), it's called **"Factitious disorder by proxy"**. *Harm a dependent to assume role. Jailed.*

Treatment

Psychotherapy is the standard treatment for alleviation. When the clinician suspects factitious disorder, be alert of the therapist's countertransference. If a "factitious disorder by proxy" is suspected, the child protective authority should be contacted for the child's protection.

Differentiation

Malingering: *any sx. intentional w intent to deceive. 2° gain.*

It's a condition characterized by the **conscious fabricating symptoms and signs for an obvious secondary gain** (money, sick leave, etc). Individual tends to complain many subjective, exaggerated symptoms and is concerned more with rewards than with alleviation of symptoms. It's more common in men in factories, jails, and the army. Diagnosis is generally made when there is a discrepancy between the patient's complaints and the actual results of physical examination and lab tests. **It is not considered a mental disorder. Treatment:** Apply skilful doctor-patient relationship to therapies. If medical evaluation reveals malingering, then skilfully confront the patient with the results and try to save the patient's self-respect. If confronted harshly, the patient may become angry and tougher to deal with.

Illness Anxiety Disorder (Hypochondriasis)

It refers to excessive preoccupancy or worry about having a serious illness despite constant reassurance by the physician. The belief is not delusional but affects the individual's level of functioning. Most onset ages are 20-30 years and duration > 6 months. *egodystonic, don't wanna feel this way. looking for-yr help.*

Treatment

Make frequent, regular schedules with the patient for psychotherapy—cognitive-behavioral therapy (CBT), to help patient relieve stress and deal with illness. If it's not effective, antidepressants such as SSRIs may be needed.

Undifferentiated Somatoform Disorder (by ICD-10 and DSM-IV)

When somatoform complaints are multiple, varying and persistent, but the complete and typical clinical picture of somatization disorder is not fulfilled, it's considered "Undifferentiated somatoform disorder".

(Persistent Somatoform) Pain Disorder

It's a condition of chronic pain experienced by a patient in one or more areas, and is thought to be caused by psychological stress. It's more common in middle-aged females.

Essentials of diagnosis

1. Symptoms more than signs: Pain exists in more than one anatomic site and causes distress to the patient. Usually there is no faked pain or acts seeking secondary gain involved. Patient usually has stressful events, a long medical history, many physicians, and poor effects with standard analgesic therapies.

2. Conditions such as dyspareunia, somatic symptoms disorder, conversion disorder, or mood disorders can eliminate pain disorder as a diagnosis. Diagnosis depends on the ability of physicians to explain the symptoms and on psychological influences.

Persistent Somatoform Pain Disorder

Treatment

1. Individual psychotherapy helps explore the psychological origin and emotional content of the pain for alleviation.

2. NSAIDs, antidepressants (SSRIs, TCAs), venlafaxine, biofeedback, and hypnosis may be helpful.

Mix: Chronic Fatigue Syndrome (CFS)

Also known as systemic exertion intolerance disease, CFS is a debilitating and complex disorder characterized by **profound fatigue for longer than 6 months** that is not improved by bed rest and that may be worsened by physical or mental activity. Most patients experience partial recovery and relapses within 2 years; female > male. **Clinical fatigue** (generalized weakness, easy fatigability, and mental fatigue) should be distinguished from somnolence, dyspnea, and muscle weakness. Chronic fatigue refers to symptoms lasting over 6 months but does not imply the presence of chronic fatigue syndrome.

Etiology

Unknown. It may be associated with viral infections, immunologic, neurologic, or endocrine dysfunctions.

Essentials of diagnosis

1. Unexplained fatigue that is not alleviated by rest, is not due to exertion, and significantly affects quality of life. Symptoms may affect several body systems and include weakness, muscle and joint pain (without redness/swelling), impaired short-term memory and/or mental concentration, insomnia, headache, sore throat, tender lymph nodes, depression, and reduced daily activities.

2. Lab tests: Usually normal and may be needed for exclusion diagnosis—CBC, LFTs, serum electrolytes, TSH, HIV, etc. **Diagnosis of CFS is made by exclusion**.

Differential diagnosis (Also good for USMLE Step 2 CS!)

1. **Psychiatric disorders**: major depressive disorder (No.1 cause), anxiety disorder, somatisation, etc.

2. **Endocrine disorders**: hypothyroidism, poorly controlled diabetes, Addison disease, hypercalcemia (hyperparathyroidism), hypopituitarism.

3. **Metabolic disorders**: chronic renal failure, hepatic failure.

4. **Hematologic diseases**: severe anemia, occult malignancy.

5. **Cardiopulmonary diseases**: CHF, obstructive sleep apnea.

6. **Infectious diseases**: viral hepatitis, endocarditis, myocarditis, mononucleosis, CMV infection, HIV infection, TB, syphilis, parasitic disease, Lyme disease.

7. **Medications**: anti-hypertensive medicines (clonidine, methyldopa), beta-R blockers, hypnotics, antihistamines, antidepressants (amitriptyline, doxepin, and trazodone with sedating effect), drug use or withdrawal.

Others: fibromyalgia, sleep disorders, etc.

Chronic Fatigue Syndrome

Treatment

1. Treat known underlying cause and provide support and reassurance.

2. Cognitive behavioral therapy (exercise, behavioral modifications), antidepressants, or/and NSAIDs can be helpful. CBT combined with graded exercise program has been effective in some patients with CFS and with idiopathic chronic fatigue. The long-term prognosis may be better than the short-term.

SUBSTANCE-RELATED AND ADDICTIVE DISORDERS

Substance Abuse disorder = related to impairment

Substance abuse: It refers to maladaptive pattern of substance use that leads to loss of control and increased use of the substance. It includes tolerance, dependence and withdrawal, and is associated with serious medical, social, or emotional consequences. Mostly it occurs among young adults and teenagers, by millions per year in the U.S.

obligations, r'ships & Activities

Health, legal | complications
too much, cutting down, too much time, cravings | risk ③
Hazardous | sex, driving
Physical ④ | Tolerance withdrawal

Intoxication: It's reversible experience with a substance that leads to harmful psychological or physiological changes.

Withdrawal: It refers to cessation or reduction of a substance leading to either psychological or physiological changes.

Dependence: It refers to maladaptive pattern of substance use that leads to tolerance. There is withdrawal reaction(s) when the patient reduces doses. Patient spends most of his time obtaining and using drugs and recovering from drug use. The drug abuse is continued despite adverse consequences.

Prevalence of substance use (abuse) by order

1. Alcohol; 2. smoking; 3. marijuana; 4. opioid; 5. cocaine; 6. others.

Etiology and risk factors

1. Family history of alcohol abuse, childhood physical or sexual abuse, poor parenting, exposure to drug use through peers or drug dealers, and social isolation.

2. Psychiatric disorders: Depression, conduct disorder, ADHD, and low self-esteem.

3. Self-drug motivation: Patient may intend to use substance to alleviate some psychological symptoms (e.g., alcohol for depression).

Diagnostic guidelines   *dx dx & screening (next page)*

1. Maintain an extent of suspicion, be ready for denial from abusers, and try to obtain more history from close family members or friends, including familial and social function. P/E should be focused on signs of drug use (burns, needle marks, and skin infections/injury) and poor hygiene and nutrition.

2. **Diagnostic lab tests:**

For **alcohol abuse:** serum GGT, AST (SGOT), ALT (SGPT), and LDH levels.

For **IV drug abuse:** HIV, hepatitis B, hepatitis C, and TB testing.

Substance Abuse disorder

Therapeutic guidelines

1. **Preventive programs:** Teach adolescents how to resist social pressures to use drugs and to enhance other social and personal skills.

2. **Detoxification**: Substance-specific therapies, usually taking 5-10 days in hospital to assure safety.

3. **Drug rehabilitation:** Stop drug abuse and develop new coping skills that make relapse less likely, usually taking one month or more. Self-help groups (e.g., **Alcoholics Anonymous**) have been the most effective treatment for many adult substance abusers, both for rehabilitation and relapse prevention.

SUBSTANCE-RELATED DISORDERS

N/V, coma

Intox: AMS, disinhibition, slurred speech, cerebellar dysfxn

Alcohol Use Disorder

Dx screen:
2-3 mild
4-5 mod
≥6 severe
Cut down
Anger
Guilt
Eye-opener

Alcohol use disorder in DSM-5 replaces **alcohol abuse and alcohol dependence** (alcoholism) in DSM-IV. **Alcohol use disorder refers to a pattern of drinking that results in social dysfunctions, physical, or legal problems**. It can be specified as mild, moderate, or severe. Alcohol dependence in DSM-IV is best represented by moderate to severe alcohol use disorder in DSM-5; alcohol abuse is similar to the mild subtype of alcohol use disorder. The prevalence is about 10% in adults. **It's the No.1 substance of abuse, male > female.** More than 85,000 deaths a year in the US are directly attributed to alcohol use; the annual economic cost of alcohol use is estimated to be over $185 billion. Excessive alcohol use is associated with increased risk of automobile accidents, cirrhosis, pancreatitis, heart disease, major depressive disorder, and many other diseases, in addition to enormous alcohol-related economic costs in.

Adolescents ?
Car - while drives
Relax
Alone
Friendship trouble
Forget stuff
Trouble w Law parents Teacher

Alcoholics Anonymous: **The largest source of alcohol treatment** in the US. It is believed to be the **most successful** treatment by providing substitute dependency, social support, inspiration, hope, and aversive pressure against alcohol drinking. **Al-Anon** is also for families and friends of alcoholics.

Screening test

CAGE-questionnaire—any two positive answers to the following four questions (or to the last question "d" alone) are suggestive of alcohol use disorder.

a. Have you ever felt that you should **cut** down your drinking?

b. Have you ever felt **annoyed** by others' criticism of your drinking?

c. Have you ever felt **guilty** about your drinking?

d. Have you ever had a morning drink (**eye-opener**) to feel easier?

Diagnostic criteria

(1) Recurrent drinking resulting in failure to fulfil role obligations; (2) Recurrent drinking in hazardous situations; (3) Continued drinking despite alcohol-related social or interpersonal problems; (4) Evidence of tolerance; (5) Evidence of alcohol withdrawal or use of alcohol for relief or avoidance of withdrawal; (6) Drinking in larger amounts or over longer periods than intended; (7) Persistent desire or unsuccessful attempts to stop or reduce drinking; (8) Great amount of time spent obtaining, using, or

recovering from alcohol; (9) Important activities given up or reduced because of drinking; (10) Continued drinking despite knowledge of physical or psychological problems caused by alcohol; (11) Alcohol craving.

Disorder severity—the severity of alcohol use disorder at the time of diagnosis can be specified as a subtype based on the number of symptoms present:

Mild: Two to three symptoms;

Moderate: Four to five symptoms;

Severe: Six or more symptoms.

Intoxication: Disinhibition, talkative, slurred speech, moody, ataxia, aggression, blackouts, hallucinations, impaired memory and judgment, coma. **Intoxication treatment:** B1, folate, anti-seizure (carbamazepine); avoid neuroleptics.

Withdrawal: Tremor, tachycardia, hypertension, agitation, seizure, delirium tremens (DTs). **Treatment:** Long-acting benzodiazepines (BZs, chloradiazepam, lorazepam) for sedation (especially for DTs); diazepam for prevention of seizure; beta-R blocker and clonidine for hypertension, etc.

Alcohol dependence and abuse (Alcoholism): (1) Physiologic dependence as manifested by evidence of withdrawal when intake is interrupted. (2) Tolerance to the effects of alcohol. (3) Evidence of alcohol-associated diseases. (4) Continued drinking despite strong medical and social contraindications and life disruptions. (5) Impairment in social and occupational functioning. (6) Depression, blackouts, etc.

Complications: GI—gastritis, esophagitis, pancreatitis, alcoholic liver disease, Mallory-Weiss tears; CVD—alcoholic cardiomyopathy, essential hypertension; CNS—Wernicke encephalopathy, Kosakoff psychosis; pulmonary—pneumonia, aspiration; sexual function—impotence, loss of libido; psychiatric—depression, anxiety, insomnia; nutritional—vitamin (B1, etc.) deficiencies and GI cancers.

Anti-abuse: Disulfiram can induce short of breath, flushing, tachycardia, headache, and nausea/vomiting shortly after alcohol intake. Naltrexone helps reduce the craving for alcohol.

Cannabis (Marijuana)

Cannabis is the most commonly used illegal psychoactive substance worldwide. Cannabis use disorder is a persisting pattern of cannabis use that results in clinically significant functional impairment in two or more fields within a year.

Typical manifestations of the disorder: Impairment in school or work function, giving up of previously enjoyed social and recreational activities, and use of cannabis in potentially hazardous situations. Brief screening can be started with the single question: "How often have you used marijuana in the past year?"

Intoxication: Euphoria, slowed sense of time, impaired judgement and motor coordination, social withdrawal, increased appetite and sexual impulse, dry mouth, conjunctival congestions, hallucinations,

Cannabis

anxiety, and paranoia. Drug testing for delta-9-tetrahydrocannabinol (THC) in urine only indicates cannabis use but not its recency.

There is **no obvious withdrawal or dependence** because cannabis withdrawal is usually mild and self-limited.

Treatment: First-line treatment for cannabis use disorder is cognitive-behavioral therapy (CBT) or/and motivational enhancement treatment (MET). If it's not effective, it is treated with addiction of counselling and referral to a mutual help group (support) such as Marijuana Anonymous. Augmentation of psychosocial treatment with N-acetylcysteine (young patients) or gabapentin (adult) may be a plus. Benzodiazepines are only used for acute agitation and paranoid delusion.

Cocaine

Cocaine is among the most commonly used illicit recreational drugs worldwide. Cocaine use, even casually, may be associated with acute or chronic cardiovascular toxicity. Acute coronary syndromes (ACS), aortic dissection and rupture, arrhythmias, myocarditis, and vasculitis are potential toxicities related to cocaine ingestion.

Intoxication: Psychosis, agitation, euphoria, pupil dilation, tachycardia, hypertension, seizures, stroke, panic, paranoia, hallucinations, violence, and sudden death. *psychomotor* *Psychosis, HTN crisis*

Treatment: (1) Treat symptoms—benzodiazepines (diazepam) or dopamine receptor (R) blocker (bromocriptine or haloperidol) for severe agitation; anti-hypertensive medicines. Beta-R blocker should be avoided for potential worsening of ACS. (2) Treat cocaine-associated ACS as for ACS by most other causes—aspirin, nitroglycerin, diltiazem or verapamil, early reperfusion, coronary angiography, and primary percutaneous coronary intervention (rather than fibrinolysis).

Withdrawal: The symptoms are predominantly psychological—depression, anxiety, anhedonia, cocaine craving, and increased sleep. Most symptoms are self-limited and resolve within one to two weeks without treatment. Significant post-use "crash" includes hypersomnolence, depression, craving, angina, nightmare, and suicidality. The severe craving may strongly contribute to compulsive use. Disulfiram (for alcohol use disorder) has shown promise for cocaine use disorder. *— cocaine bugs, tactile hallucinations*

Amphetamines

psychosis   *fever, overheating*

Intoxication: Psychomotor agitation, euphoria, pupil dilation, tachycardia, hypertension, impaired judgment, **prolonged wakefulness** and attentiveness, hallucinations, and seizure. *Water intoxication*

Treatment: Diazepam or haloperidol for severe agitation; anti-hypertensive medicines, etc. Psychosocial interventions have proven efficacy in reducing stimulant use in patients with stimulant use disorder, but these treatments alone are insufficient for many patients. Antidepressants and Disulfiram may be helpful in some patients.

Withdrawal: Post-use "crash" (hypersomnolence, depression, lethargy, stomach cramp, nightmare).

Opioids

[handwritten: heroin]

[handwritten top: HIV / Rx pills => Heroin - HCV / infective endocarditis]

[handwritten right: No tolerance to pupil constriction]

Intoxication: Euphoria then apathy, CNS and respiratory suppression (lethal), pupil constriction, constipation. *[handwritten: coma] [handwritten: Miosis] [handwritten: Tx is naloxone]*

Treatment: Medication treatment is effective for opioid use disorder. Buprenorphine is preferred. Methadone may have longer and better capacity but it has a higher risk of lethal overdose, and thus is a second-line medicine after buprenorphine. If an opioid agonist is prohibited, naltrexone can effectively block opioid-R and reverse effects. *[handwritten: Acute]*

[handwritten right: Tx: Chronic: - Narcotics Anon - Medical Assisted Tx - methadone - suboxone]

—**Withdrawal:** Dysphoria, insomnia, anorexia, myalgia, fever, lacrimation, diaphoresis, dilated pupils, rhinorrhea, piloerection, nausea, vomiting, stomach cramps, diarrhea, etc. **Treatment:** Short action: clonidine; long-term: methadone or buprenorphine. *[handwritten: pain] [handwritten: yawning] [handwritten: mydriasis]*

[handwritten left: Dx clue - Utox - naltrexone challenge]

[handwritten: ↓anxiety, restlessness HTN. loperamide for diarrhea. Baclofen for muscle cramps]

PCP (Phencyclidine)

[handwritten: Aggressive psychosis]

Phencyclidine is a dissociative anesthetic that is abused primarily for its hallucinatory effects. Significant toxicity is rare but potentially serious. The drug carries a rapid onset of action but a short duration.

Intoxication: Assaultiveness, belligerence, **violence**, psychosis, agitation, impulsiveness, impaired judgement, nystagmus/ataxia, tachycardia, hypertension, hallucination, and delirium. *[handwritten: vertical + horizontal]*

Treatment: Reassurance; diazepam or haloperidol for severe PCP-related psychomotor agitation. *[handwritten: 2°] [handwritten: ① Lorazepam /BZDs]*

LSD—Hallucinogen

Intoxication: Marked anxiety or depression, delusion, visual hallucinations, flashbacks, pupil dilation, impaired judgement, diaphoresis, tachycardia, hypertension, and heightened senses.

Treatment: Supportive counselling; diazepam or haloperidol for severe psychomotor agitation; antipsychotics or anxiolytics.

Withdrawal: Recurrence of intoxication symptoms due to GI reabsorption. Sudden onset of severe violence may occur.

Barbiturates

Barbiturate use can lead to both addiction and physical dependence, and as such they have a high potential for abuse. The GABAA receptor, one of barbiturates' main sites of action, is thought to play a pivotal role in the development of tolerance to and dependence on barbiturates.

Intoxication: CNS inhibition and life-threatening respiratory depression. The physical dependence is treated by stabilisation on the long-acting barbiturate phenobarbital followed by a gradual titration down of dose. *[handwritten: coma.]*

[handwritten: - redistribute to fat]

Barbiturates

Withdrawal: Anxiety, seizures, delirium, lethal CVS and respiratory inhibition. **Treatment:** Short-acting diazepams.

Benzodiazepines (BZDs)

BZD prescriptions and overdoses have been steadily increased in recent years.

Intoxication: Interactions with alcohol; slurred speech, incoordination, ataxia, <u>amnesia</u>, *abuse* somnolence, nystagmus, stupor or coma, diuresis, arrhythmia, and respiratory depression. The presence of depressive and anxiety disorders may increase the risk of benzodiazepine use disorder in patients prescribed benzodiazepines. *Delirium in elderly*

Testing: BZDs are NOT detected in standard urine screening tests of drug abuse. The liquid chromatography-tandem mass spectrometry can detect use of BZDs more accurately.

same as EtOH withdrawal   *Diastolic HTN*

withdcan &   **Withdrawal:** Rebound anxiety, nausea or vomiting, seizure, tremor, insomnia, and hypertension.
Tx: Flumazenil   **Treatment:** Short-acting diazepam.   *EtOH → GABA → ↓ Activity*
but it ↓ seizure threshold. only   *potentiation*
use if certain its BZD.   *chronic → ↓↓ GABA rec to maintain Activity levels*
                                         ∅ + ↓↓ => ↓ inhibition = ↑Activity = seizures en shit

Caffeine

Caffeine is the most consumed stimulant in the world. There is insufficient evidence for promoting or discouraging coffe/tea use. Short-term benefits include increased mental alertness and certain cognitive performance, etc. **Long-term use is associated with beneficial effects of reduced risk of Parkinson disease, Alzheimer disease, alcoholic cirrhosis, and gout, but also increased risks of caffeine use disorder and generalized anxiety disorder.**
excess amounts (energy drinks)   *sympathetic hyperactivity, anxiety, jitterness*
Intoxication: Restlessness, insomnia, diuresis, muscle twitching, arrhythmia (tachycardia), agitation.

Withdrawal: headache, lethargy, depression, weight gain, irritability, and craving. Caffeine withdrawal is more evident than dependence.

Nicotine

Cigarette smoking and chronic nicotine intoxication has been associated with increased risks of COPD, CAD, stroke, peripheral vascular disease, multiple malignancies, etc., and is the leading preventable cause of mortality.

Intoxication: Restlessness, insomnia, anxiety, arrhythmia. *Vtach if OD.*

Treatment: Smokers should be managed with a combination of behavioral support and medication therapy. First-line medicines for smoking cessation include nicotine replacement therapy, varenicline, and bupropion.   *cravings*
Withdrawal: Irritability, headache, anxiety, weight gain, bradycardia, and distractibility.

NON-SUBSTANCE-RELATED DISORDERS

Gambling Disorder

Formerly known as "**Pathological gambling in impulse control disorders**", it is a disorder characterized by **persistent and recurrent gambling behavior**, including a preoccupation with gambling, a need to gamble with more money, attempts to stop gambling or to win back losses, illegal acts to finance the gambling, or loss of normal relationships due to gambling. Individuals usually appear overconfident, with histories of multiple arrests, suicide attempts, alcohol abuse, loss of a loved one, poor parenting, mood disorder, etc. Prevalence is males > females.

Treatment

Gamblers Anonymous group or organization is the most effective treatment. It involves public confessions, peer pressure, and sponsors.

FEEDING AND EATING DISORDERS

Anorexia Restriction

Anorexia Nervosa

It's an eating disorder characterized by **failure to maintain a normal eating habit and body weight**, fear and preoccupation [*Anxiety*] with overweight. Patient has an unrealistic self-evaluation as overweight and disturbed body image, and usually loses weight by maintaining strict caloric control, excessive exercise, purging, fasting, and abusing laxative and diuretics. It mostly occurs in young females (**F:M = 10:1**). Average onset age is 17 years; the later the onset, the worse the prognosis. *No insight.*

Etiology and risk factors

They may be associated with some genetic factors, emotional conflicts with contraception and sexuality, and a cultural emphasis on thinness.

Essentials of diagnosis (criteria)

↓ calorie intake, ↑ calorie expenditure, excess exercise

1. Restriction of energy intake that leads to a low body weight (body mass index <18.5), given the patient's age, sex, developmental trajectory, and physical health.

2. Intense fear of gaining weight or becoming fat, or persistent behavior that prevents weight gain, despite being underweight.

3. Distorted perception of body weight and shape, undue influence of weight and shape on self-worth, or denial of the medical seriousness of one's low body weight.

Patient typically restricts food intake and maintains diets of low-calorie foods to lose weight; it may be accompanied with exercise and purging (self-induced vomiting or laxation); over-concerns with appearance and overweight; has **amenorrhea ≥ 3 cycles**; denies emaciated conditions; may have OCD or depression. Symptoms are usually > 3 months.

S/Sx: Malnourished
hypothyroid but thin → lanugo, amenorrhea
cold intolerance
emaciated

Anorexia Nervosa

There are two subtypes:

(1) **Restricting type**—Marked by weight loss through dieting, fasting, and excessive exercise without recurrent episodes of binge eating or purging.

(2) **Binge eating and purging**—Marked by episodes of binge eating and purging.

P/E results: **Body weight is ≥ 15% below expected weight**; emaciation, hypotension, bradycardia, lanugos (fine hair on the trunk), and peripheral edema. Signs of purging: eroded dental enamel and scarred/scratched hands. **Lab** tests may show electrolyte disturbances (Hypo-KCl alkalosis, metabolic acidosis, etc).

Hospitalize @ extreme — *electrolytes abn*
— leukopenia
— bradycardia, HoTN
BMI <16 ~ <85% IDW

Treatment

1. First hospitalize the patient and correct metabolic imbalance to prevent dehydration, starvation, electronic imbalances, and death. *Force feed, IVF*

2. Weight gain is the target. It's important to have psychotherapy and behavior therapy (with rewards or punishments) based on weight, and family therapy to reduce conflicts with parents. Antidepressants (SSRIs) may have some effects on promoting weight gain. Patient is usually not distressed by the disorder and may be **resistant to treatment**. *Tx w Antipsychotics, olanzapine & CBT*

3. Prognosis/outcome: The course is fluctuating; long-term mortality rate of hospitalized patients is 10%, resulting from the effects of starvation (electrolyte disorders) and purging or suicide. *f/u if comorbid OCD/MDD >> SSRI or SNRI*

Bulimia Nervosa   *Bulimia Purge*

Purge: emesis
- dental erosions
- dorsal hand
* scar*
- parotid swelling
- ↓K+, ↓mg2+, ↓Cl-
- metab alkalosis
- tachycardia, HoTN
Purge: laxatives
- diarrhea
- metab acidosis

It's an eating disorder characterized by frequent **binge-eating and purging and normal body weight, with the self-image unduly influenced by shape and weight and lack of control of overeating episodes.** It mostly occurs among **young females**. It may be in chronic or intermittent course with high remittances. *Binge = anxiety. ⊕ insight.*

Risk factors

Psychological conflicts (guilt, helplessness, etc.) and mood disorders. Worse prognosis is predicted if substance abuse is co-existent. *— ↓ energy, irreg menses, bloating, constipation*
— dry skin, ↓K+ from renal K+ loss in Alkalosis setting

Essentials of diagnosis

1. The most common symptoms are lethargy, irregular menses, abdominal pain and bloating, and constipation. Typical behaviors include recurrent episodes of binge-eating associated with emotional stress and followed by feelings of guilt, self-recrimination, and inappropriate compensatory behaviors of self-induced vomiting or laxation, fasting, or excessive exercise to avoid weight gains.

2. Attempts to conceal binge-eating or purging, or lies about the behavior. It may be accompanied by symptoms of depression, substance abuse, or personality disorder.

3. P/E results: Evidence of purging and/or laxative/diuretic abuse (on hands, teeth, etc).

Differential diagnosis

Binge-eating disorder, anorexia nervosa, atypical depression, borderline personality disorder.

Bulimia Nervosa

Treatment

Cognitive and behavioral therapy is the major treatment. It's more effective if combined with psychodynamic psychotherapy and antidepressants (SSRIs). Patient is usually distressed by the disorder, willing to be treated, and thus easier to treat. *SNRIs + CBT. Never use bupropion = ↑Seizure risk.*

Binge-Eating Disorder (BED)

BED is an eating disorder characterized by **binge eating without subsequent purging episodes.**

Essentials of diagnosis

1. Each binge consists of eating an amount of food much larger than most people would eat in a similar period of time under similar circumstances, and is accompanied by a feeling of discomfort, nausea/vomiting, and loss of control. **It occurs at least once a week for 3 months.**

2. The binge eating is not associated with the recurrent use of appropriate compensatory behavior and does not occur exclusively during the course of "Bulimia Nervosa or Anorexia Nervosa".

3. The person is seriously worried about the binge eating, feeling disgusted, depressed, or guilty after binge eating. These conditions may be **associated with obesity, which is present with 2/3 of people** with BED, although most people with obesity don't have BED.

Treatment

Strategies are similar to those for bulimia nervosa. Effects are usually good because patient is willing to be treated.

Pica (Disorder)

Pica is characterized by an appetite for substances largely **non-nutritive, such as ice, clay, chalk, dirt, or sand**. To be **diagnosed** as a disorder, it must persist for **more than 1 month** at an age where eating such objects is considered developmentally inappropriate, not part of culturally sanctioned practice and sufficiently severe to warrant clinical attention. The consumption of ice is common and harmful as there is a high risk of tooth cracking, enamel deterioration, jaw joint strain, and GI lesion. Anemia and lead and zinc poisoning are common complications. Pica is more commonly seen in women and children.

Treatment

It may vary by patient and suspected cause (e.g., child, disabled, pregnant or psychotic) and may emphasize psychosocial, environmental, and family-guidance approaches. Iron deficiency may be treatable though iron supplement.

Rumination Disorder (Syndrome)

Also called **Merycism**, it is an under-diagnosed **chronic motility disorder characterized by effortless regurgitation of most meals** following consumption, due to the involuntary contraction of the muscles around the abdomen. There is no retching, nausea, heartburn, odor, or abdominal pain associated with the regurgitation, as there is with typical vomiting. Other findings include acid-induced erosion of

Rumination

the esophagus and enamel, halitosis, malnutrition, severe weight loss, and an unquenchable appetite. Cycles of ingestion and regurgitation can mimic the binging and purging of bulimia.

Treatment

There is no known effective therapy for rumination. Treatment is different for different ages and conditions. Biofeedback and relaxation techniques may be tried for adults.

Avoidant/Restrictive Food Intake Disorder (ARFID)

Also known as **Selective Eating Disorder** (SED), it is an eating disorder that prevents the consumption of certain foods. It is often viewed as a phase of childhood that is generally overcome with age. Some people may continue to be afflicted with ARFID throughout their adult lives.

Diagnostic criteria include: (1) Disturbance in eating or feeding certain foods; (2) Substantial weight loss or absence of expected weight gain; (3) Nutritional deficiency; (4) Dependence on a feeding tube or dietary supplements; (5) Significant psychosocial interference; (6) Excluding other disorders.

Treatment

Most children can benefit from a 4-stage "4R" treatment program at home based on systematic desensitization—Record, Reward, Relax, and Review. Most adults' symptoms eventually disappear without treatment.

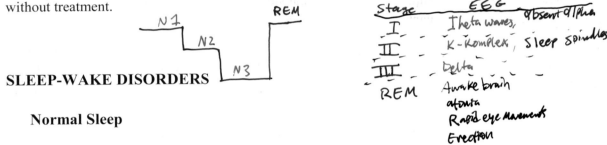

Stage	EEG	
I	Theta waves,	Absent alpha
II	K-Komplex,	Sleep spindles
III	Delta	
REM	Awake brain atonia, Rapid eye Movements, Erection	

SLEEP-WAKE DISORDERS

Normal Sleep

Two major stages

1. **Nonrapid eye movement sleep (NREM):** Characterized by slowing of the EEG rhythms, high muscle tone, and absence of eye movements and thought activity. In this stage the brain is inactive while the body is active. It consists of 4 sub-stages:

Stage-1: EEG shows alpha and theta waves. Stage-2 (45%, longest): Kappa (k)-complex and sleep spindles. *Most restful* Stage-3: Delta-waves (slowest, "slow wave sleep"). Stage-4: Continuation of delta-waves.

2. **Rapid eye movement sleep (REM):** 25%, with aroused EEG patterns (sawtooth waves), sexual arousal, rapid eye movements, generalized muscle atony, and dreams (nightmares). In this stage, the brain is active and the body is inactive. ↑nighttime sleep onset latency ↓REM latency, slow wave sleep

Changes in sleep patterns from infancy to old age

Total sleep time and REM% decrease. Stages 3 and 4 tend to vanish.

Changes in neurotransmitters during sleep

There are increased 5-HT and ACh, and decreased NE (noradrenaline) and DA (dopamine).

Sleep latency: *time* Bed → N1
↑insomnia
↓ deprivation

REM latency: time Bed → REM
90 min
↑narcolepsy, sleep depr, REM depr - alcohol

REM rebound:
amount of REM you get ↑↑ when you deprive the body of REM sleep
OSA

↑ 5-HT = ↑ sleep
↓ ACh = ↑ dream
↑ NE = ↑ arouse
↑ DA = ↑ awake

↓GABA = ↓ Sleep latency
ETOH, B2O, ↑ N3
BZD
↓REM / Zolpidem helps sleep

628

Sleep Disorders

Sleep disorders are very common. The International Classification of Sleep Disorders (ICSD-3) and DSM-5 have the following similar categories of sleep disorders:

1. Insomnia (disorder); 2. Breath-related sleep disorders (Sleep-related breathing disorders); 3. Hypersomnolence disorder and central disorders of hypersomnolence; 4. Narcolepsy; 5. Parasomnias; 6. Sleep-related movement disorders; 7. Circadian rhythm sleep-wake disorders; 8. Others.

Insomnia (Disorder)

It's a disorder characterized by difficulties in initiating or maintaining sleep followed by frequent yawning and tiredness during the day, not due to physical or mental causes. It commonly affects up to 30% of the population at the level of functioning and is exacerbated by anxiety. It must be present ≥ 3 times/week for 1 month for diagnosis. Acute or transient insomnia is usually due to psychological stress or travel over time zones. Chronic causes can be various from psychiatric, medical, medicinal, and primary. _[mood]_

Treatment
Bed for sleep & sex only.

1. **Good sleep hygiene techniques:** Establish regular sleep schedule; avoid daytime naps, evening _[exercise]_ stimulation (including CNS stimulants, alcohol). Treat underlying cause if possible.

2. If it fails, try benzodiazepines (short-term—triazolam; intermediate—estazolam, lorazepam, temazepam; long-acting—flurazepam, quazepam), non-BZ (zolpidem), melatonin agonist (ramelteon), or diphenhydramine shortly (< 2-3 weeks). _[diphenhydramine, trazodone, quetiapine, zolpidem]_

Breath-related Sleep Disorders (Sleep-related Breathing Disorders)

These are characterized by abnormal respiration during sleep, occurring in both adults and children. There are **four major types: (1) Central sleep apnea syndrome; (2) Obstructive sleep apnea (hypopnea) syndrome; (3) Sleep related hypoventilation disorder; (4) Sleep related hypoxemia disorder.**
They can be further divided according to their etiology.

Sleep apnea syndrome is a disorder with cessation of airflow at the nose or mouth during sleep. These apneic episodes usually last longer than 10 sec/each, characterized by a loud snore followed by a heavy pause. During the apneic episodes, O_2 saturation decreases, and pulmonary pressures increase. It's considered pathologic if it's more than 5 episodes/hour or > 30 episodes per night. It may be associated with depression and daytime sleepiness. **Risk factors** include obesity, family history, alcohol or sedative intake, hypothyroidism, and structural abnormalities.

Clinical features, subtypes, and diagnosis

1. Mostly seen in **obese, middle-aged males**. Patient usually presents with **somnolence with loud snoring and apnea during the day or at night, accompanied with dry mouth, fatigue, headache.**

Spouse complains of being interfered during the night. Patient may develop arrhythmias, hypoxemia, pulmonary hypertension and sudden death (especially infant and elderly). _opiates._

2. **Central sleep apnea (CSA)**: There is no central respiratory effort during the pause in breathing. After the episode of apnea, breathing may be faster (hyperpnea) for a period of time as a respiratory compensation. CSA can be primary (idiopathic) or secondary (#1 associated with Cheyne-Stokes breathing). _CO_2 retention._

daytime somnolence. Snoring.

3. **Obstructive sleep apnea/hypopnea (OSA, 95%)**: OSA is characterized by repetitive, intermittent episodes of airflow reduction (hypopnea) or cessation (apnea) due to upper airway collapse during sleep, including adult type and pediatric type. The airway collapse is due to muscle atonia in oropharynx or nasal, tongue, or tonsil obstruction. Each apneic period usually lasts 20 to 30 seconds and results in hypoxia, which arouses the patient from sleep. This occurs multiple times overnight.

4. **Diagnosis: Sleep test** (polysomnography) is the most accurate means of diagnosis. It can record decreased O2 saturation and distinguish OSA from CSA, seizures, etc. _≥ 15 apneas/hr_ _or_ _≥ 5 apneas + snoring_ _hr_ _} OSA_

Treatment

↑ PEEP

1. **CSA**: Try to target underlying cause. (1) Continuous positive airway pressure (CPAP) is usually tried first (especially with Cheyne-Stokes breathing). (2) If failed, adaptive servo-ventilation (ASV) is tried. (3) If both CPAP and ASV are failed, bi-level positive airway pressure (BPAP) is tried with a backup respiratory rate. (4) If these cannot be tolerated, medications (acetazolamide, zolpidem, or triazolam) can be tried (if no risk factors for respiratory depression).

2. **OSA**: (1) Mild to moderate cases: patient education and behavior therapy—weight reduction (for obese people), avoidance of alcohol/sedatives intake and supine position during sleep.

(2) Severe OSAHS (>20 apneic episodes with arterial oxygen desaturations) —continuous (fixed) positive airway pressure (CPAP) is the main therapy, which can prevent occlusion of the upper pharynx. If not tolerated, BPAP is an option. If this fails, uvulopalatopharyngoplasty (to remove redundant tissue in oropharynx) or an upper airway stimulation system may be tried.

(3) Children—surgery for tonsillar/adenoidal hypertrophy.

Central Disorders of Hypersomnolence and Hypersomnolence Disorder

These disorders refer to excessive daytime sleepiness that is not due to disturbed sleep or misaligned circadian rhythms. In ICSD-3, Central Disorders of Hypersomnolence include narcolepsy type 1 and type 2, idiopathic hypersomnia, and Kleine-Levin syndrome (KLS, recurrent hypersomnia). **KLS** is a rare disorder that starts during adolescence and has a male gender preference. The patients have recurrent episodes of hypersomnia, which are often associated with compulsive overeating and hypersexuality.

Hypersomnolence Disorder

It is characterised by excessive daytime sleepiness that is not due to medical or mental conditions, drugs, poor sleep hygiene, insufficient sleep, or narcolepsy. It occurs at least three times per week for at

Hypersomnolence

least 3 months and causes significant distress or impairment in social or occupational functioning. This disorder is less well-defined and lack of REM sleep and other features of narcolepsy.

Treatment

Psychostimulants (methylphenidate or amphetamine) is the choice of treatment. SSRIs may be helpful in some patients.

Narcolepsy

Also known as hypnolepsy, it is a chronic neurological disorder involving the loss of the brain's ability to regulate sleep-wake cycles normally, characterized by **excessive daytime sleepiness and abnormalities of REM sleep for more than 3 months**, causing significant impairment in social or occupational functioning. It's an inherited disorder of variable penetrance. REM sleep usually occurs in less than 5 min. Patients feel refreshed upon awakening.

Clinical features and diagnosis

1. Involuntary "**sleep attacks**": Most common symptoms—frequent **irresistible sleeping** at any time of day (during any activity) that lasts several min, **refreshed upon awakening**, and falling asleep quickly at night.

2. **Cataplexy** (70%)—**pathognomonic sign**: **Sudden loss of muscle tone**, which may have been precipitated by a loud noise or intense emotion. – *laughing*

3. **Hypnagogic and hypnopompic hallucinations: Dreaming while awaking**; it occurs as the patient is going to sleep and is waking up from sleep, respectively.

4. **Sleep paralysis:** Patient **cannot move when waking up.**

Treatment   Dx: polysomnography
                        ↓ hypocretin (orexin) in ⊘ CSF

1. Forced naps at a regular time of day is usually helpful.

2. A psychostimulant (methylphenidate or amphetamine) is the main medical treatment. TCAs can be used if cataplexy is present.   *Modafinil,*

Parasomnias

Parasomnias are undesirable physical events (movements, behaviors) or experiences (emotions, perceptions, dreams) that occur during entry into sleep, within sleep, or during arousals from sleep. The behaviors can be complex and appear purposeful; however, the patient is not consciously aware of the behavior. The sub-category includes:

(1) NREM related parasomnias: they are disorders of arousal including confusional arousals, sleepwalking, sleep terrors, and sleep related eating disorder

(2) REM related parasomnias: involve the intrusion of the features of REM sleep into wakefulness (eg, sleep paralysis), exaggeration of the features of REM sleep (eg, nightmare disorder), etc.

(3) Other parasomnias without specific relationship to sleep stage: exploding head syndrome, sleep related hallucinations, sleep enuresis, and drug-associated parasomnias.

Nightmare (disorder): It occurs commonly in 50% of the population. Patient can remember the event upon awakening. It increases during times of stress. There is no special therapy required but adjustment of stress. ⓟ REM, will remember. Any age. ↓ stressor.

Night terror: Awakened by scream or intense anxiety. Patient usually has no memory of the event the following day. It's more common in boys and with family history. No special treatment is needed. If severe, limited use of BZs may be considered. NIII, Active behaviors while asleep.   Tx reassurance
↑ ⓟtone, "awake", inconsolable

Sleepwalking: It occurs during stage 3-4 of sleep, with sequencing behaviors during sleep without full consciousness; ends in waking embarrassment without remembering anything. It's more common in young boys and may be associated with neurologic diseases. **Treatment**: First assure patient's safety. If it occurs frequently, give BZs to suppress stage 3-4 sleep.

Sleep-related Movement Disorders

These are characterized by simple, stereotypic movements that disturb sleep and cause related symptoms (daytime sleepiness, fatigue, etc.). Patients may or may not be aware of the movements.

The classic disorders include restless legs syndrome, periodic limb movement disorder, sleep related leg cramps, sleep related bruxism (teeth grinding), and sleep related rhythmic movement disorder.

Circadian Rhythm Sleep-Wake Disorder

It's characterized by chronic or recurrent sleep disturbance due to misalignment between the environment and an individual's sleep-wake cycle. People with the disorder are unable to sleep and wake at the times required for normal work, school, and social needs. They are generally able to get enough sleep if allowed to sleep and wake at the times dictated by their body clocks. The quality of their sleep is usually normal. There are several types of circadian rhythm disorders:

1. **Shift work disorder and jet lag disorder** are the most common types, although most of these cases do not come to medical attention.

2. **Delayed sleep-wake phase disorder** is characterized by sleep and wake times that are habitually delayed compared to conventional times, more common in a younger patient.

3. **Advanced sleep-wake phase disorder** is characterized by sleep and wake times that are habitually early compared to conventional time, more common in the elderly.

4. **Irregular sleep-wake rhythm disorder** is characterized by lack of a clearly defined circadian rhythm of sleep and wake. This disorder is commonly associated with developmental disorders in children and with neurodegenerative diseases such as Alzheimer disease, Parkinson disease, and Huntington disease.

Treatment

1. Jet-lag disorder: It usually resolves in 2-7 days without treatment.

2. Shift-work disorder: Light therapy may help.

3. Delayed sleep-phase disorder: Taking oral melatonin 30 min before bedtime may help.

SEXUAL DISORDERS

Terminology of Human Sexuality

Sexual identity: Based on a person's secondary sexual characteristics.

Gender identity: Based on a person's sense of maleness or femaleness, mostly established by age 3.

Gender role: Based on a person's external patterns of behavior that reflect the inner sense of gender identity.

Sexual orientation: Based on a person's choice of love object, which can be heterosexual (most population), homosexual, bisexual, or asexual.

Sexual Function Changes with Aging

Interest in sexual activity usually does not decrease with aging, but sexual functions do.

Male: It requires longer time for the genital stimulation and reaching orgasm, and has longer refractory period before next orgasm. Intensity of orgasm is mostly decreased.

Female: Menopause and decreased estrogen cause vaginal dryness and discomfort during coitus, which can be treated with hormone replacement therapy (HRT) or vaginal creams (estrogen). Increased orgasm after 30-35 y/a is common.

SEXUAL DYSFUNCTIONS

Sexual dysfunction disorders refer to disturbances in sexual arousal, desire, orgasm, or pain with sexual intercourse. They may be classified into the related four categories—sexual desire disorders, arousal disorders, orgasm disorders, and sexual pain disorders. Sexual dysfunction requires a person to feel extreme distress and interpersonal strain for a minimum of 6 months (excluding substance or medication-induced sexual dysfunction).

Sexual dysfunctions can have a profound impact on an individual's perceived quality of sexual life. The prevalence is up to 30-40% and it occurs at least once in a lifetime. **2/3 of all cases are due to bio-medical factors**. 1/3 of cases are due to psychological conditions (known as "psychosexual disorders").

I. Sexual Desire Disorders

Also known as hypoactive sexual desire disorder or decreased libido, it is characterised by a lack or absence of sexual desire for sexual activity or of sexual fantasies for certain period of time. The condition may have started after a period of normal sexual functioning or the person may always have had no/low sexual desire. It's **more common in women** with heavy burdens of dual duty of work and home care.

General **causes** may include aging, **stress, fatigue**, pregnancy, medications (such as antidepressives, antihypertensives, antipsychotics, antiparkinson drugs, and lithium), psychiatric conditions (such as depression, anxiety disorders, and panic disorder), or decrease in normal estrogen in women or testosterone in both men and women.

Treatment

Target underlying cause. Reduce work load and stress. Discontinue related medicines. Give psycho-therapy when indicated.

II. Sexual Arousal Disorders

Previously known as **frigidity in women and impotence in men**, they are now corrected as sexual arousal disorders (including **erectile dysfunction**). These conditions can manifest themselves as an aversion to, and avoidance of, sexual contact with a partner. In men, there may be partial or complete failure to attain or maintain an erection, or a lack of sexual excitement and pleasure in sexual activity.

Causes may include medications (such as antidepressives, antihypertensives, antipsychotics, antiparkinson drugs, and lithium), chronic diseases (such as diabetes and cardiovascular disease causing decreased blood flow to the genitalia), surgical or traumatic injury to the nervi erigentes, etc), and psychological conditions (including relationship between the partners).

Erectile dysfunction (ED), also known as impotence, it is a sexual dysfunction characterized by the inability to develop or maintain an erection of the penis. The causes may be psychological or physical (as stated above). It is estimated that up to 50% of all men between the ages of 40 and 70 have some form of ED; 80% of cases are organic.

Treatment

It includes psychological and medical therapies according to underlying cause. Sildenafil as a vasodilator is the effective remedy for ED. Be aware of its adverse effect or risk for cardiac ischemia.

III. Premature Ejaculation

It refers to the condition when ejaculation occurs before the partner achieves orgasm or a mutually satisfactory length of time has passed during intercourse. Generally, premature ejaculation is thought to occur when ejaculation occurs in less than 2 minutes from the time of the insertion of the penis. It is **the most common presentation of male sexual dysfunctions** (30-40% of cases).

Causes: Although historically attributed to psychological causes (#1 is anxiety), new studies suggest an underlying neurobiological cause may also lead to premature ejaculation.

Diagnosis: The patient must have a chronic history of premature ejaculation, poor ejaculatory control, and the problem must cause feelings of dissatisfaction as well as distress the patient, the partner or both.

Treatment: Psychotherapy and behavioral modification techniques (pause and penile squeeze, etc).

IV. Orgasm Disorders

These refer to persistent delays or absence of orgasm following a normal sexual excitement phase. The disorder can have physical, psychological, or pharmacological origins, and more common in females.

Causes: Medications (such as antidepressives, antihypertensives, antipsychotics, antiparkinson drugs, and lithium) are a common medical cause, as they can delay orgasm or eliminate it entirely. Other causes may include chronic diseases (CVD, endocrine-metabolic), mental disorders, and substance abuse, etc.

Treatment

Treat underlying conditions, change medications, and give cognitive behavioral therapy, etc.

V. Sexual Pain Disorders

The disorders are also known as **dyspareunia** (painful intercourse) or **vaginismus** (an involuntary spasm of the muscles of the vaginal wall that interferes with intercourse) and **affect women** almost exclusively.

Causes: Fear and anxiety about sex; insufficient vaginal lubrication (due to insufficient excitement and stimulation, or due to hormonal changes caused by menopause, pregnancy, breast-feeding, or contraceptive creams and foams); genital inflammation; past sexual trauma (such as rape or abuse), etc.

Treatment

Treat underlying condition. Vaginismus is treated with psychotherapy and dilator therapy.

Further diagnostic guidelines for sexual dysfunctions

(1) **No.1** factor of diagnostic **evaluation** is **detailed history.**

(2) **P/E**: A digital rectal examination (DRE) and neurologic examination should be done. Assess for signs of peripheral vascular disease.

(3) **Lab tests**: CBC, chemistry panel, fasting glucose, and lipid profiles. If hypogonadism is suspected, serum testosterone, prolactin and thyroid profile should be tested.

(4) **Nocturnal penile tumescence**: If normal erection occurs during sleep, a psychogenic cause is suspected; if it does not occur, an organic cause is likely.

(5) Psychological testing may be appropriate in some cases.

Further therapeutic guidelines for sexual dysfunctions

Specific treatment is determined by the specific cause.

(1) For most organic causes, address atherosclerotic risk factors.

(2) If it's a case of abrupt sexual dysfunctioning, psychotherapy is effective.

(3) If it's traumatic erectile dysfunction, pudendal artery revasculation may be needed.

Sexual Dysfxns

(4) For hypogonadism, hormone replacement is the therapy.

(5) Sildenafil (Viagra) can dilate arterioles and promote penile smooth muscle relaxation and erection. New studies indicate that it may be helpful in patients with atherosclerotic causes, and may also promote recovery from ischemic stroke, neurologic injury, and neurodegenerative disorders. Relative contraindications include heart diseases and simultaneous use with nitrates.

Gender Dysphoria

Identity ≠ assignment AND causes distress in life.
> 6 months. Desire to be or be treated like opposite sex.
Get rid of 2° sexual characteristics
believe they're opposite sex. som like delusion, is n

- internal belief, ident-ity.
Transgender!
I D is incongruent w Assignment
Mind ≠ body
dx: clx

Previously known as "**Gender Identity Disorder**", it is a disorder in which the individual has strong, persistent cross-gender identity and discomfort (dysphoria) with one's biological sex or gender role without intersexual disorders. Patient usually has a history of dressing like the opposite sex, using toys assigned to the opposite sex, playing with opposite-sex children at a young age, taking sex hormones, or/and seeking surgeries to change the gender. It's more common in males, and may be associated with depression, anxiety disorder, substance abuse, and personality disorder.

Assignment Phenotype XX or XY?

-D made switch. A social and/or A body
Transsexualism refers to the people with gender dysphoria having a strong and persistent desire to live according to their gender identity (opposite sex), rather than their biological (anatomic) sex.

Transvestism refers to a person occasionally wearing clothes typically associated with the opposite gender (cross-dressing) for a variety of reasons. *NOT transgender.*
sexual arousal. borderline paraphilia

Kids. reject same roles
accept or opposite Roles

Treatment

First give patient education and counselling about culturally acceptable values and patterns, and then supply supportive psychotherapy. *prior to gender reass- surg.*

PARAPHILIC DISORDERS

These are also classified as **Sexual Arousal Disorders, Disorders of Sexual Preference,** or Disorders of Adult Personality and Behavior.

Paraphilias refers to powerful and persistent sexual interest and arousal to objects, situations, or individuals that are not part of normative stimulation and that may cause serious social distress or consequences for the paraphiliac or associated individuals. A paraphilia involves sexual arousal and gratification towards extreme sexual behavior, mostly seen in men.

Specific types

Pedophilic disorder: Sexual preference for children (boys or girls or both) and recurrent urges involving sexual activities with prepubertal or early prepubertal children.

Exhibitionistic disorder: Recurrent urges or sexual arousal from exposing the genitalia to strangers (usually of the opposite sex), without inviting closer contact. This is usually followed by sexual excitement and masturbation.

Paraphilic Disorders

Voyeuristic disorder: Recurrent urges or sexual arousal from observing unsuspecting person's unclothed or sexual activities. This usually leads to sexual excitement and masturbation.

Frotteuristic disorder: Sexual arousal from rubbing one's genitalia against a nonconsenting person in crowded public places.

Fetishistic disorder: Recurrent urges or sexual arousal from nonliving objects or nongenital body parts (leather, silk, underwears, feet, etc).

Transvestic disorder: Recurrent urges of cross-dressing for sexual arousal.

Sexual sadism disorder: Recurrent urges or sexual arousal from inflicting suffering (pain, bondage, or/and humiliation) on sexual partner.

Sexual masochism disorder: Recurrent urges or sexual arousal from being hurt, humiliated, bound, or abused by sexual partner.

Sadomasochism: A preference for sexual activity that involves the infliction of pain or humiliation, or bondage. If the subject prefers to be the recipient of such stimulation this is called masochism; if the provider, sadism. Often an individual obtains sexual excitement from both sadistic and masochistic activities.

Multiple disorders of sexual preference: Sometimes more than one abnormal sexual preference occurs in one person and there is none of first rank. The most common combination is fetishism, transvestism, and sadomasochism.

Therapeutic guidelines for paraphilic disorders

1. Individual psychotherapy.

2. Behavioral modifications: aversive conditioning may help.

3. Antiandrogens or SSRIs can reduce sexual drive.

NEUROCOGNITIVE DISORDERS

See Chapter 9: Diseases of the Nervous System and Special Senses.

MIX: SUICIDALITY AND DEATH

Suicidality

Suicide is the act of a human being intentionally causing his or her own death. Major risk factors include psychiatric disorders, hopelessness, and prior suicide attempts or threats.

Over one million people commit suicide every year. The World Health Organization estimates that it is the 13th-leading cause of death worldwide. It's rated the 6-8th cause of death in the US. It is a leading cause of death among teenagers and adults under 35, and rates are higher in males than females. There are an estimated 10 to 20 million non-fatal attempted suicides every year worldwide.

Views on suicide have been influenced by varieties of cultures, values, religions, and beliefs.

Risk factors

Men, older adults, social isolation, financial or interpersonal distress, psychiatric or organic disorders—depression, bipolar disorder, schizophrenia, alcoholism, substance abuse, late-stage disease (such as cancer), other adverse situations, and previous attempts. High impulsivity and alcohol/substance abuse increases the risk that suicidal impulses will be carried out.

Presentation

Recent suicide attempt; complaints of suicide thought; admission of suicide thought; evidence of suicide behavior—collecting sleeping pills, writing a will, giving away possessions, buying weapons, etc.

Management

1. Guidelines: hospitalize patient at risk; prevent with serious safety procedures; treat with support, necessary medicine, and psychotherapy.

2. Recommendations: (1) Patients suspected to be at risk for suicide should be evaluated for suicidal ideation, intent, and prevention. (2) Patients at imminent risk for suicide require immediate psychiatric care and continuous monitoring. (3) After patient's safety is ensured, underlying factors of psychiatric disorders, precipitating events, and on-going life circumstances should be addressed with medications, counselling, and involvement of friends, family, and religious/community groups as appropriate. (4) For patients with mood disorders who remain at risk for suicide following proper cares, lithium maintenance +/- other medications and/or psychotherapy is recommended. (5) Patients are at increased risk for suicide soon after discharge from psychiatric inpatient care. After a suicide attempt, psychotherapy may prevent subsequent attempts, and patient should be monitored closely with follow-ups. Please note that after a suicide, friends, family, and coworkers may be at increased risk for suicide and for posttraumatic stress disorder and depression.

Death and Dying

Based on the dying stages defined by Elisabeth Kubler-Ross, dying patients do not follow a simple, regular series of responses; most patients experience the following common stages of death reactions (may not be in this order).

Stage 1. Shock and denial: "No, impossible!"

Stage 2. Anger: "Why me?"

Stage 3. Bargaining: "If you…… then I will……"

Stage 4. Depression: Silent and down.

Stage 5. Acceptance: Cooperative.

Chapter 16: High-yield Questions (HYQ)

1-3: Match the following clinical scenarios with the most likely diagnosis (Dx).

A. Autism spectrum disorder   B. Conduct disorder   C. ADHD

D. Intellectual disability   E. Hearing impairment

F. Oppositional defiant disorder (ODD)

G. Learning disorder   H. Antisocial personality disorder

1. A 10 y/o boy has frequent temper outbursts, arguments with his male teacher and working mother, and difficulties following their instructions. He has no known father. He was once reported to his mother by his teacher for a violation, and he spits on the teacher. His scores at school are very low. There are no other abnormal findings.

2. A 10 y/o boy has frequent difficulties following instructions and fulfilling his school work. His scores for each subject are poor. He's shy and often has social and behavioral disturbances, but can take care of his daily life. He has a divorced mother with a low income. He usually listens to his mother carefully.

3. A 5 y/o boy has frequent difficulties following instructions to finish anything properly. His preschool test scores are poor. He rarely talks. He plays by himself most of the time, usually with the toys. He listens to his parents but has difficulties repeating all that is said. He had a head injury after a fall three years ago.

4-8: Match the following clinical scenarios with the most likely diagnosis.

A. Normal (Nl) grief   B. Acute stress disorder (ASD)

C. Major depressive disorder   D. Dysthymia   E. PTSD

F. Bipolar disorder   G. Cyclothymic disorder

4. A 50 y/o woman is seeing the physician after her son's death half a year ago. She has been sad, irritable, and sleepless. Psychological exams reveal that she has depressed energy and mood, and feelings of helplessness. Her thinking seems logical. There are no other abnormal findings.

5. A 40 y/o woman complains of poor appetite, sleep, and energy that affect her work performance for the past 2 years. She denies any major life events or suicidal ideas. P/E results are unremarkable.

6. A 20 y/o man is seeing an expert after failing several exams at school. He often has multiple social activities and dating with conflicting schedules, but he doesn't care and manages poorly. He usually studies and works late. Psychological exams reveal that he has vigorous speech and psychomotor agitation.

7. A 35 y/o woman is seeing an export with her husband. She has periods of feeling great with increased appetite, sexual drive, and euphoric mood, followed by periods of feeling irritable with insomnia, fatigue, and low desires. This history has been over 2 years. There are no other abnormal findings.

8. A 30 y/o woman complains of sadness, anxiety, insomnia, irritability, fatigue and no desires for the past 2 months. She often dreamed of the car accident in which her husband died by her side 3 months ago, and tried to wake up to avoid the flashbacks. She admits she has performed poorly in her work and housekeeping management.

9. A 48 y/o woman is wandering in the street crying for thinking of hurting herself. She feels very sad and down since her husband and son died in a vehicle accident half a year ago. P/E shows a cut on her wrist. She is conscious but psychologically agitated. What's the most appropriate next step?

A. Refer to a psychiatrist   B. Conduct electroconvulsive therapy

C. Evaluate the suicidal ideas   D. Give fluoxetine   E. Give haloperidol

10. A 30 y/o woman is sent to the clinic because she was found wandering in the street yelling out her husband's name. She appears disheveled, talking illogically. Her husband died in vehicle accident a month ago but she said she kept hearing his voices all the times. Psychological exams reveal that her responses are from internal impulses. What's the most likely diagnosis?

A. Acute stress disorder   B. Normal grief   C. PTSD

D. Brief psychotic disorder   E. Adjustment disorder

11. For the above patient, what's the most appropriate treatment?

A. Haloperidol   B. Clozapine   C. Lorazepam

D. Risperidone   E. Phenazine

12. If the above patient's symptoms continue for more than 3 months, she will be at greatest risk of developing

A. schizotypal personality disorder   B. schizophrenia

C. schizoaffective disorder   D. schizophreniform disorder   E. delusional disorder

13. A 28 y/o woman is naked wandering in the street. When she is caught and questioned by the police, she replies, "I heard a voice from the sky telling me to do so to attract people." When she talks, she frequently changes topics, with euphoric and labile affect. She denies having similar history in the past. What's the most likely diagnosis?

A. Schizophrenia   B. Schizophreniform disorder   C. Delusional disorder

D. Schizoaffective disorder   E. Brief psychotic disorder

14-18: Match the following clinical scenarios with the best choice of medicines.

A. Lorazepam   B. Bentropine   C. Dantrolene

D. Propranolol   E. Diphenhydramine   F. NaHCO3

G. Sertraline   H. Fluoxetine   I. Bupropion

J. Buspirone

14. A 35 y/o woman complains of continuous depressed mood, irritability, and helplessness for the past 2 months after giving birth to the 2nd child. She was prescribed improperly with a more toxic TCA, nortriptyline, for 6 weeks. Now she's in the ER with occasional convulsions, hypotension, and arrhythmia (prolonged QRS on ECG).

15. A man with schizophrenia has been treated with fluphenazine for the past 3 months and suddenly presents with high fever, muscle rigidity, and autonomic instability. There are no other abnormal findings. What's the first medicine of choice?

16. After the above treatment, the same patient still has ataxia, tremor, and rigidity. What's the best medication now?

17. A 50 y/o man complains of continuous depressed mood, irritability, and helplessness for the past 2 months after losing the job. He has a history of "heart disease", alcohol drinking, and smoking for the past few years. There are no other abnormal findings.

18. A 50 y/o man complains of continuous depressed mood, irritability, and helplessness for the past 2 months after losing the job. He has a history of "vasculitis", decreased memory, alcohol drinking, and smoking for the past few years, and the physician advises him to to stop alcohol drinking and smoking.

19. A 45 y/o man comes to the ER on a rainy night, and says a voice is telling him to kill himself in the hospital. When asked about the past history, he cannot give much detailed information. He also refuses all examinations and medicines. There are no other abnormal findings. What's the most likely diagnosis?

A. Alcohol intoxication   B. Brief psychotic disorder   C. Malingering

D. Factitious disorder   E. Delusional disorder

20. A 50 y/o man is brought by his wife for evaluation. The man is laid off as a major manager in a big company recently, and his wife has good income and a stable relationship with him. For the past 3 months he frequently complains of stomach pains and always believes his wife has put poison in the food to kill him for his money. His thoughts seem logical. He denies taking any medicines. P/E results are normal. The most likely diagnosis is

A. Schizophreniform disorder   B. Delusional disorder   C. Somatization disorder

D. Brief psychotic disorder   E. Acute stress disorder

21. A husband brings his wife to the physician for "many complaints." For the past year, she has visited several doctors who can't confirm any disease, taken lots of medicines, but still feels the same symptoms. Today she has dizziness, headache, chest pain, abdominal pain, headache, and fatigue. P/E results are unremarkable. What's the most likely diagnosis?

A. Hypochochiasis   B. Delusional disorder   C. Somatic symptom disorder

D. Factitious disorder   E. Chronic pain syndrome

22. A 25 y/o female becomes angry and bitter after her longtime boyfriend left her for another woman. She soon quit her job without giving notice and began drinking alcohol and smoking heavily, often threatening to kill her boyfriend and herself. What's the most likely diagnosis?

A. Acute stress disorder   B. Adjustment disorder   C. PTSD

D. Alcohol-induced mood disorder   E. Borderline personality disorder

23. An 18 y/o female complains of fatigue, headache, abdominal pain, and lack of menses for the past 3 months. Careful history taking reveals that she has a history of binge-eating and laxative-induced diarrhea, and she always worried about gaining weight. P/E shows her body weight is below normal limit. What's the most likely diagnosis?

A. Anorexia nervosa   B. Bulimia nervosa   C. Major depressive disorder

D. Somatic symptom disorder   E. Chronic pain syndrome

24-29: Match the following clinical scenarios with the most likely type of personality disorders.

A. Schizotypal   B. Schizoid   C. Paranoid

D. Histrionic   E. Narcissistic   F. Borderline

G. Antisocial   H. Avoidant   I. Dependent

J. Obsessive-compulsive

24. A 50 y/o man works as a small-group supervisor in a company. He frequently has conflicts with his colleagues, and always criticizes them with arrogance for small issues. He's been commented as "self-centred" by his colleagues. There are no other abnormal findings.

25. A 28 y/o female lives alone without much social life. She works as a receptionist in an office. She often ignores invitations from colleagues for social activities, and has no outside interests. She is otherwise fine.

26. A 35 y/o man is mostly preoccupied with computer manipulations at home. He enjoys assembling and dissembling his computer repeatedly, often talking and laughing to himself. He spends most of his time alone, and has no history of illogical speech and behavior.

27. A 28 y/o female is visiting a manager, dressing improperly in a seductive way. She keeps asking the manager to comment on her dress. When the manager refuses, she becomes upset and walks out. There are no other abnormal findings.

28. A 30 y/o stressful financial broker complains of hard family life after losing his job, and blames his wife for it. He has a history of work-rule and traffic violations, substance abuse, and several conflicts with colleagues.

29. A singing star walks away from the stage when the conductor points out some mistakes for her during the practice, and states she won't come back unless the conductor apologizes to her publicly. There are no other abnormal findings.

30. A 45 y/o obese man complains of fatigue, headache, and sleepiness during the day for the past month. These symptoms usually follow episodes of waking up in the middle of the night recently. He's missed several days of work due to the sleep problem. The most likely diagnosis is

A. Narcolepsy   B. Insomnia disorder   C. Sleep apnea

D. Hypersomnolence disorder   E. Chronic fatigue syndrome

31. A 10 y/o boy suddenly falls down without losing consciousness. P/E finds decreased muscle tone on the limbs. There are no other abnormal findings. He does not have a special medical history. The most likely cause is

A. Sleep paralysis   B. Cataplexy   C. Syncope

D. Hypoglycemia   E. Sleep attack

32. Which of the following is the most common cause of impotence due to a medical condition?

A. Alcohol   B. CAD   C. Drugs

D. Diabetes   E. Hypertension

33. A 22 y/o man with labile mood was brought to the ER by a family member. The family member informed the physician that he's been on lithium for his "bipolar disorder" for the past one month. In the ER, the patient became combative. The most appropriate next step of management is to

A. prescribe olanzapine   B. add valproic acid   C. add fluvoxamine

D. test the lithium level   E. admit into psychiatric unit

34-35. 34. A 66 y/o man is brought to the clinic by his son. He feels lack of interests, appetite and energy, sleepless, helpless, and hopeless since his wife died 4 months ago. He says he wishes to die with his wife. The most appropriate next step of management is

A. fluoxetine   B. supportive psychotherapy   C. brief psychotherapy

D. phenelzine   E. evaluation for suicidal risk

35. After the diagnosis is confirmed, the above patient is on fluoxetine and trazodone (for his sleep disorder). Against the physician's advice, the patient keeps alcohol drinking. The next day he is brought to the ER with agitation, confusion, sweating, hyperthermia, tachycardia, shivering, and tremors. The most appropriate next step of management is

A. propranolol therapy   B. supportive therapies   C. cyproheptadine therapy

D. alcohol cessation   E. fluoxetine and trazodone cessation

36. A 55 y/o man is brought to the ER after a car accident. He is suffering from multiple fractures of the limbs and skin bruises, and is on oxycodone. The next day after his admission, he presents with confusion and tremors in both hands. He also complains of "seeing bugs on the bed." The most likely cause for his symptoms is

A. brief psychotic disorder   B. traumatic brain injury   C. oxycodone intoxication

D. flumazenil withdrawal   E. alcohol withdrawal

37. A 30 y/o woman assistant manager presents with "weird" behaviors revealed by her colleagues for the past 6 months. She believes that the company will face a radical change very soon, and "a major manager's position will be replaced by me." She states that she has dreamed of this several times and her dream "has always come true." During her routine work of 5 days a week, she has certain conflicts with some colleagues because of her wayward behaviors. Physical and psychiatric examination results are unremarkable. What is the most likely diagnosis?

A. Delusional disorder   B. Schizophrenia   C. Brief psychotic disorder

D. Schizophreniform disorder   E. Paranoid personality disorder

Answers and Explanations

1. (F). This is similar to but a milder form of conduct disorder. The Key treatment (Tx) is to spend more time with the child and care for him, especially in a single-parent family lack of the model and love of the father. 'B' is a repetitive violation in four areas (aggression, destruction, cheating/theft, and rule-breaking) lasting > 6 months (mo) in a patient < 18 y/a; > 18 y/a it's 'H'.

2. (G). He has learning disabilities, poor self-esteem and social-maturity, and school failure. It can be diagnosed by IQ, academic achievement tests, and excluding hearing disorder and intellectual disability (IQ < 70, significantly decreased intellectual function and adapting to demands in daily lives).

3. (A). The boy has most symptoms of autism: defects in social-behavior, communication, speech, and mentality. Poor outcome is associated with intellectual disability and speech failure. Hearing deficits is possible but the 5 y/o child could have finished something well without listening to the parents carefully.

4. (C). She has most symptoms of major depression.

5. (D). This resembles "mild depression" for a course of 2 years.

6. (F). This is in the state of acute mania.

7. (G). A milder form of bipolar II disorder: many periods of depressed mood and hypomanic mood for > 2 years.

8. (E). A situation of a life disaster + depression + maladaptation; < 1 month, it is ASD; > 1 month, it is PTSD.

9. (C). First choose 'C' to prevent suicide, then 'E' for anti-psychosis, followed by 'A' or 'D' (anti-depression). 'B' is indicated for severe depression with high risk of suicide.

10. (D). Brief psychotic disorder: acute psycho-symptoms after a big disaster for 1 month.

11. (E). Phenazine is the best choice here (with relatively less S/E), because 'A' as a typical antipsychotic and "B and D" as atypical ones all carry many S/E.

12. (D). The duration is crucial: < 6 months, it's schizophreniform disorder; if symptoms persist > 6 months, it's schizophrenia.

13. (D). Schizoaffective disorder = Illogical thinking and association + labile affect, but not consistent with the criteria of schizophrenia.

14. (F). This is a case of TCA intoxication. Stop the TCA and give IV NaHCO3.

15. (C). This is neuroleptic malignant syndrome. Stop fluphenazine and give dantrolene or bromocriptine along with IV fluid.

16. (B). Common extrapyramidal S/E and best treated with bentropine. "A and E" are 2nd choices.

17. (G). Only sertraline here is safe for patient with CVD.

18. (I). Bupropion is the drug of choice for depression with confusion and alcohol/smoking cessation. It also helps improve cognition (as with sertraline, selegiline, and Vit-E). Buspirone is good for most anxiety disorders (especially refractory ones).

19. (C). Typical malingering for the secondary gain (a free night in the hospital). It's not considered a mental disease.

20. (B). This is most likely caused by drug abuse (such as cocaine). 'E' usually doesn't cause delusion.

21. (C). Typical somatization disorder. 'A' is an irrational belief in having some specific disease despite constant reassurance by the physician. 'E' is "chronic pain only."

22. (B). Maladaptive reactions to an identifiable psychosocial stressor occurring within 3 months of the stressor and lasting 1-6 months. 'A' is < 1 month; 'C' is > 1 month; both focus on "trauma and stress" reactions.

23. (A). It's the binge-eating type disorder. Lower body Wt and lack of menses are key to Dx.

24. (C). Paranoid type: Distrust and suspiciousness, taking other's motivation as malevolent, emotionally cold and odd, often with social isolation.

25. (B). Schizoid type: Detached and isolated "loners" with restricted and distant emotionality.

26. (A). Schizotypal type: Odd thought, behavior, and appearance but not to the standard of schizophrenia.

27. (D). Histrionic type: Colorful, exaggerated behavior, emotions and appearance to draw attention.

28. (F). Borderline type: Unstable affect, mood, relationships, and self-image; chronic feelings of emptiness; marked impulsivity, etc.

29. (E). Narcissistic type: Sense of self-importance, grandiosity, and entitlement.

30. (C). Sleep apnea. 'A' —excessive daytime sleepiness and patient feels refreshed upon awakening.

31. (B). Cataplexy: sudden loss of muscle tone without sleep. Sleep attacks: falling asleep quickly at night. Sleep paralysis: patient is unable to move while awakening.

32. (D). Diabetes. Alcohol and drugs are also very common causes, but they are not "medical conditions."

33. (A). The patient is presenting with acute mania and an antipsychotic is the drug of choice. If symptoms persist or get worse, you can enrol him into the psychiatric unit. Testing the lithium level may not be helpful because the patient most likely did not comply with the medicine.

34. (E). The patient has depressed symptoms after losing a loving wife that are severe enough for the Dx of major depression. He needs a first-line antidepressant ("A") after being evaluated for suicidal risk. Supportive psychotherapy is best for bereavement and PTSD. A brief psychotherapy is best for acute stress disorder and adjustment disorder. Phenelzine is the best Tx for atypical depression with brief psychosis and phobia, etc.

35. (E). This is a typical life-threatening serotonin syndrome, occurring during therapeutic use of SSRIs with inadvertent interactions between medications with serotonic nature. The first step of management is cessation of SSRIs, followed by supportive therapies, a beta-R blocker ("A"), or/and a serotonin antagonist ("C"), as well as alcohol cessation.

36. (E). This patient presents with typical alcohol withdrawal—visual hallucinations and tremors on the 2nd day of hospitalization. "B" should have a direct head injury and more neurologic signs. "D" may have similar symptoms but there is no history of benzodiazepine or flumazenil use. Adverse effects of the analgesic oxycodone include disturbing nightmares, memory loss, constipation, etc.

37. (A). This patient has most features of delusional disorder—delusional but still functional for regular work, although she may also have some symptoms of other disorders. Psychotic disorders are characterized by impaired thinking and affection, and differentiated mainly by the duration of psychotic symptoms: brief psychotic disorder (1 day—1 month), schizophreniform disorder (1 month—6 months), and schizophrenia (more than 6 months). Paranoid personality disorder—pervasively distrustful or mistrustful, suspicious, socially isolated, and emotionally cold.

Chapter 17

EPIDEMIOLOGY, PREVENTIVE MEDICINE,

BIOSTATISTICS, AND MEDICAL ETHICS

EPIDEMIOLOGY

BASIC CONCEPTS

Epidemiology: Study of patterns of disease in populations and the determinants of these patterns of disease. It's the "study of epidemics".

Epidemic: Occurrence of disease in excess of the expected rate in certain area, e.g., the rapid rise in cases of AIDS in Africa in recent years.

Pandemic: A worldwide epidemic, e.g., the multinational outbreak of "atypical pneumonia" in 2005.

Endemic: The usual, expected rate of disease over time, e.g., the long-term, stable rate of colon cancer as a "flat" pattern.

Epidemic curve: A visual description of an epidemic curve as disease cases plotted against time. The classic epidemic feature is a "spike" in time.

ASSESSMENT OF DISEASE FREQUENCIES

Rates

Rate: It is the frequency of occurrence of epidemiologic events in populations. Rates are used to directly compare epidemic events per identical number of people in the two or more populations, and events occurring in a single population assessed at several points in time.

Rate = (Numerator/Denominator) X Multiplier.

Multipliers

1. For **major vital statistics** (birth rate, death rate, etc.), the preferred multiplier is 1,000. The result is expressed as a "**rate per 1,000**".

2. For **individual disease**, the commonest multiplier is 100,000. The result is expressed as a "**rate per 100,000**".

Essential rule: **Always match** the numerator with the denominator on person, place, and time.

Prevalence (Rate) *all people who have the dz Right now*

It's the proportion of people with existing disease at a point in time (**point prevalence**) or during a period of time (**period prevalence**). It refers to **all cases** and focuses on **chronic diseases**.

Incidence (Rate) *all new dz this year*

It is the rate of **new diseases in a population during a period of time**, not at a single point. The focus is on **acute conditions and new cases only**.

Relationship: Prevalence = Incidence X Duration (conceptually)

Increase in incidence or duration will increase prevalence. Changes in prevalence can be determined by monitoring incidence, recovery, and mortality rate over time.

Vital Statistics

Birth rate: Live births per 1,000 population in a year.

Fertility rate: Live births per 1,000 women of childbearing age in a year.

Mortality rate: Deaths per 1,000 population in a year; also as death rate, crude death rate.

Infant mortality rate: Infant deaths (< 1 year of age) per 1,000 live births during the same year; equals to neonatal mortality rate + postneonatal (< 1 year) mortality rate.

Neonatal mortality rate: Infant deaths prior to day 28 per 1,000 live births.

Postneonatal mortality rate: Infant deaths from day 28 through day 365 per 1,000 live births.

Maternal mortality rate: Maternal deaths per 100,000 live births during the same year.

Case fatality rate (ratio): Proportion of cases that end in death within a specified time period.

Cause specific mortality rate: Deaths from a specific cause per number of people with the disease.

ASSESSMENT OF DIAGNOSTIC TESTS

Screening Tests

Screening tests are used to offer early detection of risk factors and the disease, and thus early diagnosis and treatment. They are usually applied to apparently "healthy" people. The test results are classified as "positive" (+) or "negative" (-), and displayed by the standard "2 X 2 table".

Table: 17-1: Screening Test 2 X 2 Table

	Disease (+)	Disease (-)
Test (+)	A (TP)	B (FP)
Test (-)	C (FN)	D (TN)

It displays the distribution of the screening measurements separately for people with disease and people without disease.

True Positives (TP): Diseased people who are correctly classified as positive.

True Negatives (TN): Well people who are correctly classified as negative.

False Positives (FP): Well people who are misclassified as positive.

False Negatives (FN): Diseased people who are misclassified as negative.

Measures of Screening Test Performance

rarely miss disease, but have RFPates

Sensitivity $= \frac{TP}{TP+FN}$ *snnouT, ↑sensitive, when neg, rules out a dz*

Sensitivity = A/(A+C): True (+) per all people with disease (= TP + FN).

False negative ratio = 1 – sensitivity.

High sensitivity is desirable to rule out disease in a screening test because it will rarely miss people with the disease.

confirm dx after ①screen test

Specificity $\frac{TN}{FP+TN}$ *SP PIN, ↑specific, when positive, rules in a dz*

Specificity = D/(D+B): True (-) per all well people (= TN + FP).

False positive ratio = 1 – specificity.

High specificity is desirable to rule in disease in a confirmatory test because it will rarely include a patient who does not have the disease.

Positive Predictive Value (PPV) $\frac{TP}{TP+FP}$, *with ↑prevalence → ↑PPV*

True positive per all people with a positive test result = A/(A+B)

Negative Predictive Value (NPV) $\frac{FN}{FN+TN}$ '

True negative per all people with a negative test result = D/(C+D)

Reliability *Reliable PRecise repeatability*

It refers to the ability of a test to measure the consistency or repeatability.

Validity (Accuracy) *Valid accurate*

It refers to the degree to which a test measures what is intended to measure. Reliability is a necessary, but insufficient, condition for validity.

In the 2 x 2 Table, **Accuracy** is the proportion of **all screened people who are correctly classified** by the screening test. **Accuracy = (TP + TN)** per all screened people.

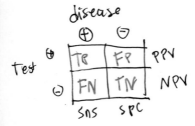

PEARLS— Fig. 17-1: Relationship between Sensitivity & Specificity (Courtesy of drcoplan.com)

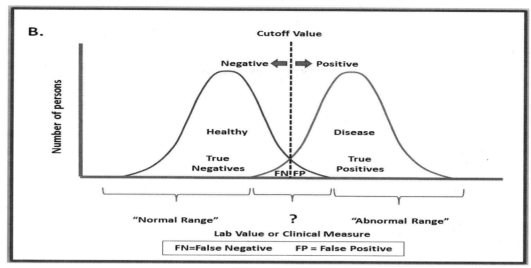

ASSESSMENT OF RISK
don't   *have interventions*

Observational and Experimental Studies

Observational studies refer to observation of the relationships between exposures and the disease outcome in specific populations. In these studies, the natural course is followed without intervention.

Experimental studies aim at minimizing the disease-producing exposures and optimizing health-promoting factors. In these studies, there is an intervention and the results assess the effects of the intervention.

Case report: A brief, objective report of a clinical case.

No intervention **Case series report:** An objective report of a series of clinical cases. There is no control group.
~ qualitative data.

Observational Studies

Cross-sectional study
a bunch of cross sectional studies on same group over time = longitudinal study. assesses change in prevalence

The disease and variables are determined in a representative sample **at a single point in time**.
Features: It determines disease **prevalence** but not the incidence and sequence of cause (effect), because risk factors and the disease cases are collected simultaneously.

Case-control study

It's a retrospective study to assess a group of people with the disease and compares them with a comparable group without the disease. *dz status*

Advantages: Small number of subjects, short time period, and low cost; can help determine causal relationships; very useful for studying conditions with low incidence or prevalence.

Limitations: It cannot assess incidence or prevalence of disease, and may contain **recall bias**.

[handwritten: exposure status, do they develop the dz?]
[handwritten: compare to]
[handwritten: yes   No]

Cohort study

A prospective study to assess the populations with and without the exposure following the risk factors over time.

Advantages: It can give incidence and causality; can assess a single risk factor that affects many diseases; give relative risk (RR) and attributable risk (AR) to estimate the risk of disease.

Limitations: Large number of subjects, longer time period, and higher cost; cannot give prevalence; only works with disease with high incidence; must follow population long enough for incidence to appear; may contain **selection bias**.

PEARLS—Table 17-2: Important Differentiation of Observational Studies

Study type	Time differentiation	Analysis method and result	Major bias
Case-Control	Retrospective	Group analysis; Odd's ratio (OR)	Recall
Cross-Sectional	At one moment in time	Chi-square; Prevalence	Multiple
Cohort	Prospective	RR, AR; Incidence rate; Causality	Selection
Clinical study	Prospective	Group analysis; Efficacy; Safety	Selection; Observation.

[handwritten left margin: Probability: event / events + nonevents / sof if (r)in(d)p of are / ers hauled]

Risk Ratio and Relative Risk

Risk ratio or relative risk (they mean the same thing and are both abbreviated as RR) is simply the risk of the event in one group divided by the risk of the event in the other group.

Table 17-3: Risk Ratio 2 X 2 Table

	Disease Develops (+)	No Disease (-)
Exposure (+)	A	B
Exposure (-)	C	D

"A+B" means prospective cohort, with common characteristics.

"C+D" means control: Source of comparison; not receive the intervention under study.

"A+C" means retrospective study (case-control).

"B+D" has no meaning.

Relative risk (RR)

It's a comparative probability, the ratio of the chance of developing a disease among a group of population exposed to a factor compared with a similar group not exposed to the factor. In many cases the relative risk is modified by the duration or intensity of exposure to the causative factors.

RR = [A/(A+B)] / [C/(C+D)] = (Incidence rate of exposed group) / (Incidence rate of the unexposed group).

E.g., RR = 1 for Null hypothesis (Ho), RR = 0.7 means the risk is decreased by 30%. If infant mortality in Group A is 10 per 1,000 live births and 20 in Group B, then RR in Group B against A is 20/10 = 2.0, meaning Group B infants are twice as likely to die compared to Group A.

Odds ratio (OR)

It focuses on the increased odds of getting a disease with exposure to a risk factor against non-exposure to that factor.

In the 2 x 2 table: **OR = AD/BC = (Odds of exposure for cases) / (Odds of exposure for controls)**. For a rare disease, OR is close to RR, giving similar conclusion. For a common disease, OR > RR.

Attributable risk (AR)

It's also a comparative probability, asking "How many more cases of diseases death in one group compared to the other group?"

In the 2 x 2 table: **AR = [A/(A+B)] - [C/(C+D)] = (Incidence of disease or death of exposed group) — (Incidence of disease or death of the unexposed group)**.

Using the same example as above, AR = 20-10 =10. It means that out of 1,000 of Group B infants, there are 10 more deaths than that of Group A.

Attributable risk percentage (ARP) = (Risk of exposed group – risk of unexposed group) / Risk of exposed group X 100%.

E.g., if RR = 4, ARP = (4-1)/4 = 75%.

Absolute risk reduction (ARR)

It refers to arithmetic differences between two groups—the treated and untreated groups. E.g., 20 patients with the disease, 5 died out of the 10 treated ones, 7 died out of the 10 untreated ones, then ARR = 7/10 – 5/10 = 2/10.

Number needed to treat (NNT)

NNT asks "How many people in general population need to be treated to prevent one case?" **It is the inverse of the incidence rate or 1/ARR.**

E.g., from the above ARR case, NNT = 1/ARR = 1 / (2/10) = 5; thus 5 patients need to be treated to prevent one death.

Clinical trial (Intervention Study)

It's a **prospective**, experimental study in which patients are designed to a treatment group or a control group, to evaluate the safety and efficacy of a test or treatment. Clinical trials can: (1) Test new treatments to see if they help with certain diseases or conditions better than the current treatments; (2) Test treatments or lifestyle changes to see if they prevent or lower the chance of getting certain diseases; (3) Test new ways of finding out if people have certain diseases. Clinical trials that test new treatments, such as medicines, fall into three types/phases.

Three phases of clinical trials

These must be approved by the US Food and Drug Administration (FDA) before clinical applications.

Phase 1: Testing safety in healthy volunteers.

Phase 2: Testing protocol and dose levels in small group of patient volunteers.

Phase 3: Testing efficacy and occurrence of adverse effects in larger group of patient volunteers. This is the definitive phase of test.

Study designation rules

(1) **Randomization** to eliminate selection bias and to balance prognostic factors;

(2) **Double-blind** to prevent observer bias on the performers.

Advantages: Scientifically it is the most rigorous study. It can control many potential confounders with careful exclusion and inclusion. It also can potentially prove causality.

Limitations: It's very costly in time and money, and a single clinical trial, even a large one, is seldom sufficient to provide a confident answer to a clinical question.

Systemic Review and Meta-analysis

A systematic review is a comprehensive summary of all available evidence that meets predefined eligibility criteria to address a specific clinical question or range of questions. Systematic review and meta-analysis are methods to synthesize the available evidence using an explicit, transparent approach that considers the strengths and weaknesses of the individual studies, the populations and interventions, and specific outcomes that were assessed. Organizations that develop guidelines can use the results of systematic reviews and meta-analyses to provide evidence-based recommendations for care.

Mega-analysis is a systemic analysis is a statistical method that quantitatively combines the results from different types of studies, usually based on literature search. It can provide an overall estimate of the net benefit or harm of an intervention, as well as an overall quantitative estimate of other parameters such as diagnostic accuracy, incidence, or prevalence. **Meta-regression and network meta-analysis** are enhancements to traditional meta-analysis. **Advantages:** It can obtain greater statistical power; may also solve conflicting issues in the clinical literature. **Limitations:** Within limitations of different studies in methodology and statistics.

DEFECTS IN STUDY DESIGNS

Confounding Variables

Variables in a study that are associated with each other, thus may obscure the effects of these variables, leading to erroneous conclusions. It's **a study flaw rather than a bias**, and can be decreased or **fixed by:**

(1) **Randomization; (2) Matching (case-control); (3) Restriction; (4) Multivariate analysis.** E.g., alcohol is a variable associated with increased risk of liver cancer in a study; if smoking affects both alcohol drinking and liver cancer, it is a confounding variable.

Bias

Bias is any process that is deviated from the truth of inferred results systematically. Good scientific research requires potential bias to be minimized. **Types of bias include:**

Lead-time bias: It occurs when using an earlier diagnosis to give a false survival rate. E.g., patients with certain cancer seem to live longer after it is diagnosed by a new screening test.

Length bias: The tendency of a screening test to detect a disproportionate number of slow or chronic disease and to miss rapidly progressive disease, leading to overestimation of the test efficacy.

Selection bias (sampling bias): It occurs when the sample selected does not represent the population. E.g., People enrolled in a study are different from those who are not enrolled (not comparable). The bias can be fixed with a random, independent sampling.

Measurement bias: Methods used in the measurement or data collection are different in different study groups, leading to distorted data. It occurs when there is no control group in a prospective study. E.g., Subjects' behavior is altered because they are being studied ("**the Hawthorne effect**"). This type of bias can be fixed with a control group.

Recall bias: In a retrospective study, subjects fail to accurately recall events in the past. Fix the bias by confirming information with other sources. *'sick pts remember more" out of eagerness to explain their illness*

Experimenter expectancy (Pygmalion effect): It occurs when the experimenter's expectations are improperly communicated to subjects and causes them to produce the desired effects. This effect can be avoided by double-blind design. *observer effect*

Late-look bias: It occurs when patients with severe disease die before they are taken into a survey. Stratify the cases by severity to fix bias.

Other Factors

Generalizability: It means external validity—how applicable the results are to other populations. E.g., middle-aged study results may not be applied to all patients.

Effect Modification: It's present when the effect of the main exposure on the outcome is modified by the level of another variable. **It's not a bias or flaw**; it's a natural phenomenon. E.g., Estrogen's effect on the venal thrombosis is modified by smoking.

Open label study = no blind, ↑ bias
single blind study = less bias
*   pt*
2x blind study = least bias

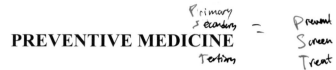

PREVENTIVE MEDICINE

TYPES OF PREVENTION

1. **Primary prevention** *Prevent onset dz, VX*

It refers to all health-promoting activities at both the individual and the community level that facilitate **health-enhancing behavior**, prevent risky behavior, and diminish exposure to environmental hazards. **Primary prevention decreases disease incidence.** E.g., Educational programs on smoking cessation decrease the incidence of lung cancer and CVD.

screen's intervene — 2. **Secondary prevention** *delay progression dz . -↑sensitivity tolerate FP so we don't miss FN.*

It refers to the screening for risk factors and supplying **early diagnosis and effective treatment** of diseases. Secondary prevention **decreases disease prevalence**, for example, timely screening of BP and lipids for early diagnosis and treatment of CVD.

3. **Tertiary prevention** *preventing dz complications, TX*

It refers to all efforts to **reduce** long-term impairment and **disability, and to prevent disease recurrence.** E.g., early exercise programs to help patient's recovery from injury.

STATISTICAL DATA OF DISEASES

—Adapted Data from the U.S. Centers for Disease Control and Prevention (CDC) (http://cdc.gov)

Mandatory Reportable Diseases and Rank

1. Chlamydia; 2. Gonorrhea; 3. Chicken pox; 4. AIDS; 5. Syphilis; 6. Salmonella; 7. Hepatitis A; 8. Tuberculosis; 9. Lyme disease; 10. Hepatitis B; 11. Pertussis; 12. Hepatitis C; 13. Legionnaires; 14. Mumps; 15. Rubella; 16. Measles.

Table 17-4: Reportable Infectious Diseases

STDs	HIV (+), AIDS, syphilis, gonorrhea, chlamydia, chancroid, and HCV (+).
Water/food-borne diseases	Cholera, botulism, shigellosis, shiga toxin-producing E. coli, salmonellosis, giardiasis, legionnaires, trichinellosis, and typhoid.
Vaccine-preventable diseases	Diphtheria, tetanus, pertussis, measles, mumps, rubella, polio, varicella (death), Hepatitis A, Hepatitis B, HIB, and meningitis.
Potential bio-weapons	Anthrax, smallpox, and plague.
Tick-borne diseases	Lyme disease, Rocky mountain spotted fever, and Ehrlichiosis.
Zoonotic diseases	Tularemia, psittacosis, brucellosis, and rabies.
Mix	Toxic shock syndrome, TB, leprosy, severe acute respiratory syndrome (SARS), West Nile virus infection, MRSA infection, VRSA infection, coccidioidomycosis, and cryptosporidiosis.

Most Common Acute Medical Problems

1. Upper respiratory infections
2. Influenza
3. Injuries

Main Reasons for Seeing a Physician

1. General well-being
2. Upper respiratory infections
3. Diagnosis and treatment of hypertension or hyperlipidemia

Leading Causes of Death

Summary: <1 year: Congenital Anomalies; 1-44 years: Unintentional Injury; 45-64 years: Malignant Neoplasms; 65+ years: Heart Disease; All ages: 1. Heart disease; 2. Cancer; 3. Stroke; 4. Chronic lower respiratory disease; 5. Accident; 6. Diabetes.

PEARLS — Table 17-5: Leading Causes of Death by Age*

Age	Major Causes of Death
0-1 month:	Perinatal conditions.
2-12 months:	1. Congenital anomaly, 2. SIDS (Sudden infant death syndrome), 3. Low birth weight, maternal complications.
1-14 years:	1. Injury, 2. Others: congenital anomaly, neoplasms, homicide.
15-24 years:	1. Injury, 2. Others: neoplasm, congenital anomaly, homicide, suicide.
25-44 years:	1. Injury, 2. Others: neoplasm, heart disease, suicide, homicide, HIV.
45-64 years:	1. Cancer (lung), 2. Heart disease, 3. Injury, stroke, diabetes, chronic lower respiratory disease.
> 65 years:	1. Heart disease, 2. Cancer, stroke, COPD, influenza and pneumonia, diabetes.

*Adapted from the National Center for Health Statistics, USA.

Statistical Data of Malignancies in the U.S.

PEARLS — Table 17-6: Top Ten Cancers*

Gender	Incidence Rates
Male	1. Prostate; 2. lung & bronchus; 3. colon & rectum; 4. urinary bladder; 5. melanoma of the skin; 6. non-Hodgkin lymphoma; 7. kidney; 8. oral cavity & pharynx; 9. leukemia; 10. pancreas.
Female	1. Breast; 2. lung & bronchus; 3. colon & rectum; 4. corpus and uterus, NOS; 5. thyroid; 6. melanoma of the skin; 7. non-Hodgkin lymphoma; 8. ovary; 9. kidney; 10. pancreas.

Gender	Death Rates
Male	1. **Lung & bronchus; 2. prostate; 3. colon & rectum**; 4-10 (the order may vary): liver, esophagus, pancreas, urinary bladder, stomach, leukemia, non-Hodgkin lymphoma.
Female	1. **Lung & bronchus; 2. breast; 3. colon & rectum**; 4-10 (the order may vary): ovary, pancreas, esophagus, non-Hodgkin lymphoma, leukemia, uterus, and stomach/liver.

*Adapted from http://apps.nccd.cdc.gov

POPULATION HEALTH

Population health is defined as **the health outcomes of a group of people and its distribution**. It is an approach to health that aims to improve the health of an entire human population. It has been described as consisting of three components—health outcomes, patterns of health determinants, and policies and interventions. An important aspect of it is to reduce health inequities among different population groups due to the social determinants of health (SDOH), which include all the factors (social, environmental, cultural and physical) that the different populations are born into and grow up with throughout their lifetimes which potentially have a measurable impact on the health. Both WHO and USA have reported that SDOH were the major causes of health disparities and avoidable mortality in all countries.

From a population health perspective, **health** has been defined not simply as a state free from disease but the capacity of people to adapt to, respond to, or control life's challenges and changes, and **a state of complete physical, mental, and social well-being**.

Population health management (PHM): It is a health-improving method to utilize a variety of individual, organizational and cultural interventions to help improve the morbidity patterns and behavior health. A good example is the intensive care management for individuals at the highest level of risk. Another example is that family planning programs (including contraceptives and healthy sexuality education) as a cost-effective medicine play a major role in population health. It saves lives and money by reducing unintended pregnancy and STDs significantly.

Suggested approaches for effective population health management include precise patient registries and their numerators, determination of patient-provider attribution, measurement of clinical and cost metrics, following basic clinical practice guidelines, engagement in risk-management outreach, good communication and coordination between care team and patient, and patient education.

Patient Safety

Patient safety is a discipline that emphasizes safety in health care through the prevention, reduction, reporting, and analysis of medical error that often leads to adverse effects. Patient safety has been supported by an immature yet developing scientific framework, with improvement efforts such as applying lessons learned from business, adopting innovative technologies, educating providers and consumers, enhancing error reporting systems, and developing new economic incentives.

Effective communication is essential for ensuring patient safety, including provisioning of available information on any operational site especially in mobile professional services.

Causes of healthcare error include human factors, medical complexity, complicated technologies, powerful drugs, intensive care, prolonged hospital stay, system failures, etc.

Patient Education

Patient education regarding regular exercise, healthy and safe eating and sexuality, and cessation of smoking, alcohol abuse, and substance abuse, combined with routine physical examination, have been proved effective in improving population health and outcomes.

Smoking and Smoking Cessation

Cigarette smoking is the leading preventable cause of mortality, responsible for over six million deaths worldwide and 400,000 deaths in the US annually. If current trends continue, tobacco will kill more than eight million people worldwide each year by the year 2030. Most smokers begin before age 21. The three major causes of smoking-related deaths are atherosclerotic cardiovascular disease, lung cancer, and chronic obstructive pulmonary disease (COPD).

Health risks associated with cigarette smoking

1. COPD: Increased risk in a dose-dependent manner.

2. Cardiovascular disease: Increased risk of CAD, stroke, and peripheral vascular disease (including Buerger disease) in a dose-dependent way.

3. Malignancy: Increased risk of carcinoma of the lungs, oral cavity, esophagus, larynx/pharynx, bladder, cervix, and pancreas. People who smoke two packs/day have a risk of lung cancer 20 times higher than the normal population.

4. Other risks: Peptic ulcer disease (PUD), osteoporosis, premature skin aging, adverse effects during pregnancy (spontaneous abortion, neonatal death), depression, impotence, infertility, automobile accidents, etc.

Smoking cessation

Smokers who stop smoking reduce their risk of developing and dying from tobacco-related illnesses significantly. Screening all smokers and providing them with behavioral counseling and intervention programs to stop smoking are among the most valuable preventive services in health care.

Patient education, behavioral counseling and pharmacotherapy (nicotine gum/patch, continuous nicotine delivery) can effectively help smokers quit. The patient should not continue to smoke while using the patch, due to increased risk of myocardial infarction. Bupropion is helpful in both smoking cessation (similar as nicotine patch) and depression.

After cessation: Risk of lung cancer decreases significantly but still remains 2 times higher than non-smokers; risk of other cancers drops to level of non-smokers 10-15 years after cessation; risk of CAD drops to the level of non-smokers in < 2 years.

Alcohol Use Disorder

See "SUBSTANCE-RELATED AND ADDICTIVE DISORDERS".

Obesity

See "Digestive and Nutritional Diseases".

Health Care Screening

Health care screening is very **important in promoting early diagnosis and treatment** of diseases, especially malignancies.

PEARLS — Table 17-7: Recommended Cancer Screening Measures by Age*

Screening Measure	Age and Interval
CXR	Not recommended as a screening test.
Breast self-exam	Every month after age 20.
Breast exam by a physician	20-40: every 3 yrs; after 40: every year.
Mammography	Every 1-2 yrs after 40-50 (depending on risk factors).
Pap smear (cytology)	21-30: every 3 yrs; 30-65: screened every 5 yrs with cytology and HPV testing.
Pelvic exam	20-40: every 1-3 yrs; after 40: every year.
Endometrial sampling	Indicated for postmenopausal bleeding.
Prostate exam	Recommended together with PSA only with risk factors (after age 50).
DRE (digital rectal exam)	Screening is non-beneficial.
FIT/iFOBT (fecal immunochemical test)	Every year after 50, plus colonoscopy if with family history.
Flexible sigmoidoscopy	Every 5 yrs after 50, with FOBT every 3 yrs; for high-risk patients: starts at 40.
Colonoscopy	Every 10 yrs after 50, or CT colonography every 5 yrs after 50.

*From U.S. Preventive Services Task Force (USPSTF).

[handwritten margin notes: til age 68; 3 consecutively normal paps or TAH; don't screen, lead time bias; or FOBT Q1y; N 10 yrs before relative's dx age]

Table 17-8: Health Care Screening by Age

Age	Screening Measure
At birth	Height (Ht) and weight (Wt), phenylalanine, TSH, and T4.
1-24 yrs	Height and weight, BP, vision, hemoglobin (in high-risk population), lead level (before 6 yrs), Pap smear, rubella serology or vaccination (females before pregnancy), alcohol abuse, Chlamydia and gonorrhea (if sexually active; culture or enzyme immunoassay).

[handwritten notes at bottom: Lung Ca: 55-80, 3 5 pack-yr, quit < 15 years ago, annually = Lo-dose CT, til age 80, or quit over 15 years ago; Ovarian — screen only if BRCA ⊕]

25-64 yrs	Height and weight, BP (every 2 yrs), cholesterol (>35 yrs), Pap smear, FOBT (fecal occult blood test), sigmoidoscopy or colonoscopy (>50 yrs), clinical breast exam/mammography (50-69 yrs), and screen for alcohol abuse and depression.
>65 yrs	Height and weight, BP, FIT, clinical breast exam/mammography, sigmoidoscopy, Pap smear, screening for vision, hearing, alcohol abuse, and depression.

Note: Refer to specific diseases for details of screening and surveillance.

MAJOR RISK FACTORS OF IMPORTANT DISEASES

Please refer to specific diseases for details.

IMMUNIZATION AND VACCINATION

Definitions and classifications

A **vaccine** is a suspension of attenuated live or killed microorganisms administered to induce active immunity.

Active immunity: Antibody (Ab) is produced in the body in response to a vaccine or toxoid (usually effective for long years).

Passive immunity: Preformed antibody is given (IV IG) to supply temporary immunity (for several months).

Herd immunity: The resistance of a group to attack by a disease to which a large proportion of the members are immune. It occurs when enough persons are immunized to prevent transmission of disease to unimmunized persons.

Attenuated live virus vaccines: MMR, OPV (polio), influenza, and yellow fever. Never give it to pregnant or immunodeficient patients. Zoster

Attenuated live bacteria vaccines: Typhoid, BCG. Never give it to pregnant or immunodeficient patients.

Inactivated virus vaccines: Polio, rabies, influenza (IIV), and HBV. It may be given to pregnant or immunodeficient patients.

Inactivated bacteria vaccines: H. influenza (Hib), pneumococcus (PCV), meningococcus (MCV, serotypes A, C, W-135, and Y), pertussis, cholera, and typhoid. It may be given to pregnant or immunodeficient patients.

Toxoid vaccines: Modified or reduced bacterial toxins that can stimulate formation of antitoxins, including DTaP (diphtheria, tetanus, and acellular pertussis), IPV (inactivated poliovirus), Hib (H. Inf), PP(S)V (pneumococcal polysaccharide vaccine, Pneumococcus spp. -heptavalent), and HBV vaccines.

Immunization rules

1. Inactivated vaccines may be given simultaneously at separate sites (except cholera, typhoid, and plague).

2. Live virus vaccines given on different days should be separated by 1 month. Pneumococcus and whole virus influenza vaccines can be given at the same time but different sites.

3. If egg hypersensitivity exists, avoid egg with MMR, influenza, and yellow fever vaccines. Neomycin/streptomycin is contained in MMR and IVP. *Not a thing anymore*

4. Give as many vaccines as possible; skip any missed vaccines. For a premature child, give vaccines at the chronological age.

5. Conditions that are not contraindicated to vaccines: A mild, acute illness in an otherwise well child; with previous DPT fever < 40.5°C; redness, soreness, and swelling; concurrent antimicrobial therapy; a family history of seizures.

6. Special vaccines:

PP(S)V: It is recommended for adults 65 y/a or older, anyone with immunodeficiency or serious chronic diseases or without spleen (function), and smokers.

Varicella vaccine: More than 90% of patients are immune, and titers should be tested in adults before the vaccine is given. A history of chickenpox is a strong evidence not to test or give the vaccine.

PEARLS — Table 17-9: Important Immunization Schedules for All (USA)

Vaccine	Birth	2M	4M	6M	12-15M	2Y	4-6Y	11-12Y	Sum
HAV					1st	2nd			2 doses
HBV	1st	2nd		3rd					3 doses
DTaP		1st	2nd	3rd	4th (15-18M)		5th		+ Td per 10Y
IPV		1st	2nd	3rd			4th		4 doses
Rotavirus		1st	2nd						2 doses
Hib		1st	2nd	(3rd)	3-4th				3-4 doses
MMR					1st		2nd		2 doses
Varicella					1st		2nd		+ Shingles at 60Y
Influenza (IIV)				1st					Annually
PCV		1st	2nd	3rd	4th				+ PPSV at 65Y
MCV								1st	Booster at 16Y
HPV	2 doses with 6M gap under 15Y; 3 doses over 24 weeks above 15Y.								

Handwritten annotations:
- *DTaP is for kids for kids*
- *much higher Dose than Tdap*
- *new give 13 & 23 @ same time*
- *+ Td per 10Y for 3 life dose time*
- *everyone every yr*
- *everyone age 9-26*

Applications of vaccinations

See related chapters.

BIOSTATISTICS

IMPORTANT CONCEPTS

Measure of Central Tendency

It is a general term for several characteristics of the distribution of a set of observed values around a value at or near the middle of the set.

Mean ("Average"): The summary of the observed values divided by the number of observations. It is especially **sensitive to an outlier**, and shifts toward it.

Median: The middle point of a set of observations that divides the group into two halves. The **50th percentile** is the measurement below which half the observations fall.

Mode: The most frequent value in a set of observations. The mode and median are both resistant to an outlier.

Normal Distribution

It is the continuous frequency distribution of an infinite range defined by a specific math-function. It carries the following features:

1. **A continuous, symmetrical distribution; both tails extend to infinity.**
2. The arithmetic **mean, mode, and median are identical**.
3. The **shape** is **determined by** the **mean** and standard deviation (**SD**).

Probability of the normal distribution curve:

Between the mean and the value of 1 SD from the mean in either direction there will be 32% of the cases; there will be 68% of the cases between the score at 1 SD above and 1 SD below the mean. Within 2 SD of the mean there are 95.5% of the cases. Within 3 SD of the mean there are 99.7% of the cases.

Figure 17-2: Normal Distribution Curve (Courtesy of www.ntl.bts.gov)

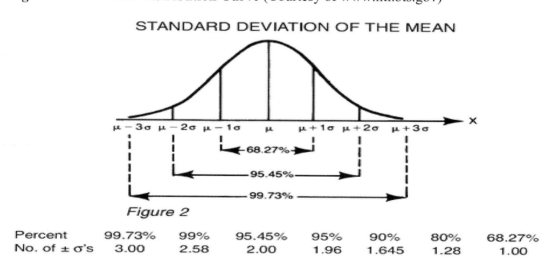

Percent	99.73%	99%	95.45%	95%	90%	80%	68.27%
No. of ± σ's	3.00	2.58	2.00	1.96	1.645	1.28	1.00

Indices of Variation

Variance

A measure of the variation shown by a set of observations, defined by the summary of the squares of deviations from the mean divided by the number of degrees of freedom in the set of observations.

Standard deviation (SD)

SD = Positive square root of the variance; it's stated in score units and is the most widely used measure of dispersion of a frequency distribution. SD summarizes the extent of disbursement values around the center, whereas the mean tells where the group of values is centered.

Standard error (SE)

SE = SD/n, the standard deviation of the sample in a frequency distribution.

Inferential Statistics

Generalization
—From a sample to the population as a whole.

The purpose of inferential statistics is to determine **how likely it is that a given finding is simply the result of chance**. Because we cannot typically observe and study entire populations, we can only try to select samples that are the best representative of an entire population so that we can generalize the results from the sample to the population.

Confidence Interval (CI)

It's a way to indicate the reliability of an estimate and to admit that any measurement from a sample is only an estimate of the population. It specifies how far a sample-based value lies above or below the population value within a given range.

Applications: For a "95% CI", there is a 95% chance that the interval contains the true value of the parameter closest to the interval center. If the CI is wide, the power is low. The level of confidence is set by the researcher, not determined by data. If a corresponding hypothesis test is performed, the confidence level corresponds with the level of significance, i.e. a 95% confidence interval reflects a significance level of 0.05. If the confidence interval contains 1.0, it means there is no statistically significant effect of exposure.

Standard Error of the Mean (SEM)

It's the SD divided by the square root of the sample size. The larger the SD is, the greater the chance of error in the estimate is; the larger the sample size is, the lower the chance of error in the estimate is.

Confidence Interval of the Mean (CIM)

It contains two parts:

(1) SEM: an estimate of the quality of the sample for the estimate;

(2) Standard or Z-score: the confidence degree provided by the interval specified.

In comparison of two groups, any overlap of confidence intervals means the groups are not significantly different.

Probability (p)

Combined probabilities

1. For independent events, use simple multiplication. If the chance of having disease A is 0.4 and the chance of having disease B is 0.3, the chance of having both disease A and B is 0.4 x 0.3 = 0.12 (or 12%).

2. If events are non-independent, then multiply the "p" of one event times that of the second, given that the first has occurred.

3. For mutually exclusive events (one event precludes the occurrence of the other), use addition. E.g., if you flip a coin, the chance that it will be either heads or tails is 0.5 + 0.5 = 1.0 (or 100%).

4. If two events are not mutually exclusive, the combination of "p" is obtained by adding the two together and then subtracting the product "p". E.g., if the chance of having hypertension is 20% and the chance of being obese is 30%, then the chance of meeting someone who is obese or has hypertension is 0.2 + 0.3 - (0.2 times 0.3) = 0.44 (or 44%).

Logic of Statistical Inference

Statistics are the most important references of logic in scientific research. Basic steps of statistical inference are:

1. Define the research question. What do you want to show?

2. Define the **null hypothesis (Ho)**: Generally, the opposite of what you hope to show, e.g., the chance the drug will not work.

3. Differentiate between the two types of Ho.

(1) One-tailed, i.e., directional or "one-sided", such that one group is either > or < the other.

(2) Two-tailed, i.e., non-directional or "two-sided", such that two groups are not the same.

Hypothesis Testing

At this point, data are collected and analyzed by the appropriate statistical test. Be prepared to explain the statistical results in the test question.

p-Value

A p-value is a calculated result and standard for interpreting output from a statistical test. Classical p-value criterion is set at 0.05 or less. If $p \leq 0.05$, then there is statistical significance for the null hypothesis (Ho). Generally speaking, the smaller the p value, the better (significance).

Meaning of the p-value

1. Provides criterion for making decisions about the Ho: If $p \leq 0.05$, reject the Ho (has reached statistical significance). If $p > 0.05$, do not reject the Ho (your test has not reached statistical significance).
2. Quantifies the chance that a decision to reject the Ho will be wrong.
3. Tells statistical significance, not clinical significance or likelihood.

Types of Errors

When we reject the Ho, we are not fully certain that we are correct. For some reason, the results given by the sample may not be consistent with the whole population. If this is true, any conclusion we have on the basis of the sample could be in error. There are two possible types of errors:

1. Type I (α) error:

Rejecting the Ho when it is really true, i.e., assuming a statistically significant effect on the basis of the sample when there is none in the population. The chance of a Type 1 error is given by the p-value. If $p = 0.05$, then the chance of a Type 1 error is 5 in 100, or 1 in 20.

2. Type II (β) error:

Failing to reject the null hypothesis when it is really false, i.e., declaring no significant effect on the basis of the sample when there really is one in the population. Type 2 error cannot be directly estimated from the p-value.

Power = 1 - β error. Power is the capacity to detect a difference if there is one. Increasing sample size (n) increases power.

Definition of Statistical Tests

Meta-Analysis

It's a statistical method of combining the results of many studies from different sources to produce one overall, powerful conclusion. It's a mathematic literature review.

Correlation analysis

It ranges from -1 to +1. A positive value means that two variables go together in the same direction (positively related), for example, years of alcohol drinking and incidence of cirrhosis. A negative value means that two variables go in the opposite direction (negatively related), e.g., regular exercise and incidence of cardiovascular disease. The further from zero, the stronger the relationship. A zero correlation means that two variables have no linear relationship. Correlation does not mean causation by itself.

Types of correlations

There are two types of correlations. Pearson correlation compares two interval level variables, and the Spearman correlation compares two ordinal level variables.

Graphing correlations using scatter plots

A scatter plot will show points that approximate a line. Be prepared to interpret scatter plots of data: positive slope, negative slope, and which plot set indicates a stronger correlation, etc.

ANOVA (Analysis of variance)

It is to analyze the variation shown by a set of observations. The output from an ANOVA is one or more "p" statistic.

One-way ANOVA

It compares means of many groups (>2) of a **single nominal variable** using an interval variable. p-value < 0.05 (or 0.01) means that at least two of the tested groups are different.

Two-way ANOVA

It compares means of groups generated by **2 nominal variables using an interval variable**. It can test effects of several variables at the same time.

Repeated measures ANOVA

Multiple measurements of the same group of people over time. Interval: 1, nominal: 1; used for > 2 groups.

t-Test

It is to compare the means of two groups for an interval variable to see whether the groups are different. The output of a t-test is a "t" statistic value, applied only for two groups; interval: 1; nominal: 1.

1. **Pooled t-test**: Regular t-test, assuming the variances of the two groups are the same.

2. **Matched pairs t-test**: If each person in one group is matched with a person in the second. Applies to linked data of two groups before and after measurements. It is more sensitive than the regular t-test to yield a significant P value.

Chi-Square

It's the test method to see whether two nominal variables are independent, e.g., to analyze the efficacy of a new drug by comparing the number of patients with certain disease who recover after taking the drug with the number who recover without taking the drug. It's for nominal data only and can be used in any number of groups. Interval: 0; nominal: 2.

MEDICAL ETHICS

Ethical Legal Rules In the U.S. Healthcare System

1. Autonomy is essential.

Autonomy is more important than the beneficence that the patient may have in the health care. Following patient's wishes is more important than the intention of helping the patient.

Competent patients (with autonomy) have the right to refuse medical treatment.

Limitations on patient's rights:

(1) Preserve life in incompetent/altered mental status.

(2) Prevent suicide or protect third parties.

(3) Protect the ethical standard of the health professional.

In reality, patients have almost absolute rights to control their bodies and to refuse treatment. Competent patients with mental disorders retain their rights (to refuse treatment or command the court to determine "mental status", etc.).

Incompetent patients may also have the rights to refuse treatment via a surrogate. Assume that the patient is competent unless clear behavioral evidence indicates otherwise. Generally speaking, competence is a legal issue rather than a medical issue. In contested cases, only courts can decide the competence, not the physician.

Clear behavioral **evidence of incompetence** includes:

(1) Patient attempts suicide.

(2) Patient is significantly psychotic and dysfunctional.

(3) Patient's physical or mental state prevents simple communication and understanding.

In those situations, a psychiatric evaluation of the patient is important. It is mostly your duty, not the patient's, to prove or deny the patient's competence. If you are unsure, assume the patient is competent. If patient is incompetent, physician may rely on advance directives (oral or written).

2. Informed consent is always necessary.

A physician cannot expose a patient's information to anyone without the patient's permission. Getting a confidential consultation from a professional is permitted. Be careful not to be overheard by others. If you get a court subpoena, go to the court but only disclose necessary information of the patient.

Exceptions: If the patient is a lethal threat to self or others, the physician must break the confidentiality. These include suicide, homicide, gunshot, knife wound, child/elder abuse, major contagious disease, intoxicated drivers, etc. Detain patient to protect the patient and others if necessary.

3. Always obtain informed consent.

The person doing the procedure must obtain consent from the patient. Full informed consent requires that the patient has received and has understood **five pieces of information**:

(1) Nature of procedure; (2) Purpose; (3) Benefits; (4) Risks; (5) Options.

There are **four exceptions**:

(1) Emergency; (2) Waiver by patient; (3) Patient is incompetent; (4) Therapeutic privilege (unconscious, confused, physician taking patient's autonomy away in interest of health).

The consent is effective in the oral (including telephone) or written form if it's given out of the patient's understanding. Written consent can be verbally revoked by the patient at any time.

4. A patient should never be abandoned for financial or uncertain reasons.

5. Prevent **risky health care professionals** who have infectious or psychiatric diseases from contacting or working with patients.

6. Ethics committee is important when a patient has lost the decision-making capacity and the advance directive is missing or unclear.

7. Court order:

It's important when the patient is incapable of understanding and the family is in disagreement. E.g., the patient has no capacity and no healthcare proxy (agent); the family is split about the decision; caregivers wish to withdraw care and the ethics committee is split about the decision.

Avoid going to court. Make the decision in the clinical setting if possible. Court approval of the decision to terminate life support is rarely required. Consider going to court only if:

(1) There is intractable disagreement about a patient's competence, and about who should be the surrogate or make the decision on life support.

(2) You perceive a serious conflict of interest between surrogate and patient's interests.

8. Life-ending issues:

(1) **Physician-assisted suicide is always unethical and wrong for the physician, even if it may be legal to do so. Thus never actively assist the patient to die sooner. Euthanasia**--giving patient a lethal agent to end sufferings and life, **is highly controversial** and not allowed by law and ethics in most countries. However, it is acceptable to administer pain medication even if there is a risk of shortening the patient's life. E.g., giving opiates to a patient with end-stage pulmonary disease (pain-relieving but risky of respiratory suppression) is acceptable.

(2) **The physician decides when the patient is dead (legal brain death)** and has no obligation to provide futile treatment when: a) the patient is brain dead; b) maximal treatment is failing or has failed; c) there's no pathophysiologic rationale for treatment or treatment will not achieve the goals of care.

9. Advance directive and living will:

An advance directive informs the caregivers what care the patient wishes. A living will is a written advance directive that expresses the patient's wishes in specific situations, e.g., DNR ("Do not resuscitate") or DNI ("Do not intubate"). Even with DNR or DNI, patients should still receive maximal other life-saving treatments. Both the advance directive and the living will can be changed by the patient at any time, and the patient's last wishes (oral or written) must be honored.

Durable Power of Attorney (DPOA) is a written advance directive that legally designates a person as the medical care decision maker if the patient can't make the decision. It's more flexible than a living will. The designated person should make best decisions consistent with the patient's stated wishes.

10. Surrogate:

When patients cannot make decisions on their medical treatment and no living will or DPOA exists, decisions should be made by persons clearly familiar with the patient's wishes: (a) close family members; (b) close friends; (c) personal doctors. They should use the following criteria and in this order:

(1) Subjective standard: Actual intent, advance directive. What did the patient say in the past?

(2) Substituted judgment: Who best represents the patient if he or she could decide?

(3) Best interests standard: Burdens versus benefits on the patient's side.

11. Good Samaritan Laws:

It protects physicians by limiting liability when physicians voluntarily help in non-medical situations (such as roadside help). A physician is not required by law to stop and help.

12. Special rules for children or minors:

(1) Children < 18 y/a are minors and are legally incompetent. Exceptions are emancipated minors (marriage, military service, etc.). Minors do not have decision-making capacity and cannot consent to or refuse medical treatment. Only the parents or legal guardian can consent or refuse. Exceptions include contraception, prenatal care, STD, HIV/AIDS, substance abuse treatment, etc.

(2) Children between 13-18 years and living independently are treated as adults.

(3) Parents can refuse vaccines for minors, but cannot refuse necessary treatment for STD, drug abuse, pregnancy, and life/limb-saving procedures for their children. If it's not life/limb-saving treatment, one parent's refusal is not effective; if both parents refuse treatment, try to get a court order.

(4) Mother has the right to refuse necessary treatment for the fetus because it's considered part of her body.

13. Organ and tissue donation:

Payment for organ donation is not acceptable, but payment for renewable tissues (such as sperms and eggs) is acceptable. The organ donation organization should ask for consent for the organ donation instead of the physician, who may have an ethical conflict of interest and more refusals. The patient's family can refuse organ donation even if the patient has left an organ donor card when alive.

Physician-Patient Relationship Rules

1. Patient's interest and safety are the No.1 priority.

A physician's obligation is to serve the patient well, not to think too much about legal protection for self. A physician is not obligated to accept every patient coming to him/her. The physician has the right to end the physician-patient relationship but must give the patient sufficient time to find another physician.

2. It is essential to build up a trustful, long-term relationship with the patient.

Small gifts from patients are acceptable as long as they are not tied to a specific request. Commercial gifts from industry (such as drug companies) are never acceptable. Romantic or sexual relationship between current patients and their physicians is never acceptable.

3. Good communication is highly important.

Be sure you understand the patient's concerns and questions before acting. Start with open-ended questions (allow broad answers), then change to closed-ended questions (limit answer to yes/no).

You should make eye contact and let the patient know what you are doing. Talk to the patient, not colleagues. Always be an advocate and provider for the patient. Always respond to the patient in time. Answer any question asked. Listen, reflect, encourage. Take time to listen to the patient before you or colleagues. Tell the patient everything possible for his/her interests if the patient is willing or ready to know. Let information pass from the patient to the family, not the reverse direction. Express empathy, and then control the situation when facing grieving or angry patients or family members, e.g., "I understand you are suffering, and I'm doing my best to help you."

4. Let the patient make medical decisions from the doctor's suggestions.

Negotiation is always better than orders.

5. Admit to the patient when you make a mistake and take responsibility.

Do not blame it on the resident, student, or nurse. Do not deceive to protect a colleague. Never lie or manipulate patients.

6. Be responsible for patient referral.

In most cases, you have to do something within your duties before referring the patient to a specialist, except for certain emergencies and specialties (such as ophthalmology). The key is not only what you do to the patient, but also how well you do it.

How to Break Bad News

1. Make sure the patient is in a comfortable and relatively private environment.

2. Ask the patient how much he/she knows about the condition, and how much he/she wants to know.

3. If the patient wants to know the truth, give the patient a warning sign, then break the news.

4. Tell the patient the prognosis, but always give options to make the rest of life enjoyable.

5. Try to explain everything clearly and simply.

6. If family members already know it and ask the physician not to tell the patient, you should ask "why" to explore important information like suicide. Ask the same question if the patient refuses treatment.

7. If the patient is confirmed with a contagious disease such as AIDS but does not wish to tell the spouse, first encourage the patient to do it; if patient still refuses, it's the doctor's moral duty to inform the spouse and the local health authority directly.

8. If the patient has a non-contagious disease but does not wish to tell the spouse, first encourage the patient to do so; if patient still refuses, keep confidentiality for the patient.

ABUSE

Elder Abuse

It is a mandatory reportable offense, including neglect and physical, psychological, or financial cruelty toward the elderly. Prevalence is 1-3%. Caretakers and spouses are the most likely abusers. You can report the elderly abuse against the patient's consent, because the abused elders may be too weak to protect themselves. Elderly abuse should be treated ethically like child abuse.

The elderly people have lower incidence of all psychiatric disorders compared with younger adults, but more memory impairment. The elderly are usually not alone and about 80% of them keep frequent contact with their children. The family is the major social support resource for the elderly with illness. About 85% of the elderly have at least one chronic illness; 50% have some limitation to activities; 5% are homebound.

Child Abuse

It's a mandatory reportable offense up to age 18, including **neglect (most common)**, battery, tissue damage, sexual exploitation, and/or mental cruelty. **Failure to report it to a legal authority is a criminal offense**. If a case is reported in error, the physician is protected from legal liability because it's the physician's duty to protect the child (to be kept away from the abuser) and to report. Each year in the US, it's reported that millions of children are abused and thousands are killed by abuse. It is estimated that most cases of child abuse go unreported in many countries.

Typical clinical signs (<u>Image 121</u>)
1. Unusual broken bones in first year of life.
2. STDs in young children, or evidence of genital bleeding, swelling, or discharge.
3. > 90% of injuries are soft tissue injuries (bruises, burns, lacerations). 5% have no physical signs.
4. Non-accidental burns (not on arms and hands, or on arms but not hands): Usually associated with poor outcome.
5. "Shaken baby syndrome": Typical broken blood vessels may be found in the eyes.
6. Abused children are more likely to be aggressive, hostile, despised at school, or with higher rate of withdrawal from school (more for girls).
7. Children at risk for abuse are: < 1 y/a, premature, defective, very active, step-children, and parent's history of child abuse.
8. Be careful not to mistake acceptable cultural practices (e.g. "coining") as child abuse, but consider female circumcision as abuse. Try to get clues by discussing with the parents how they treat the child.

Child Sexual Abuse

Most victims are 9-12 y/o girls and 50% abusers are the family members and relatives. Most likely abusers are stepfathers, uncles, and older male siblings or friends.

Risk factors: Single-parent families, marital conflict, history of physical abuse, and/or social isolation. > 25% adult females report being sexually abused as a child (defined as sex experience before age 18 with a person 5 year older); 50% by family members; 50% told no one.

Sexually abused women are more likely to have numerous sexual partners, more PIDs, learning disabilities, and obesity.

Spousal Abuse

In the US, millions of women are beaten each year and about 2000 are killed by their abusers. It is **not a mandatory reportable offense and can only be reported with the patient's consent**. It's the physician's obligation to give the victim helpful counseling and information about local protective organizations.

Domestic Violence

It is **not a mandatory reportable offense and can only be reported with the patient's consent**. It's the **No.1 cause of injury to women** (for man, motor vehicle accident is the No.1 cause), occurring in all racial and cultural backgrounds and socioeconomic status. Once it occurs, more events are likely to follow. Both the patient and physician (or social worker) should be prepared for it (prevention).

Risk factors for a male abuser: Low education level, alcoholism, jealous or possessive sense, and being verbally insulted.

Risk factors for a female to be abused: Growing up in a violent home (about 50%), married at a young age, dependent personality (disorder), in the last-trimester of pregnancy, etc. Abused spouses tend to blame themselves for the abuse. Thus physician's protective consultation is a great help to the victim.

Chapter 17: High-yield Questions (HYQ)

1-5: In a study of traumatic brain injury (TBI), head MRI scan is used as the main diagnostic tool. Among the 100 patients enrolled with TBI, 90 are MRI (+). Among the 100 non-TBI volunteers, 5 are MRI (+).

A. 75%	B. 80%	C. 85%	
D. 90%	E. 95%	F. 9	G. 18

1. The sensitivity of MRI diagnosis (Dx) is

2. The specificity of MRI Dx is

3. The (+) predictive value (PPV) of MRI Dx is

4. The (-) predictive value (NPV) of MRI Dx is

5. The likelihood ratio for positive MRI in TBI is

6. A total of 500 TBI patients are enrolled and randomized by age, sex, and other conditions. 250 patients receive recombinant human growth hormone therapy and 250 receive placebo at the investigator's discretion. Head MRI scan is used to compare the morphologic changes in the brain now and 6 months later. This study design may have a major defect of

A. self-selection bias	B. observer bias	C. recall bias
D. effect modification	E. confounding variables	

7. In a study of 100 patients with CLL (chronic lymphocytic leukemia), 50 received a new drug and 50 received placebo. Three months later, 20 of the 50 receiving the new drug developed a decrease in WBC, but in the placebo group only 1 developed decrease WBC. What's the relative risk of developing decrease WBC on the new drug?

A. 0.5   B. 2   C. 10   D. 15   E. 20

8. In a study of the relationship between vasculitis and smoking, patients with vasculitis were matched with controls by age and sex. The quantities of cigarettes smoked were compared between the two groups. What can we get from this study?

A. Attributive risk	B. Relative risk	C. Odds ratio
D. Prevalence	E. Incidence	

9-16: Match the following important concepts or questions with the choices below.

A. 2.5%	B. 16%	C. 0.15%
D. 25%	E. Standard deviation (SD)	F. Standard error (SE)
G. Mean	H. Median	I. Type I error
J. Type II error	K. Accuracy	L. Reliability
M. Regression to the mean	N. Power	O. Mode
P. 32%	Q. 1%	R. 5%

9. In the normal distribution curve, what percent of cases is less than 1 SD below the mean?

10. In the normal distribution curve, what percent of cases is less than 3 SD below the mean?

11. A summary of how widely dispersed the values are around the center.

12. For two independent events, if the probability of event 1 (p1) = 0.5 and event 2's p2 = 0.5, what's the chance of having both events 1 and 2?

13. A clinical study shows a statistical result with a p-value = 0.05. Hence, we assume that the result is significant, with a 5% chance that we are making an incorrect conclusion. What type of error it is?

14. The degree to which the results of a test correspond to the true state of the phenomenon.

15. In a screening study, four measurements of a single patient's mean arterial pressure (MAP) are 100, 94, 93, and 92 mmHg. What does the progression of values represent?

16. In Q15, the MAP (BP) value of 100 will affect which of the above choices most?

17-22: Match the following clinical scenarios with the most beneficial screening choice.

A. CXR   B. FOBT (fecal occult blood test)   C. Serum cholesterol test

D. Pap smear   E. Mammography   F. Pelvic examination

G. PSA (prostate specific antigen)   H. DRE (digital rectal exam)   I. FOBT plus sigmoidoscopy

J. FOBT plus colonoscopy   K. Rubella serology   L. Chest CT

M. Screening for depression   N. Screening for alcohol use disorder O. Chlamydia and gonorrhea

17. A 39 y/o man complains of fatigue, mild weight loss, insomnia, poor appetite, and irritability for the past 2 months. There are no other abnormal findings.

18. A 34 y/o obese man comes for his annual health examination. He has a history of smoking and alcohol use for the past 5 years. He denies history of abnormal urine or stool.

19. A 35 y/o female presents with fatigue, nausea, and amenorrhea for the past month. She has been married to her husband for 5 years. She denies any history of abnormal urine or stool. Last year's Pap smear result was normal.

20. A 45 y/o man comes for his annual health examination. He has a 5-year history of smoking, alcohol use, and hyper-Chol. Careful history taking also reveals that his uncle died of "GI cancer."

21. A 48 y/o female with fatigue comes for her annual health examination. She has no history of chronic diseases, nor family history of cancers. Her mammography result from last year and Pap smear from the past 3 years were normal (Nl). She has no habit of smoking or alcohol use, while her husband smokes and drinks for several years at home.

22. A 50 y/o man comes for his annual health examination. He has a 5-year history of smoking. Careful history taking also reveals that his uncle died of prostate cancer at age 60. His CXR, FOBT and DRE results from last year were normal.

23. A 50 y/o man comes for a health examination. He has a 5-year history of smoking and alcohol drinking. His uncle died of "heart disease." His P/E results are unremarkable. Lab results: total fasting cholesterol (Chol) = 270 mg/dL, LDL = 140 mg/dL, triglyceride (Trig) = 250, and HDL = 45 mg/dL. The best next step is

A. dietary modification and exercise

B. starting pravastatin

C. starting niacin

D. re-testing lipid fraction in 3 months

E. cessation of smoking and alcohol use

24. Continued from Q 23: The above patient comes back for the re-evaluation a year later. He claims he has "followed the dietary modification and exercise for a couple of months." Lipid fraction testing shows total fasting cholesterol = 280 mg/dL, LDL = 150 mg/dL, triglyceride = 260 mg/dL, and HDL = 38 mg/dL. Now the best next step of treatment is

A. dietary modification and exercise

B. starting pravastatin

C. starting niacin

D. re-testing lipid fraction in 3 months

E. cessation of smoking and alcohol use

25. Hepatitis B vaccination should be given to all the following groups of people **EXCEPT**:

A. all newborns

B. all adolescents

C. all elderly patients

D. patients with chronic liver diseases

E. individuals with risks

F. those with two shots

26. All the following are reportable infectious diseases **EXCEPT**:

A. chlamydia

B. shigellosis

C. salmonellosis

D. toxin-producing E. coli

E. legionnaires

F. HCV (+) status

G. HBV (+) status

H. chancroid

I. toxic shock syndrome

J. rubella

K. Lyme disease

L. tularemia

27-28: 27. A 45 y/o female comes for a routine health examination. She is generally healthy and her medical and family history is unremarkable. P/E results are normal. Which of the following cancer screening method is likely to benefit the patient most?

A. Colonoscopy now

B. Colonoscopy at age 50

C. Pap smear now

D. Pap smear at age 50

E. Mammography now

F. Mammography at age 50

28. For the above woman in Q27, careful history taking finds out that her loving mother died of breast cancer at age 60. Now which of the following is likely to benefit the patient most?

A. Monthly breast self-exam

B. BRCA test

C. HER-2/neu test

D. Tamoxifen ingestion

E. Annual mammography

F. Estrogen and progesterone receptor tests

29. Colorectal cancer carries the 3rd mortality among all cancers in both male and female. Which of the following is likely to benefit the patient most?

A. Annual barium enema after age 50

B. Digital rectal examination (DRE) after age 50

C. Annual fecal occult blood test (FOBT) after 50

D. Colonoscopy per 10 years after age 45

E. Colonoscopy per 10 years after age 50

F. Sigmoidoscopy per 3-5 years after age 50

30-34: Match the following clinical scenarios with the correct choice of vaccination.

A. Tetanus   B. Pneumococcus   C. Influenza

D. H. Inf.   E. MMR   F. Varicella

G. Inactivated HAV   H. HAV-IG   I. Bacillus Calmette-Guerin (BCG)

J. HBV vaccine   K. No vaccination   L. HBV vaccine and HBIG for the newborn

M. HBV vaccine and HBIG for the patient

30. A 66 y/o man with history of smoking, chronic cough, and dyspnea is diagnosed with COPD. His symptoms are relieved after proper treatment. He was vaccinated for both Pneumococcus and Influenza last year.

31. A 30 y/o man from the countryside presents with non-productive cough for the past month. Examination results are normal except PPD (+). CXR is unremarkable. He is prescribed INH with Vit-B6 for 9 months.

32. A 45 y/o physician will be traveling in 2 weeks to a developing nation to lead a series of disease prevention programs. He has received regular vaccines for hepatitis B and tetanus, but not others. He is in good general heath.

33. A newly employed nurse accidentally sticks her finger with the needle after injecting a patient who is known as HBV (+). She has never been vaccinated for HBV and asks for the right vaccine.

34. A pregnant patient is found to be HbsAg (+) and HbeAg (+) 3 months after a blood transfusion. She is now at 28 weeks of gestation and in generally good health.

35. An anxious father brings a 4 y/o boy to the physician after a fall. The boy is crying. P/E reveals bilateral swollen knees and arms with bruises and tenderness. The joints have restricted range of motion. There are no other abnormal findings. What's the best next step?

A. Multiple X-rays   B. Report to the child protective authority

C. Symptomatic treatment   D. Physical therapy

E. Restriction of movement

36. A 35 y/o female comes to the doctor crying for help. She recently discovered that her husband was having an affair with another woman. Since then, she has been beaten by her husband on several occasions. P/E finds multiple bruises on the arms, chest, and legs. CXR reveals a soft rib fracture. What's the most appropriate next step?

A. Symptomatic treatment

B. Give counseling and information about protective organizations

C. Advise the victim to divorce for long peace

D. Report to a protective organization

E. Psychological counseling

37. A 75 y/o man at the end stage of a chronic disease is in a coma. The physician has made best efforts for treatment and advises that continued treatment is now futile. Among the patient's three sons, two insist on continuing treatment but one wishes "Let it go." What's your decision?

A. Stop the treatment   B. Continue the treatment

C. Ask for a court order   D. Ask for the hospital's decision

E. Ask the three sons to reconsider the decision

38. A 10 y/o girl is sent to the ER after a car accident. She is in life-threatening ischemic shock due to a suspected rupture of her spleen that requires emergent blood transfusion and surgery, but the parents and girl all refuse transfusion. While preparing for the operation, what's your immediate next step?

A. Perform the blood transfusion

B. Do not perform blood transfusion

C. Call for an urgent court order

D. Start urgent parent counseling to get consent

E. Administer other fluids available

39. A 16 y/o girl who lives independently from her divorced parents has 2-3 sexual partners. Now she is found to have an STD that requires immediate treatment. She asks you not to inform her mother of the disease or treatment. What should you do before the therapy?

A. Obtain consent from her mother

B. Obtain consent from her closest friend of her wish

C. Obtain consent from her closest relative of her wish

D. Obtain consent from herself

E. Refer her to an expert.

40. A 20 y/o female is brought to the ER after a major traffic accident 30 min ago. She is in a state of hypovolemic shock from a suspected severe internal hemorrhage. She is conscious and fully understands your explanations that an immediate surgery is absolutely necessary to save her life, but she clearly rejected it. Her parents both strongly demand the surgery. The patient has signed an agreement of "Will comply with necessary medical treatment" at admission. What's the best next step to do?

A. Psychiatric consultation

B. Emergency court order or ethics committee

C. Follow her written agreement and perform surgery

D. Follow her oral wish of "No surgery"

E. Try other therapies first and perform surgery if she's in a coma

Answers and Explanations

Q1-5 Keys: These questions require a 2x2 (or 3x3) table. Be sure you understand how to use a 2x2 table.

	Patients with TBI	Patients without TBI
MRI (+)	a=90	b=5
MRI (-)	c=10	d=95
Totals	100	100

1. (D). a/(a+c) = 90%.

2. (E). d/(d+b) = 95%.

3. (E). PPV = a/(a+b) = 90/95 or 95%.

4. (D). NPV = d/(c+d) = 95/105 or 90%.

5. (G). [a/(a+c)]/[b/(b+d)] = 18.

6. (B). It can be prevented by a double-blinded study design. 'A' is due to a patient's selection of his/her own treatment strategy in a study. 'C' is found in retrospective and case-control studies. "D and E" are not biases and potential effects can be minimized by randomization, restriction, and matching.

7. (E). Make a simple 2x2 table:

a: 20	b: 1
c: 30	d: 49

It's a cohort (prospective) study. RR = [20/(20+30)] / [1/(1+49)] = 20. Larger RR implies higher risk.

8. (C). This is a case-control (retrospective) study used to calculate an odds ratio.

9. (B). 68% of cases are within 1 SD of the mean.

10. (C). 99.7% of cases are within 3 SD of the mean, or 0.3%/2 = 0.15% of cases are less than 3 SD below the mean. 95% of the cases are within 2 SD of the mean, or 2.5% of cases are less than 2 SD below the mean.

11. (E). SD = positive square root of the variance. SE = SD/n; the SD of the sample in a frequency distribution.

12. (D). 0.5 x 0.5 = 0.25.

13. (I). It's caused by rejection of the null Ho when it is actually true. Type II (beta) error is from failure to reject the null Ho when it is actually false. Increasing sample size can increase power (= 1 – beta error) by decreasing beta error.

14. (K). Accuracy = validity; Reliability = reproducibility.

15. (M). Regression to the mean implies that patients with very high or very low test results (outliers) are expected to move closer to the center of the distribution (Nl or Gaussian) when the test is repeated.

16. (G). The mean is especially sensitive to an outlier, whereas the median and mode are resistant.

17. (M). Depression is the most likely diagnosis given his age and symptoms. Alcohol abuse would be more likely if < 25 y/a. Cholesterol tests also need to be performed if they have not been done yet.

18. (C). This man has > 2 risk factors for CAD (obesity, alcohol, and smoking), and thus needs Chol test.

19. (K). She's most likely pregnant and requires rubella serology or vaccination as well as beta-hCG and glucose tests.

20. (J). He has high risk for colorectal cancer and requires early colonoscopy with FOBT (fecal occult blood test).

21. (A). This patient may be a victim of 2nd-hand smoking (more harmful than first-hand smoking) and thus has increased risk of lung carcinoma. CXR should be done first although it's not a routine screening method for lung cancer. If a suspected mass is found, a chest CT-guided biopsy is indicated. Annual mammography after age 50 is also beneficial for her breast cancer screening.

22. (G). All men > age 40 should have annual DRE and prostate examination after age 50. PSA screening among healthy men is not routinely done but clearly indicated in this man with two risk factors (smoking and family history) for his best benefit. CXR, FOBT and DRE will be less beneficial to him than PSA.

23. (A). This patient has more than two risk factors for CAD (coronary artery disease). As a preventive measure for CAD, the best screening test is fasting lipid profile at 35 in males and 45 in females (with LDL-C and HDL levels as the most important). If total fasting cholesterol is < 200 and no risk factors, evaluate the 10-year risks for CAD. If LDL = 130-159 with > 2 risk factors, LDL > 160, or LDL = 100-129 with CAD: borderline risk; treat with dietary modification and exercise. Cessation of smoking and alcohol use is a good initial step but inadequate.

24. (C). The patient's triglyceride is > 250 mg/dL and HDL is < 40 mg/dL, he should be treated with niacin or gemfibrozil. If LDL > 130 plus CAD, LDL > 160 plus 2 risk factors, or LDL > 190, he is treated with pravastatin.

25. (C). Hepatitis B vaccination should be given to all newborns (except those whose body weights are < 2 kg) and adolescents, and all adults with risks. Patients with chronic hepatic diseases will be particularly benefited. Elderly patients with low risks should not be administered with this vaccine. It requires a series of three vaccinations for the patient to develop immunity.

26. (G). Please review Table 17-4 again. Hepatitis A and hepatitis B are both reportable infectious diseases but HBV (+) status is not.

27. (F). The most benefit that the patient may get is the mortality reduction from the screening. Because breast cancer after 50 y/a carries the highest morbidity and mortality among others, mammography at or after age 50 will benefit the patient most. Screening 100 women at age 50 will detect more breast cancer than screening at age 45.

28. (D). This asymptomatic patient has a high risk because a first-degree relative died of breast cancer, and thus preventive treatment of the selective estrogen receptor modulator (tamoxifen) will most likely reduce the morbidity and mortality of breast cancer she may have. "A, E" is inadequate. BRCA (+) may indicate increased risk. HER-2/neu is helpful in guiding the anti-cancer use of trastuzumab, but not as prophylaxis. "F" is useful to guide the anti-cancer therapy as well.

29. (E). Colonoscopy after age 50 is the best of all the colon cancer screening methods for most people with risks. Sigmoidoscopy may miss the 40% colon cancers proximal to the sigmoid colon. Barium enema (+) or FOBT (+) must be followed by colonoscopy for polyp removal and biopsy. DRE may not help much.

30. (C). Influenza vaccine is recommended per year for people after age 50 or with risks. Pneumococcus should be given to all patients with chronic Cardio-pulmonary diseases and asplenia, and any patient > 60 y/a. It is effective for 5-7 years. Hib is only needed in risky patients.

31. (K). He is suspected of TB infection and needs 9-12 months of INH but no vaccination at this time. BCG is only recommended for disseminated TB.

32. (H). Inactivated HA vaccine is recommended for all travelers to endemic areas. It is given 4 weeks in advance in order to be effective (95%). If one has to travel within 1-3 weeks, give one anti-HAV-IG shot.

33. (M). HBV vaccine is indicated for all newborns and high-risk people (per 10 years)—healthcare workers and chronic liver diseases, with 95% protection. This patient has been exposed to HBV and has not been vaccinated

yet. Therefore, she needs HBIG + vaccine within 24 hours, and the total vaccine 3 times. If the patient has been exposed to HBV and had no response to a previous vaccine, she only needs HBIG within 24 hours.

34. (L). This pregnant patient is at high risk for hepatitis B, but unfortunately it is too late for vaccination. After delivery, give the newborn HBIG and HBV vaccine immediately followed by an additional 2 vaccines on schedule.

35. (A). This is most likely an ordinary fall injury—common sites, extent, and age of injuries. Multiple X-ray films are needed to exclude fractures of the knees and arms (and the spine if suspected). If the spine is fractured or there are other injuries of unusual sites and nature, child abuse should be suspected.

36. (B). Spouse abuse is not a mandatory reportable offense; neither is it the physician's job to advise the victim to divorce her husband (it may be the job of a psychologist or social worker). A physician has the obligation to give the victim counseling and information on how to seek protection. If the victim's life is at risk, the physician should call the police immediately. "A and E" are needed after 'B'.

37. (B). The majority of legal surrogates decide treatment for an incompetent patient.

38. (A). Parents cannot refuse a life-saving treatment for a child, and the child has no right to determine treatment. If the refusal refers to a life-threatening condition but not an immediate emergency (like diabetic coma), you can ask for a court's permission to treat.

39. (D). A 16 y/o person that lives independently is not considered "underage" and has the right to decide the treatment of an STD confidentially. If it's threatening to this person's life or others' health (such as AIDS), the legal surrogate (parent) has to be notified, but treatment is determined by the physician. A physician should never "refer" ("transfer") a patient to another doctor if the patient's care is within the physician's own duty and ability!

40. (D). Physicians must follow the conscious adult patient's last known wishes, oral or written. Any previous wishes or agreement can be reversed by the last wishes. Psychiatric consult is unnecessary if the patient clearly understands the risks and makes the decision. An emergency court order or ethics committee decision has no legal effects on an adult capable of understanding. It's wrong to go against a patient's wishes after the patient loses consciousness.

Normal Laboratory Values of Importance

Hematology Reference Values

Note: Reference values for commonly applied laboratory tests are listed in traditional units and in SI units.
The tables are a guideline only. Values are method-dependent and may vary between laboratories.

Determination	Normal Reference Value	
Blood, Plasma or Serum	**Conventional units**	**SI units**
Ammonia (NH3) - diffusion	20-120 µg/dL	12-70 µmol/L
Amylase	35-118 IU/L	0.58-1.97 µkat/L
Anion gap (Na^+- [Cl^- + $HCO3^-$]) (P)	7-16 mEq/L	7-16 mmol/L
Bicarbonate		
Arterial	21–28 mEq/L	21–28 mmol/L
Venous	22–29 mEq/L	22–29 mmol/L
Bilirubin		
Conjugated (direct)	≤ 0.2-0.4 mg/dL	≤ 4-7 µmol/L
Total	< 1.5 mg/dl	< 20 µmol/L
Calcitonin	< 100 pg/ml	< 100 ng/L
Calcium		
Total	8.6–10.3 mg/dL	2.2–2.74 mmol/L
Ionized	4.4–5.1 mg/dL	1–1.3 mmol/L
Carbon dioxide content (plasma)	21–32 mmol/L	21–32 mmol/L
Chloride	95–110 mEq/L	95–110 mmol/L
Coagulation screen		
Bleeding time	< 9 min	< 540 sec
Clotting time	5-15 min	5-15 min
Prothrombin time	10–13 sec	10–13 sec
Partial thromboplastin time (activated)	22–37 sec	22–37 sec
Glucose, fasting	65–115 mg/dL	3.6–6.3 mmol/L

Glucose Tolerance Test (Oral)

	(mg/dL)		(mmol/L)	
	Normal	Diabetic	Normal	Diabetic
Fasting	70–105	> 140	3.9–5.8	> 7.8
60 min	120–170	≥ 200	6.7–9.4	≥ 11.1
90 min	100–140	≥ 200	5.6–7.8	≥ 11.1
120 min	70–120	≥ 140	3.9–6.7	≥ 7.8

Hematologic Tests		
Fibrinogen	200–400 mg/dL	2–4 g/L
Hematocrit (Hct)		
female	36%-44.6%	0.36–0.45 fraction of 1
male	40.7%-50.3%	0.4–0.5 fraction of 1
Hemoglobin A $_{1c}$	5.3%-6.5% of total Hgb	0.053–0.065
Hemoglobin (Hb)		
female	12.1–15.3 g/dL	121–153 g/L
male	13.8–17.5 g/dL	138–175 g/L
Leukocyte count (WBC)	3800–9800/µL	3.8–9.8 x 10^9/L

Erythrocyte count (RBC)		
female	$3.5–5 \times 10^6/\mu L$	$3.5–5 \times 10^{12}/L$
male	$4.3–5.9 \times 10^6/\mu L$	$4.3–5.9 \times 10^{12}/L$
Mean corpuscular volume (MCV)	$80–97.6 \text{ mcm}^3$	80–97.6 fL
Mean corpuscular hemoglobin (MCH)	27–33 pg/cell	1.66–2.09 fmol/cell
Mean corpuscular hemoglobin concentrate (MCHC)	33–36 g/dL	20.3–22 mmol/L
Erythrocyte sedimentation rate (sedrate, **ESR**)	$\leq$30 mm/hr	$\leq$30 mm/hr
Reticulocytes erythrocytes	0.5%-1.5%	0.005–0.015
Platelet count	$150–450 \times 10^3/\mu L$	$150–450 \times 10^9/L$
Erythrocyte enzymes		
Glucose 6-phosphate dehydrogenase (G-6-PD)	$250–5000 \text{ IU}/10^6$ cells	250–5000 µIU/cell
Iron:		
Female	30–160 µg/dL	5.4–31.3 µmol/L
Male	45–160 µg/dL	8.1–31.3 µmol/L
Ferritin	10–383 ng/mL	23–862 pmol/L
Iron binding capacity	220–420 µg/dL	39.4–75.2 mcmol/L
Folic acid: normal	>3.–12.4 ng/mL	7–28.1 nmol/L
Vitamin B$_{12}$	223–1132 pg/mL	165–835 pmol/L
Lactate dehydrogenase	100–250 IU/L	1.67–4.17 µkat/L
Lactic acid (lactate)	6–19 mg/dL	0.7–2.1 mmol/L
Lead	$\leq$ 50 µg/dL	$\leq$ 2.41 µmol/L
Lipase	10–150 IU/L	10–150 IU/L
Magnesium	1.3–2.2 mEq/L	0.65–1.1 mmol/L
Osmolality	280–300 mOsm/kg	280–300 mmol/kg
Arterial Blood Gas (ABG)		
Oxygen saturation (arterial)	94%-100%	0.94 -fraction of 1
PCO$_2$, arterial	35–45 mmHg	4.7–6 kPa
pH, arterial	7.35–7.45	7.35–7.45
PO$_2$, arterial:		
Breathing room air	80–105 mmHg	10.6–14 kPa
On 100% O$_2$	> 500 mmHg	
Potassium	3.5–5 mEq/L	3.5–5 mmol/L
Prostate specific antigen	0–4 ng/mL	0–4 ng/mL
Protein:		
Total	6–8 g/dL	60–80 g/L
Albumin	3.6–5 g/dL	36–50 g/L
Globulin	2.3–3.5 g/dL	23–35 g/L
Rheumatoid factor	< 60 IU/mL	< 60 kIU/L
Sodium	135–147 mEq/L	135–147 mmol/L
Testosterone		
Female	6–86 ng/dL	0.21–3 nmol/L
Male	270–1070 ng/dL	9.3–37 nmol/L
Thyroid Hormone Function Tests:		
Thyroid-stimulating hormone (TSH)	0.35–6.2 µU/mL	0.35–6.2 mU/L
Thyroxine-binding globulin capacity (TBG)	10–26 µg/dL	100–260 mcg/L 1.2–3.4 nmol/L

Total triiodothyronine (T3)	75–220 ng/dL	51–142 nmol/L
Total thyroxine by RIA (T4)	4–11 µg/dL	0.25–0.38 fraction of 1
T3 resin uptake	25%-38%	
Transaminase:		
AST (SGOT)	11–47 IU/L	0.18–0.78 µkat/L
ALT (SGPT)	7–53 IU/L	0.12–0.88 µkat/L
Urea nitrogen (BUN)	8–25 mg/dL	2.9–8.9 mmol/L
Uric acid	3–8 mg/dL	179–476 µmol/L

	Urine	
Determination	**Conventional units**	**SI units**
Calcium	50–250 µg/day	1.25–6.25 mmol/day
Catecholamines, 24-hr	< 110 µg	< 650 nmol
Creatinine:		
Female	0.6–1.5 g/day	5.3–13.3 mmol/day
Male	0.8–1.8 g/day	7.1–15.9 mmol/day
pH	4.5–8	4.5–8
Protein		
Total	< 150 mg/24h	< 0.15 g/day
Phosphate	0.9–1.3 g/day	29–42 mmol/day
Potassium	25–100mEq/day	25–100 mmol/day
Sodium	100–250 mEq/day	100–250 mmol/day
Specific gravity, random	1.002–1.030	1.002–1.030
Uric acid, 24-hr	250–750 mg	1.48–4.43 mmol

MAIN REFERENCES

Current Medical Diagnosis and Treatment, current editions
Kaplan Medical USMLE Step 2 CK, Step 3 books, current editions
First Aid for the USMLE (Step 2 CK, Step 3), current editions
www.uptodate.com
www.usmleworld.com (Notes from the Qbank)

INDEX

ABBREVIATIONS

A

A-a: alveolar-arterial (oxygen gradient)
ABG: arterial blood gas
ACE-I: angiotensin-converting enzyme inhibitor
ACTH: adrenocorticotropic hormone
ADH: antidiuretic hormone
ADHD: attention-deficit hyperactivity disorder
AF, A-fib: atrial fibrillation
AFP: alpha-fetoprotein
AKP: alkaline phosphatase
ALL: acute lymphocytic or lymphoblast leukemia
ALS: amyotrophic lateral sclerosis
ALT: alanine aminotransferase, SGPT
AML: acute myeloid leukemia
ANA: antinuclear antibody
ANCA: anti-neutrophil cytoplasmic antibody
aPTT: activated partial thromboplastin time
ARDS: acute respiratory distress syndrome
ARF: acute renal failure
ASA: acetylsalicylic acid (aspirin)
5-ASA: 5-aminosalicylic acid
ASD: atrial septal defect
ASO: antistreptolysin O
AST: aspartate aminotransferase
ATN: acute tubular necrosis
A-V: atrioventricular; artey-vein
AZT: azidothymidine (zidovudine)

B

BCL: bronchoalveolar lavage
BM(B): bone marrow (biopsy)
BMI: body mass index
BPM (bpm): beat per minute
BT: bleeding time
BUN: blood urea nitrogen
BZ: benzodiazepam

C

CaEDTA: edetate calcium disodium
CABG: coronary artery bypass grafting
CAD: coronary artery disease
CBC: complete blood counts
CEA: carcinoembryonic antigen
CHD: coronary heart disease
CHF: chronic/congestive heart failure
Chol: cholesterol
CHOP: cytoxan, adriamycin (doxorubicin), oncovin (vincristine), prednisone
CIN: cervical intraepithelial neoplasia
CIS: carcinoma in situ
CK: creatine kinase
CLL: chronic lymphocytic/lymphoblastic leukemia
CML: chronic myelocytic/myelogenous leukemia
CMV: cytomegalovirus
CN: cranial nerve
CNS: central nervous system

CO: carbon monoxide; cardiac output
COMT: catechol-O-methyltransferase
COPD: chronic obstructive pulmonary disease
COX-I: cyclo-oxygenase inhibitor
Cr: creatinine
CPK: creatine phosphokinase
CPR: cardiopulmonary resuscitation
CRF: chronic renal failure
CVD: cardiovascular disease
CVA: cerebrovascular accident (stroke)
CVP: central venous pressure

D

D&C: dilation and curettage
DDAVP: 1-deamino (8-D-arginine) vasopressin
DDI: dideoxyinosine (HIV medication)
DES: diethylstilbestrol
DEXA: dual-energy x-ray absorptiometry
DI: diabetes insipidus
DIC: disseminated intravascular coagulation
DIP: distal interphalangeal (joint)
DKA: diabetic ketoacidosis
DLCO: diffusing capacity of carbon monoxide
DMD: Duchenne muscular dystrophy
DMSA: 2,3-dimercaptosuccinic acid, succimer
DNase: deoxyribonuclease
DNI: do not intubate
DNR: do not resuscitate
DRE: digital rectal examination
DTaP: diphtheria, tetanus, acellular pertussis vaccine
DTR: deep tendon reflex
DTs: delirium tremens
DUB: dysfunctional uterine bleeding
DVT: deep venous thrombosis

E

EBV: Ebstein-Barr Virus
ECG, EKG: electrocardiography
ECT: electroconvulsive therapy
EF: ejection fraction
EEG: electroencephalogram
EGD-scopy: esophagogastroduodenoscopy
ELISA: enzyme-linked immunosorbent assay
EMG: electromyogram
ENT: ears, nose, and throat
ER: emergency room; estrogen receptor
ERCP: endoscopic retrograde cholangio-pancreatography
ESR: erythrocyte sedimentation rate

F

FAP: familial adenomatous polyposis
FDP: fibrin degeneration product
FEV1: forced expiratory volume in 1 second
FFP: fresh frozen plasma
FNA (FNB): fine needle aspiration (biopsy)
FOBT: fecal occult blood test

FSH: follicle-stimulating hormone
FTA-ABS: fluorescent treponemal Ab-absorption
FVC: forced vital capacity

G
GA: gestational age
GBM: glomerular basement membrane
G-CSF: granulocyte colony-stimulating factor
GERD: gastroesophageal reflux disease
GFR: glomerular filtration rate
GGT: gammar-glutamyltranspeptidase
GH: growth hormone
G6PD: glucose-6-phosphatase deficiency
GnRH: ganodotropin-releasing hormone
GTD: gestational trophoblastic disease
GTT: glucose tolerance test

H
HbA1c: glycosylated hemoglobin
HbO_2: hyperbaric oxygen
HBcAb/Ag: hepatitis B core antibody/antigen
HBeAb/Ag: hepatitis B e-antibody/antigen
HBIG: hepatitis B immunoglobulin
HBsAb/Ag: hepatitis B surface antibody/antigen
Hep-A/B/C/D/E: hepatitis A/B/C/D/E
HHNK: hyperosmolar hyperglycemic nonketotic
HCTZ: hydrochlorothiazide
hCG: (beta) human chorionic gonadotropin
HDL: high-density lipoproteins
HHV: human herpesvirus
5-HIAA: 5-hydroxindoleacetic acid
HIDA: (Tech[99]) hepatobiliary immodiacetic acid
HLA: human leukocyte antigen
HMG-CoA: hydroxymethylglutaryl-CoA
HNPCC: hereditary nonpolyposis colorectal cancer
HPV: human papillary virus
HRT: hormone replacement therapy
HSV: human herpes virus
HUS: hemolytic uremic syndrome

I
IBD: inflammatory bowel disease
IBS: irritable bowel syndrome
ICD-15: international classification of diseases-2015
ICH: intracranial hemorrhage/hematoma
ICP: intracranial pressure
IL: interleukin
IFN: interferon
IG: immunoglobulin
IGF: insulin-like growth factor
INH: isoniazid
INR: International Normalized Ratio
IOP: intraocular pressure
IPV: inactivated poliovirus vaccine
ITP: idiopathic thrombocytopenic purpura
IU: international units
IUD: intrauterine device
IUGR: intrauterine growth retardation
IVC: inferior vena cava

IVDA: intravenous drug abuse
IVP: intravenous pyelogram

J
JVD(P): jugular venous distention (pressure)

L
LAD: left anterior descending
LBBB: left bundle branch block
LBO: large bowel obstruction
LCA: left coronary artery
LCL: lateral collateral ligament
LDH: lactate dehydrogenase
LDL: low-density lipoproteins
LES: lower esophageal sphincter
LFTs: liver function tests
LH: luteinizing hormone
LLQ: left lower quadrant
LMN: lower motor neuron
LMP: last menstrual period
LMWH: low-molecular-weight heparin
LP: lumbar puncture
LRS: lactated Ringer's solution
L:S: lectine:sphingomyeling ratio
LSD: lysergic acid diethylamide
LUQ: left upper quadrant
LVH: left ventricular hypertrophy

M
MAC: mycobacterium avium-intracellulare complex
MAI: mycobacterium avium-intracellulare
MAOI: monoamine oxidase inhibitor
MCA: middle cerebral artery
MCHC: mean corpuscular hemoglobin concentration
MCL: medial collateral ligament
MCP: metacarpopharlangeal (joint)
MCV: mean corpuscular volume
MEN: multiple endocrine neoplasia
MHC: major histocompatibility complex
MMR: measles, mumps, rubella (vaccine)
MRA: magnetic resonance angiography
MRSA: methycillin-resistent Staph. Aureus
MS: multiple sclerosis
MSAFP: maternal serum α-fetoprotein
MTP: metacarpopharlangeal (joint)
MuSK: muscle-specific kinase
MVA: motor vehicle accident

N
NF: neurofibromatosis
NG: nasogastric
NKH: nonketotic hyperglycemia
N-M: neuromuscular
NPH: isophane insulin suspension
NPO: nothing by mouth
NPV: negative predictive value
NS: nervous system; normal saline
NSAID: nonsteoroidal anti-inflammatory drug
NSCLC: non-small cell lung cancer

O

OCP: oral contraceptive pill
OPV: oral poliovirus vaccine
ORIF: open reduction and internal fixation
P
PaO2: partial pressure of oxygen in arterial blood
PAS: periodic acid-Schiff
PCKD: polycystic kidney disease
PCOS: polycystic ovary syndrome
PCP: pneumocystis carinii pneumonia
PCR: polymerase chain reaction
PCWP: pulmonary capillary wedge pressure
PDA: patent ductus arteriosus
PE: pulmonary embolus
PEEP: positive end-expiratory pressure
PFTs: pulmonary function tests
PG: penicillin G; prostaglandin
PID: pelvic inflammatory disease
PIP: proximal interphalangeal (joint)
PIV: parainfluenza virus
PMI: point of maximal impulse
PML: progressive multifocal leukoencephalopathy; promyelocytic leukemia
PMN: polymorphonuclear (leukocyte)
PMR: polymyalgia rheumatic
PMS: premenstrual syndrome
PPD: purified protein derivative (TB test)
PPI: proton pump inhibitors
PPSV: pneumococcal polysaccharides vaccine
PPV: positive predictive value
PR: progesterone receptor
PSA: prostate-specific antigen
PT: prothrombin time
PTCA: percutaneous transluminal Cor-angioplasty
PTD: parathyroidism
PTH: parathyroid hormone
PTSD: post-traumatic stress disorder
PTT: partial thromboplastin time
PUD: peptic ulcer disease
PVC: premature ventricular contraction
PVR: peripheral vascular resistance
R
RA: right atrium; rheumatic arthritis
RAIU: radioactive iodine uptake
RBBB: right bundle branch block
RDW: red blood cell distribution width
REM: rapid eye movement
RF: rheumatic factor
RhoGAM: Rh immune globulin
RLQ: right lower quadrant
RPR: rapid plasma reagin (for syphilis)
RR: respiratory rate; relative risk
RSV: respiratory syncytial virus
RTA: renal tubular acidosis
RUQ: right upper quadrant
RV: residual volume; right ventricle
S

SAH: subarachnoid hemorrhage
SBO: small bowel obstruction
SBP: spontaneous bacterial peritonitis
SCD: sickle cell disease
SCID: severe combined immunodeficiency disease
SCLC: small cell lung cancer
SD: standard deviation
SEM: standard error of the mean
SIADH: syndrome of inappropriate ADH
SIDS: sudden infant death syndrome
SS: somatostatin, such as octreotide
SSRIs: serotonin-selective reuptake inhibitors
STD: sexually transmitted disease
SVC: superior vena cava
SvO2: systemic venous oxygen saturation
SVR: system vascular resistance
SVT: supraventricular tachycardia
T
T3RU: T3 resin uptake
TAH/BSO: total abdominal hysterectomy and bilateral salpingo-oophorectomy
TBG: thyroxine-binding globulin
3TC: dideoxythiacytidine (lamivudine)
TCA: tricyclic antidepressant; trichloroacetic acids
Td: tetanus-dyphtherial (booster vaccine)
TEE: transesophageal echocardiography
TEN: toxic epidermal necrolysis
TG: triglyceride
TGV: transposition of great vessels
TIA: transient ischemic attack
TIBC: total iron-binding capacity
TIPS: transjugular intrahepatic portosystemic shunt
TMP/SMX (Z): trimethoprim-sulfamethoxazole
TNM: tumor, node, metastasis (staging)
TORCH: toxoplasma, others, rubella, CMV, herpes
tPA: tissue plasminogen activator
TPN: total parenteral nutrition
TRH: thyroid-releasing hormone
TSH: thyroid-stimulating hormone
TTP: thrombotic thrombocytopenic purpura
V
VDRL: Venereal Disease Research Lab test
VLDL: very low density lipoprotein
VIPoma: vasoactive intestinal peptide tumor
VMA: vanillylmandelic acid
V/Q: ventilation/perfusion (ratio)
VSD: ventricular septal defect

y/a: years of age
y/o: year-old
$1°$: primary
$2°$: secondary
$3°$: tertiary
(+): positive
(-): negative
+/-: positive or negative; with or without

A

B

C

D

HIGH-YIELD CLINICAL IMAGES

(Courtesy images reorganized from www.images.google.com & related websites for public sharing)

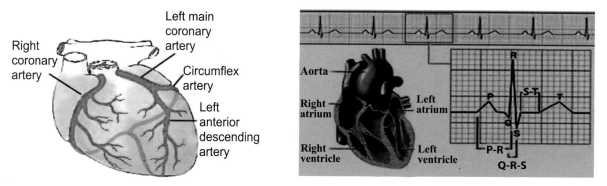

Image 1-2. Normal heart anatomy and ECG (EKG): SA and AV nodes are supplied mostly by the right coronary artery (RCA), which supplies the inferior portion of the LV (via the posterior descending artery). Most coronary A. occlusions occur in the LAD (L-anterior descending A.), which supplies the anterior inter-ventricular septum.

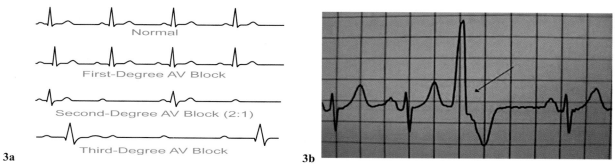

3a.
3b.

3a. A-V block: 1⁰: P-R interval >0.02s; 2⁰: P wave occurs without QRS; 3⁰: No P before QRS, escape rhythm.

3b. Premature Ventr-contraction: early, wide QRS complex without a preceding P followed by a compensatory pause.

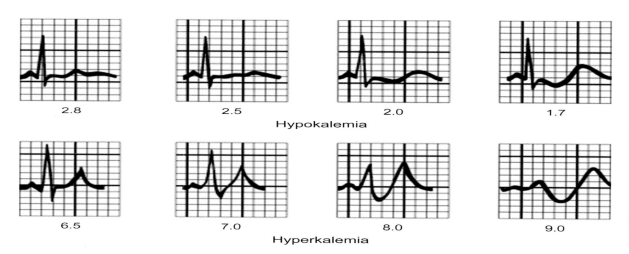

4. Hypo-K and hyper-K: flat T wave vs peak T wave. QRS complex can be irregular with severe hyper-K.

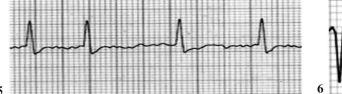

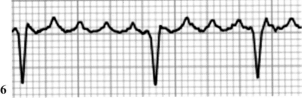

5. **Atrial fibrillation:** wavy baseline without discernible P waves; variable QRS response

6. **Atrial flutter:** regular rhythm; "sawtooth" P waves; varying A-V conduction (5:1 and 4:1)

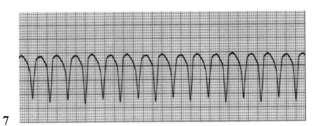

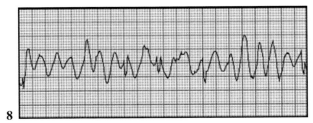

7. **Ventricular tachycardia:** ≥ 3 consecutive PVCs; regular, rapid wide-complex rhythms

8. **Ventricular fibrillation:** totally erratic tracing, requiring emergent defibrillation to save life

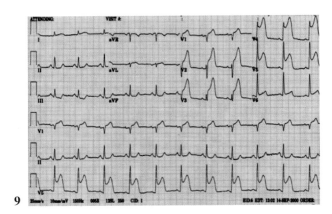

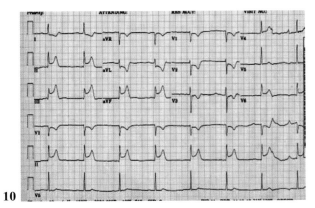

9. **Anterior wall MI:** ST-elevation in leads V1-V5 with reciprocal ST-T in the inferior leads (aVR, aVL)

10. **Inferior wall MI:** ST-elevation in leads II, III, and aVF with reciprocal ST-T in the anterior leads (V1-V3)

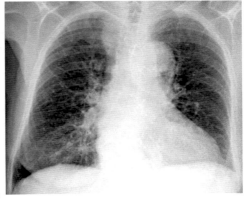

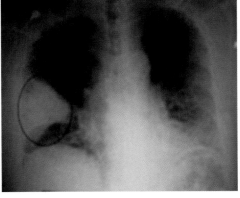

11. **Chronic bronchitis:** thickening of bronchial walls, increased linear markings + enlarged cardiac shadow

12. **Lobar pneumonia:** lobar consolidation and air bronchograms

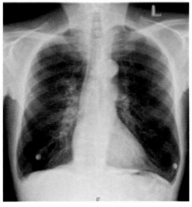
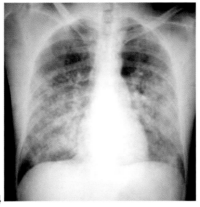
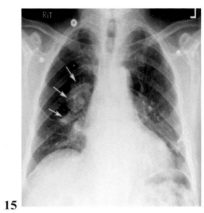

13   14   15

13. **Asthma, emphysema, and bronchiectasis:** hyperinflated lungs and flattened diaphragm indicating asthma and emphysema; streaky shadowing and bronchial wall thickening in both lungs indicating bronchiectasis

14. **Cardiogenic pulmonary edema (CHF):** increased vascular shadows in all lobes + enlarged left atrium

15. **Pneumoconiosis:** multiple small irregular opacities and interstitial densities

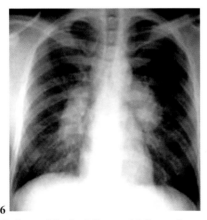
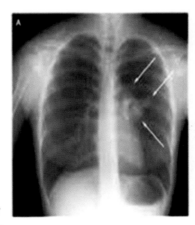
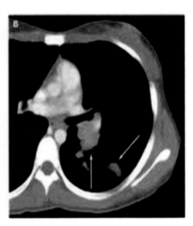

16   17

16. **Sarcoidosis:** bilateral hilar adenopathy

17. **Small-cell lung cancer with lymphadenopathy:** CT confirms enlarged left hilum and mediastinum

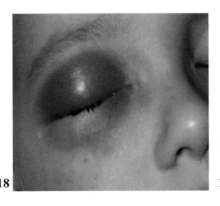
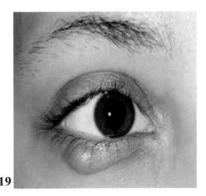
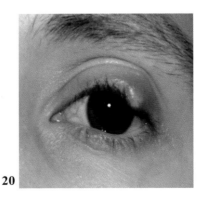

18   19   20

18. **Orbital cellulitis:** proptosis, painful eyes, decreased eye movement, and red swollen eyelids

19. **Chalazion:** meibomian gland lipogranuloma

20. **Hordeolum (Stye):** "Horrible Staph"—eyelid infection

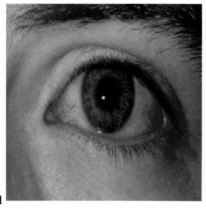 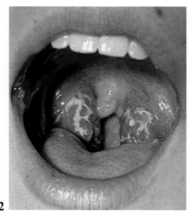 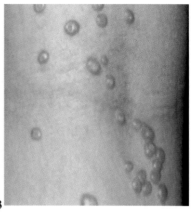

21. **Infectious conjunctivitis ("Pink eye"):** viral—severe ocular irritation, copious watery discharge from the eye, and pre-auricular lymph mode (LN) swelling (Differentiation: Bacterial –purulent discharge)

22. **Strep-pharyngitis:** fever, sore and red throat with exudates, and tonsil and cervical lymph node swelling

23. **Molluscum contagiosum:** painless, fleshy, pearly, oval papules

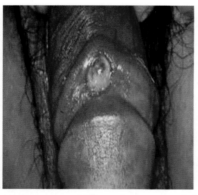 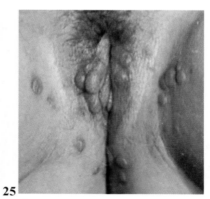 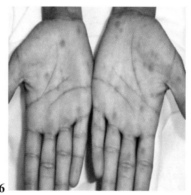

24. **Primary syphilis—chancre:** painless ulcerated papule(s) with clear base and raised borders

25. **Secondary syphilis: condyloma lata:** pinkish or pigmented papules

26. **2nd syphilis:** erythematous rash

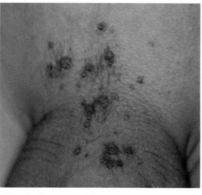 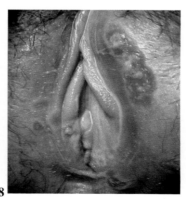 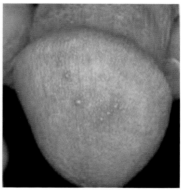

27. **Genital warts (Condyloma acuminata):** cauliflower-like papules or nodules with velvety or white color on the genitoanal area

28. **Chancroid:** irregular, deep, painful genital papules or ulcers; by H. ducreyi

29. **Herpes simplex (Type II):** red, painful vesicles with ulcers in the anogenital area

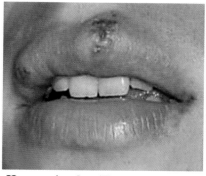
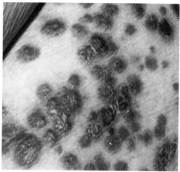
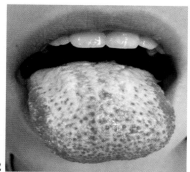

30. **Herpes simplex (Type I):** red, painful vesicles +/- erosive vesicular gingivostomatitis

31. **Kaposi Sarcoma:** caused by HHV8 with AIDS; multiple red-purple nodules and surrounding pink-red macules or multicentric vascular macules

32. **Oral candidiasis—thrush:** white patches of exudates on the tongue or buccal mucosa

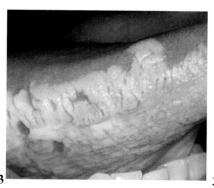
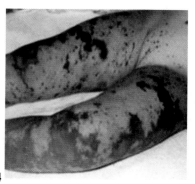
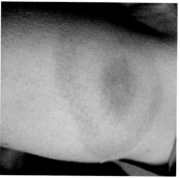

33. **Oral hairy leukoplakia:** a hairy, whitish, painless patch on the tongue; associated with EBV and HIV infections

34. **Purpura fulminans/gangrenosa:** associated with pediatric sepsis, DIC, etc.

35. **Lyme disease:** circular, expanding erythema chronicum migrans

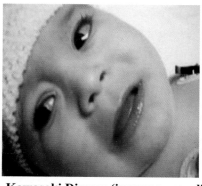
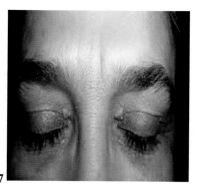
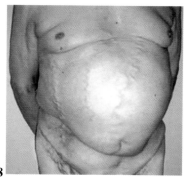

36. **Kawasaki Disease (immune vasculitis):** painful red swelling of the skin, membranes, conjunctiva, and LN; cracked or bleeding lips, strawberry tongue; multi-form, purple rash on the trunk, palms, and soles; +/- MI

37. **Hypercholesterolemia—xanthelasmas:** fatty depositions of yellowish cholesterol-rich material under the skin or in tendons

38. **Cushing syndrome:** "moon face", "buffalo hump", truncal obesity, and cutaneous striae and easy bruisability

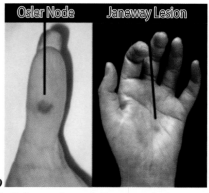
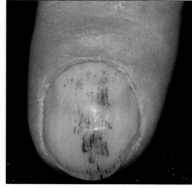
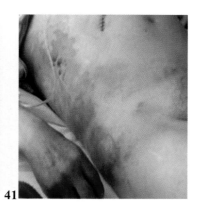

39. Osler node and Janeway lesion: endocarditis, immune complex deposition

40. Splinter hemorrhage: endocarditis, vasculitis, connective tissue disease

41. Grey-Turner's sign—blue discoloration in the flank area: seen in ruptured aortic aneurism and severe acute pancreatitis

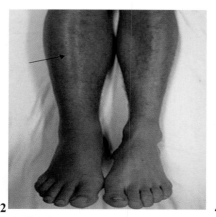
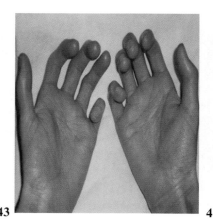
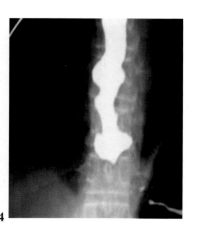

42. DVT: in the right leg, with swelling and redness

43. Scleroderma: symmetric skin thickening in the face and sclerodactyly in distal extremities

44. Diffuse esophageal spasm: Ba X-Ray shows a wobbly shape "corkscrew esophagus". Differentiation: Nutcracker esophagus is high-amplitude all-esophageal contractions.

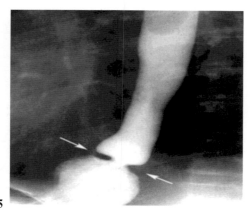
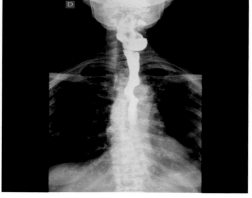

45. The Schatzki ring: a weblike mucosal ring proximal to LES, a supra-sphincter obstructive ring

46. Zenker diverticulum: a hypopharyngeal pouching of mucosa (a false diverticulum)

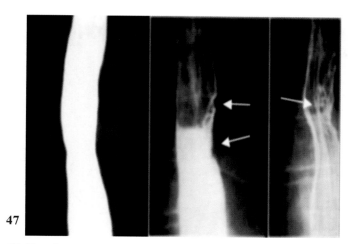
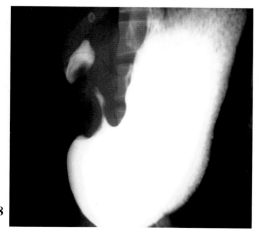

47. Esophageal carcinoma (early): (1) Lesion is not visible on single contrast esophagram; (2) air-contrast esophagram shows surface irregularity (arrows) indicating a small mucosal lesion.

48. Gastric carcinoma: upper GI series Ba X-ray shows a filling defect in the antrum

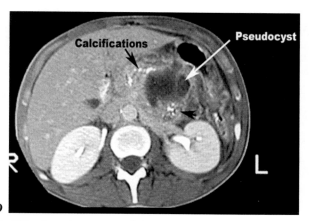
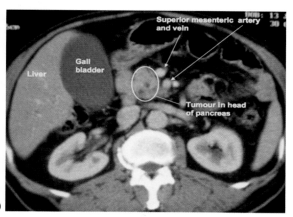

49. CT: chronic pancreatitis + pseudo cyst + calcifications; note hyper- & hypo- mass density in pancreas

50. Pancreatic (head) carcinoma: CT/MRI is sensitive; high CA19-9 level is highly specific.

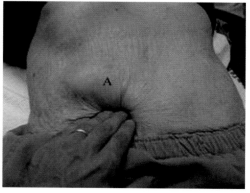
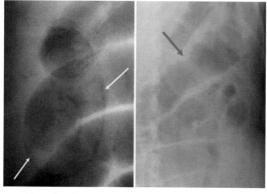

51. Courvoisier sign—palpable, nontender gallbladder with jaundice: indicating a late-stage malignancy of the gallbladder or pancreas

52. Mesenteric ischemia: AXR shows thumb printing (red arrow), ileus, and pneumatosis (white arrows).

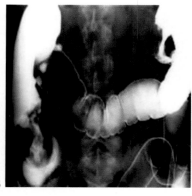
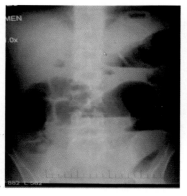
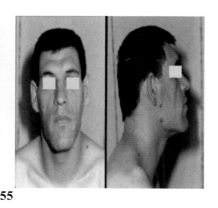

53. Ba X-ray: colon carcinoma: "apple-core" filling defect

54. Small bowel obstruction: upright AXR demonstrates multiple air fluid levels.

55. Acromegaly: enlarged hands, feet, facial organs, bones, and soft tissues, plus enlarged internal organs

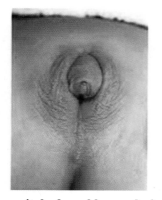
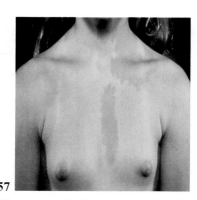
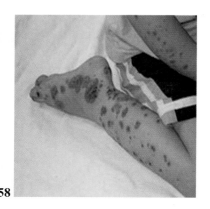

56. Congenital adrenal hyperplasia: ambiguous genitalia

57. GIPP and café au lait spot: The girl has gonadotropin-independent precocious puberty plus café au lait macules with McCune-Albright syndrome and neurofibromatosis-1. Café a. l. spot can also exist in Nl persons

58. Henoch-Schonlein purpura: palpable purpura; systemic vasculitis

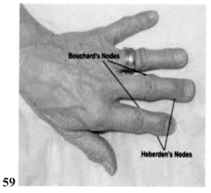
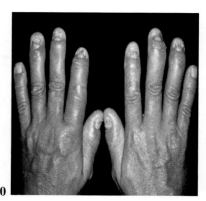
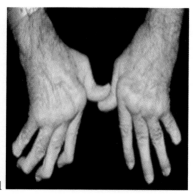

59. Osteoarthritis: Osteophytes--Bouchard's (PIP) & Heberden's (DIP) nodes

60. Psoriatic Arthritis: pitting, onycholysis, and "oil spots"; "sausage fingers"

61. Rheumatoid arthritis: MCP and PIP joint hypertrophy & deformities

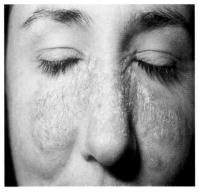 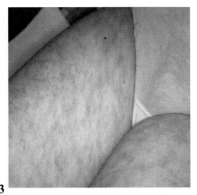 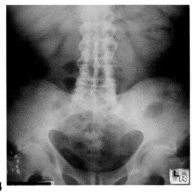

62   63   64

62. SLE: Malar (butterfly) rash, discoid rash, non-erosive arthritis, serositis, and multi-systemic manifestations

63. Livedo reticularis: a mottled, lace-like, purplish discoloration of the skin, usually on the legs.

64. Ankylosing spondylitis: fusion of both sacroiliac (SI) joints and thin, symmetrical syndesmophytes bridging the intervertebral disc spaces

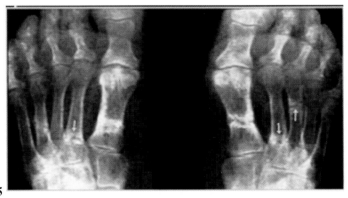 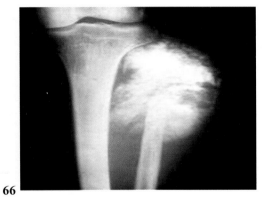

65   66

65. Bilateral fractures plus osteoporosis (showing osteopenia) indicate osteomalacia (showing "looser zones"), which is due to Vit D deficiency (rickets)

66. Osteosarcoma: erosive "sunburst" pattern of neoplastic bone or "Codman's triangle", with periosteal new bone formation and inflammatory reaction, and osteolytic lesion

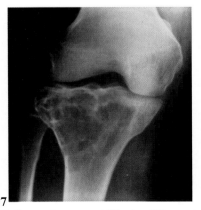 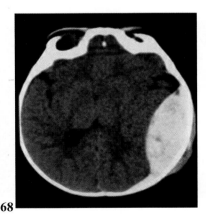 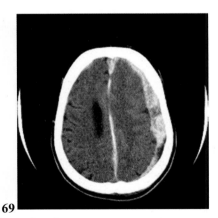

67   68   69

67. Osteoclastoma (Giant cell bone tumor): "soap bubble" sign in the epiphyseal end

68. CT: Epidural hematoma: A biconvex, lens-shaped lesion

69. CT: Subdural hematoma: a semilunar, crescent-shaped lesion

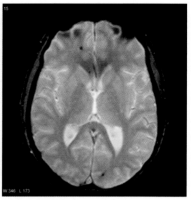 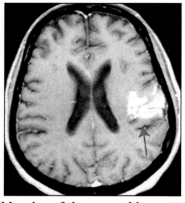 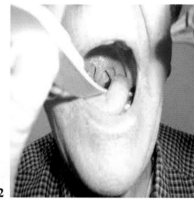

70. MRI: Diffuse axonal injury—diffuse blurring of the gray-white matter interface

71. MRI: a bright lesion in an ischemic stroke

72. Left CN IX/X lesion: posterior 1/3 of the tongue and palate/uvula deviating to the right side (decreased gag reflex on the lesion side)

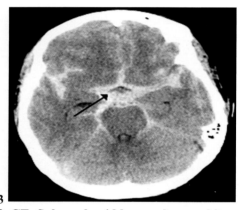 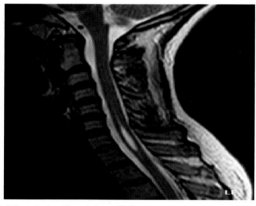

73. CT: Subarachnoid hemorrhage: white center stretching into the side sulci

74. MRI: Syringomyelia: an idiopathic syrinx. Note the thin light grey shape (filled with spinal fluid) inside the spinal cord, placed at center in the bottom half of the above image.

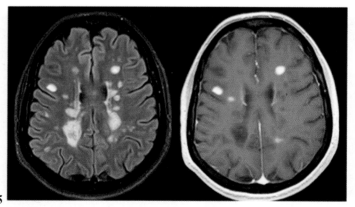 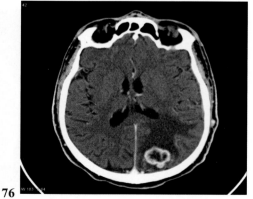

75. Multiple sclerosis: Axial T2-weighted MRI demonstrates multiple white matter plaques in a callosal and pericallosal white matter distribution.

76. CT: Metastatic carcinoma to the brain with cerebral edema: a well-demarcated lesion in the brain parenchyma, with vasogenic edema around metastasis

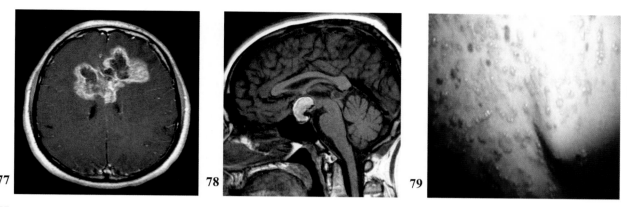

77. 77. MRI: Glioblastoma multiforme (Grade 4 astrocytoma): a poorly demarcated lesion with irregular shape in the brain parenchyma

78. MRI: Craniopharyngioma: a benign pituitary tumor above the sella turcica, with calcification +/- "cyst of oil"

79. Dermatitis herpetiformis: chronic; itching blisters with fluid

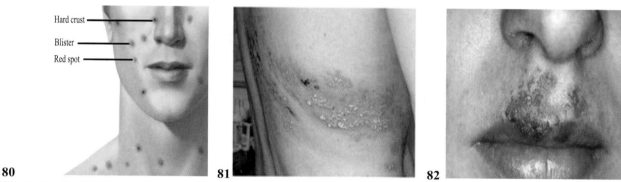

Hard crust
Blister
Red spot

80. Varicella (Chickenpox): generalized, pruritic, teardrop-like vesicles usually at different stages of healing

81. Herpes zoster (Shingles): painful erythematous segmented vesicles/blisters +/- scars

82. Impetigo: maculopapules to vesiculo-papules, by Staph-A with ulcers in the mouth/facial area or Strep-B

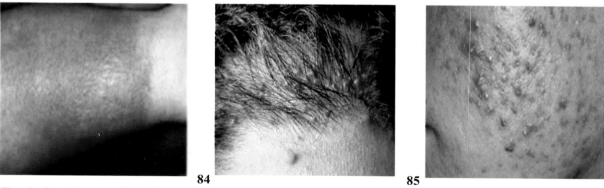

83. Erysipelas: the superficial form of cellulitis; by Strep. pyogenes; red, swollen, painful vesicles/petechiae with a sharply-demarcated border

84. Folliculitis: tiny pustule(s) at the hair follicle opening with a penetrating hair; can develop into a painful or pruritic furuncle or abscess

85. Acne vulgaris: non-inflammatory comedo, closed comedones (whiteheads)

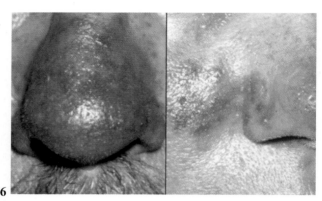 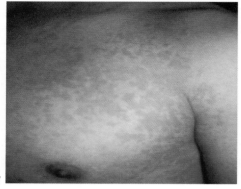

86   87

86. (Acne) Rosacea (adult acne): erythema, papules, pustules, red nose, flushing face, teleangiopathy, or rhinophyma

87. Tinea (Pityriasis) versicolor: multiple hypo-, hyperpigmented scaly patches that vary in color

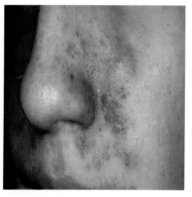 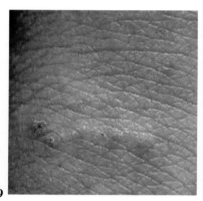 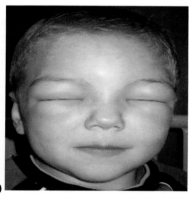

88   89   90

88. Seborrheic dermatitis (dandruff): scaly, flaky, itchy, red patches around the ears, eyebrows, nasolabial fold, midchest, and scalp

89. Scabies: pruritus, erythematous and excoriated papules, and burrows on flexural surfaces of the skin

90. Angioedema: Abrupt swelling of the face, eyes, or/and tongue with stridor following minor physical Inj.

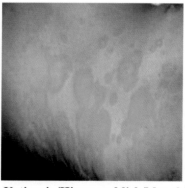 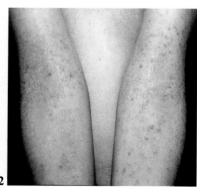 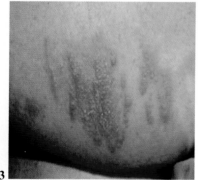

91   92   93

91. Urticaria/Hives: reddish/blanching, elevated papule/plaque (wheal) with variable sizes; type I hypersensitivity reaction

92. Atopic dermatitis: dry, itchy, scaly patches, and plaques with red edema, blisters, crusting, and white dermatographism

93. Poison Ivy—contact dermatitis: allergic or irritant type, erythematous vesicles and crusted patches grouped in geometric shapes

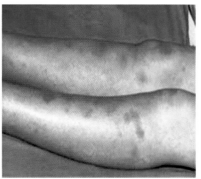
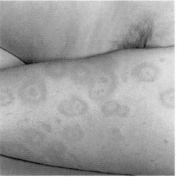
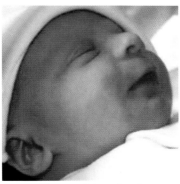

94. **Erythema nodosum:** tender, erythematous nodules on the lower legs, slowly spreading and turning brown

95. **Erythema multiforme:** multiple target-like erythematous macules on the skin and mucous membranes

96. **Erythema Toxicum:** autoimmune rash with small red or yellow papules or pustules on an erythematous base

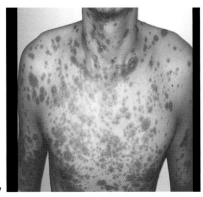
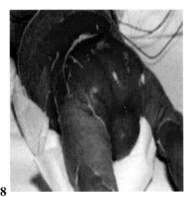
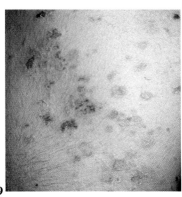

97. **Stevens-Johnson syndrome:** widespread erythematous maculopapular rash; a milder form of TEN

98. **Staph scalded skin syndrome (SSSS):** widespread blisters with fluid and thin wall, Nikolsky's sign (+); superficial damage of the epidermis only

99. **Pemphigus vulgaris:** autoimmune lesions involving the skin and mucous membrane--erosions, crusting, and weeping; Nikolsky's sign (+); acantholysis

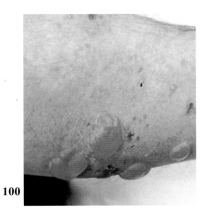
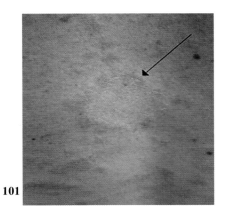
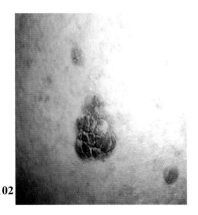

100. **Bullous pemphigoid:** urticaria + erythematous blisters; Nikolsky's sign (-)

101. **Pityriasis rosea:** a "herald patch" followed by smaller satellite papules and plaques

102. **Seborrheic keratosis ("senile wart"):** multiple exophytic, waxy, brown papules, nodules, and plaques

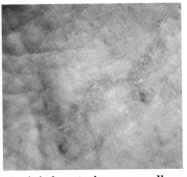
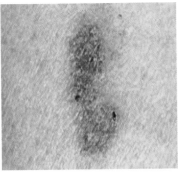
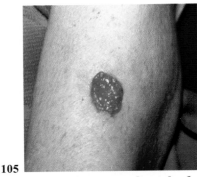

103

104

105

103. Actinic keratosis: a premalignancy, erythematous, thick, scaly, crusty, and sharply demarcated patch of skin, mostly on sun-exposed areas

104. Bowen disease: SCC in situ; well-demarcated erythematous plaque with an irregular border and surface crusting or scaling

105. Basal cell carcinoma (BCC): a superficial fleshy nodule with "pearl" surface, can be ulcerated, sclerosing, and pigmented

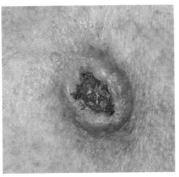
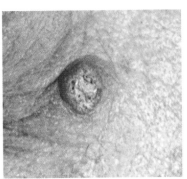
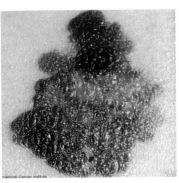

106

107

108

106. Squamous cell carcinoma (SCC): an irregular exophytic nodule with scaling, erosion, or ulceration

107. Keratoacanthoma: a "well-differentiated SCC"; a firm, flesh-colored "volcano" nodule of about 1 cm², with a sharp rising edge and kerato-debris in the crater center

108. Melanoma: "ABCD" features: Asymmetric, Border and Color irregularity, and Diameter > 6 mm

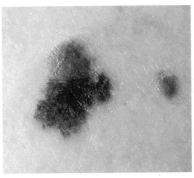
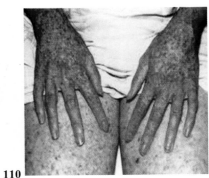
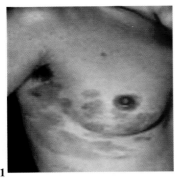

109

110

111

109. Atypical mole (Dysplastic nevus): a pigmented mole-like lesion on sun-exposed areas, with irregular borders and colors and a flat shape; can be multiple

110. Xeroderma pigmentosum: solar keratosis-- scaly, dry skin, irregular dark spots on the skin with freckling, painful eyes, spidery blood vessels, hair growth on chest and legs, and increased skin malignancies

111. Cutaneous T-cell lymphoma (Mycosis fungoides): pruritic, palpable, patchy, psoriatic plaques, or/and multicentric, reddish-brown nodules on the skin +/- enlarged lymph nodes, liver, and spleen

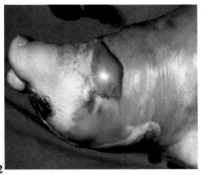
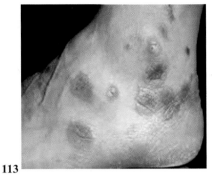
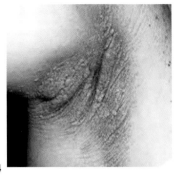

112   113   114

112. Gas gangrene: caused by anaerobic Clostridium perfringens infection after injury or surgery; swelling with pallor, dark redness, and crepitus

113. Lichen planus: pruritic, violaceous, flat-topped, polygonal papules; may have white stripes and ulceration

114. Acanthosis nigricans: hyperkeratotic and hyperpigmented skin with velvety appearance; associated with obesity or endocrinopathy

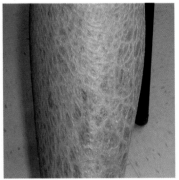
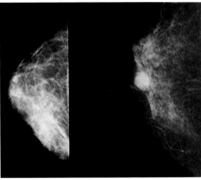
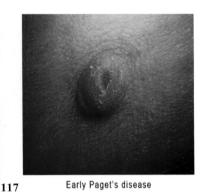

Early Paget's disease

115   116   117

115. Ichthyosis vulgaris: Nl skin at birth, gradually growing dry, rough, and scaly, like "lizard skin"

116. Mammograms: left--normal breast; right—cancerous (increased density with microcalcifications and irregular borders)

117. Paget disease of the breast: nipple CIS, with redness, itching, burning, and erosion of the nipple

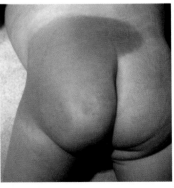
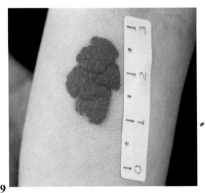
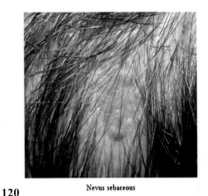

Nevus sebaceous

118   119   120

118. Congenital dermal melanocytosis: a benign, flat, gray-blue, congenital birthmark with wavy borders and irregular shape, disappearing in the first few years of life; to be differentiated from child abuse.

119. Capillary hemangiomas: bright red, strawberry-like macules, disappearing with time

120. Nevus sebaceous (scalp): yellow-orange, hairless plaques located on the scalp resembling flat warts; with malignant potential

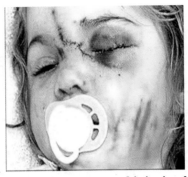
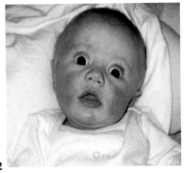
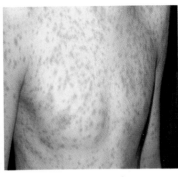

121. **Child abuse**: unusual injuries, bruises, bleeding, swelling, fractures, etc. in atypical places (the face, genitalia, thighs, etc.). It's a mandatory reportable offense up to age 18!

122. **Erythema infectiosum**: "slapped face" by erythrovirus (parvovirus B19)

123. **Measles**: erythematous, maculopapular spots spreading from the head down

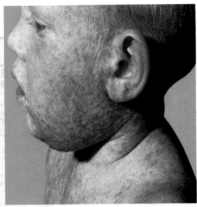
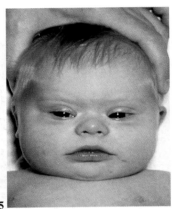
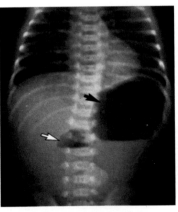

124. **Rubella (German measles)**: "3-day measles" —erythematous, maculopapular, tender spots; starting on the face and spreading distally

125. **Down syndrome**: a flat facial profile (a flat nasal bridge, thin upper lip), small chin, large tongue, slanted eyes, prominent epicanthal folds, simian crease, wider space between the eyes and No.1&2 toe

126. **Duodenal Atresia**: X-ray shows typical "double bubble" sign.

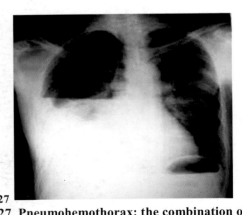
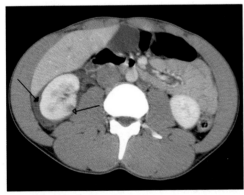

127. **Pneumohemothorax**: the combination of pneumothorax and hemothorax; CXR shows increased lucency of the right hemi-thorax with a liquid level, and mediastinal shift to left side.

128. **Abdominal trauma** resulting in a right kidney contusion (open area) and blood surround the kidney (closed arrow) as seen on CT.

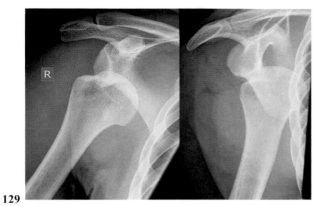

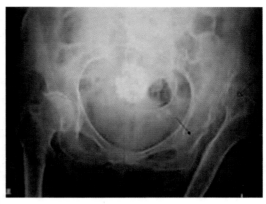

129   130

129. Anterior shoulder dislocation: Two position XR shows the humeral head is (always) displaced anteriorly and medially, with a large Hill–Sachs lesion.

130. Developmental dysplasia of the hip

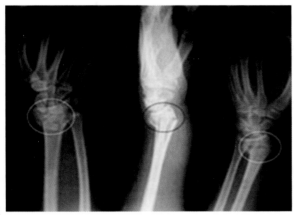

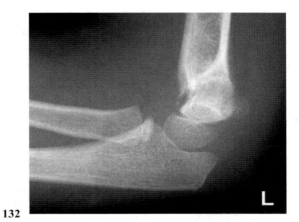

131   132

131. Colles fracture: radius fracture & angulation

132. (Distal) Supracondylar humerus fracture

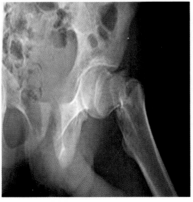

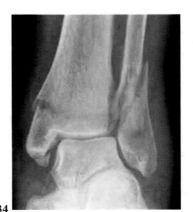

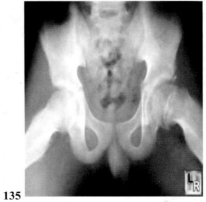

133   134   135

133. Hip fracture: intertrochanteric hip fracture and displaced femoral neck fracture in a young male

134. Foot-ankle fracture & dislocation

135. Slipped capital femoral epiphysis

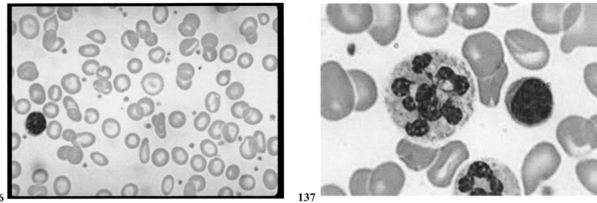

136. Iron deficiency anemia: microcytic, hypochromic RBC ("doughnut cells")

137. Folate and Vit-B12 deficiency: megaloblastic anemia, macro-oval RBC and hypersegmented neutrophils

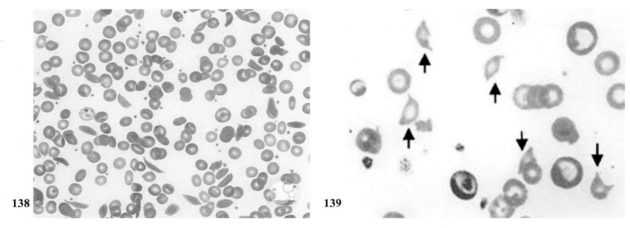

138. Sickle cell disease: RBC sickling-- changed shape to long, thin sickle forms

139. Schistocytes as fragmented cells: hemolysis, DIC, etc.

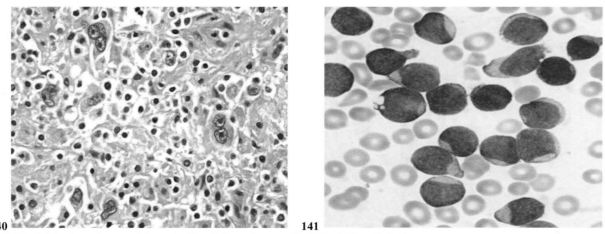

140. Hodgkin lymphoma (biopsy): Reed-Sternberg cells ("Owl Eye Cells")

141. Acute lymphoblastic leukemia (ALL): large, uniform lymphoblasts in blood smear

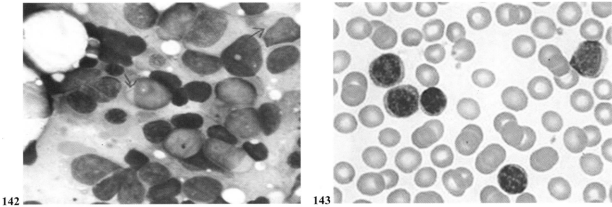

142. Acute myelocytic leukemia: large myeloblasts with notched nuclei and Auer rod/bar in blood smear
143. Chronic lymphocytic leukemia: numerous, small, mature LC and "smudge cells" in blood smear

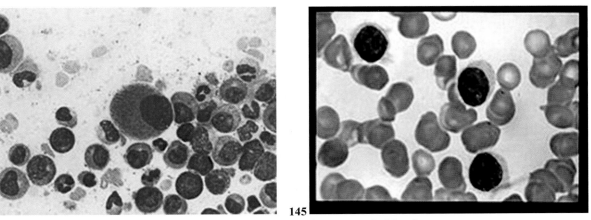

144. Chronic myeloid leukemia: a small, hypolobated megakaryocyte in blood smear
145. Hairy cell leukemia: hair-like cytoplasmic projections from B-cells in blood smear

Hypertensive Retinopathy - Grade 4

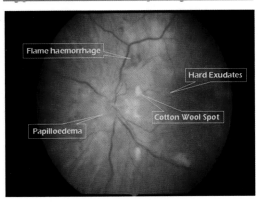

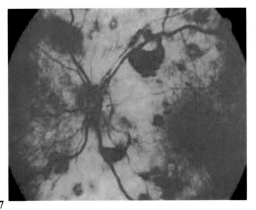

146. Hypertensive retinopathy (Funduscopy): papilledema (blurred disc margins), cotton wool spot, hard exudates, flame hemorrhage
147. Retinal (flame) hemorrhage: Roth's spots, seen in HTN, endocarditis, shaken baby syndrome, etc.

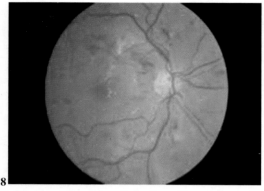
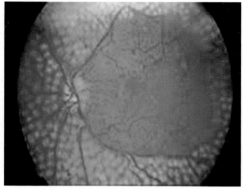

148. **Non-proliferative diabetic retinopathy:** with microaneurysms, exudate, hemorrhages, and edema

149. **Proliferative diabetic retinopathy:** formation of new fragile vessels, edema, hemorrhages, and scarring

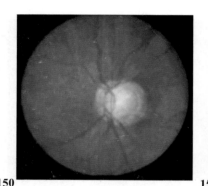
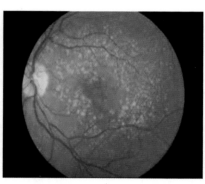
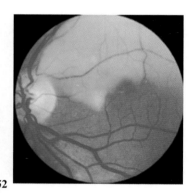

150. **Glaucoma:** disc cupping-- atrophy of the optic disc

151. **Aging:** macular degeneration + central vision loss

152. **Central retinal artery occlusion:** the pale edema of optic disc and ischemic area vs the normal color of the retina

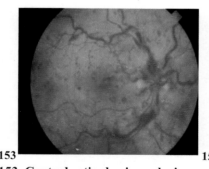
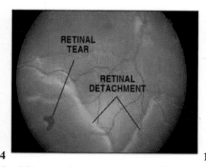
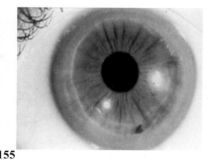

153. **Central retinal vein occlusion:** retinal hemorrhage, cotton wool spots and fundus edema

154. **Retinal detachment:** gray-cloudy or dark-red retina debris hanging in the vitreous humor

155. **Wilson disease:** The Kayser-Fleischer ring—copper deposition in part of the cornea. (END)